LANCHESTER LIBRARY

3 8001 00518 4522

LANCHESTER LIBRARY

£40
4/05

Ballistic Trauma
Second Edition

WITHDRAWN

D1614800

WITHDRAWN

Ballistic Trauma

A Practical Guide

Second Edition

Edited by
Peter F. Mahoney, James M. Ryan, Adam J. Brooks
and C. William Schwab

Project Coordinators
Miranda Dalrymple and Cara Macnab

With 161 Illustrations

Foreword by Martin Bell

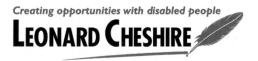

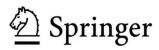

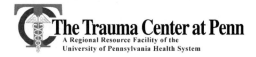

Peter F. Mahoney, OStJ, TD, MSc, MB BS, FRCA, FFARCSI, FIMC RCSEd, DMCC, RAMC
Defense Medical Service and Leonard Cheshire Centre, Royal Free and University College Medical School, Academic Division of Surgical Specialities, London, UK

James M. Ryan, OStJ, MB, BCh, BAO, MCh, FRCS, DMCC, FFAEM
Leonard Cheshire Centre, Royal Free and University College Medical School, Academic Division of Surgical Specialities, London, UK

Adam J. Brooks, MB, ChB, FRCS (Gen Surg), DMCC, RAMC(V)
Department of Surgery, University of Pennsylvania School of Medicine, Division of Traumatology and Surgical Critical Care, Hospital University of Pennsylvania, Philadelphia, PA, USA

C. William Schwab, MD, FACS, FRCS (Glasg)
Department of Surgery, University of Pennsylvania School of Medicine, Division of Traumatology and Surgical Critical Care, Hospital University of Pennsylvania, Philadelphia, PA, USA

British Library Cataloguing in Publication Data
Ballistic trauma : a practical guide.—2nd ed.
 1. Gunshot wounds 2. Penetrating wounds
 I. Mahoney, Peter F.
 617.1'45
 ISBN 185233679X

Library of Congress Cataloging-in-Publication Data
Ballistic trauma : a practical guide/Peter F. Mahoney . . . [et al.].
    p. ; cm.
  Rev. ed. of: Ballistic trauma: clinical relevance in peace and war. 1997.
  Includes bibliographical references and index.
  ISBN 1-85233-678-1 (hardcover : alk. paper)—ISBN 1-85233-679-X (softcover : alk. paper)
  1. Gunshot wounds. I. Mahoney, Peter F.
  [DNLM: 1. Wounds, Penetrating—diagnosis. 2. Wounds, Penetrating—therapy. WO 700 B193 2004]
  RD96.3.B355 2004
  617.1'45—dc22   2004050435

ISBN 1-85233-678-1 (hardcover)   ISBN 1-85233-679-X (softcover)   Printed on acid-free paper

©2005 Springer-Verlag London Limited

First edition, Ballistic Trauma: Clinical Relevance in Peace and War (0340581144), published by Arnold, 1997.

Apart from any fair dealing for the purposes of research or private study, or criticism, or review, as permitted under the Copyright, Designs and Patents Act 1988, this publication may only be reproduced, stored or transmitted, in any form or by any means, with the prior permission in writing of the publishers, or in the case of reprographic reproduction in accordance with the terms of licenses issued by the Copyright Licensing Agency. Enquiries concerning reproduction outside those terms should be sent to the publishers.
The use of registered names, trademarks, etc., in this publication does not imply, even in the absence of a specific statement, that such names are exempt from the relevant laws and regulations and therefore free for general use.
Product liability: The publisher can give no guarantee for information about drug dosage and application thereof contained in this book. In every individual case the respective user must check its accuracy by consulting other pharmaceutical literature.

Printed in the United States of America (BS/EB)

9 8 7 6 5 4 3 2 1   SPIN 10887535 (hardcover)   SPIN 10887543 (softcover)

Springer Science+Business Media
springeronline.com

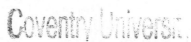

Foreword

This is a book first and foremost for surgeons and those who work with them in the management of ballistic trauma and treatment of its victims. But the book is also of value to others with front-line experience and an interest in the issue of harm reduction, whether in war or "peace," on the field of battle or at the scene of a crime. These pages can also be studied fruitfully by politicians, most of whom lack medical or military expertise, in helping them understand the real world consequences of the decisions that they make. (My own special interest, cheerfully declared, is that of a beneficiary—having once been hit by mortar fire as a war reporter, I am grateful for the care of the surgeons and nurses who so expertly put me back together again and returned me to front-line duty).

I believe that we live in the most dangerous times since the global warfare of the mid-twentieth century. Appropriately, the editors of this book have set their remit wider than the most recent advances in the relevant fields of medical science—necessary advances—to keep pace with those in ballistic science, as man finds ever more ingenious ways of killing and maiming his own kind.

Napoleon III is reputed to have declared, "The history of artillery is the history of progress in the sciences, and is therefore the history of civilization." I wonder, where does that leave us in the early twenty-first century? Nowhere very civilized, for sure.

In their preface to the first edition, in 1997, the editors noted: "The lesson of history is that you cannot take the experience of an urban hospital onto the battlefield. It also can be said, that you cannot do the reverse, and nowadays there is further confusion from the deployment of troops to peacekeeping duties performed under the scrutiny of the media. The latter is not the same as war."

A great deal has happened since then, including the events of 11 September 2001, to change or qualify that judgment. Civilian and military targets are attacked, not only by insurgent and revolutionary forces, without distinction, discrimination, or regard to the Geneva Conventions. The front lines are everywhere and all around us, as much in the concrete defences of the Palace of Westminster as the contested streets of Najaf or the abandoned villages of Darfur. Nor is there any monopoly of virtue—or realistic concept of one side which observes the rules, against another which violates them. This book properly draws attention to the use by the Western powers of the cluster bomb—a weapon that has the properties of an aerially sown antipersonnel mine. The APM is banned by international treaty. The cluster bomb is not. Yet international law prohibits any weapon "of a nature to cause superfluous injury or unnecessary suffering."

One of the most controversial issues covered here is the distinction between civilian and military casualties—insofar as it exists, or indeed if it exists at all. The impact on the human frame and human tissue of a high-velocity bullet or a mortar fragment will be exactly the same, whether the victim is clad in combat fatigues or jeans and a T-shirt. In his firsthand analysis of the circumstances of the siege of Sarajevo from 1992 to 1995 (p. 583) John P. Beavis puts the ratio of civilian to military casualties at 63% to 37%. In the war in Iraq (2003–?) the ratio is probably higher, although the figures are politically sensitive, and therefore not divulged. In other conflicts, such as the wars in Angola and the Drina Valley of Bosnia, I would suggest that a 90% to 10% ratio would be nearer the mark. So much for the advance of civilization through the enlightening power of the artillery shell.

Professionals in the field of ballistic trauma will learn much from each other in this new edition. A more general conclusion they will draw, I hope, is that the present epidemic of global violence is not an acceptable outcome of continuing failures of politics and diplomacy. I am with Robin M. Coupland on this (p. 132): "Armed violence resulting in ballistic trauma should be considered for what it is—a global health issue." Those who deal with the effects of ballistic trauma surely have the least reason to be indifferent to its causes.

There are certain ways of expressing this in plain English, admittedly nonmedical and nonspecialist. One is religious: that we are all members one of another. The other is political: that politics is too important to be left to the politicians.

Martin Bell
London 2004

Preface to the Second Edition: Why This Book, Why Now?

In 1997, Professor J.M. Ryan and others produced the reference work *Ballistic Trauma: Clinical Relevance in Peace and War* (Arnold, 1997). Much of this is still valid, but a number of concepts in care of the ballistic casualty have changed. These include developing ideas on fluid resuscitation and refinement of field protocols based on operational experience.

Authors, editors, and colleagues expressed the view that there was a need for a practical guide encompassing these developments, along the lines of *Conflict and Catastrophe Medicine* (Springer, 2002). The aim was to distill real-life practice and try to capture that which often is lost or diluted in traditional texts.

With 9/11, the world changed. Since then, major conflicts have occurred in Afghanistan and Iraq, and operations are still ongoing. Many of the authors and editors deployed to these conflicts with nongovernmental organizations, Aid Agencies, and the military. Others are working with these injuries on a day-to-day basis at one of the USA's busiest trauma centers.

This has delayed the production of *Ballistic Trauma: A Practical Guide*, but means that people are writing with recent experience of managing ballistic injury. Colleagues returning from deployment have emphasized the need for clear guidance on managing ballistic injury, especially as more and more military reservists are being deployed and their day-to-day work may not include managing these types of injury.

Authors have been given a relatively free hand in structuring their chapters so they would be unconstrained by the book's style and be able to pass on their lessons unhindered.

Finally, our request is that this book be a "living" document. Give us feedback. Record what treatment works and what treatment does not. Use this knowledge to improve the care of the ballistic casualty.

Peter F. Mahoney
James M. Ryan
Adam J. Brooks
C. William Schwab

Preface to the First Edition, *Ballistic Trauma: Clinical Relevance in Peace and War*

This book aims to bring together the science behind and the management of ballistic trauma. It is directed at the surgeon, though perhaps not an expert, who might find him or herself having to deal with patients suffering from penetrating trauma in environments as diffuse as a late twentieth-century hospital or the arduous conditions of a battlefield.

The book also brings together the views of UK and US experts from military and civilian backgrounds. This composite view was deliberate, as it was recognized that these potentially diverse views reflected the complexity of an international problem that increasingly impinges on the practice of surgery in today's world.

The UK editors were the joint professors of military surgery to the three armed services and the Royal College of Surgeons of England, along with a medical scientist with an international reputation in the field of ballistic science. The US editor is Professor and Chairman of the Department of Surgery at the Uniformed Services University of the Health Sciences and has extensive experience in the management of ballistic trauma.

Though the book is influenced heavily by the military background of many of the authors, it is directed at a much wider audience, particularly those who may have to deal unexpectedly with the consequences of the trauma seen in an urban environment. It compares and contrasts the differing civil and military management viewpoints and goes on, where relevant, to debate the areas of controversy in the specialized fields of the relevant authors.

The subject of ballistic trauma is controversial in part because its management depends so much upon the situation in which it occurs. Thus, there often is confusion and a misunderstanding that emanates from the failure to recognize that the location of surgical facilities, the number of injured, and whether the injuries are sustained during peace or war may have a profound effect on the way patients are treated. The lesson of history is that you cannot take the experience of an urban hospital onto the battlefield. It also can be said that you cannot do the reverse, and nowadays there is further confusion from the deployment of troops to *peace-keeping* duties performed under the scrutiny of the media. The latter is not the same as war.

The book has four sections. The first section is on the science behind understanding ballistic trauma; it also adds to its declared remit by including a chapter on blast injury. The second section is on general principles of assessment and initial management. The third section deals with management from a regional perspective, and the fourth section is on more specific but general problems. The intention is to provide surgeons with an understanding of the fundamentals of ballistic trauma, the mechanisms and some insight into the significance of new weapons, as well as the variations on the principles of management.

The book acknowledges that no single viewpoint can address the management of patients sustaining ballistic injuries and does not fall into the trap of recommending rigid and single guides unless there is a convergence of opinion. Its approach has been to provide a greater understanding so that the clinician facing the clinical problem feels sufficiently informed as to make coherent choices appropriate to the circumstances.

J.M. Ryan
N.M. Rich
R.F. Dale
B.T. Morgans
G.J. Cooper
1997

Contents

Section 2   Clinical Care

Contributors

Neil Arya, BASc, MD, CCFP
Environment and Resources Studies, University of Waterloo and Faculty of
Health Sciences McMaster University, Hamilton, ON, Canada

Toney W. Baskin, MD, BS
Trauma and Critical Care Service, Brooke Army Medical Center, United
States Army Institute of Surgical Research, San Antonio, TX, USA

John P. Beavis, MB BS, DMCC, FRCS
Leonard Cheshire Centre, Royal Free and University College Medical
School, Academic Division of Surgical Specialties, London, UK

Kenneth D. Boffard, BSc, MB BCh, FRCS, FRCPS, FACS
Department of Surgery, Johannesburg Hospital, University of the
Witwatersrand, Johannesburg, South Africa

Douglas M. Bowley, FRCS
Department of Surgery, University of the Witwatersrand Medical School,
Johannesburg, South Africa

Benjamin Braslow, MD
Division of Traumatology and Surgical Critical Care, Department of
Surgery, University of Pennsylvania School of Medicine, Philadelphia, PA,
USA

Adam J. Brooks, MB, ChB, FRCS (Gen Surg), DMCC, RAMC(V)
Department of Surgery, University of Pennsylvania School of Medicine,
Division of Traumatology and Surgical Critical Care, Hospital University of
Pennsylvania, Philadelphia, PA, USA

Neil Buxton, MB ChB, DMCC, FRCS
Department of Neurosurgery, Walton Centre for Neurology and
Neurosurgery, Royal Liverpool Children's Hospital, Liverpool, UK

Mark Byers, MB BS, MRCGP, DA, DipIMC RCS Ed, DRCOG
16 Close Support Medical Regiment, Royal Army Medical Corps, Colchester, UK

Ian Civil, MBE, ED, MB ChB, FRACS, FACS
Trauma Services, Auckland Hospital, Auckland, New Zealand

Jonathan C. Clasper, DPhil, DM, FRCS, DMCC
Department of Orthopaedic Surgery, Frimley Park Hospital, Frimley, UK

Graham Cooper, OBE, PhD
Biomedical Sciences, Defence Science and Technology Laboratory, Salisbury, UK

Bryan Cotton, MD
Division of Traumatology and Surgical Critical Care, Department of Surgery, University of Pennsylvania School of Medicine, Philadelphia, PA, USA

Robin M. Coupland, FRCS
Legal Division, International Committee of the Red Cross, Geneva, Switzerland

Wendy L. Cukier, MA, MBA, PhD, DU, LLD, MSC
School of Information Technology Management, Ryerson University, Toronto, ON, Canada

Pauline A. Cutting, FRCS, FFAEM
Emergency Department, Gwynedd Hospital, Bangor, UK

Elias Degiannis, PhD, MD, FRCS, FCS, FACS
Department of Surgery, University of the Witwatersrand Medical School, Johannesburg, South Africa

Richard A. Donaldson, MSSc, BSc, MB, FRCS
Department of Urology, Belfast City Hospital, Belfast, UK

Jay J. Doucet, CD, MD, FRCSC, FACS
Division of Trauma, Burns and Critical Care, University of California Medical Center, San Diego, CA, USA

Paul Dougherty, MD
Department of Surgery, Orthopedic Surgery Program, William Beaumont Army Medical Center, El Paso, TX, USA

James M. Ecklund, MD
National Capital Consortium (Walter Reed Army Medical Center, National Naval Medical Center), Washington, DC, and Division of Neurosurgery, Uniformed Services University of the Health Sciences, Bethesda, MD, USA

Spiros G. Frangos, MD, MPH
Section of Trauma/Surgical Critical Care, Yale University, New Haven, CT, USA

Heidi Frankel, MD, FACS
Section of Trauma/Surgical Critical Care, Yale University, New Haven, CT, USA

Marilee Freitas, MD
Section of Trauma/Surgical Critical Care, Yale University, New Haven, CT, USA

Stephen C. Gale, MD
Department of Surgery, Hospital of the University of Pennsylvania, Philadelphia, PA, USA

Philip Gotts, BSc
Defence Clothing Research and Project Support, Defence Logistics Organisation, Ministry of Defence, Bicester, UK

Vicente H. Gracias, MD, FACS
The Trauma Center at Penn, Department of Surgery, Division of Traumatology and Surgical Critical Care, University of Pennsylvania, Philadelphia, PA, USA

Jenny Hayward-Karlsson, SRN
Health Services Unit, International Committee of the Red Cross, Geneva, Switzerland

Walter Henny, MD
Department of Surgery, Erasmus Medical Center, University Hospital, Rotterdam, The Netherlands

John B. Holcomb, MD, FACS
Trauma and Critical Care Service, Brooke Army Medical Center, United States Army Institute of Surgical Research, San Antonio, TX, USA

Adriaan Hopperus Buma, MD, PhD, DMCC
Medical Service, Royal Netherlands Navy, Naval Base Den Helder, The Netherlands

David B. Hoyt, MD, FACS
Division of Trauma, University of California Medical Center, San Diego, CA, USA

Donald Jenkins, MD, FACS
59 MDW/Wilford Hall Medical Center, Lackland AFB, TX, and Uniformed Services University of the Health Sciences, Bethesda, MD, USA

Alan R. Kay, FRCS, RAMC
Defence Medical Service and South West Regional Burn Centre, Frenchay Hospital, Bristol, UK

Ari K. Leppäniemi, MD, PhD, DMCC
Department of Surgery, Meilahti Hospital, University of Helsinki, Helsinki, Finland

Geoffrey S.F. Ling, MD, PhD
Departments of Anesthesiology, Neurology, and Surgery, Uniformed Services University of the Health Sciences, and Departments of Neurology, Critical Care Medicine and Neurosurgery, Walter Reed Army Medical Center, Washington, DC, USA

Peter F. Mahoney, OStJ, TD, MSc, MB BS, FRCA, FFARCSI, FIMC RCSEd, DMCC, RAMC
Defense Medical Service and Leonard Cheshire Centre, Royal Free and University College Medical School, Academic Division of Surgical Specialities, London, UK

Chris J. Neal, MD
Department of Neurosurgery, Walter Reed Army Medical Center, Washington, DC, USA

Ian P. Palmer, MB ChB, MRCPsych
Former Tri Service Professor of Defence Psychiatry, Her Majesty's Armed Forces, London, UK

Graeme J. Pitcher, MB BCh, FCS
Department of Paediatric Surgery, University of the Witwatersrand, Johannesburg, South Africa

John P. Pryor, MD
Division of Traumatology and Surgical Critical Care, Department of Surgery, University of Pennsylvania Medical Center, Philadelphia, PA, USA

Matthew J. Roberts, MA, BM BCh, FRCA
Department of Anesthesiology, University of Colorado Health Sciences, Denver, CO, USA

Malcolm Q. Russell, MB ChB, DCH, DRCOG, MRCGP, FIMCRCS Ed
Helicopter Emergency Medical Service, The Royal London Hospital, London, UK

James M. Ryan, OStJ, MB, BCh, BAO, MCh, FRCS, DMCC, FFAEM
Leonard Cheshire Centre, Royal Free and University College Medical School, Academic Division of Surgical Specialities, London, UK

Hendrik Johannes Scholtz, MBChB, MMed Path
Division of Forensic Medicine, School of Pathology, University of the Witwatersrand, Johannesburg, South Africa

C. William Schwab, MD, FACS, FRCS (Glasg)
Department of Surgery, University of Pennsylvania School of Medicine, Division of Traumatology and Surgical Critical Care, University Hospital Pennsylvania Medical Center, Philadelphia, PA, USA

Martin D. Smith, MB BCh, FCS
Department of Surgery, University of the Witwatersrand, Chris Hani Baragwanath Hospital, Johannesburg, South Africa

Michael E. Sugrue, MD, FRCSI, FRACS
Trauma Department, Liverpool Hospital, Liverpool, Sydney, NSW, Australia

Nigel R.M. Tai, MBBS, MS FRCS (Eng)
Trauma Unit, Johannesburg Hospital, Johannesburg, South Africa

Jeanine Vellema, MBBCh, FCPath
Division of Forensic Medicine, School of Pathology, University of the Witwatersrand, Johannesburg, South Africa

Paul D. Wallman, MB ChB, FRCS, FFAEM
Department of Emergency Medicine, Homerton University Hospital, London, and Department of Emergency Medicine, The Royal London Hospital, London, UK

Stephen Westaby, PhD, MS, FETCS
Oxford Heart Centre, John Radcliffe Hospital, Oxford, UK

David J. Williams, MB BS, FRCS, MD
Department of Vascular Surgery, The Bristol Royal Infirmary, Bristol, UK

Paul R. Wood, MB BCh, FRCA
Department of Anaesthesia, University Hospital Birmingham NHS Trust, Selly Oak Hospital, Birmingham, UK

Section 1
Introduction, Background, and Science

Introduction

This first section of *Ballistic Trauma* considers wider issues surrounding firearms injury. This includes firearms use and misuse in different countries and cultures, as well as the legal treaties and restrictions that attempt to limit the damaging effects of weapons. These issues are addressed in the chapters on small-arms control and international humanitarian law.

Many health-care professionals have little experience of how firearms and munitions work; this is addressed in the chapters on "Guns and Bullets" and "Bombs, Mines, Blast, and Fragments."

Health-care professionals need to know that the injuries produced by firearms and fragments can be modified by helmets and body armor, as outlined in the chapter on "Ballistic Protection."

The management and handling of the ballistic casualty has associated legal, as well as clinical, implications, and some of the procedures and pitfalls are considered in the "Forensics" chapter.

1
The International Small Arms Situation: A Public Health Approach

Neil Arya and Wendy L. Cukier

Introduction

Whether emergency room physicians, trauma surgeons, psychiatrists, pediatricians, or family doctors, physicians throughout the world bear witness to the terrible consequences of small arms on human health. A physician stemming a bleed in the chest of a gunshot victim is not concerned with whether the shooting was a suicide, an accident or a homicide, whether it took place in a conflict situation or in peacetime, or whether the perpetrator was a gang member, a soldier, a non-state actor, or a law-abiding gun owner. What matters to the physician is whether bullet struck bone, whether bone shattered, whether metal and bone splinters punctured vital organs or blood vessels, or severed the spinal cord—in short, whether the patient will survive and if so, what his or her future health will be.[1] Medical treatment has advanced in the last decade, but physicians have long recognized that preventing death and injury in times of war[2] or peace[3] can produce more significant benefits than an exclusively treatment-based approach.

Public health approaches to the small-arms issue based on evidence and science involve various disciplines of expertise, including epidemiology, but also psychology, sociology, criminology, economics, education, and medicine. A harm-reduction approach begins with the premise that the weapons, by their very nature, are designed to kill, harm, or threaten other beings. Given the accepted utility of legal firearms in society, the goal is typically not a ban, as was the case with antipersonnel mines, but regulation or "harm reduction."

This public health approach to injury might begin with a careful analysis of the epidemiology and etiology of the injury and concentrates on the causal factors that produce the injury. The injury-prevention model examines the interactions between the environment (both physical and social), the host (the victim), the agent (the firearm), and the vector (the ammunition). The focus is on understanding the causal chain and breaking the chain at its weakest link with "fact-based" interventions.[4] Interventions may address the underlying factors, for example, programs to improve the social and economic conditions that give rise to violence. Interventions may focus on reducing the severity of violence—efforts focused on supply of weapons, for example, which attempt to control exports or access to small arms. Finally, interventions may focus on "treatment", trauma care, rehabilitation, and reintegration.[5]

This model is a useful one for understanding the problem of small arms and the approaches to reducing their negative effects on health. This chapter will consider:

1. Basic Concepts
2. The Health Effects of Small Arms
3. Causal Factors
4. Proliferation of Legal and Illegal Small Arms
5. Interventions
6. Evaluations
7. Conclusions

Basic Concepts

What Are Small Arms?

Broadly speaking, small arms are those weapons designed for personal use. They are lightweight and would include "man-portable" weapons such as personal and police firearms such as revolvers and self-loading pistols, rifles and carbines, light machine-guns, sub-machine guns. (e.g., The Uzi of Israel, and the HK MP5 of Germany) and assault rifles (e.g., the Russian AK-47 "Kalashnikov, the US M-16, the Belgian FAL, and the German G-3).[6]

Light weapons are those designed for use by several persons serving as a crew. Light weapons include heavy machine-guns, hand-held under-barrel and mounted grenade launchers, portable anti-aircraft guns, portable anti-tank guns, recoilless rifles, portable launchers of anti-tank missile and rocket systems, portable launchers of anti-aircraft missile systems, and mortars of calibers of less than 100 mm. Ammunition and explosives form an integral part of small arms and light weapons used in conflicts, and include cartridges (rounds) for small arms, shells and missiles for light weapons, anti-personnel and anti-tank hand grenades, landmines, explosives, and mobile containers with missiles or shells for single-action anti-aircraft and anti-tank systems.

The Small Arms Survey estimates there to be stockpiles of at least 688 million small arms and light weapons in the world, of which about 59% are in legal civilian possession, 38% are in the arsenals of national armed forces, 3% are held by police forces, and, most surprisingly, far less than 1% are in the hands of insurgent groups.[7]

People generally believe that military, law enforcement, and selected security officials need weapons in order to protect society. Civilian firearms ownership is also considered by many to be legitimate for sports, recreation, and wildlife control, including such activities as target-shooting and managing pests. Aboriginal peoples (Native Americans) in North America see hunting as a tradition, a way of life, and, for many, even livelihood. When law enforcement is unable to adequately defend certain individuals, possession of handguns might be considered as acceptable for purposes of self-defense. In most developed countries, however, this is rare. The United States is the notable exception.

In conflict and in crime, small arms may be used by those wishing to use force to achieve their aims. Small arms are easily available and cheap. AK-47s, for instance, are manufactured in over 40 countries and can be purchased for as little as $10–12 in Afghanistan and Angola.[7] They are durable, easy to produce, easy to operate. and often may be concealed easily and trafficked past legal restrictions where these exist. Most importantly, they are extremely deadly and provide the user with a high capacity for killing. A single gunman with an assault rifle can slaughter dozens of people in a matter of minutes.[8]

It is important to note that the reliability of weapons-availability data varies considerably. In highly regulated states, official estimates of legally licensed firearm owners and registered firearms may be reasonably reliable, but estimates of illegal weapons in circulation are difficult. In other cases, estimates are based on surveys such as the International Crime Victimization Survey, but these estimates can vary significantly for a single country.[9] Apart from surveys, it has been suggested that, in industrialized countries, one of the most reliable ways to estimate firearm ownership is to examine suicide data.[10] The Small Arms Survey considers there to be about 230 million weapons in the US, 98% of which are in civilian possession, 0.3% in police possession, and 2% in military possession.[11]

In less developed countries, the capacity for collecting consistent, reliable, and relevant data on small arms for evaluation, is limited by various cultural, economic, infrastructural, and logistical factors, especially in conflict and post-conflict situations. In many post-conflict countries in Central America and Africa, where only a tiny percentage of guns are registered, estimates of the total in circulation vary widely. The Small Arms Survey cites many examples of wild projections of number of arms, in particular, local claims in Mozambique of 6 million AK-47s in circulation, and widely reported figures of the wildly implausible 60 million weapons manufactured in Yemen.[10]

The Health Effects of Small Arms

Overview

An estimated 300000 people die annually due to firearms used in armed-conflict situations. Together with the estimated 200000 people who die each year from firearms used in non-conflict situations,[12] these deaths would amount to almost one death each and every minute. Putting these 500000 deaths per annum in a public health context ranks them ahead of the mortality and morbidity caused by landmines and only slightly behind other public health priorities in terms of damage, such as HIV/AIDS (2.9 million), tuberculosis (1.6 million), and malaria (1.1 million).[13] They represent about a quarter of the 2.3 million deaths due to violence,[14,15] of which 42% are suicides, 38% are homicides, and 26% are war related.[16,17]

The limitations of the data concerning the mortality and morbidity of small arms have been noted. In developed countries, different data sources yield different results; for example, Emergency Room (ER) Codes often produce different data than the Uniform Crime Reporting (UCR) Codes. In addition, while homicide is one of the more reliably reported crimes, other crimes (or injuries) involving firearms may not be reported or recorded accurately, even in highly developed countries.[18] Language might play a role in this—the definition of homicide in Spanish includes involuntary manslaughter. Even US and Canadian definitions differ. Hospital records may be unreliable if coding is not a priority. In under-developed countries, reporting of injuries or deaths may be affected by fear of authorities. Cultural factors may come into play; for example, suicides are under-reported when there is a religious taboo against them, whereas "accidents" may be over-reported. Domestic violence in many settings is still not considered a crime and injuries that result from domestic violence may be un-reported or reported as self-inflicted wounds or accidents.[19]

Reporting of death and injury in conflict zones is even more unreliable. Nevertheless, it is maintained that small arms and light weapons remain the weapons of choice in the vast majority of the world's conflicts.[20] International Committee of the Red Cross (ICRC) personnel working in conflict zones claim that these weapons are responsible for more than 60% of all weapons-related deaths and injuries in internal conflicts—far more than landmines, mortars, grenades, artillery, and major weapons systems combined.[21]

The costs of small arms in conflict are reinforced by research undertaken by the World Health Organization (WHO). Because the victims are often the youngest and healthiest of society, it is important to calculate the impact of disability-adjusted life years (DALYs) of the survivors, as well as the impact of the number of deaths. Krug estimates that, whereas war may have ranked 16th in 1990, by 2020 war may be the 8th leading cause of DALYs.[22] Many of the deaths caused by small arms are considered to be preventable, making this *pandemic* a major concern for public health professionals.

Health and Well Being

Death and injury are the most obvious consequences of small arms. Acute injuries may include damage to major organs or vital structures, rupture of major vessels, shattering of bones, trauma to the brain, or severing of the spinal cord. Psychological consequences also take their toll on survivors, the families of victims, whether they survive or not, and on the perpetrators. These include post-traumatic stress disorder, emotional detachment, social withdrawal, suspicion, and recurrent nightmares. In the longer term, there may be rehabilitative issues. What health professionals may fail to appreciate are the many indirect effects.

Social and Environmental Costs

The presence of a large number of weapons in society may foster a climate of fear, whether or not an armed conflict is raging. Increased incidence of crimes involving the use of weapons, such as robberies and assaults, has been shown in societies with a large number of arms.[23] Instability may result in the creation of refugees and internally displaced peoples (IDPs).

Social instability makes protecting the environment essentially impossible and even irrelevant to victim and perpetrator alike. Natural resources are destroyed in armed conflicts exacerbated by small arms. People, forced to flee their homes, eat or burn whatever they can find in order to survive.

Economic Impacts

In many areas of the world, the economic well being of populations is significantly affected by small arms use and possession. The direct effects include the cancellation of direct medical care and rehabilitative services, the disruption of basic human services, the negative impacts on property values and tourism, and the undermining of responsible governance. The indirect effects include economic downturns, lost growth, and reduced productivity. The Inter-American Development Bank estimated the direct and indirect cost of violence for Latin America at $140–170 billion US per year.[10] In Colombia, violence primarily related to small arms has been calculated as costing up to 25% of the country's gross domestic product (GDP).[24]

In First World, non-war situations, the impact is also significant. The direct cost of deaths and injuries due to firearms in the US has been calculated at $14 000 for each fatal gunshot and $38 000 for each injured person. The total impact goes much further than emergency medical care and rehabilitation, to psychological support for victims and their families, to children growing up without parents, and to those relations and contacts who continue to live in fear. Societal financial costs extend to police services and to lost productivity. Ted Miller has estimated costs of firearm-related damage as being $195 per person per year in Canada and $495 in the US.[25] These figures have been criticized on the grounds that they assign monetary values to substantially unquantifiable factors, such as pain, burden of suffering, loss of livelihood, and quality of life.

Humanitarian Relief Efforts

Gun violence depletes health-care resources, such as blood supplies, in the field and in emergency rooms. Victims may occupy hospital beds or take the time of rehabilitative personnel. When the damage is extensive, it makes careful testing of blood for HIV and other viruses impossible. Armed violence promotes the flow of IDPs and refugees. Within refugee camps, assaults and injuries further strain the resources of humanitarian aid agencies, UN peacekeepers, and the international community, decreasing access to basic services.

International relief operations are disturbed and may be suspended when aid workers themselves become targets of attack or require additional costs for security. More than twice as many ICRC personnel were killed in Chechnya and Rwanda alone in the 1990s than in all other conflicts since the Second World War.[9]

The nightly show of armed conflicts and their consequences on our television screens may lead to a perceived need for a quick remedy in these zones, diverting resources from more enduring treatments of the underlying ills of poverty, deprivation, lack of access to education, and social injustice. During the 1990s, international relief aid for regions in conflict increased from $1 billion to $5 billion a year, while at the same time, long-term development aid dropped.[9]

Effects on Women and Children

Men, who are overwhelmingly the perpetrators of violence and the users of small arms, represent the vast majority of direct casualties. In war situations, however, noncombatants may account for more than 35% of casualties. Among these, women and children often are represented disproportionately.[26,27]

Women's experience of small-arms violence is different than men's. In many parts of the world, women are more at risk from guns in the hands of their intimate partners than they are at risk from strangers or combatants. Women also may be more vulnerable to the secondary effects of small-arms violence, which include psychological, social, and sexual assaults. Studies in post-conflict societies have shown that women's perception of security differs considerably from men's: women more often experience the presence of small arms in the household as threatening, while many men feel more secure in the presence of a weapon.[28]

Children are made victims when they die, lose a parent, lose limbs, or suffer sexual violence. Yet the incredible firepower of modern weapons also allows children to become combatants and victimizers. In West Africa in particular, demobilization of these child soldiers has become a major issue. Yet even these children, who may have committed terrible atrocities, are victims in another way. They have been robbed of their childhoods, have lost their ties to their family, and often know little else other than war. They may have become addicted to drugs and may have become accustomed to a certain lifestyle that may be difficult to achieve without violence. As United Nations' Deputy Secretary-General Louise Frechette[29] has noted:

Small children have big dreams. Small arms cause big tragedies. Clearly, the two do not mix. And yet, from war zones to inner city streets to suburban classrooms, this combustible blend is wreaking havoc and ruining lives.

Regional Perpectives

North America

The US has more than 28 000 deaths per year from small arms—accidents, suicides, and homicides—by far the highest rate in the developed world.[30] The Centers for Disease Control (CDC) data show that gun-related deaths have now dropped slightly behind motor-vehicle accident (MVA) deaths in the 15–24 age category, after three years in the mid 1990s, when gun deaths actually exceeded MVA deaths. In the US, 38% of firearm deaths are due to homicide; this is similar to patterns found in Third World countries such as Colombia, Brazil, and Jamaica, where firearm homicide rate is comparable to or surpasses the firearm suicide rate. This is the opposite of the pattern in most industrialized countries, where the firearm suicide rate is approximately 5 times the firearm homicide rate.[10]

Each year in Canada, approximately 1000 people die as a result of firearms and a comparable number suffer injuries requiring hospitalization.[31] The bulk of the deaths, over 80%, are suicides. There are about 150–175 firearm homicides each year and less than 50 accidental deaths.[31] Despite media portrayals of gun violence as an urban phenomenon, the murder rate in communities in Canada with populations greater than 500 000 is half that of rural locations, where there are more guns.[32]

Europe

Britain's rates of firearm death are much lower than those in other countries. England and Wales have a firearm suicide rate of

Continued

0.2 per 100000, a total suicide rate of 7.0, a firearm homicide rate of less than 0.1, and a total homicide rate of 0.6.[33] Rates in other western-European countries are somewhat higher.

Finland has a much higher rate of firearm death, with firearm homicides at 0.4 per 100000, firearm suicides at 5.2, and total firearm deaths at 5.7. It should be noted that the high firearm suicide rate represents less than 20% of total suicides.[34] Alcohol often plays a role.

Estonia, though next door, has a much different pattern of firearm death, perhaps because of the influence of gangs and organized crime. Its firearm suicide rate is 3.7 (one tenth of the total suicide rate), and its firearm homicide rate is 6.3 (about a third of the total violent homicide rate).[35]

Africa

Shortly before the end of 1989, Charles Taylor invaded Liberia with 100 poorly trained soldiers equipped only with small arms: AK-47 assault rifles, a few machine guns, and some hand grenades. Within a matter of months they had seized several mines, using the profits to purchase additional light weapons. In less than a year, Taylor was able to overthrow the government of President Samuel Doe (himself no paragon of virtue). Less than two years later, rebels, aided by Taylor, repeated the same "success" story next door in Sierra Leone. Weapons originating in Bulgaria and Slovenia, arriving by way of Senegal, from the Ukraine by way of Burkina Faso, and from Liberia, continued to fuel this war. By the time of a ceasefire in July of 1999, the death toll was greater than 50000 people; another 100000 were deliberately injured and mutilated.[9]

The triumphant tale of the South-African transition to a multiracial democracy is remarkable in that, in the end, it occurred with relatively little violence. Unfortunately, the toll of overtly "political" conflict is dwarfed by the costs of other forms of violence: 25000 South Africans were murdered in 1997 alone compared with 15000 people killed between 1990–1998 in acts deemed "political". Handguns have been the weapon of choice, rather than military-issue rifles such as the infamous AK-47s. Violence in South Africa remains a major impediment to the provision of basic health-care, diverting resources from other health and social services. It has been identified as a great threat to human rights, economic and social development, and perhaps to democracy itself.[36]

South and Central America

In Brazil, there are about 45000–50000 murders per year, of which 88% are committed with firearms. These have increased about 320% since 1979.[36] Firearms account for the majority of deaths in the 15–19 age category. Interestingly, Brazil reports ten times as many injuries as fatalities from firearms, whereas most industrialized countries, such as Canada and Finland, report approximately equal proportions.[18] This may reflect the fact that in Brazil, in contrast to highly industrialized countries, firearms are more likely targeted at others than at one's self.

In Colombia, there was an increase of 366% from 1983 to 1993. By 1998 there were 18000 firearm murders per year (a rate of about 50 per 100000),[37] accounting for 80% of total homicides.[36] A large proportion of these remain in the nation's capital, Bogota, as well as in the cities of Cali and Medellin, historic centers of the cocaine trade.

It is calculated that in 1998–1999, the number of violent deaths from small arms in Nicaragua, El Salvador, and Guatemala exceeded those that had occurred in the respective civil wars.[7] During the civil wars in Nicaragua, Honduras was a transit point for arms, and weapons, including AK-47s, could be purchased cheaply (for less than $20) and easily along the border. Honduras' murder rate is about 45 per 100000, and a strong majority of these homicides (36 of the 45 per 100000 in 1999) are committed with firearms.[38] Guatemala's murder rate is similar and El Salvador's is somewhat higher. Over 75% of El Salvador's murders are committed with firearms, and more than 60% of violent deaths in total are caused by firearms or explosives. Seven percent of 9 to 13 year olds admitted to carrying a gun to school. The vast majority of weapons in the country are pistols and revolvers.[39]

The Causal Factors

"[T]he root causes of ethnic, religious and sectarian conflicts around the world are quite complex and varied, typically involving historical grievances, economic deprivation, inequitable distribution of resources, human rights abuses, demagogic leadership and an absence of democratic process."[9] Socioeconomic factors such as poverty, family disruptions (separation, death, divorce), alcoholism, mental illness, history of violence, and illicit drug use all serve as predictors of individual and group violence, both in first- and third-world settings. Yet research indicates that households and societies with these problems and without guns do not have the same rate of death and injury.[40]

Social conditions have a significant impact on the desire to obtain weapons. Individuals or groups who feel chronically marginalized may be driven by political desperation or domestic despair. Individual criminals and crime organizations may see user-friendly, cheap, and readily accessible weapons as a dramatic and speedy means to gain access to political or economic control.

Child psychiatrist Joanna Santa Barbara's *Cycle of Violence* illustrates how the weaponization of states or communities with pre-existing social conditions undermining stability can ignite, fuel, prolong, or exacerbate armed conflicts.[41] Societal and economic conflicts may spin out of control; political conflicts in individual states may be transformed into armed conflicts that cross borders.

The greater insecurity generated throughout society may in itself lead to a spiraling demand for, and use of, firearms and small arms. States may lose their monopoly on the use of force, leading to progressive privatization of security forces and spreading weapons throughout civilian society. Glorification of weapons on television and in movies may fuel demand further. A population may become acculturated to violence and intractable conflict may develop, sustaining a demand for weapons that may be accelerated simply by their availability.

The development of a culture of firearm violence certainly would hamper efforts towards non-violent conflict resolution, impede peace-building processes, and inhibit the establishment of civil society and stable models of governance.

A number of scholars have maintained that while the proliferation of small arms does not cause violence, it increases the lethality of violence.[42] Studies undertaken by the ICRC, for example, provide evidence that if small arms remain in circulation after political "conflicts" have ceased, violence among warring factions is replaced by interpersonal violence. Afghanistan in the mid 1990s illustrates the problems faced by armed societies once the fighting has stopped. Meddings compared the circumstances and rates of weapons-related injuries in Kandahar for 5 years before the region came under uncontested control by the Taliban, and the first year-and-a-half in peace after the Taliban's establishment of control (after a six month hiatus allowing for some semblance of stability). Weapons injuries declined only 20–40%, while the rate of gun deaths actually increased. In this "peaceful" post-conflict region, there was a high rate of non-combat injury and 80 deaths per 100000; 50% of these were firearm related. Meddings attributed the failure to reduce injury and death more substantially to two factors: a) after peace was established, there was no disarmament and the weapons remained in circulation, and b) although this one area of the country was at peace, there were armed conflicts between factions in other parts of the country.[43]

There is similar evidence from developed countries "at peace." The famous *New England Journal of Medicine* comparison of Seattle, WA, and Vancouver, Canada, showed that murder rates vary between cities just a few kilometers apart and in many other ways similar.[44] In terms of total firearm deaths, Cukier found that the US rate (11.4 per 100000) is about three-and-a-half times that of Canada's rate, roughly correlating to the number of firearms per capita. While the murder rate without guns in the US is roughly equivalent (1.3 times) that of Canada, the US murder rate with handguns is 15 times the Canadian rate.[45] Zimring and Hawkins compared transnational patterns of violent crime and concluded that while assault rates in Canada, New Zealand, and Australia are higher than in the US, American rates of *lethal* violence dwarf other industrialized countries.[46] Similarly, suicides attempted with firearms are more likely to succeed. A study of more than 20 developed countries demonstrated that this direct correlation of the percentage of households with firearms and firearm death rates held true across linguistic, cultural, and geographic boundaries.[47,48] Miller and Cohen added England and Wales, the US, and Australia to the mix and still found that over 90% of variance in death rate could be explained by access to firearms in those areas. This would suggest that a 1.0% increase or decrease in the number of households with guns in Canada would be associated with a 5.8% increase or decrease in the death rate.[49]

Some have argued that, to the contrary, possession of firearms decreases violence by allowing citizens to protect themselves.[50,51] For example, widely publicized studies conclude that Americans save thousands of lives each year possessing, using, or threatening the use of firearms. Published estimates of the number of times that a gun is used in the United States for protection in a single year have ranged from 62 000 to 23 million. One study, which asked for details about gun use, estimated that, in 1993, about 400 000 adults felt that they had saved a life by using a gun.[52] Such studies have been critiqued, however, because of the unreliability of self-reported data, flaws in the research design, and lack of corroborating evidence in, for example, police reports.[53]

Others have maintained that relaxing controls on firearms improves public safety; for example, the well-known thesis of John Lott states that with more guns there is less crime, and that the right to carry concealed weapons deters criminals.[50] However, these claims have, on balance, not received support in the medical literature.[54]

In many situations, pre-meditation might be an issue; in others, there is an element of impetuosity. Chapdelaine has noted that gunshot wounds have 5 to 15 times the mortality rate of knife wounds.[32] Guns are the most lethal means of attempting suicide, with a 92% mortality rate per attempt, in comparison with hanging at 78% and drug overdosing at 23%.[32] Suicide attempts may represent a cry for help or a long-term plan. Impulsivity often plays a role in both violence and suicide, particularly involving youth. Guns often represent a permanent solution to a temporary problem.

A gun in the home is far more likely to be involved a fatal or non-fatal accidental shooting, criminal assault, or suicide attempt than to be used to kill or injure in self-defense. Controlling for such confounding factors as sex, race, and age, households with firearms have three times the number of homicides[55] and five times the number of suicides[56] (due to all causes) compared to similar households in the same neighborhoods. Mental illness, illicit drug use, alcohol, and domestic violence also are predictors of death.

Recent purchasers of handguns may be the most at risk.[57] Similarly, risk-assessment instruments for domestic violence in the United States have indicated that firearm ownership is one of the strongest predictive factors of intimate partner femicide.[58]

The Proliferation of Legal and Illegal Small Arms

The value of legal trade in small arms accounts for perhaps $7.4 billion US, a relatively small proportion of the roughly $850 billion spent on military forces annually worldwide.[7] The major arms producers and exporters in the world include the US, China, Russia, and many western and eastern European nations. These countries are economically and politically influential and include all five permanent Security Council members, who have veto power at the UN over any significant action. They view guns as legitimate items of commerce and thus might be reluctant to embrace any measures that would restrict their trade. According to information provided by 77 counties to the UN *International Study on Firearms Regulation*, 45 countries acknowledged that firearms, components, or ammunition were produced legally on their territories.[59] In 1999, the UN Group of Governmental Experts estimated that arms were produced by at least 385 companies in 64 countries.[10,60] The Small Arms Survey[7] has calculated more recently that 98 countries produce or have the capacity to produce weapons, and over 1000 companies are involved. Perhaps the most successful weapon on record is the Kalashnikov or AK-47: designed in 1941, mass produced in 1947, now has licensed production in more than 19 countries, and numbers worldwide are estimated at between 70–100 million.[10]

While most of these weapons end up in the hands of state forces, a significant number are found in the hands of irregular armies, communal factions, crime and drug syndicates, and individuals.

Despite its opposition to regulation on an international level, the US, remarkably, has some of the strictest controls on exports and documentation of transfers. Yet figures for small-arms transfers vary. The 2001 Small Arms Survey placed the value of the small-arms and ammunition trade in the US as being worth about $1 billion of that country's total $20 billion in arms exports.[10] The US exports $367 million of firearms annually through customs (whereas the UK exports about $57 million).[10] Total sales or transfers of small arms and ammunition in 1998 were considered to be worth $463 million; these were to 124 different countries.[9] Of these 124 countries, about 30 were at war or experiencing persistent civil violence in 1998; in at least five, US or UN soldiers on peacekeeping duty have been fired on or threatened with US-supplied weapons.[9] This particularly ironic situation has been termed the "boomerang" effect. Yet the general perception within the US remains that the arms industry makes a positive contribution to employment and the economy because of these exports. Recent public awareness of the weapons the US supplied to Osama Bin Laden and Saddam Hussein in the late 1980s and early 1990s may finally change this perception.

Canada is the world's 9th largest arms exporter. Small-arms exports permits increased in value from $1.5 million (Canadian) in 1990 to 29.3 million by 1996. In the same year, the number of countries authorized to receive weapons increased from 18 to 50.[61] During the 1990s, Canada exported military items to at least 17 countries engaged in armed conflict and many more regimes with undemocratic rule or human-rights abuses.[62] Six percent of Canada's 292 million arms exports are small arms and ammunition.[63]

Virtually all illegal small arms begin as legal small arms, whether in the hands of insurgents or criminals. While arms are supplied through a complex global system, their transfer may be summarized as being channeled through the licit, illicit, and "gray" markets. Legally manufactured and traded weapons may be misused by their owners or others, including the State, in human-rights violations. They also represent the vast majority of gun suicides.

The so-called "gray" area weapons transfers are those that involve legal weapons that are stolen by, given to, or sold to criminals or allied paramilitary forces (the state, police or military could be the donor party). Such transfers often exploit loopholes to circumvent national policies or laws and involve the most significant proportion of criminal misuse.

The experience of police forces throughout the world shows that the illegally manufactured and traded weapons represent only a small minority of those used in the commission of suicides or homicides.

Lines between civilian and military markets, and between domestic and international markets, often are unclear. Lora Lumpe tracks the flow of these weapons in *Running Guns*, showing how weapons may be misappropriated on a massive scale from First World producers through a shadowy network of straw purchases to conflict zones. The different supply networks interact, sharing personnel, transportation, and banking infrastructure.[64] When one network is constrained, for example, by political forces, another network may assume some of the distribution function. If an arms embargo is imposed on a country, the illicit trade may increase as governments and non-state actors resort to covert transfers. An individual state's attempts to constrain legal access to firearms may be undercut by weaker controls in neighboring countries. Since the end of the Cold War, the role played by private interests has increased. However, regulatory efforts are not futile because the growth in illegal markets seldom offsets the decline in legal markets.

The US, with few domestic constraints, is often the source of weapons in other countries. In 1994, for example, foreign governments reported 6238 unlawfully acquired firearms that had originated in the US to the US Bureau of Alcohol, Tobacco and Firearms. Over 3000 of these were found in Mexico. Most (60–70%) of the handguns used in crime in Canadian cities are imported illegally, mainly from the US. Many of these go from Canada to the US and back again. In Japan, most (60%) of the firearms recovered by police are smuggled in from the US (30%) and China (30%).[65]

The Right to Bear Arms?[66]

Rights arguments have been prominent in the ongoing debate over firearms controls. However, rather than any notion of a collective right to safety, the rights that tend to be emphasized are the purported rights of individual citizens to keep and bear arms free from state intervention. The principal source of this argument is, of course, the powerful gun lobby in the United States. On a recent visit to Canada, the president of the National Rifle Association, actor Charlton Heston, referred to the right to bear arms as "God-given," telling a group of supporters that "You may not be absolutely free by owning a firearm. . . . but I guarantee that you will never be free when you can't."[67] This conception of rights and freedom generally is propounded by those opposing restrictions on firearm ownership and use. However, there is no right to bear arms under any instrument guaranteeing international human rights. The United States appears to be the only national jurisdiction in which such a right may have any semblance of a legal or constitutional basis. Even in that country, the existence of such a right is contested. Even a literal reading of the Second Amendment to the US Constitution reveals that the provision relates to the possession of arms by organized protectors of the people, not individuals: A well-regulated Militia, being necessary to the security of a free State, the right of the people to keep and bear Arms, shall not be infringed.[68] In addition to this, US courts have repeatedly and unanimously held that the United States Constitution does not guarantee individuals the right to possess or carry guns; the Second Amendment only protects the right of the state to maintain *organized* military forces.[69] It does not impede local, state, or national legislatures from enacting or enforcing gun-control laws.[70] While controversy may remain over the interpretation of the American Second Amendment, the notion that a right to bear arms exists has been dismissed in other countries. The issue of gun control was comprehensively revisited in the United Kingdom in the public inquiry following the Dunblane massacre. In the inquiry report, Lord Cullen declared, "The right to bear arms is not a live issue in the United Kingdom."[71] The New Zealand High Court has stated, "It should be emphasized, that there is no general right to bear arms in this country such as is safeguarded—if that is the appropriate term for it—under the United States Constitution."[72] In Canada, in a case dealing with legislative controls on automatic weapons, the Supreme Court has stated that Canadians "do not have a constitutional right to bear arms. Indeed, most Canadians prefer the peace of mind and sense of security derived from the knowledge that the possession of automatic weapons is prohibited."[73]

International Law

Even in the absence of formal treaties, international law regulates the flow of arms. The UN Charter and customary international law prohibit the use of force and interference in the domestic affairs of another country. It forbids states and non-state actors from assisting in terrorism, human-rights violations, and genocides with arms transfers. It also prevents states from assisting other states in illegal action even if the assistance itself is legal. Human-rights law to protect the physical integrity and dignity of the governed from states is guaranteed by the 1948 Universal Declaration of Human Rights.

Security Council Resolutions also have the force of law and are binding on all UN states. The Council may decide to enforce regional embargoes, such as the one on the former Yugoslavia, as it seemed to do on an increasing basis in the last decade. Embargoes are designed to reduce tensions. One drawback cited is that the weak and dispossessed may not be allowed the means to combat rights abuses with a more powerful opponent with greater resources at its disposal.

International humanitarian law is meant to protect non-combatants and may be applied to restrict weapons that cause damage disproportionate to the war aims. This was seen most spectacularly with the landmines signing treaty. Whole classes of weapons such as assault weapons and weapons of war (grenades, rocket launchers, etc.) could be banned from civilian possession, just as landmines and other indiscriminately harmful weapons have been banned from military and civilian use.

Article 36 of the 1977 Additional Protocol I of The Geneva Convention bans proposed weapons, which, by its design, causes effects on health that may constitute "superfluous injury or unnecessary suffering." The SirUS (Superficial Injury and Unnecessary Suffering) project, sponsored by the Red Cross and supported by numerous medical and humanitarian organizations, is a major appeal to practical recognition of these principles.

Other UN Resolutions

Effective national regulation on the possession of small arms has been affirmed by the United Nations, including the UN Security Council Resolution 1209 (1998) and the Report of the Disarmament Commission adopted at the General Assembly (1999).[36]

Continued

Universal Declaration of Human Rights[66]

All human beings have the right to life, liberty, and security of the person under Article 3 of the *Universal Declaration of Human Rights*. Furthermore, the preamble of the *Universal Declaration* states that freedom from fear is one of the highest aspirations of the common person. Freedom from physical or psychological violence is a prerequisite to the enjoyment of fundamental human rights. War is said to be, by definition, a means of violating human rights.[74] Peace itself has been identified as a human right, with the United Nations Charter providing the foundation for this right.[75]

Interventions

The best preventative strategies, whether aimed at cancer or violence, strike at the roots of the disease. Consequently, the importance of long-term primary prevention strategies that address the root causes of violence at the community and individual levels are critical. Demand-reduction approaches include a broad array of development and democracy-building measures, as well as measures aimed at reducing the "culture of violence."

As noted above, the extensive work that establishes the strong link between mortality and morbidity and the proliferation of small arms provides general support for measures aimed at improving controls over legal small arms in order to reduce the risk of misuse and diversion.

There are a number of international resolutions and agreements that are aimed at reducing the illicit trade in small arms. These include:

- The United Nations Convention on Transnational Organized Crime (UN A/REC/55/25, 2000) which establishes standards for import, export, transfer, marking, and tracing of firearms (excluding state to state transfers).
- The Protocol against the Illegal Manufacturing of and Trafficking in Firearms, Their Parts, Components, and Ammunition (A/RES/55/255, 2000), part of the UN Convention on Transnational Organized Crime, which regulates commercial shipments of firearms. It is legally binding and requires both export and import licenses, marking and tracing standards, and provisions for confiscation, seizure, and deactivation.
- A Program of Action (PoA) established by the UN 2001 Conference on the Illicit Trade in Small Arms in All Its Aspects which provides a framework for focusing on stemming the flow of illegal weapons to conflict zones.

The PoA stops short of measures supported by many nongovernmental organizations (NGOs),[76,77] which have maintained that much more needs to be done to prevent the proliferation and misuse of small arms. In addition to encouraging states to ratify existing international agreements, a number of other measures are being promoted. Given the nature of the illicit trade and the misuse of these weapons, the proposed measures are similar, regardless of whether the concern is conflict, crime, injury, or terrorism. These measures include:

- Strengthening export and import license authorizations; for example, ensuring that there are reciprocal measures so that both the importing and exporting country must approve transactions;
- concluding a legally binding global agreement on the marking and tracing of weapons to include systems for adequate and reliable marking of arms at manufacture and/or import;
- adequate record keeping on arms production, possession, and transfer;
- agreeing on international definitions of arms brokers and shipping agents and developing legally binding controls on their activities;
- establishing, on an international basis, a set of standards and measures to strengthen controls governing the legal transfer of weapons to both state and non-state actors in order to prevent the transfer of weapons that might be used for repression or aggression, or contribute to the escalation of conflicts or regional destabilization.

Despite continued opposition within the US,[79] it is clear that strong domestic regulation of civilian possession and use is critical.[77] Measures that allow legitimate civilian uses of small arms, but reduce the risk that small arms will be misused or diverted from legal to illegal markets, include licensing, regulation, standards for safe storage and, for example, the ban on civilian possession of fully automatic military assault weapons, which usually would not be needed for legitimate sporting activities.[66] The purposes for which guns may be acquired vary, and the standards for screening applicants differ, but clearly norms are emerging worldwide.[80] The efforts of the international community to establish norms for domestic regulation have been blocked consistently by the United States, owing largely to the influence of the National Rifle Association. The draft Program of Action for the UN 2001 Conference on the Illicit Trade in Small Arms in All Its Aspects contained measures to encourage states to ensure adequate regulation of the civilian use and possession of small arms; it also suggested a prohibition on the civilian possession of military assault weapons. However, the United States forced removal of any reference to the responsibility of states to adequately regulate civilian possession of firearms from the final Program of Action.[81]

In addition to the international agreements, which are notoriously difficult to develop and even more difficult to implement, there has been considerable activity at the regional level to address the problem of small arms.

Efforts are underway to develop multilateral agreements to curb the trade in small arms to human-rights abusers. Nongovernmental organizationss have attempted to incorporate the best of existing treaties with international law. In 1997, a group of 18 Nobel Peace Laureates, including both

{To

.-

TABLE 1-1. Regional approaches

European Union Program for Combating and Preventing Illicit Trafficking in Conventional Arms[82]

In 1993, the Organization for Security and Cooperation in Europe developed criteria for arms transfers, including small arms.[83] These criteria consider a recipient state's human rights record, record of compliance with international commitments and the cost of the arms in question in proportion to the economic circumstances of the recipient state. The European Union later expanded on this with a Code of Conduct, which entered into force in 1997. To the criteria above, it adds the requirement of respect of international sanctions and further consideration of the internal situation of a country, the country's efforts to preserve regional peace and security, stability, international security, the recipient country's attitude towards terrorism and the risk of diversion or re-export. Individual European countries may have additional national restrictions on transfers. Though comprehensive, the Code of Conduct's one major drawback is its non-binding nature.

OAS: Inter-American Convention Against the Illicit Manufacturing and Trafficking in Firearms, Ammunition, Explosives, and Other Related Materials[84]

The Organization of American States (OAS), recognizing the close link between illicit arms sales, drug trafficking, and violent crime, adopted a convention that requires member states to criminalize the unauthorized production and transfer of firearms, ammunition, and related materials, and to cooperate with one another in suppressing the black-market trade. This requires that countries develop and implement domestic laws and regulations setting out procedures for the legal manufacture, importation, and exportation of these materials. This agreement is binding on individual countries. However, only half of the countries have ratified the treaty; Canada and the US have yet to do so.

ECOWAS: Moratorium on the Import, Export, and Manufacture of Small Arms[85]

Even in war zones, individual countries or communities of nations can help curb the trade. West Africa, the locale of several of the most horrific conflicts of the 1990s, adopted a renewable, three-year voluntary moratorium on the import, export, and manufacture of small arms and light weapons in 1998. Major credit must be given to the president of Mali, Alpha Oumar Konaré, who spearheaded this effort in the Economic Community of West-African States (ECOWAS). States are allowed to apply for exemptions because of re-training or replacement of outdated weapons from the international regulatory body. This agreement represents the first time that a block of states that import large numbers of light weapons has adopted a measure of this kind, and it stands as an important model that other regions can emulate. The moratorium has been largely observed by member states.

Other regional agreements have been developed in the Great Lakes Region and the Horn of Africa, in Latin America, in the South Africa Development Community (SADC), and the Organization of African Unity.

---

individuals and organizations, began a campaign for a more responsible arms trade. It incorporates the best of the comprehensive European approach and of the binding OAS approach. Like-minded countries and NGOs are in the process of developing a new Framework Convention based on these principles.[86]

Attention also has been focused on measures to collect and destroy surplus weapons. International standards have been proposed for the destruction of confiscated or surplus small arms and light weapons.

Weapons-collection programs in post-conflict areas are critical to the establishment of lasting peace—otherwise the risk of high levels of violence remains.[21] The value of weapons-collection programs in other contexts varies from region to region. In some cases, particularly where they are mandatory and accompanied by incentives and/or criminal sanctions—for example, in Australia or Great Britain—these programs have resulted in large numbers of weapons being collected and destroyed. In other settings, their impact appears to be largely educational and associated with efforts to build a culture of peace. In Canada, a volunteer amnesty in 1991 netted 50000 firearms; this has been criticized as of little utility because many of them were just old hunting rifles.[80] In the US, collection programs have been initiated in many inner cities, and in Brazil, on 24 June 2001, just prior to the UN Conference on Illicit Small Arms, more than 100000 weapons were collected and destroyed. In post-conflict areas, NGOs often are helpful with collection and destruction programs to disarm paramilitaries.

Improvements to record keeping, tracing, information exchange, and enforcement also have been emphasized by the international community. There has been renewed emphasis on local measures; for example, more strictly controlling access to small arms in public places. Some countries, such as South Africa, have legislated "gun-free zones" to reduce risk.

There also have been efforts directed at manufacturing "smart guns," which can only be activated with codes or biometric information, and at developing technologies to reduce the impact of bullets (kevlar vests are a notable example).

From a public health perspective, injury prevention also must be supported by injury control. Timely and appropriate treatment of injuries due to small arms can significantly reduce mortality. Consequently, improved emergency services, training, etc., are critical parts of any strategy.

Evaluation

One of the most important steps in implementing an injury-prevention strategy is evaluation. Given the complex interaction of factors thought to produce or exacerbate violence, evaluation of particular interventions is notoriously difficult.[5,87,88] With the differences in the causes of firearms injury among specific populations, and given the multiple factors involved much of the research, particularly in the US, has focused on the impact on certain populations of particular interventions—for example, legislation concerning safe storage. Extensive research also has been conducted on the factors influencing crime rates; for example, social and economic inequality, culture and values, the political environment, substance abuse, and other high-risk behaviors have been identified as important factors.[47] The interactions between these variables are complex, and they are not all easy to measure or control for in longitudinal studies. While the diminishing proportion of males between the ages of 15 and 24 has been identified by some researchers as a key factor in the decline in crime rates in many countries,[89] a number of studies have pointed to stronger legislation as at least partly responsible for reductions in firearm-related deaths. For example, in Canada, firearm deaths and injuries have declined significantly with stronger legislation, and, more significantly, the rates of firearm homicide with rifles and shotguns—the focus of the legislation—have declined by more than 60% over a 10-year period, while murders with handguns (often illegally imported from the US) remained relatively flat.[90] Australia also has reported significant decreases in fire-arm violence following a nationwide agreement on firearms.[91] Even in Colombia, a ban on carrying handguns in Bogota and Cali on certain days, coupled with strict enforcement, has been linked to a significant decline in homicides.[92]

The impact of legislative changes seems clearest in industrialized countries with high incomes, stable political environments, and effective policing and judicial systems.[12] While there is limited research suggesting that interventions focused on controlling access to firearms may have an impact in other countries, such as Colombia,[92] it is clear that a wide range of variables shape demand for and use of firearms in the South, including criminal activity, drug use, parental factors, and religious beliefs.[93] It has been observed that some developing and newly democratic nations with relatively strict laws on the books—such as Brazil,[94] Estonia,[95] Jamaica,[59] and South Africa[96]—have large numbers of illicit firearms in circulation and high rates of lethal violence. More study is needed, but this appears to be the result of strong social, economic, and political conditions fuelling demand, coupled with a lack of effective enforcement capacity and well-established sources of illicit weapons.

It also is interesting to note that the politically charged nature of the question of firearms regulation—especially in the US—appears to have placed a burden of proof on researchers that is much higher than that normally required to support other public health or safety interventions.[97] Yet criminologist Neil Boyd,[90] in a study of Canadian law, has concluded that there is more evidence to support the efficacy of gun-control legislation in reducing death and injury than for most other legislative interventions.

The results of amnesties, buybacks, and weapons-collection programs are variable. In some cases there is limited evidence of significant short-term impact on weapons availability, although there appears to be an important educative function involved In response to massacres at Dunblane and Port Arthur, the United Kingdom and Australia both tightened regulations; the former banned handguns, and the latter, semi-automatic rifles. British citizens voluntarily turned in 200–250000 weapons, while the Australian buyout program netted 750000.[98] The empirical evidence from Australia suggests that, in the short term at least, firearm homicides have declined. In Great Britain, the evidence is less clear. It seems that an increase in illegal gun trafficking may have offset some of the gains. However, female firearm homicides have declined dramatically.[7]

Conclusions

Mainstream health-care organizations throughout the world—including the US—universally support measures to strengthen controls over firearms and to treat the global problem of small arms. The American Academy of Pediatrics, the American College of Physicians, the American Society of Internal Medicine, the American Academy of Child and Adolescent Psychiatry, and the American Medical Association are members of the Handgun Epidemic Lowering Plan (HELP) Network.[99] The Canadian Public Health Association, the Canadian Association of Emergency Physicians, the Canadian Paediatric Society, the Trauma Association of Canada, and the National Emergency Nurses Affiliation also support stricter laws.[100] Many law-enforcement officials outside of the US believe that licensing firearm owners and registering firearms are essential to prevent the diversion of legal guns to illegal markets. In Canada, the Canadian Association of Chiefs of Police and the Canadian Police Association have been strong supporters of gun-owner registration.[101] In Britain and Western Europe, the societal consensus for controls on private firearms is even stronger. Similar coalitions have emerged in the South as well, as evidenced by the diverse range of regional initiatives that have emerged.

While it is true that more research is needed on the impact of small arms, particularly in some regions, and on the effectiveness of particular interventions, it is critically important that health-care professionals avoid the "paralysis of analysis." As Austin Bradford Hill remarked in 1965 on the need to control tobacco products, "All scientific work is incomplete . . . All scientific work is liable to be upset or modified by advancing knowledge. That does not confer upon us the freedom to ignore the knowledge we already have or to postpone the action that it appears to demand at any given time."[102]

Resources

Web sites

IANSA: http://www.iansa.org/
Small Arms Survey: http://www.smallarmssurvey.org/
SAFER-Net: http://www.ryerson.ca/SAFER-Net/
HELP: http://www.helpnetwork.org/
WHO Injury and Violence Prevention: http://www5.who.int/violence_injury_prevention

Johns Hopkins: http://www.jhsph.edu/gunpolicy/
Physicians for Social Responsibility: http://www.psr.org/violence.html
IPPNW: http://www.ippnw.org
Arias Foundation: http://armslaw.org/fccomment.html
Coalition for Gun Control (Canada): http://www.guncontrol.ca/
Gun Control Network (UK): http://www.gun-control-network.org/
Gun Control Alliance (South Africa): http://www.gca.org.za/
Guncite (US): http://www.guncite.com/

Acknowledgments. The authors would like to acknowledge the contributions of Amelie Baillargeon, Justyna Susla, Katherine Kaufer Christoffel, Philip Alpers, John Loretz, Matt Longjohn, Roland Browne, Greg Puley, Alison Kooistra, Antoine Chapdelaine and Robert Muggah in the preparation and development of this article.

Amelie and Justyna contributed significantly to information gathering and fact checking while Katherine, Philip, John, Matt, Roland and Antoine each contributed to development of concepts, information on specific countries and editing of documents on which this article was based.

Country Comparison http://www.ippnw.org/MGS/V7N1Cukier.html

Canada/US Comparison

Firearms Death (Rate per 100000)*		Canada	US	US/Canada
Accidental deaths with Firearms	1999	0.1	0.3	2.6x
Suicides with Firearms	1999	2.6	7.1	2.7x
Total Firearms Deaths	1999	3.3	10.7	3.2x
Crime Statistics (Rate per 100000)		Canada	US	US/Can
Murders with Firearms	2001	0.55	3.6	6.5x
Murders with Handguns	2001	0.35	2.8	8.0x
Murders without Guns	2001	1.23	2.0	1.6x
Robberies with Guns	2001	14	62	4.4x
Robberies without Guns	2001	74	87	1.2x

Fewer firearms are being used in crimes in Canada—for example, the rate of firearm robberies has declined significantly by over 50% since 1991, including a 12% decline in 2001, the lowest rate since 1974. The Government of Canada firmly believes that the Firearms Program is making an essential contribution to our efforts to sustain this reduction.
Sources:
Statistics Canada (Canadian Center for Justice Statistics): Homicide Survey
Statistics Canada (Canadian Center for Justice Statistics): *Canadian Crime Statistics*
US Department of Justice: *Sourcebook of Criminal Justice Statistics*
Prepared by:
Department of Justice Canada
January 2003

References

1. Arya N. Speech before UN General Assembly, United Nations Conference on the Illicit Trade of Small Arms and Light Weapons in All Its Aspects; July 2001. Available at: http://www.un.org/Depts/dda/CAB/smallarms/statements/Ngo/ippnw.html.
2. Jenssen C. Medicine against war. In: Taipale I, et al., eds. *War or Health*. London: Zed Books; 2002:7–29.
3. Rivara FP. An overview of injury research. In Rivara FP, Cummings P, Koepsell TD, Grossman DC, Maier RV, eds. *Injury Control: A Guide to Research and Program Evaluation*. New York: Cambridge University Press, 2001.
4. Chapdelaine A, Maurice P. Firearms injury prevention and gun control in Canada. *Can Med Assoc J*. 1996:155(9):1285–1289.
5. Bonnie RJ, Fulco C, Liverman CT, eds. *Reducing the Burden of Injury: Advancing Treatment and Prevention*. Washington: National Academy Press, 1999.
6. *Report of the Panel of Governmental Experts on Small Arms*. New York: United Nations General Assembly; August 27, 1997. Report A/52/298.
7. Graduate Institute of International Studies (GIIS). *Small Arms Survey 2002: Counting the Human Cost*. Geneva: Oxford University Press; 2002.
8. Boutwell J, Klare MT. A scourge of small arms. *Sci Am*. 2000;282(6):48–53.
9. Smithies A. Ten myths about gun control. Canadian Shooting Sports Association. Available at: http://www.cdnshootingsports.org/tenmyths.html.
10. Hemenway D, Miller M. Firearm availability and homicide rates across 26 high income countries. *J Trauma*. 2000;49:985–988.
11. Graduate Institute of International Studies (GIIS). *Small Arms Survey 2001: Profiling the Problem*. Geneva: Oxford University Press; 2001:66.
12. Cukier W. Firearms/small arms: finding common ground. *Can Foreign Policy*. 1998;6:73–87.
13. World Health Organization (WHO). Statistical annexes. *World Health Report 2001*. Geneva: World Health Organization; 2001. Available at: http://www.who.int/whr2001/2001/main/en/pdf/annex2.en.pdf.
14. Krug EE, ed. *World Report on Violence and Health*. Geneva: World Health Organization; 2002. Available at: http://www5.who.int/violence_injury_prevention/main.cfm?p=0000000675#Appendix%204.
15. United Nations Development Programme (UNDP). *UNDP Human Development Report 2000*. New York: Oxford University Press; 2000:36. Available at: http://hdr.undp.org/reports/view_reports.cfm?year=2000.
16. Reza A, Mercy JA, Krug EE. Epidemiology of violent deaths in the world. *Inj Prev*. 2001;7:104–111. Available at: http://www.injuryprevention.com.
17. World Health Organization (WHO). Small arms and global health. Paper prepared for SALW talks. Geneva: July 2001. Available at: http://www5.who.int/violence_injury_prevention/download.cfm?id=0000000158.
18. United Nations (UN). *International Study on Firearm Regulation*. New York: United Nations; 1998.
19. World Health Organization (WHO). Collaborating Center for Safety Promotion and Injury Prevention. International Workshop on Small Arms and Firearms Injury: Finding a Common Ground for Public Health. Québec City, February 7, 1998.

20. Project Ploughshares. *Armed Conflicts Report 1996*. Waterloo, Ontario: Institute of Peace and Conflict Studies, 1996. Available at: http://www.ploughshares.ca/imagesarticles/ACR02/ACRmonitorSpring02.map.pdf.
21. International Committee of the Red Cross (ICRC). *Arms availability and the situation of civilians in armed conflict.* Geneva: International Committee of the Red Cross; 1999.
22. Krug EE, Powell KE, Dahlberg LL. Firearm-related deaths in the United States and 35 other high- and upper-middle-income countries. *Int J Epidemiol.* 1998;27:214–221.
23. Van Dijk, JJM. Criminal victimisation and victim empowerment in an international perspective. Paper presented at: Ninth International Symposium on Victimology. August 25–29, 1997; Amsterdam.
24. Vieira O. Workshop on International Small Arms/Firearms Injury Surveillance and Research; Ryerson Polytechnic University, Toronto; June 18, 1998.
25. Miller T. Costs associated with gunshot wounds in Canada in 1991. *Can Med Assoc J.* 1995;153:1261–1268.
26. International Committee of the Red Cross (ICRC). *Arms transfers and international humanitarian law*. Geneva: International Committee of the Red Cross; 1997.
27. Meddings D. Protecting children from armed conflict: Are most casualties non-combatants? *BMJ.* 1998;317:1249.
28. Cukier W, Anto M, Kooistra A. Gendered perspectives on small arms proliferation and misuse: Effects and policies. In: Farr VA, Gebre-Wold K, eds. *Brief 24: Gender Perspectives on Small Arms and Light Weapon*. Bonn: BICC; July 2002:25–39.
29. Frechette L. Speech quoted in United Nations Daily Highlights, Deputy Secretary-General opens exhibit highlighting impact of small arms proliferation on children; 20 July 1999. Available at: http://www.hri.org/news/world/undh/1999/99-07-20.undh.html.
30. See preliminary 2000 figures in Centers for Disease Control (CDC), National Vital Statistics 2001;49(12). Available at: http://www.cdc.gov/nchs/data/nvsr/nvsr49/nvsr49_12.pdf.
31. Canadian Center for Justice Statistics (CCJS). *Homicide Survey*. Ottawa: Statistics Canada; October 2001.
32. Chapdelaine A, Samson E, Kimberley MD, Viau L. Firearm-related injuries in Canada: Issues for prevention. *Can Med Assoc J.* 1991;145:1217–1223.
33. *England and Wales*. Available at: http://www.ryerson.ca/SAFER-Net and http://www.helpnetwork.org/.
34. *Finland*. http://www.ryerson.ca/SAFER-Net and http://www.helpnetwork.org/.
35. *Estonia*. Available at: http://www.ryerson.ca/SAFER-Net and http://www.helpnetwork.org/.
36. Cukier W, Chapdelaine A. Global trade in small arms: Public health effects and interventions. International Physicans for the Prevention of Nuclear War (IPPNW) and Small Arms/Firearms Education and Research Network (SAFER-Net); March 2001.
37. *Colombia*. Available at: http://www.ryerson.ca/SAFER-Net.
38. Castellanos J. Quoted in Godnick W, Muggah R, Waszink C. *Stray Bullets: The Impact of mall Arms Misuse in Central America*, Small Arms Survey, Occasional Paper No. 5, Geneva: Small Arms Survey; Oct. 2002:23.

39. Cruz JM, Beltrán MA. Las armas en El Salvador: Diagnóstico sobre su situación y su impacto. University Institute of Public Opinion (IUDOP), Central American University for the Arias Foundation for Peace and Human Progress. Available at: http://www.arias.org.cr/fundarias/cpr/armasliv.
40. Kellermann AL, Lee RK, Mercey JA, Banton J. The epidemiologic basis for the prevention of firearms injuries. *Ann Rev Public Health*. 1991;12:17–40.
41. Arya N. Healing our planet: Physicians and global security. *Croat Med J*. 2003;44:139–147. Available at: http://www.cmj.hr/index.php?D=/44/2/139.
42. Zimring FE, Hawkins G. *Crime is Not the Problem: Lethal Violence in America*. Oxford: Oxford University Press, 1997; or Lab, SP. *Crime Prevention: Approaches, Practices and Evaluations*. Cincinatti: Anderson; 1997.
43. Meddings D. Weapons injuries during and after periods of conflict: Retrospective analysis. *BMJ*. 1997;315:1417–1420.
44. Sloan JH, Kellermann AL, Reay DT. Handgun regulations, crime, assaults, and homicides: A tale of two cities. *N Engl J Med*. 1988;319:1256–1262.
45. Cukier W. Firearms regulation: Canada in the international context. *Chronic Dis Can*. 1998;19:25–40.
46. Zimring F, Hawkins G. *Crime is Not the Problem: Lethal Violence in America*. New York: Oxford University Press; 1997.
47. Killias M. Gun ownership, suicide and homicide: An international perspective. Understanding Crime, Experiences of Crime and Crime Control. Rome: UNICRI, 1993:289–302.
48. Killias M. Gun ownership, suicide and homicide: An international perspective. In: Alvazzi del Frate A, Zvekic Uvan Dijk JJM, eds. *Understanding Crime Experiences of Crime and Crime Control*. Rome: UNICRI; 1993:289–302.
49. Miller T, Cohen M. Cost of gunshot and cut/stab wounds in US with some Canadian comparisons. *Accid Anal Prev*. 1997;29:329–341.
50. Lott J. *More Guns, Less Crime: Understanding Crime and Gun-Control Laws*. Chicago: University of Chicago Press; 1998.
51. Mauser GA. Armed self defense: the Canadian case. *J Crim Just*. 1996;24:393–406.
52. Hemenway D. Survey research and self-defense gun use: An explanantion of extreme overestimates. *J Crim Law Criminol* 1997;87:1430–1445.
53. Cummings P, Koepsell TD. Does owning a firearm increase or decrease the risk of death? *JAMA* 1998;280:471–473.
54. Webster DW, Vernick JS, Ludwig J. No proof that right-to-carry laws reduce violence. *Am J Public Health* 1998;88:982–983.
55. Kellermann AL, Rivara FP, Rushforth ND. Gun ownership as a risk factor for homicide in the home. *N Eng J Med* 1993;329:1084–1091.
56. Kellermann AL, Rivara FP, Somes G, Reay DT, Franciso J, Banton JG. Suicide in the home in relation to gun ownership. *N Eng J Med* 1992;327:467–472.
57. Wintemute GJ, Parham CA, Beaumont JJ, Wright M, Drake C. Mortality among recent purchasers of handguns. *N Engl J Med* 1999;341:1583–1589.
58. Campbell JC, Webster D, Koziol-McLain J, Block CR, Campbell DW, Gary F, McFarlane JM, Sachs C, Sharps PW, Ulrich Y, Wilt SA, Manganello J, Xu X, Schollenberger J, Frye V. Risk factors for femicide in abusive relationships: Results from a multi-site case control study. *Am J Public Health* 2003;93:1089–1097.

59. United Nations (UN). *International Study on Firearm Regulation*. Updated database; 1999. Available at: http://www.uncjin.org/Statistics/firearms/index.htm.

60. A note by the Secretary-General containing the report of the Group of Governmental Experts established pursuant to Assembly resolution 54/54 V of 15 December 1999, entitled *Small Arms* (Document A/Conf.192/2). New York: United Nations; 2000. Available at: http://ods-dds-ny.un.org/doc/UNDOC/GEN/N00/622/52/PDF/N0062252.pdf.

61. Coalition to Oppose the Arms Trade (COAT). Canadian military exports and international human rights. *Press for Conversion*. March 1998;32.

62. Coalition to Oppose the Arms Trade (COAT). Canadian military exports and international human rights. *Press for Conversion*. April 2000;40.

63. Project Ploughshares. Arms deliveries to the Third World. Available at: http://www.ploughshares.ca/imagesarticles/ACR00/map_arms_deliveries_3rd2a.pdf.

64. Lumpe L, ed. *Running Guns: The Global Black Market in Small Arms*. London: Zed; 2000.

65. Cukier W, Shropshire S. Domestic gun markets: The licit/illicit links. In: Lumpe L, ed. *Running Guns: The Global Black Market in Small Arms*. London: Zed; 2000.

66. Cukier W, Sarkar T, Quigley T. Firearm regulation: International law and jurisprudence. *Can Crim Law Rev* 2000;6:99–123.

67. Mickleburgh R. Moses brings gun gospel north. *Globe and Mail*. 14 April 2000; A8.

68. U.S. Const. amend II.

69. *United States v. Cruikshank,* 92 U.S. 542 (1875); *United States v. Mille*, 307 U.S. 174 (1939); *Lewis v. United States,* 445 U.S. 55 (1980), all of which hold that the Second Amendment of the American Constitution does not guarantee any individual the right to possess firearms. For a more complete discussion, see Ingram JD, Ray AA. The right (?) to keep and bear arms. *N Mex Law Rev* 1997;27:491.

70. Stephens OH Jr. Scheb JM II. *American Constitutional Law*. Minneapolis/St. Paul: West; 1993 at 473.

71. Lord Cullen. Public enquiry into the shootings at Dunblane Primary School. 1996. Available at: www.official-documents/co/uk/document/scottish/dunblane/dunblane.htm

72. *Police v. David Goodwin* (High Court, Hamilton, NZ), unreported AP 107/93.

73. *R. v. Hasselwander* (1993), 81 C.C.C. (3d) 471, 20 C.R. (4th) 277, [1993] 2 S.C.R. 398 (S.C.C.) at 479 [C.C.C.].

74. Tomasevski K. The right to peace. In: Claude RP, Weston BH, eds. *Human Rights in the World Community* Philadelphia: University of Pennsylvania Press; 1989:168.

75. Alston P. Peace as a human right. In: Claude RP, Weston BH, eds. *Human Rights in the World Community: Issues and Action*. 2nd ed. Philadelphia: University of Pennsylvania Press; 1992:201. See also *United Nations Declaration on the Right of Peoples to Peace*, GA Res. 39/11, 39 GAOR Supp. (No. 51), UN Doc. A/39/51 (1985), which states that "... the preservation of the right of peoples to peace and the promotion of its implementation constitute a fundamental obligation of each State." (Article 2).

76. International Action Network on Small Arms (IANSA). *Focusing Attention on Small Arms: Opportunities for the UN 2001 Conference on the Illicit Trade in Small Arms and Light Weapons*. International Action Network on Small Arms; 2000.
77. Cukier W, Bandeira A, Fernandes R, Kamenju J, Kirsten A, Puley G, Walker C. Combating the illicit trade in small arms and light weapons: Enhancing controls on legal transfers. *Biting the Bullet* [Briefing 7]. London: International Alert, Saferworld, BASIC; 2001.
78. Goldring N. A glass half full. Paper present at The UN Small Arms Conference, Council on Foreign Relations, Roundtable on the Geo-Economics of Military Preparedness, 26 September 2001.
79. Cukier W, Sarkar T, Quigley T. Firearm regulation: International law and jurisprudence. *Can   Crim   Law   Rev*. 2000:6:99–123. See also http://www.ryerson.ca/SAFER-Net.
80. Meek S. *Buy or Barter: History and Prospects for Voluntary Weapons Collection Programmes*. Institute for Security Studies; Monograph No. 22; March 1998.
81. United Nations Foundation. *Despite US Resistance, States Agree on Pact*. July 27, 2001.
82. Norwegian initiative on small arms transfers. Available at: http://www.nisat.org/EU/European_Union_theme_page.htm Small Arms Survey http://www.smallarmssurvey.org/RegionalDocs.html
83. Organization for Security and Co-operation in Europe. *Principles governing conventional arms transfers*, Nov. 25, 1993 Available at: http://www.osce.org/docs/english/pia/epia93-3.pdf
84. OAS Inter-American Convention Against the Illicit Manufacturing and Trafficking in Firearms, Ammunition, Explosives, and Other Related Materials, 1997. Available at: http://www.oas.org/juridico/english/sigs/a-63.html.
85. Small Arms Survey. Available at: http://www.smallarmssurvey.org/Regional-Docs.html
86. For an article-by-article defense of the legal arguments behind the Framework Convention on International Arms Transfers, see: http://armslaw.org/fccomment.html.
87. Clarke RV, ed. *Situational Crime Prevention: Successful Case Studies*. Albany, NY: Harrow and Heston; 1992.
88. Christoffel T, Gallagher SS. *Injury Prevention and Public Health: Practical Knowledge, Skills and Strategies*. Gaithersburg, Maryland: Aspen; 1999.
89. Foot D, Stoffman D. *Boom, Bust and Echo 2000: Profiting from the Demographic Shift in the New Millenium*. Toronto: Stoddart; 2001.
90. Boyd N. *A Statistical Analysis of The Impacts of the 1977 Firearms Control Legislation: Critique and Discussion*. Ottawa: Department of Justice; 1996.
91. Mouzos J. Firearm-related violence: The impact of the nationwide agreement on firearms. *Trends and Issues in Crime and Criminal Justice*. Australian Institute of Criminology, May 1999.
92. Villaveces A, Cummings P, Espitia V, Koepsell T, McKnight B, Kellermann A. Effect of a ban on carrying firearms on homicide rates in 2 Columbian cities. *JAMA*. 2000;283:1205–1209.
93. Falbo G, Buzzetti R, Cattaneo A. Homicide in children and adolescents: a case control study in Recife, Brazil. *Bull World Health Organ*. 2001;79:2–7.

94. Logan S "Under the Gun in Rio", Brazzil, Nov. 2003. http://www.brazzil.com/
2003/html/news/articles/nov03/p118nov03.htm
95. *Estonian Human Development Report*, 2000. Available at: http://www.undp.ee.
96. World Bank. Controlling the Jamaican crime problem: Peace building and
community action. *World Bank Report*. 2000.
97. Kellermann AL. Comment: Gunsmoke—Changing public attitudes towards
smoking and firearms. *Am J Public Health* June 1997;87:910–913.
98. Faltas S, McDonald G, Waszink C. Removing small arms from society: A review
of weapons collections and destruction programmes. *Small Arms Survey*,
Occasional Paper No. 2. Geneva: Small Arms Survey; 2001.
99. See the Handgun Epidemic Lowering Plan (HELP) Network web site. Available at: http://www.helpnetwork.org/.
100. See the Coalition for Gun Control (CGC) website. Available at:
http://www.guncontrol.ca.
101. Griffin D. Executive Officer of the Canadian Police Association, Testimony
before the Senate's Standing Committee on Lagal and Constitutional Affairs.
February 6, 2003: 2nd Session, 37th Parliament, 140(33). Available at:
http://www.parl.gc.ca/37/2/parlbus/chambus/senate/deb-e/033db2003-02-06-
E.htm?Language=E&Parl=37&Ses=2. See also MacLeod, E. (Chief), Canadian
Association of Chiefs of Police. Don't Cop Out on the Gun Registry. Comment,
Globe and Mail, Thursday January 15, 2004.
102. Dab W. Cited in: Cukier W, Chapdelaine A. Global trade in small arms: Public
health effects and interventions. International Physcians for the Prevention of
Nuclear War (IPPNW) and Small Arms/Firearms Education and Research
Network (SAFER-Net); March 2001.

2
Guns and Bullets

Part 1—How Guns Work
MARK BYERS, JAMES M. RYAN, and PETER F. MAHONEY
Part 2—The Effects of Bullets
DONALD JENKINS and PAUL DOUGHERTY

Introduction

This chapter is written for clinical staff with little or no previous exposure to firearms. Although one must "treat the wound and not the weapon," a knowledge of how firearms work should lead to a better understanding of how bullets and other projectiles cause injury. The chapter is in two parts—Part 1 describes how guns work and Part 2 gives an introduction to the effects of bullets.

Part 1—How Guns Work

MARK BYERS, JAMES M. RYAN, and PETER F. MAHONEY

History

Nearly all firearms work the same way. An explosive force is applied to a projectile that is propelled down a tube to fly towards its target. The first guns were cannons, the first propellant was black powder, and the first projectiles were cannon balls. Gunpowder was placed in the barrel, the cannon ball rolled in, and then the gunpowder was ignited. The hot gases produced by the burning gunpowder pushed the cannon ball up and out of the barrel.

The 19th century saw the development of the cartridge. The cartridge packaged the bullet, propellant, and primer/detonator within a case. This allowed the development of repeating firearms, such as the bolt-action rifle.

Small Arms—Revolvers and Pistols

Some of the first modern small arms were revolvers (Figure 2-1). Cartridges are loaded into a chamber, the chamber revolves, lines up with a fixed barrel, and then the cartridge's primer is struck by a hammer. The propellant ignites and the cartridge expands within the cylinder, blocking it and forcing all the gases forward, which accelerates the bullet down the barrel. Grooves in the barrel spin the bullet, which imparts stability to the bullet in flight and improves accuracy.

The original revolvers needed to have their hammer manually pulled back until it caught. The trigger then could be pulled, and the hammer was released (the "single-action" revolver). "Double-action" revolvers can be used the same way. Alternatively, by exerting continued pressure on the trigger, the hammer moves back and compresses a spring housed in the handle. A lever attached to the trigger causes a ratchet to turn the cartridge cylinder to align the next bullet with the barrel. When the hammer is all the way back, further pressure on the trigger releases it and it is pushed forward by the spring.

Revolvers are robust, simple, and rarely malfunction. Revolvers do have disadvantages. They need frequent reloading, and the empty cases need to be ejected manually from the cylinder.

The modern pistol has a magazine that holds more cartridges than the revolver cylinder and is capable of self-loading as the magazine itself is spring loaded (Figure 2-2). The magazine spring pushes a cartridge into place, which is loaded, fired, and then automatically ejected. There are two methods for self-loading. The simplest method employs the reaction forces of the fired cartridge to push back a heavy breech block against a breech spring. The empty casing is discarded and the breech block is pushed forward by the breech spring, collects the next bullet (forced into place by the magazine spring), and loads it into the barrel. The trigger then can be pulled; the cartridge is fired and the process repeats itself.

Rifles and Carbines

Modern rifles have long barrels cut with a spiral groove to spin the bullet. The spin imparts stability to the bullet in flight. Carbines are shorter and lighter (Figure 2-3). The first breech-loaded rifle appeared in the 1830s. Individual cartridges were loaded by a bolt, which cocked and housed the firing pin. By the 1880s, the Swiss, French, and Germans had developed a bolt-action rifle with a magazine using full metal-jacketed bullets. The more bullets that can be housed in the magazine, the more that can be individually loaded and fired using the bolt action before the magazine is empty and has to be changed.

Similar advances occurred in rifles as had occurred in pistols, and semiautomatic and automatic rifles were developed. Semiautomatic rifles work

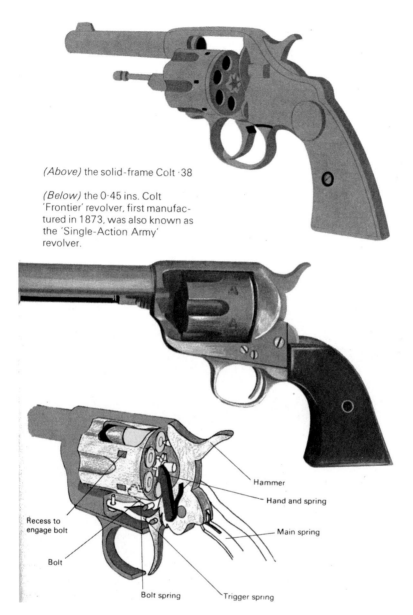

(Above) the solid-frame Colt ·38

(Below) the 0·45 ins. Colt 'Frontier' revolver, first manufactured in 1873, was also known as the 'Single-Action Army' revolver.

Hammer

Hand and spring

Recess to engage bolt

Main spring

Bolt

Bolt spring

Trigger spring

FIGURE 2-1. The mechanism of the Colt "Frontier" revolver. (Reprinted from Frederick Wilkinson, *Guns*, Copyright 1970, Hamlyn, p. 121).

Italy
BERETTA MODELLO 84

The well-known Italian firm of Beretta has been making good quality self-loading pistols since 1915 and the particular model illustrated may be taken as a reasonably typical example of a simple blow-back mechanism without any positive locking device, but relying entirely on the weight of the slide and the power of the spring. As a normal 9mm cartridge would probably be somewhat too powerful for this basic mechanism a special short cartridge is used. This works well but is rather under-powered for normal military use. This pistol has an external hammer; others have internal ones, but the principle on which they work is very much the same.

(Full specification of the Beretta Modello 1934 on page *203*.)

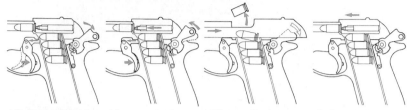

1 *The first round is loaded manually by pulling back the slide to its fullest extent and then allowing the spring to carry it forward. This cocks the hammer and feeds the top round into the chamber.*

2 *Pressure on the trigger releases the hammer which springs forward to strike the rear end of the firing pin, thus driving it onto the cap of the cartridge in the chamber and firing it.*

3 *The gases drive the bullet forward and also force the empty case back, the pressure being sufficient to operate the slide as already described. This action also ejects the empty case.*

4 *The forward action is then repeated. The next round in the magazine, having been forced upwards by the magazine spring, is fed into the chamber and the pistol is ready for the next shot.*

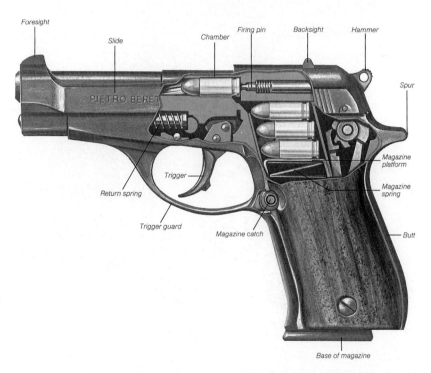

FIGURE 2-2. Diagram of semiautomatic pistol, Beretta Modello 84. (With permission, Myatt F. *Modern Small Arms.* Copyright 1978, London, Salamander Books, p. 195).

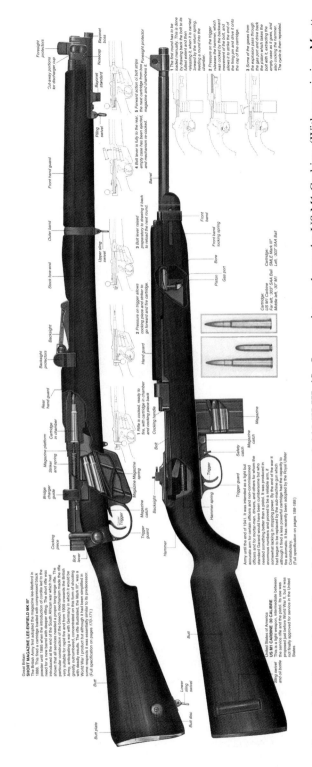

FIGURE 2-3. Upper picture shows the bolt action Lee Enfield MK III rifle. Lower picture shows the US M1 Carbine. (With permission, Myatt F. *Modern Small Arms*. Copyright 1978, London, Salamander Books, pp. 154–157).

in a similar manner to semiautomatic pistols. Gases from firing a bullet are used to re-cock and reload the weapon with the next bullet from the magazine, but the trigger has to be pulled again to fire the next bullet.

To achieve higher rates of fire, manufacturers developed the machine gun.

Machine Guns

A machine gun (Figure 2-4) is an automatic weapon. The term includes automatic rifles, "assault rifles," and submachine guns. They are belt or magazine fed, and theoretically keep firing for as long as the trigger is depressed or until the ammunition runs out.

Shotguns

Shotguns, developed for sport or combat, fire a cartridge containing shot (Figure 2-5). Shotguns may be single barrelled or double barrelled. If double barrelled the barrels may be next to each other (side by side) or one on top of the other (under and over). Working mechanisms include semi-automatic and pump action (Figure 2-6). Shotgun calibres are measured by the number of spherical lead balls, of the same diameter as the barrel, that make up a pound of lead.

For instance, an 8-bore has the same diameter as a 2-ounce ball of lead ($8 \times 2\,oz = 16\,oz$ or $1\,lb$). The 12-bore has a diameter the same as a 1.33-ounce ball of lead ($12 \times 1.33\,oz = 16\,oz$ or $1\,lb$). The smaller the bore number of the gun, the larger the diameter of the barrel and the cartridge.[1]

Cartridges contain primer, propellant, and shot. The choking of the gun determines how much the shot spreads on discharge. A fully choked gun has a narrower barrel than a gun with true cylinders. Choking gives constrictions ranging from 3- to 40-thousandths of an inch towards the muzzle end of the barrel. The constriction means that the shot is kept closer together as it leaves the end of the barrel. The other feature that affects the spread of shot is the length of the barrel. A short barrel allows the shot to spread out earlier after discharge than a long barrel. A "sawed-off" shotgun is a shotgun with its barrels cut off, thus shortening the weapon and allowing early and wide spread of the shot. In the US, the legal barrel limit is 20 inches.

Combat shotguns are designed to be quick to load and relatively short barrelled. They are commonly "slide-loaded" or pump action, have a magazine under the barrel, and gain their effect from the ammunition they use. Where as sporting shotguns use small loads with many hundreds of pellets per shell (for example No. 7 shot for a 12-bore shotgun has 361 pellets per shell), combat shotguns use shells such as the double 00 buck, which are loaded with nine balls each. Shotguns have an effective range of between 30 and 50 meters. Beyond this distance, the velocity falls off and the spread increases markedly. Combat shotguns are being developed that will have longer ranges.

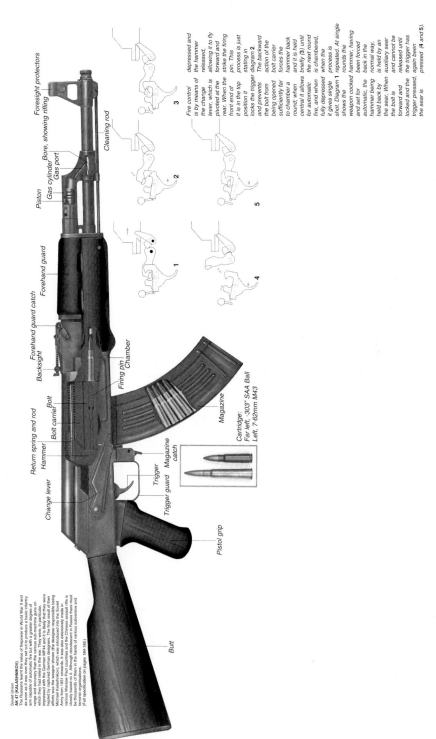

Soviet Union
AK 47 (KALASHNIKOV)
The Russians learnt the value of firepower in World War II and as soon as it was over they set out to produce a basic infantry arm capable of automatic fire but with a greater degree of range and accuracy than the various sub-machine guns on which they had relied in the war. They were, in particular, impressed with the German MP44 and it is likely that they were headed by captured German designers. The final result of their efforts was the weapon shown (the designer responsible being Michael Kalashnikov), which was introduced into the Soviet Army from 1951 onwards. It was also extensively made in various Warsaw Pact countries and the Chinese assault rifle is closely based on it. Although obsolescent in Russia there must be thousands of them in the hands of various subversive and terrorist organisations.
(Full specification on pages 164–165.)

Butt

Change lever

Return spring and rod
Hammer

Bolt
Bolt carrier

Trigger guard
Trigger

Pistol grip

Magazine catch

Magazine

Cartridge:
Far left, .303" SAA Ball
Left, 7.62mm M43

Firing pin
Chamber

Backsight
Forehand guard catch

Forehand guard

Piston
Gas cylinder
Gas port

Bore, showing rifling

Cleaning rod

Foresight protectors

Fire control is by means of the change lever, which is pivoted at the rear. When the front end of it is in the top position it locks the trigger and prevents the bolt from being opened sufficiently far to chamber a round; when central it allows for automatic fire, and when fully depressed it gives single shot. Diagram 1 shows the weapon cocked and set for automatic, the hammer being held back by the sear. When the bolt is forward and locked and the trigger pressed, the sear is depressed and the hammer released, allowing it to fly forward and strike the firing pin. This process is just starting in diagram 2. The backward action of the bolt carrier forces the hammer back and it is held briefly (3) until the next round is chambered, when the process is repeated. At single rounds the hammer, having been forced back in the normal way, is held by an auxiliary sear and cannot be released until the trigger has again been pressed (4 and 5).

FIGURE 2-4. Diagram of AK47. (With permission, Myatt F. *Modern Small Arms*. Copyright 1978, Salamander Books, pp. 158–161).

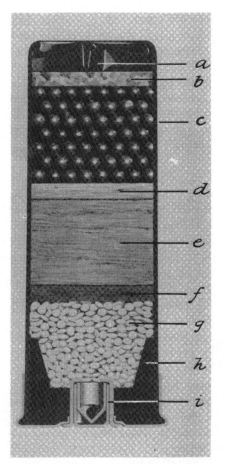

FIGURE 2-5. A modern Eley cartridge showing (a) crimp closure, (b) frangible waterproof seal, (c) plastic case, (d) under-shot card, (e) vegetable felt "Kleena" wad, (f) over-powder card, (g) doubled-based powder, (h) compressed paper base wad, and (i) cap or primer. (With permission, Thomas G. *Shotguns & Cartridges for Game and Clays*, 4th ed. Copyright 1987, Adam & Charles Black: London, England, p. 86).

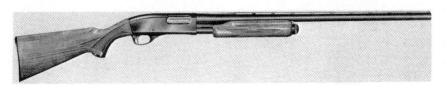

FIGURE 2-6. A typical American pump gun. The model shown is the popular Remington M 870. (With permission, Thomas G. *Shotguns & Cartridges for Game and Clays*, 4th ed. Copyright 1987, Adam & Charles Black; London, England, p. 36).

Ammunition

There is a great deal of difference between pistol and rifle ammunition. Pistol ammunition is designed to be accurate to a range of around 40 meters, whereas rifle rounds need to be capable of hitting a target up to 1000 or more meters away (Figure 2-7). Pistol ammunition usually is straight cased. Rifle ammunition is often "bottle necked," so it can contain a larger amount of propellant.

The distinction is not quite so clear, as there are pistols that fire rifle ammunition and long-barrelled weapons (including some submachine guns) that fire pistol ammunition.

There are several different sorts of bullets, such as:

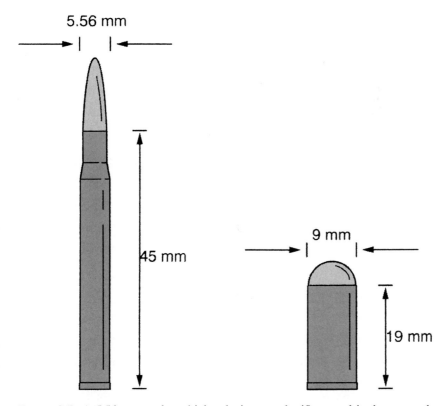

FIGURE 2-7. A 5.56 mm modern, high-velocity assault rifle round is shown on the left. Note its slender, elongated shape and sharp, pointed nose. On the right is a short, squat, blunt-nosed 9 mm low-velocity handgun round. (Ryan JM, Biant L. Gunshot wounds and blast injury. In: Greaves I, Porter KM (eds). Pre-hospital medicine: principles and practice of Immediate Care. London: Arnold 1999. Page 364. With permission).

Full Metal Jacket—A metal casing around a lead core. This produces a non-expanding, deep-penetrating round that is considered very reliable.

Jacketed Hollow Point—These bullets have an exposed, hollowed lead tip that allows expansion of the round on impact. They are likely to penetrate tissue less deeply than a full metal jacket bullet but more energy is transferred to the tissue.

Soft Point—An exposed lead tip allows the bullet to expand rapidly on impact at lower velocities. A wide wound of up to 200% of original bullet diameter is produced from the round's rapid expansion.

Altered ammunition—People alter ammunition to increase the severity of the inflicted wounds. An example is the Dum Dum, produced by cutting a cross in the soft lead tip of the bullet to ensure it that it fragments on impact. The term Dum Dum comes from the Dum-Dum Arsenal in India, which produced soft-nosed bullets for the British Army in about 1890 for the Lee Metford rifle. British troops found their weapons did not have as much stopping power with the new full metal-jacketed bullets compared to the 0.45″ Martini-Henry rifles, and this led them to modify the bullet design. An amendment to the The Geneva Convention banned such projectiles.

The laws and conventions covering bullet design are considered in Chapter 6 on International Humanitarian Law.

Rubber Bullets

Rubber bullets first were used in Northern Ireland in 1970 by the British Army. The missiles are blunt-nosed, with a low muzzle velocity, and they are designed to inflict superficial injuries only, but they have caused death.[2]

In 1989, they were replaced by plastic bullets, which were considered less dangerous. There are several variants available in many countries, including rubber-coated metal bullets, rubber plugs, and beanbag rounds (a fabric beanbag full of lead pellets).

Part 2—The Effects of Bullets*

DONALD JENKINS and PAUL DOUGHERTY

Bullets cause wounds by interacting with body tissues. The kinetic energy (KE) of a bullet is given by the formula $KE = \frac{1}{2} MV^2$, where M is the bullets mass and V is the velocity. While the formula indicates how much energy is available, it does not describe how this energy is used nor the surgical magnitude of the problem.

---

* The opinions expressed herein are the private views of the authors and are not to be construed as official or reflecting the views of the US Department of the Army, or the US Department of the Air Force, or the US Department of Defense.

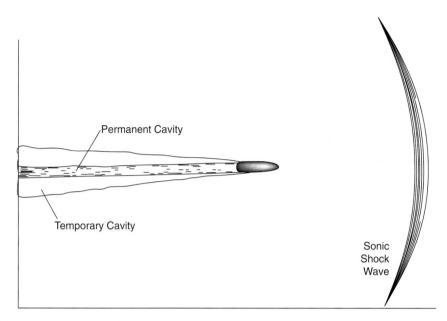

Permanent Cavity

Temporary Cavity

Sonic
Shock
Wave

FIGURE 2-8. The energy transferred to the tissues by a bullet depends upon the bullet's shape, how it impacts the tissue (point first, side first, or blunt end first). (Reprinted from *Emergency War Surgery* 2nd United States revision. NATO handbook 1988. US Government printing office, Washington, DC).

A number of factors influence the severity of the wound, including the diameter, shape, and composition of the projectile, its linear and rotational velocity, and the type of tissue struck, including intermediate targets (Figure 2-8).

Mechanism of Injury

There are two areas of projectile–tissue interaction in missile-caused wounds: the permanent and the temporary cavity. The *permanent* cavity is the localized area of cell necrosis, proportional to the size of the projectile as it passes through tissue. The *temporary* cavity is the transient lateral displacement of tissue, which occurs after passage of the projectile. *Elastic* tissue, such as skeletal muscle, blood vessels, and skin, may be pushed aside after passage of the projectile, but then rebound. *Inelastic* tissue, such as bone or liver, may fracture.

Below are some examples of the characteristics of commonly encountered firearms seen throughout the world. The illustrations are of the entire path of missiles fired consistently at 5 to 10 meters in range into ordnance gelatin tissue-simulant blocks. Variations of range and intermediate targets such as body armor and different body tissues will alter the wound seen.

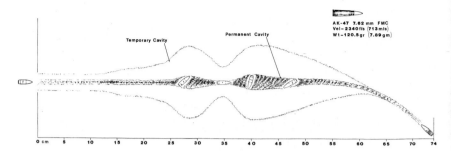

FIGURE 2-9. The AK-47 rifle in Figure 2-4 is one of the most common weapons seen throughout the world. (Reprinted from *Emergency War Surgery* 2nd United States revision. NATO handbook 1988. US Government printing office, Washington, DC.)

Examples of Different Bullet Effects

The AK-47 rifle is one of the most common weapons seen throughout the world. For this particular bullet (full metal jacketed or ball), there is a 25 centimeter path of relatively minimal tissue disruption before the projectile begins to yaw. This explains why relatively minimal tissue disruption may be seen with some wounds (Figure 2-9).

The AK-74 rifle was an attempt to create a smaller-caliber assault rifle. The standard bullet does not deform in the tissue simulant, but does yaw relatively early (about 7 centimeters of penetration) (Figure 2-10).

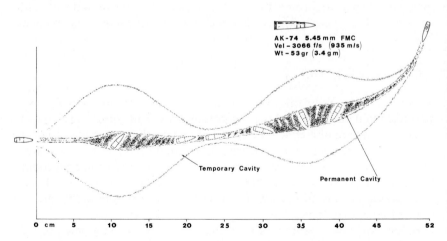

FIGURE 2-10. The AK-74 rifle was an attempt to create a smaller caliber assault rifle. (Reprinted from *Emergency War Surgery* 2nd United States revision. NATO handbook 1988. US Government printing office, Washington, DC.)

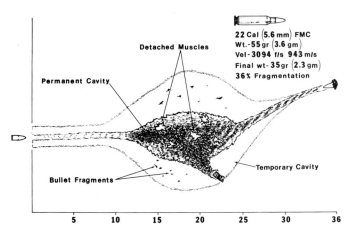

FIGURE 2-11. The M-16A1 rifle fires a 55-grain full metal-jacketed bullet (M-193) at approximately 950 meters per second. (Reprinted from *Emergency War Surgery* 2nd United States revision. NATO handbook 1988. US Government printing office, Washington, DC.)

The M-16A1 rifle fires a 55-grain full metal-jacketed bullet (M-193) at approximately 950 meters/second. The average point forward distance in tissue is about 12 centimeters, after which it yaws to about 90 degrees, flattens, and then breaks at the cannalure (a groove placed around the middle section of the bullet). The slightly heavier M-855 bullet used with the M-16A2 rifle shows a similar pattern to the M-193 bullet (Figure 2-11).

The 7.62 millimeter NATO rifle cartridge still is used in sniper rifles and machine guns. After about 16 centimeters of penetration, this bullet yaws through 90 degrees and then travels base forward. A large temporary cavity is formed and occurs at the point of maximum yaw (Figure 2-12).

The wound created by a shotgun is created by the shot. The actual size and damage done is a function of the size of shot used and the range from which the gun is fired. As a rough guide, ranges over 10 meters produce multiple superficial wounds; between 5 and 10 meters, the pellets can penetrate deeply into the tissue; and below 5 meters, the shot acts as a solid "slug." The slug can penetrate deeply, impart a great deal of energy, and produce a large high-energy transfer wound. Additionally, the wounds often are contaminated.[3]

Bullet wounds and their different characteristics are considered further in Chapter 5, on "Forensic Aspects of Ballistic Injury."

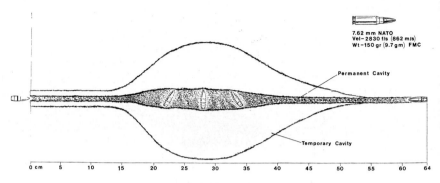

FIGURE 2-12. The 7.62 millimeter NATO rifle cartridge still is used in sniper rifles and machine guns. (Reprinted from *Emergency War Surgery* 2nd United States revision. NATO handbook 1988. US Government printing office, Washington, DC.)

Summary

All small arms work in roughly the same way. An explosive imparts a force to a missile (bullet) that is directed along a tube towards its target.

Bullets cause wounds by interacting with tissue. The factors involved with the production of a missile wound are: projectile diameter, shape, and composition; linear and rotational velocity; and the type of tissue struck.

References

1. Sedgwick NM. *The Young Shot*, 3rd Edition, London, England: Adam & Charles Black Ltd; 1975.
2. Millar R, Rutherford WH, Johnston S, Malhotra VJ. Injuries caused by rubber bullets: A report on 90 patients. Br J Surg. 1975;62:480–486.
3. Ryan JM, Biant L. Gunshot wounds and blast injury. In: Greaves I, Porter K, eds. *Pre-hospital Medicine: The Principles and Practice of Immediate Care*. London: Arnold: 1999:363–373.

3
Bombs, Mines, Blast, Fragmentation, and Thermobaric Mechanisms of Injury

TONEY W. BASKIN and JOHN B. HOLCOMB

Introduction

Once confined to the battlefield and the occasional industrial accident, the sequela of explosive force has now become all too commonplace and continues to increase as industry expands and explosive weaponry proliferates. The chaos and "fog of war" no longer can be considered the sole province of the battlefield. The ubiquitous threat of terrorism places responsibility for the care of victims not only upon the military surgeon, but upon civilian counterparts as well. The medical system, military, and civilians must understand the pathophysiology of injury induced from explosive devices, be they letter bombs, shaped warheads from a rocket propelled grenade (RPG), antipersonnel land mines, aerial-delivered cluster bombs, or enhanced blast weapons.

Urban warfare is becoming more widespread, providing both a rich environment for the bomber to strike and the ideal medium for enhanced blast weapons. The terrorist may employ pipe bombs, large high-energy car bombs, or the suicide bomber wearing several kilograms of explosive.

In the United States alone from 1990 to 1995, the FBI reported 15 700 bombings, with 3176 injuries and 355 deaths, and these numbers only continue to increase.

Primary blast injury, secondary to conventional high explosives, is uncommon in surviving casualties. This is because they would have been close to the epicenter of the explosion and are likely to have suffered lethal fragment and heat injury. With the advent of enhanced blast weapons (already populating the arms market), primary blast injury will increase in frequency, placing extreme clinical and logistical stress on the medical system.

Although antipersonnel mines were banned by the Ottawa Convention in 1997, civilian mine injuries have become even more common than military mine injuries that occur during combat, with farmers, women, and children 10 times more likely to encounter these abandoned weapons of war. The immense number of antipersonnel mines scattered throughout many parts of the world continues to plague civilization with horrible disabling injuries that, according to the International Committee of the Red Cross (ICRC), number 24,000 per year.[1]

In this chapter we will address the myriad types of explosive weapons, how they work, and the resulting patterns of injury that threaten to present as mass casualties and to severely impact the health-care system clinically, logistically, and psychologically.

Explosions

An explosive is a chemical compound or mixture that, when subjected to heat, shock, friction, or other impulse, leads to a rapid chemical reaction or combustion and an equally rapid generation of heat and gases. The consequent combined volume is much larger than the original substance.

Explosives are classified as high or low, depending upon the rate at which this reaction takes place. Gunpowder, the first explosive used in military ordnance, is an example of a low explosive. Low explosives change relatively slowly from a solid to a gaseous state, generally less than 2000 meters per second.

By comparison, high explosives (HE) react almost instantaneously, causing sudden increases in pressures and a detonation wave that moves at supersonic speed (1400–9000 meters per second). Common examples are 2,4,6-trinitrotoluene (TNT) and the more recent polymer-bonded explosives, such as Semtex and Gelignite, which are 1.5 times the power of TNT. High explosives are used commonly in military ordnance.

A detonator is a type of explosive that reacts very rapidly and is used to set off other more inert explosives. Fulminate of Mercury mixed with potassium chlorate is the most commonly used detonator. Detonators also can be equipment, which by flame, spark, percussion, friction, or pressure are used to set off a chemical detonator. Detonation refers to the chemical and exothermic reaction that creates a pressure wave propagating throughout the explosive, creating rapid production of heat and gases, resulting in a "runaway" process and producing the resulting explosion.

The rapid release of enormous amounts of energy in a high explosion results in a primary blast wave, propulsion of fragments and environmental material or debris, and often generates intense thermal radiation. The initial explosion creates an instantaneous rise in pressure, resulting in a shock wave that travels outward at supersonic speed. The shock wave is the leading front and an integral component of the blast wave. The generation and propagation of blast waves are governed by nonlinear physics.

The response of structures, including human tissues, also may be nonlinear, as evidenced by the pathophysiology of blast injuries.

This sudden variation in air pressure creates a mass movement of air known as the dynamic overpressure or blast wave. The Friedlander Relationship (Figure 3-1) illustrates the physical properties of an ideal blast

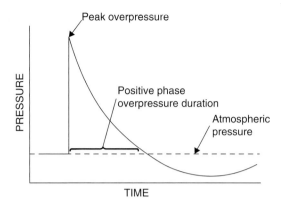

FIGURE 3-1. Friedlander relationship.

wave in open air. With the arrival of the shock wave, the pressure instantly increases to a peak overpressure, then rapidly falls and creates subatmospheric pressures before returning to normal ambient atmospheric pressure.

In reality, the reflection of the blast wave as it encounters environmental structures creates a very complex pattern of overpressures. These overpressures and an actual reversal of the blast wind in the negative phase may cause significant damage. For an in-depth discussion of the creation and propagation of blast waves and how they interact with various structures, the reader is referred to an article by I.G. Cullis.[2]

Enhanced-Blast Weapons

Ongoing research in the ordnance industry and recent technological advances in explosives and material has propagated the development of enhanced-blast weapons (EBW). There are four known types of enhanced-blast explosives:

1. metallized explosives,
2. reactive surround,
3. fuel-air,
4. thermobaric.

Once confined to fuel-air explosive (FAE) bombs, EBWs, recently proliferating the arms market, span the range of weapon systems from small grenades and hand-held weapons to large-caliber rockets (Table 3-1).

Relatively few primary blast injuries have been seen, as there are few survivors with primary blast injury from conventional HEs. Most die immediately, but this may change with the increase of EBW usage. With

TABLE 3-1. EBWs currently in use

	Fuel-air explosives	Thermobaric
United States	Fuel-air warheads • BLU-64/B (200 kg fuel) • BLUE-72B Pave Pat 2 (1202 kg ethylene oxide)	
Former Soviet Union	ODAB-500 PM (193 kg) high-speed low-level attack, can be launched from vehicle KAB-500 Kr S8-DM—3.6 kg multiple-barrel rocket launcher • SPLAV 220 mm (Uragan) BM 9P140 • SPLAV 300 mm (SMerch) BM 9A52	Guided missiles • AT-6-SPIRAL (helicopter launch)* • AT-9 (vehicle launch)* • AT-14 • METIS-M (crew-served weapon) • Khrizantema (BMP)* • TOS-1 (Burantino—mobile rocket launder) S8 unguided air-launched rocket TOS-1 Buratino—multiple-barrel rocket launcher Flame thrower RPO-A (2.1 kg) Grenade launcher GM-94 RShG-1 Multipurpose assault weapon RPG (range 900 m)*
China	250 kg bomb with 2 bomblets 500 kg bomb with 3 bomblets (800 square m)	

Note. * Denotes FAE ability as well.

conventional HEs, the blast wave decays very rapidly and is affected significantly by the environment. Enhanced-blast weapons produce a lower overpressure than conventional HE, but the period of overpressure lasts longer and reaches farther, thereby increasing the lethality zone and producing blast casualties farther from the epicenter of the detonation (Figure 3-2).

The classic EBW mechanism is illustrated best in the FAE, which has an initial small explosion that disperses a vapor cloud of ethylene oxide or other fuel. At a critical time and distance, the dispersed fuel is ignited by a second detonation, producing a uniform dynamic overpressure through the covered area. This may produce lethal overpressures as high as 2 Mpa, whereas a conventional HE would produce only 200 Kpa at a similar distance from the initiating explosion. The EBW also produces a longer-lasting fireball and may produce more energy [area beneath the curve (Figure 3-2)], resulting in more casualties with primary blast injuries combined with burns, crush, and penetrating-fragment injuries.

The blast wave from an EBW can diffract around corners, rapidly expanding and filling a structure, and is enhanced by reflection in enclosed spaces, making this an ideal weapon to defeat field defenses, soft unreinforced buildings, communication equipment, and low-flying aircraft. As an antipersonnel weapon, an EBW can be expected to rapidly produce large numbers of casualties with burns, blast injuries, fragment, translational injuries, and crush injuries from demolished buildings, placing a sudden and intense clinical and logistical strain on medical resources.

Several foreign studies have suggested that body armor enhances the effects of primary blast, creating a "behind armor blunt trauma" (BABT). Although studies by the US Army Soldier Systems Command, Natick, MA, indicated that the Interceptor Body Armor in use by US forces does not enhance the blast effect—and may actually reduce effects—when the ceramic plates are included in the armor, it is safe to say that most body armor currently in use will protect only marginally against primary blast injury and offer little, if any, protection against an accompanying thermal injury. Armor-employing decouplers or layers of material with different acoustic and mechanical properties specifically designed to maximally attenuate the shock wave needs to be designed.

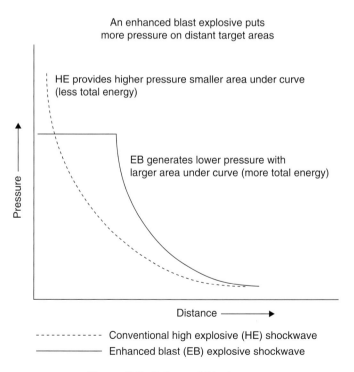

FIGURE 3-2. Enhanced blast wave.

TABLE 3-2. Classification of injury by mechanism

Class of injury	Mechanism
Primary	Interaction of blast wave (overpressure) with body, gas-filled structures being most at risk, complex stress and shear waves produce organ injury.
Secondary	Wounds produced by fragments from weapon, environmental projectiles, and debris, with penetrating injury predominating
Tertiary	Displacement of body (translational) and structural collapse with acceleration–deceleration, crush, and blunt injuries
Quaternary	All other mechanisms producing injury, burns, toxidromes from fuel, metals, septic syndromes from soil and environmental contamination (*septic meliodosis*)

It is the combination of the shock wave or leading edge, the dynamic overpressure, the secondary and tertiary effects, and the associated thermal energy that result in the characteristic injuries seen following detonation of an explosive device. These injuries may be classified according to the mechanism by which they are produced (Table 3-2).

Both conventional and terrorist weapons are designed to produce multiple wounds with the maximum number of casualties. Indeed, on today's battlefield, up to 90% of casualties are secondary to fragmentation wounds, with wounding from small arms or bullets producing generally less than 15 to 20% of battlefield casualties. Modern fragmentation weapons have a high casing-to-explosive ratio designed to produce preformed fragments, which significantly enhances the wounding radius and casualty probability. The major classes of available weapons are categorized in Table 3-3.

TABLE 3-3. Major weapon classification

Conventional	Grenades, aerial bombs, artillery, RPG. See all types of injuries with fragment wounds from preformed fragments predominating along with environmental debris
Antipersonnel mines	Point detonating mine (5 kg), traumatic amputation of foot or lower extremity, dirty, contaminated with debris, clothing, footwear, body parts, and soil Triggered mine (Claymore, Bouncing Betty), upper extremity, chest, face, and ocular injury
Enhanced blast munition	Designed to injure by blast wave, dispersed by fuel vapor, pulmonary injury, may have delayed onset, destroy and damage "soft" targets and personnel
Terrorist bombs	Letter bomb to several hundred kg, low mortality, fragment wounds, debris and crushing injury, some primary blast injury, suicide bomber with human-tissue fragments as wounding agent

Pathophysiology of Primary Blast Injury

The biological effects of the blast wave depend on the peak pressure and the duration of the dynamic overpressure and the effects of the secondary, tertiary, and quaternary mechanisms of injury.

Primary blast injury results from the interaction of the blast wave with the body or tissue, producing two types of energy: stress waves and shear waves. Stress waves produced by the interaction of the blast wave and the body surface are supersonic longitudinal pressure waves that create high local forces with small, but very rapid distortions, producing microvascular injury; they are reinforced and reflected at tissue interfaces, thus enhancing the injury potential.

Organs with heightened differences in physical properties such as the lungs, auditory system, and the gas-filled intestine are most susceptible.

Injuries from the stress waves are caused in several ways.

Pressure differentials across delicate structures such as alveoli;
Rapid compression of and subsequent re-expansion of gas-filled structures;
Reflection of a component of the compressive stress wave known as a tension wave at the interface of tissue and gas.

These myriad mechanisms result in damage originating in the mucosa and submucosa, but also reflect outward. Therefore, evidence of serosal injury may well represent full thickness damage. The interaction of these forces at the tissue interface is also known as spalling, characterized by the "boiling" effect seen at the air–water interface following an underwater explosion. A similar phenomenon most likely occurs at tissue interfaces, with resultant microvascular damage.

Shear waves are transverse waves with a lower velocity and longer duration that cause asynchronous movement of tissues. Actual damage depends on the degree to which the asynchronous motions overcome the inherent tissue elasticity, resulting in tearing of tissue and possible disruption of attachments. However, muscle, bone, and solid-organ injury is far more likely to result from the tertiary and quaternary effects of the blast than from the blast wave alone.

Thoracic

Blasts producing overpressure of less than 40 pounds per square inch (psi) generally will not cause pulmonary injury, (40 psi being produced by 20 Kg TNT exploding 6 meters away). Approximately 50% or more of casualties will sustain pulmonary damage with pressures of 80 psi or more, with overpressures of 200 psi being uniformly fatal in open-air blasts.

Blast injury to the lungs is the cause of the greatest morbidity and mortality from the blast effect alone. In the lungs, reflection of stress waves at more rigid interfaces account for the predilection of paramediastinal, peribronchial, and subpleural tissue disruption and hemorrhage. Propagation of the stress wave results in pulmonary contusions distant from the site of impact in air-filled tissues, with damage to alveolar septae. Type I and some Type II pneumocytes are disrupted structurally and dysfunctionally, with loss of surfactant production, which when combined with capillary endothelial damage and release of ecosinoids and TXA2 may lead to progressive hypoxic respiratory failure and a clinical picture resembling acute respiratory distress syndrome (ARDS).

Pathologically, when the alveola septae are disrupted, hemorrhage occurs in three distinct patterns

1. pleural and subpleural,
2. multifocal and diffuse parenchymal and alveolar hemorrhage,
3. peribronchial and perivascular hemorrhage.

These patterns of injury may range from isolated scattered petechiae to confluent, consolidated areas of hemorrhage. Subpleural cysts and lacerations of pleura may lead to hemo-pneumothorax, pneumomediastinum, or tension pneumothorax. A lethal primary blast injury potentially could present with no outward signs of trauma. In severe blast injury, immediate death may be attributed to a characteristic triad of physiologic responses of primary thoracic blast of bradycardia, apnea, and hypotension that is unrelated to hemorrhage. Immediate death also has been attributed to massive air embolism resulting from the disruption of the alveolar wall and adjacent pulmonary capillaries, with the air emboli primarily affecting cerebral and coronary vessels.

Multiple animal studies have demonstrated large alveolar–venous and broncho–venous fistulae following blast injuries. This occurs in both air and underwater blasts and is commonly found in both cerebral and coronary circulation at autopsy and in experimental animal studies. Dysrythmias, signs of neurologic injury, and retinal artery air emboli may be seen in immediate survivors. The Trendelenberg position is not advisable in these patients, as now it is thought to predispose patients to coronary air embolus. The immediate therapy is supplemental oxygen, with Hyperbaric Oxygen being the definitive treatment of systemic air embolus, although not usually available or clinically practical. Alveolar–venous fistulae are thought to resolve in 24 hours, but must be considered a continuing risk in casualties that require positive pressure ventilation, especially with application of positive end expiratory pressure (PEEP), which is commonly used for hypoxic pathophysiology.

In survivors, clinical manifestations of primary blast may be present immediately or may have a delayed onset of 24 to 48 hours.

Intrapulmonary hemorrhage and focal alveolar edema leading to ventilation perfusion (V/Q) mismatch, increased intrapulmonary shunting, and decreased compliance results in hypoxia and increased work of breathing that is pathophysiologically similar to pulmonary contusions induced by other mechanisms of nonpenetrating thoracic trauma. Chest X-rays have revealed diffuse patchy infiltrates that present in a butterfly pattern. These become more extensive over the first 48 hours, but are usually nearly resolved in seven days. Continued progression of the infiltrates after 48 hours should lead one to consider ARDS or superimposed pneumonia. Clinically, one also may see pneumothorax, hemothorax, subcutaneous and mediastinal emphysema, and even pneumoperitoneum or tension pneumoperitoneum, which may or may not be secondary to ruptured hollow viscous injury. Rib fractures should always alert one to tertiary or quaternary injury to the thorax.

Blast Lung casualties are more susceptible to pulmonary barotrauma (pneumothorax, air embolism) than other pulmonary injuries, and although early positive-pressure mechanical ventilation with the application of positive-end expiratory pressure to maintain adequate oxygenation may be required, the risk of barotrauma may be enhanced by such therapeutic requirements. Various ventilatory strategies have been proposed to lessen such risk, including Continuous Positive Airway Pressure (CPAP), Intermittent Mandatory Ventilation (IMV), and volume-controlled ventilation with low tidal volumes and permissive hypercapnia. Prophylactic tube thoracostomy should be considered if casualties must be evacuated by air or when close observation is impractical.

Fluid resuscitation should be managed judiciously, and early monitoring of hemodynamic parameters should be considered. The ideal fluid for resuscitation in blast injury is not known; however, pre-load should be optimized without overload using crystalloid with or without colloid. Patients probably should not be resuscitated to a mean arterial pressure (MAP) of greater than 60 millimeters mercury. In the absence of hemorrhage, many patients with thoracic blast manifest a prolonged hypotension for several days, with MAPs typically in the range of 50 to 60 millimeters Hg, with systolic pressure of 80 to 90 millimeters Hg and diastolic pressure of 40–50 millimeters Hg. The mechanism of this hypotension is poorly understood and may complicate management in the face of ongoing blood loss.

Auditory

The auditory system is very susceptible to blast and is the most commonly observed blast injury. Perforation in the anteroinferior part of the pars tensa is the most common manifestation of injury. Perforation occurs at 5 to 15 psi, and 33% of injuries are associated with ossicular injury, which does not occur in the absence of tympanic disruption. Cholesteatoma from embedded squamous debris is a long-term complication occurring in up to 12% of blast-perforated ears, dictating long-term follow up. Associated ossicular injury is a feature of more severe blast injury in as many as a third of reported cases. Sensorineural hearing loss associated with a high-pitched tinnitus frequently occurs immediately following a blast. Hearing loss may resolve in hours or may become permanent in greater than 50% of patients, as has been reported in some series. Although not a priority for treatment, auditory injury should be addressed in 24 hours and auditory canal cleaned of all debris. Fifty to 80% of ruptured tympanic membranes will heal spontaneously without further treatment.

Although studies have not shown perforated tympanic membranes to be a marker for blast injury, traumatic loss of an ear or ear lobe secondary to primary blast is a marker of severe primary blast injury and associated morbidity and increased mortality.

Ophthalmic

The eyes are markedly resistant to primary blast injury and more often tend to suffer to secondary and tertiary mechanisms with resultant penetrating trauma.

Intestinal

While primary blast injury to the intestine may be overshadowed by the more immediate life-threatening pulmonary and cardiovascular manifestations, a review of US Army collective animal data indicates that gastrointestinal primary blast injury may be far more prevalent and occur with equal frequency in free-field blasts. In the case of immersion blast or in enclosed spaces, primary blast injury may occur even more frequently than pulmonary injury and at less intense exposure to dynamic overpressures.

The lower gastrointestinal (GI) tract more often tends to be air filled, with the ileo-cecal area being the most susceptible to primary blast injury and the small intestine generally spared. The mechanism of injury, as discussed earlier, is varying degrees of rapid compression/decompression resulting in wall damage and immediate rupture leading to peritonitis and hemorrhage. Displacement and tearing of mesenteric and peritoneal attachments with bleeding and devascularizing injury and the reflection of stress waves and spalling at the mucosal–gas interface, resulting in submucosal to transmural injury. The characteristic injury seen is a multifocal intramural hematoma beginning in the submucosa, extending with increasing severity to large transmural confluent hematoma and may involve the mesentery and vascular supply. Serosal injury always should be considered indicative of transmural injury. Cripps identified those lesions at greater risk of perforation in experimental studies in pigs, suggesting that serosal lesions greater than 15 millimeters in the small intestine and greater than 20 millimeters in the large bowel are at higher risk of perforation and should be resected. Delayed perforation up to 14 days post injury can occur and most likely is related to progressive ischemia and necrosis with transmural injury or adjacent mesenteric injury.

Clinically, patients present with nausea, vomiting, abdominal pain, rectal and testicular pain, tenesmus, and rarely hemetemesis. Treatment is guided best by clinical judgment, with selective use of diagnostic peritoneal lavage (DPL) being the most sensitive diagnostic test for early diagnosis of GI injury in the obtunded or intubated patient. Diagnostic peritoneal lavage fluid should be examined for blood, fecal material, bile, food particles, Alkaline phosphatase >10 international units (IU), Amylase >175 IU, elevated lactate dehydrogeanse (LDH), aspartate aminotransferase (AST), and Phosphate all being suspicious for possible GI injury. Computed tomography (CT), which has not proven to be sensitive for intestinal injury, should only be used in selective cases (suspected solid organ hemorrhage) and should probably not be considered in the situation with multiple casualties. Free air and excess free fluid not characteristic of blood, when seen on CT, are considered indications for laparotomy in blunt trauma patients; however, in primary blast with pulmonary injury, free-air and even tension pneumoperitoneum without intestinal injury has been reported and should be kept in mind.

Solid Organ Injury

Liver, spleen, adrenal, kidney, and testicle injuries have all been reported in underwater blasts; solid organ injury is less common in air blasts. Such injuries are most likely the result of shear forces and present similarly to solid organ injury resulting from blunt trauma. Gallbladder, renal pelvis, and bladder injury secondary to primary blast rarely have been recorded.

Central Nervous System

Traumatic brain injury (TBI) remains a major cause of death in bombing, accounting for 71% of early and 52% of later deaths. However, TBI and death usually is due to secondary and tertiary effects, not the primary blast. Recent studies have shown that significant histologic damage and CNS dysfunction does occur with primary blast. Patients may present with prolonged periods of loss of consciousness, agitation, excitability, and irrational behavior. Long-term sequelae such as posttraumatic stress syndrome also have been related to TBI from primary blast mechanisms.

Musculoskeletal

Traumatic amputation as a result of a primary blast is a marker of injury severity that has few survivors (1.5%), but relatively more common in non-survivors. Traumatic amputation is seen in 11% of immediate fatalities in suicide bombings. Patients with traumatic amputation caused from the blast effect of a conventional bomb usually are within one meter of the detonated ordnance. Traumatic amputations of the ear lobe also should be considered a marker of injury severity and mortality. Stein, reporting in 1999 on a series of suicide bombings in Israel, noted only one survivor among traumatic amputations of the ear lobe.[9]

Thermal Blast

The flash (fireball) produced by the detonation of an explosion can reach temperatures greater than 3000 degrees centigrade. There is some controversy regarding the incidence of burns in surviving casualties, although Stein reported an incidence as high as 31%. With the increasing prevalence of FAEs and thermobaric EBWs that have a larger and longer lasting fireball, the incidence of burns may increase. Flash burns, flame burns from secondary fires, and inhalation injury from toxic substances all may be seen, complicating an already severe mechanism of injury.

Fragmentation Injury

There are a myriad of weapon systems and missiles, ranging from grenades to aerial delivered bombs weighing several tons that depending on the size and design of the weapon may deliver several thousand fragments ranging in weight from a few milligrams to many grams with an initial velocity of greater than 1500 meters per second. These fragments decline in velocity rapidly generally producing multiple low velocity incapacitating wounds. Modern fragmentation weapons are designed with preformed fragments to optimize velocity, distance, and probability of hit producing multiple casualties with multiple wounds (Figure 3-3). Body armor has altered the pattern of distribution of fragmentation injury so that the most common casualty seen on today's battlefield will have multiple extremity, head, and facial wounds (Table 3-4).

The use of antipersonnel bomblets or submunitions effectively has increased the probability of a hit and increased the lethality and wounding area of the munition. In the Israeli–Egyptian October War of 1973, each antipersonnel canister released 600 Guava bomblets (named from an Egyptian fruit with large numbers of seeds), with each bomblet containing 300 pellets. Each bomblet is released at one-meter intervals and can travel 150 meters, with an explosive lethal radius of 5 to 8 meters. Each pellet acts as a small missile of moderate velocity, striking from different angles within the lethal zone. This raised the incidence of multiple system injuries, with penetrating wounds of the extremities constituting 56% of injuries. There also was a 15% increase in head and neck injuries, with 14% of injuries to the chest and abdomen. Pellet paraplegia was a characteristic injury seen with the Guava bomblet in the Israeli–Egyptian conflict. Penetrating abdominal wounds with visceral injury proved difficult, with frequently missed visceral injury due to the small pellet size (Figure 3-4).

Improved grenade launchers with preformed fragments, laser-sighted accuracy, and precision fusing such as the US Objective Infantry Combat

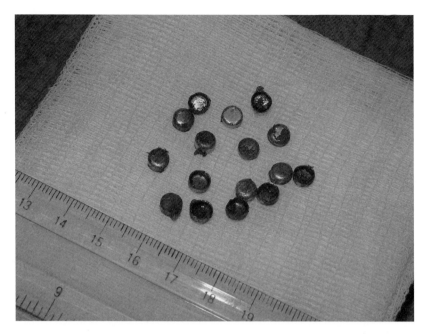

FIGURE 3-3. Preformed fragments from cluster bomblet. (Maj Scott Gering, Operation Iraqi Freedom).

TABLE 3-4. Anatomical distribution of penetrating wounds as a percent (80% fragment)

Conflict	Head & Neck	Thorax	Abdomen	Limbs
World War I	17	4	2	70
World War II	4	8	4	75
Korea	17	7	7	67
Vietnam	14	7	5	74
Northern Ireland	20	15	15	50
Israel 1975	13	5	7	40
Israel 1982	14	4	5	41
Falkland Island	16	15	10	59
Gulf War (UK)	6	12	11	71
Gulf War (US)	11	8	7	56
Afghanistan (US)	16	12	11	61
Chechnya (Russia)	24	9	4	63
Somolia	20	8	5	65
Average	15	9.5	7.4	64.6

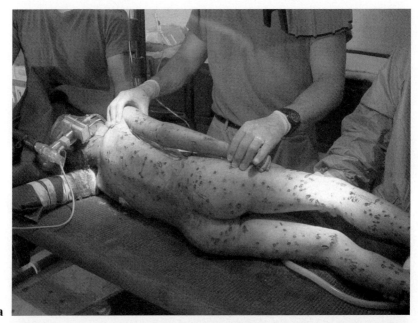

FIGURE 3-4. (a, b) Multiple fragment wounds from cluster bomblet (US) (Maj Scott Gering, Operation Iraqi Freedom). (c) Multiple fragment wounds from cluster bomblet with environmental fragments. (Maj Scott Gering, Operation Iraqi Freedom).

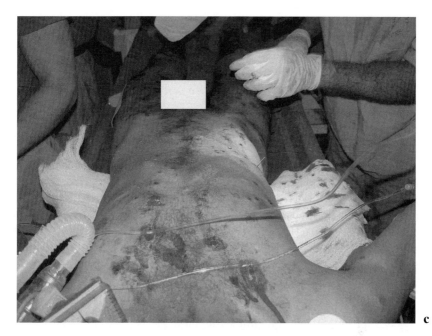

c

FIGURE 3-4. *Continued*

Weapon, with a 5.56 barrel combined with a 20-millimeter grenade launcher, will increase firepower and extend the killing range to 1000 meters. The use of flechettes, depleted uranium, and tungsten missiles capable of penetrating body armor and conventional cover may further compound the complexity of wounding with toxicities that have yet to be defined, thus increasing the impact on the medical support system.

Many of the more modern fragment munitions are designed to produce multiple preformed fragments that weigh 100 to 200 milligrams and are 2 to 3 millimeters in diameter, whereas others may weigh as much as 20 grams. Both have initial velocities of 1500 meters per second, which falls off rapidly, especially with the large, more irregular-shaped fragments. The mechanism of injury is related as much to energy transfer as to the velocity of the projectile, and the magnitude of injury is thought to depend more upon the inherent tissue characteristics of the organ involved than upon the projectile itself. The clinical impact and priority of treatment depends on the tissue or organ involved. Extremity wounds that may be innumerable usually are not life threatening and perhaps may not be immediately disabling. In contrast, wounds of the eyes or thorax are far more likely to be immediately disabling or life threatening, respectively.

Environmental debris such as glass, splinters, soil, and various structural particles are propelled with similar velocities by the blast wind and may well be the major cause of fragment wounding. The advent of the human suicide bomber brings a new dimension to fragment wounding, with human body parts acting as missile fragments and projectiles that may carry with them the specter of human immunodeficiency virus (HIV), hepatitis, and other serious and yet to be identified threats of unknown clinical consequence, thus presenting a rather complex therapeutic dilemma for the clinician.

Penetrating fragment wounds of the abdomen and thorax are no different than other penetrating wounds except that the number of pellets and the small size of visceral injuries demand meticulous attention to detail. Almost all penetrating fragment wounds of the abdomen can be closed primarily and 85% of penetrating thoracic wounds can be managed successfully by tube thoracostomy. Animal studies examining multiple colonic injuries found that colotomies closed by either one-layer interrupted absorbable suture or stainless steel skin staples were equivalent, except that the stapled anastomosis histologically healed more quickly than the sutured anastomosis, supporting definitive repair of intestinal low-velocity wounds.

All war wounds are contaminated by soil, clothing, and skin. High-velocity missiles have been shown to widely contaminate a wound track,[3] whereas low-velocity fragmentation wounds are minimally contaminated with debris. Bacterial contamination is ubiquitous in fragmentation wounds, with soil and skin organisms, Clostridia, Streptococcus, Staphylococcus, Proteus, E Coli, and Enterococcus,[4] although infection is uncommon in small low-velocity wounds of the extremity.

Although somewhat controversial, some reports in the literature support early antibiotics and nonoperative treatment of extremity wounds less than a centimeter in size in patients who show no evidence of neurovascular injury or compartment syndrome and also have a stable fracture pattern.[5] Operative debridement of these numerous wounds can lead to increased morbidity and, in general, is unnecessary.[6] However, in the authors' experience, small low-velocity wounds involving a major joint resulted in a higher incidence of infection when treated with early antibiotics and delayed operative treatment of more than 6 hours (Operation Just Cause).

Small (less than one centimeter) low-velocity wounds with no evidence of contamination that can be cleaned and dressed with early administration of appropriate broad-spectrum antibiotics may be treated nonoperatively. However, when there is question, delay in treatment greater than 6 hours, or evidence of cavitation and contamination in wounds greater than one centimeter, operative debridement should be the standard.

Land Mine

Land mines currently are deployed in 64 countries around the world and number between 84 to 100 million. Two thousand victims a month fall prey to this indiscriminate forgotten remnant of war that are ten times more likely to injure a noncombatant than a soldier. Although banned by the Ottawa Convention of 1997 and prohibited by International Humanitarian Law, mines continue to be laid across the world. It is estimated that in countries with existing mine fields such as Cambodia, Angola, and Somalia, one in every 450 persons undergoes traumatic amputation compared to United States, where amputations only number one per 22 000. It is estimated that only half of these noncombatant victims even live to reach a hospital and undergo treatment for these devastating injuries.[7]

Mines can cost no more than $3.00 apiece and can be distributed by a plethora of weapon systems to include aerial delivery and Multiple Launch Rocket Systems (MLRS) that can deliver 8000 bomblets and hundreds of mines in a matter of minutes. The American Gator mines (72 antitank and 22 antipersonnel) are delivered aerially in containers with one fighter aircraft able to deliver 600 mines in a single sortie. There is no reason to expect that the use of antipersonnel mines will cease or that the incidence of landmine injuries will decline. Mines with increased blast radius and lethality, and with fuel-air–enhanced blast technology already are in development.[8]

There are essentially three classes of conventional antipersonnel land mines based on mechanism of action—static, bounding, and horizontal-spray mines.

Static mines are implanted in the ground and vary from 5 to 15 centimeters in diameter, contain 20 to 200 grams of explosive, and most commonly are detonated by direct contact, although newer mines that detonate on motion and proximity motion are being developed.

Bounding mines, known as "Bouncing Betty," have the highest mortality. These mines propel a small explosive device 1 to 2 meters above ground then explode, dispersing multiple small preformed fragments.

Horizontal-spray or directional fragmentation mines, of which the US M18A1 Claymore AP munition mine is the best known, can be command detonated or victim detonated by means of trip wires. The Claymore fires 700 steel spheres, each weighing 0.75 grams in a 60 degree arc, resulting in multiple penetrating wounds dispersed throughout the body, creating multiple system injuries and multiple casualties. The horizontal spray and bounding mines essentially produce multiple penetrating injuries of both high and low velocity, depending on the range of the target, with a very high mortality. Thus, the mechanism of injury is no different than any other penetrating wound and surviving casualties are treated as such.

The static mine is most common throughout the world, and its mechanism of injury is unique to this weapon system. Upon contact and detonation, an instantaneous rise in pressure or shock wave is produced, which along with the products and heated air produce a blast wave or dynamic overpressure. Contact with the body produces stress waves that propagate proximally along with shear waves produced by the blast effect. These stress waves can propagate as far as the middle thigh with demyelination of nerves occurring 30 centimeters above the most proximal area of tissue injury. This, combined with fragments from the device, soil, and footwear, produces the classic land-mine injury of complete tissue destruction, distally associated with traumatic amputation at the midfoot or distal tibia (Figures 3-5 and 3-6). Proximal to the variable level of amputation there is complete stripping of tissue from the bony structures and separation of fascial planes contaminated with soil debris, microorganisms, pieces of the device, footwear, and clothing. Associated penetrating injury to contralateral limb and perineum are common.

Injuries occur in three distinct patterns. Pattern 1 injuries occur with contact of a buried mine that produces severe lower-extremity, perineal, and genital injury. Pattern 2 injuries occur with a proximity device explosion that produces less severe lower-extremity injury with less traumatic amputation. Head, thoracic, and abdominal injuries are common. Pattern 3 injuries occur with handling or clearing that produce severe head, face, and upper-extremity injury.

Ocular injuries are not uncommon with all categories of mines. The products of detonation and environmental fragments and debris producing penetrating ocular wounds are the primary mechanism and were seen in 4.5% of all antipersonnel mine injuries in Afghanistan.

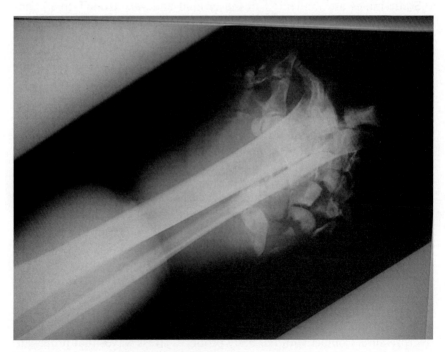

FIGURE 3-5. Boot and clothing debris from small antipersonnel land mine. (Major Scott Gering, Operation Iraqi Freedom).

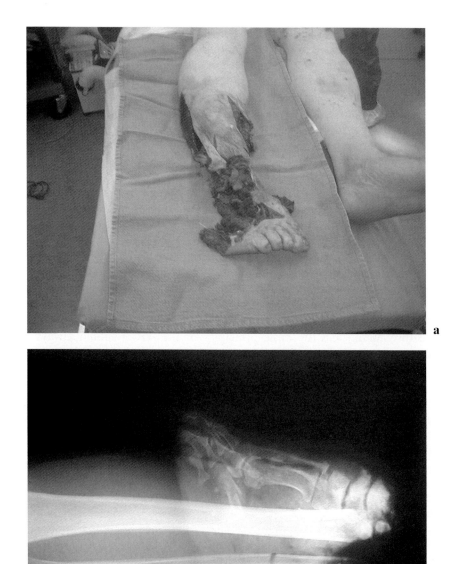

FIGURE 3-6. Injury from antipersonnel mine. (Major Darryl Scales, Kosovo, 2000).

All lower-extremity injuries need debridement or completion of amputation and many may require laparotomy, with all wounds of perineum, buttocks, back, and abdomen having a low threshold for laparotomy. Every effort should be made to conserve the contralateral limb. The primary injury is treated with excision, lavage, and exploration and lavage of fascial planes with delayed closure. All casualties should receive broad-spectrum antibiotics to cover indigenous soil spore-forming microorganisms.

Combined Injury

Combined injuries, including primary blast injury, penetrating fragment wounds, crush, burn, and inhalation injuries, are to be expected, especially in urban-warfare environments or urban terrorist bombings. With the advent of EBWs and handheld thermobaric weapons, these combined injuries are likely to become even more common, placing extreme stress on medical support systems, be they military or civilian. Triage and appropriate patient distribution may be the most critical piece of patient management. Combined blast and penetrating injuries are almost always the most life threatening and the basic principles of the ABCs should always be adhered to. Blast lung may not present for 24 to 48 hours; therefore, all patients requiring early mechanical ventilation or those going immediately to the operating room should be managed with low tidal volumes of 5 to 6 milliliters per kilogram of ideal body weight, peak inspiratory pressures of less than 25 centimeters H_2O, allowing for permissive hypercapnia. If associated TBI is present, hypercapnia should be avoided or minimized, if possible, due to the deleterious effects on intracranial hypertension. For a patient undergoing anesthesia with obvious signs of blast lung injury, there is an increased risk of barotrauma with resultant tension pneumothorax. The authors recommend consideration of bilateral prophylactic tube thoracostomy.

Patients without vascular compromise or evidence of compartment syndrome who have penetrating injuries of the extremities of one centimeter or less may be managed conservatively with early antibiotics and cleansing with frequent observation.

Penetrating injuries of the trunk associated with hemodynamic instability should undergo immediate operation. Most thoracic injuries can be managed with tube thoracostomy, and thoracotomy is rarely indicated in combined injury. Emergent thoracotomy for penetrating thoracic injury in the presence of primary blast should be considered futile and be abandoned.

Abdominal wounds with associated hemodynamic instability require immediate laparotomy once the airway is controlled.

Management of truncal penetrating injuries combined with blast should undergo, at minimum, a focused abdominal sonogram for trauma (FAST) exam if available, but the decision to operate frequently must be based on clinical judgment and a high index of suspicion. Patients with blast injury and associated blunt abdominal trauma from tertiary and quaternary mechanisms who are hemodynamically unstable should undergo immediate laparotomy, as conservative management in this scenario is not indicated at this time. However, the use of Recombinant factor VIIa and other nonoperative hemorrhage control methods may alter the clinical management of some categories of blast-injured casualties in the near future.

Retained Ordnance

An injury that is truly unique to the military is the casualty presenting with retained and unexploded ordnance. Since World War II there have been 36 documented cases with only four deaths. The deaths occurred not from the detonation of the missile, but from the moribund condition of the casualty, usually due to hemorrhage. The M79 grenade launcher (40 mm), mortars, and RPG missiles have been the most commonly reported cause of retained ordnance. A fuse or detonator that can be triggered by impact, electromagnetic energy, or time and distance normally detonates this type of ordnance. There is often a safety built into the device requiring a defined number of revolutions or a required distance and time before the missile is armed to explode. The RPG round must travel a proscribed distance before the fuse is armed to trigger on impact. All missiles that have been fired must be considered armed, and a defined and predetermined algorithm for the care of the casualty and the safety of the medical personnel should be followed.

A casualty with unexploded ordnance should be transported in the position found so as not to change the missile orientation and should always be grounded to the airframe if evacuated by air. These patients should be isolated and, in a mass casualty situation, should be treated last as the removal of ordnance is time consuming and the surgeon must attend to other casualties before placing his or herself at risk. Closed chest massage or defibrillation should never be attempted, and during removal, any equipment emanating electrical energy, heat, vibration, or sonic waves, such as the electrocautery, ultrasound, blood warmers, or power instruments, should be avoided. The patient should be placed in a protected area away from the main hospital, and all personnel in the immediate area should employ body armor or explosive ordnance disposal (EOD) equipment. Explosive ordnance disposal personnel should be involved prior to removal to help with identifying the round and fuse; a plain radiograph will help in planning the operative removal and will not cause the round to explode. The minimum anesthesia required should be used and in such a manner that the anesthesia provider need not be present during actual removal. The only personnel required during removal are surgeon and an assistant—ideally, EOD personnel. The round should be removed *en bloc* without touching the missile with metal instruments. Every effort should be employed to maintain the orientation of the missile until removed from the area by EOD. The basic guidelines for removal of ordnance are outlined in Table 3-5.

TABLE 3-5. Removal Un-exploded Ordnance

1. Notify EOD
2. No CPR or electric shock
3. Isolate to protected area (sandbagged bunker)
4. Protective equipment for medical personnel
5. Do not use cautery, power equipment, blood warmers
6. Avoid vibration, change in temperature, change in missile orientation
7. Do plain radiograph, no CT or Ultrasound
8. Minimal anesthesia, anesthesia provider to leave after induction
9. Surgeon and assistant (EOD) only personnel present during removal
10. Remove without changing orientation and hand over to EOD
11. Move casualty to Operating theater for definitive procedure

Source: Lein B, Holcomb J, Brill S, Hetz S, McCrorey T. Removal of unexploded ordnance from patients: a 50-year military experience and current recommendations. Mil Med 1999;164:163–5.

Triage

Triage of overwhelming numbers of casualties with multisystem injury from terrorist explosive munitions, once the sole province of the battlefield hospital, now threaten the urban hospital, the civilian trauma surgeon, and health systems throughout the populated world. All medical providers must bear the burden of preparing for the eventuality of casualties in overwhelming numbers, sustaining primary blast, penetrating wounds, burns, and crush injuries. We must understand the nature of the weapon and the physiologic consequences of these weapons of war and terror and be prepared to provide care that will save lives and reduce morbidity.

References

1. International Committee of the Red Cross. Available at: http://www.icrc.org/eng. Accessed Registry of mine incidents: From March 1996 until September 1996. April 23, 2003.
2. Cullis IG. Blast waves and how they interact with structure. *JR Army Med Corps.* 2001;147:16–26.
3. Ryan J. *An Enquiry into the Nature of Infection in Fragment Wounds* [master's thesis]. Dublin: University College Dublin; 1990.
4. Hill PF, Edwards DP, Bowyer GN. Small fragment wounds: biophysics, pathophysiology and principles of management. *JR Army Med Corps.* 2001;147:41–51.
5. Coupland RM. War Wounds of Limbs—Surgical Management. Oxford, England: Butterworth-Heinemann Ltd; 1993.
6. Stein M, Hirschberg A. 9th Annual Brooke Army Medical Center San Antonio Trauma Symposium, August 18–19, 2003. Henry B. Gonzales Convention Center, San Antonio, Texas, Medical consequences of terrorism. The conventional weapon threat. *Surg Clin North Am.* 1999;79:1537–1552.
7. International Committee of the Red Cross. Five years on: Anti-personnel mines reman a constant threat for millions. Available at: www.Icrc.org. April 25, 2003.
8. *Trends in Land Mine Warfare.* London, England: Janes Information Group; July 1995. Special Report.

4
Ballistic Protection*

Graham Cooper and Philip Gotts

Introduction

Personal armor is the term used to describe items that are worn or carried to provide an individual with protection from energy. In the military and law-enforcement environment, this energy is principally in the form of impact by nonpenetrating projectiles or blows, blast waves from explosions, and penetrating missiles.

Energy is the capacity to perform work. The work done on the body may produce contusion and laceration of tissues and fracture of bones. Penetrating missiles deliver energy internally during their passage through tissues. Blast waves and nonpenetrating impacts interact with the body wall, and the motion of the body wall resulting from the application of energy couples the external energy into the viscera, where it will do work. Energy may be transferred internally from the motion of the body wall by stress (pressure) waves and shear (the disparate motion of components of tissues and of organs).

Additionally, personal armor is available to offer protection from burns and the acceleration of the body surface resulting from the impact of the moving body against a rigid, unyielding surface—"bump" protection. Many types of personal armor combine protection from penetrating and non-penetrating impacts. For example, military helmets are designed to stop penetrating missiles such as bullets or fragments and offer protection against "bump" impacts arising from falls, missiles such as bricks, or obstacles at head height.

This chapter will address principally the retardation of penetrating projectiles. Penetrating projectiles encompass bullets and fragments arising from the detonation of munitions such as artillery shells, mortars, and grenades. Knives also may be considered a penetration threat, particularly to law-enforcement officers. Personal armor takes a number of forms that are designed to defeat different ballistic threats:

---

* © British Crown copyright 2003/DSTL—published with the permission of the Controller of Her Majesty's Stationary Office.

- Ballistic helmets provide protection from antipersonnel fragments or from low-energy bullets (fired from revolvers and pistols, for example). In general, ballistic helmets will not stop high-energy bullets from rifles.
- Body armor provides protection from fragments, low- and high-energy bullets, or even slash and stab from knives. The most extensive personal armor systems are Explosive Ordnance Disposal (EOD) suits, popularly known as bomb-disposal suits.
- Hand-held armor consists of ballistic shields, which are designed principally to defeat low-energy bullets.

Apart from EOD suits, there are no modern equivalents to the suit of armor of the Middle Ages. Protection over the whole body against modern ballistic threats would be too heavy for the dismounted soldier or police officer. Therefore modern personal armor covers only the most vulnerable parts of the body—the head and the torso. The helmet covers some proportion of the head, principally the brain (although not completely[1]). The face may be protected with a visor, or the eyes alone may be protected by goggles or other type of eyepiece. Most transparent armor components are not usually of a very high ballistic performance. The only exception is the visor used in conjunction with an EOD suit that is a complex, heavy, multilayered item designed to stop high-energy fragments from detonations at very close range.

General Principles of Protection

Mechanics

The technical approaches for stopping penetrating missiles and mitigating nonpenetrating impacts are different. The underlying principles of minimizing the effects of energy transfer from a projectile are:

- absorbing energy in armors by making it do work on materials before it gains access to the body—breaking materials, stretching them, or compressing them all use energy, or extend the time over which it is applied to the body;
- redistributing the energy so that other materials or the body wall are more able (due to the reduction in pressure—force per unit area) to withstand the total energy.

The helmet will serve to demonstrate the principles. In simple terms, a helmet comprises a hard shell backed with a foamed material (for example, a polymer or, historically, rubber). The helmet will stop a penetrating missile such as an antipersonnel fragment by enabling the fragment to *stretch* armor fibers in the shell, *cutting/breaking* some of them, and *compressing* layers of fibers ahead of it. The foam backing plays little part.

For a nonpenetrating missile such as a brick or for the bump of a fall, the hard shell *redistributes* the energy over a larger area of the shell, resulting in a small *deformation*, which is *absorbed* more *slowly* and further *redistributed* by the foamed liner.

The technical approaches are different, but the common themes are:

– absorb energy
– redistribute it
– extend the duration of its application.

Coverage

Body armor can be heavy and constrain movement. It is essential that the optimal balance between protection and mobility is maintained. In practice, this dictates that armor must be relevant to the principal ballistic threat and be applied to the most vulnerable areas of the body. Vulnerable in this context may with be with respect to maintaining operational effectiveness or saving life (or both). For example, the chest plainly is vulnerable to penetrating missiles. For soldiers and law-enforcement officers in static locations where it is essential that they are able to return fire, it is essential that the chest has optimal coverage. For a high-energy bullet, this would require a large, heavy ceramic plate. A mobile infantry soldier as part of a mobile platoon cannot carry such a plate and maintain agility and mobility; thus, the armor should be designed to save life, taking account of the medical facilities available. Thus, in the context of Northern Ireland, soldiers were issued with small, lightweight plates that covered only the heart and great vessels. Penetrating wounds to the lungs alone have a low mortality with immediate medical care and so the inefficient coverage over the lungs was unlikely to lead to high mortality, but significantly improved the mobility of troops by limiting the bulk and mass of ceramic plates. Thus, body coverage is an issue dictated by *clinical issues*, in addition to the *ergonomic aspects*.

Knowledge of the clinical consequences and risk to life from low- and high-energy penetrating projectiles is necessary to optimize the location of armor. Table 4-1 shows the distribution of wounds in those Killed in Action (KIA), Died of Wounds (DOW), and Wounded for Korea and Vietnam. Also shown in this Table are the presented areas for four regions of the body of a man in a combat posture. It is evident (unsurprisingly) that projectile impacts to the head and thorax are very frequent in the KIA and DOW, and are out of proportion to their presented areas. The key points emerging from these data from Korea and Vietnam are:

– the limbs make up 61% of the presented area, but limb wounds accounted for about 66 and 69% of wounded battle casualties, albeit it with a low fatality rate (around 10% of those KIA);

70   G. Cooper and P. Gotts

- the head and neck combined are about 12% of the presented area and accounted for 18 and 34% of wounded casualties, but for about 42 and 48% of deaths;
- the abdomen and thorax account for 27% of presented area, and for 37 and 51% of battlefield deaths (KIA).

It is also important to recognize that the term "head" encompasses sensory structures, the brain, and other soft/bony tissues, each of which have different vulnerabilities. For example, the eyes make up only 0.27% of the frontal presented area, but are injured in up to 10% of combat casualties.

Wounding Missile

The principal threats to law-enforcement officers are knives and low- and high-energy bullets. Military personnel are subjected to a broader range of missiles (in terms of mass, numbers, velocity, direction of attack, and intensity of fire), and the armor systems employed need to reflect this divergence. It also must be recognized that the balance of bullets and fragments in various military conflicts is different. Table 4-2 shows that in general war against other armies (e.g., World War I and World War II), fragments are the principal wounding agent, but in urban or jungle operations against irregular militia or terrorists, bullets predominate. Thus, the preferred armor for these different scenarios may be confined to flexible materials such as aramids for antipersonnel fragments, but with a threat from high-energy bullets, more substantial armors such as ceramic plates are required to counteract the threat. The heads of troops particularly are vulnerable to air-burst munitions and aimed fire of fragmentation weapons at their covert positions; thus, helmets are essential to optimize protection. Law-enforcement officers on general patrol duties are not subjected to these

TABLE 4-1. Percentage distribution of wounds by anatomical areas in Korea and Vietnam conflicts

	Head	Neck	Thorax	Abdomen	Extremities
Presented area	12		16	11	61
Korea					
KIA	38	10	23	17	11
DOW	25	7	20	30	15
Wounded who lived	7	11	8	7	66
Vietnam					
KIA	34	8	41	10	7
DOW	46	46	23	21	9
Wounded who lived	17	17	9	6	69

KIA = Killed in Action; DOW = Died of Wounds.
Source: From Carey, 1988.[2]

TABLE 4-2. Distribution of wounding agents in casualties for wars and campaigns this century (%)

	Bullets	Fragments	Other
World War I	39	61	—
World War II	10	85	5
Korea	7	92	1
Vietnam	52	44	4
Borneo	90	9	1
Northern Ireland	55	22	20
Falkland Islands	32	56	12

threats; ballistic helmets normally are not issued and the personal armor should address knife and low-energy bullet attack to the torso.

Threats and Testing

When designing or assessing personal armor, it is usual to divide the ballistic threats into three main categories: fragments, low-energy bullets, and high-energy bullets.[†]

Armors to defeat either low- or high-energy bullets usually are specified to defeat a specific bullet at a specific velocity, often its velocity at the muzzle of the weapon. The wearer would like to be assured that the armor will stop a specific bullet. The test employed is referred to as a *Complete Protection Test*. This is a pass/fail test and therefore sets a threshold that must be exceeded for the armor to pass quality-control tests. It does not provide any information about how far above the stated threshold the effective performance of the armor is.

Fragments have high velocity close to the detonation and generally low mass; consequently, their available energy usually is low. Their velocity declines rapidly as range extends. For flexible lightweight armor, it generally is not possible to protect against specific fragmenting munitions at close range. There is a much greater spread of mass, velocity, and shape of fragments from both individual munitions and between different types of munitions. Therefore, a *Complete Protection Test* is not employed. Fragmentation protective armor is specified using a criterion known as the V_{50}. The V_{50} is defined as the velocity at which 50% of the projectiles are stopped by the armor and 50% go through. This is a statistical measure and a scientific method that allows the armor designer to rank armor materials

---

[†] Bullets frequently are classed as low and high velocity. For terminal ballistics, it is more appropriate to classify projectiles by their available energy—the capacity to perform work. The kinetic energy of a projectile (Joules) is 0.5 × mass (kg) × velocity (m/s), i.e. $\frac{1}{2}mv^2$.

and systems. It does not attempt to advise the user of the armor how it will perform in the field, but only how its ballistic performance compares to another armor. Plainly, the 50% of fragments that perforate the armor are capable of producing penetrating trauma.

For armor, there is no specific velocity above which the projectile will always perforate and below which it is retarded. An example of a relationship between impact velocity and perforation of the armor, from which a V_{50} for armor is determined, is shown in Figure 4-1. It was obtained by using a series of shots that are penetrating and nonpenetrating at known velocities. From these data, an S-shaped curve can be calculated that predicts the probability of penetration with respect to the velocity of the projectile. The velocity at which the probability is predicted to be 50% is the V_{50}. Note the considerable overlap in the velocities of nominally identical projectiles that penetrated and those that did not.

In order to attempt to relate this V_{50} to the effectiveness of the armor in operational use, a Casualty Reduction Analysis model is used. The operational impact of armor with a particular V_{50} will depend upon a large number of factors that need to be encompassed within a Casualty Reduction Analysis model:

– the coverage of the armor on the body;
– the ballistic threat in terms of the number, size, velocity distribution, and trajectory of the projectiles from specific munitions (usually acquired from field trials);
– the presented area of the man and the shielding effects of the ground and structures;

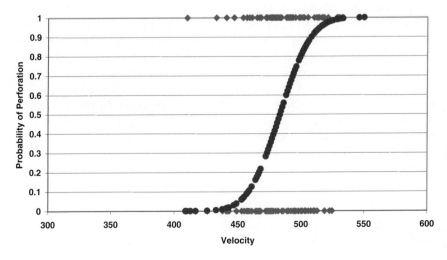

FIGURE 4-1. A V_{50} curve for an armor system.

– the incapacitation predicted from penetration of fragments through the armor or through other unprotected parts of the body.

These models enable developers to predict the benefits of trade-offs, such as between weight (i.e., coverage), anatomical location of armors, V_{50} performance, and casualty reduction. Additional Operational Analysis tools also can address the effects of a reduction in mobility arising from armor use on the success of the mission and the production of casualties. Placing armor on personnel has many ramifications—some good, some bad; these types of tools are essential to assess the operational consequences. Whether armor stops a particular piece of metal (or not) is not the pinnacle of armor design and deployment.

Materials

The materials used in personal armor depend upon the threat to be defeated and the part of the body to be protected. Similar materials are used for the defeat of fragmentation and low-energy bullets. For the torso, these will be multiple layers of woven, unidirectional, or felted textiles produced from high tensile strength fibers. The most common fibers are ballistic nylon, para-aramids (Kevlar® or Twaron®), Ultra High Molecular Weight Polyethylenes (UHMWPE) (Dyneema® and Spectra®), and Polyphenylene-2,6-benzobisoxazole, (PBO), (Zylon®). The materials also can be encapsulated within a resin matrix and pressed into a rigid composite structure. These rigid composites are used for helmets.

Composite materials also can be used for protection from high-energy bullets. Composites used for high-energy bullet protection are most usually combined with a ceramic strike face, particularly if the threat projectile contains a steel core, rather than only lead. Figure 4-2 shows a ceramic-faced high-energy bullet protective plate that has been struck by a 7.62-millimeter caliber North Atlantic Treaty Organization (NATO) bullet. The damage to the ceramic strike face is evident over a greater area than the bullet strike location.

The most challenging items of armor are those that are required to be transparent. They require the ballistic resistance, but also good optical quality. The materials used for transparent armor include polycarbonate, polyurethane, acrylic, glass, and glass-ceramics.

Mechanisms of Projectile Defeat

Some projectiles can be defeated using flexible textile materials and some require a rigid structure. When any projectile of a mass m, travelling at a velocity v, impacts a target, it possesses kinetic energy ($KE = \frac{1}{2} mv^2$). The

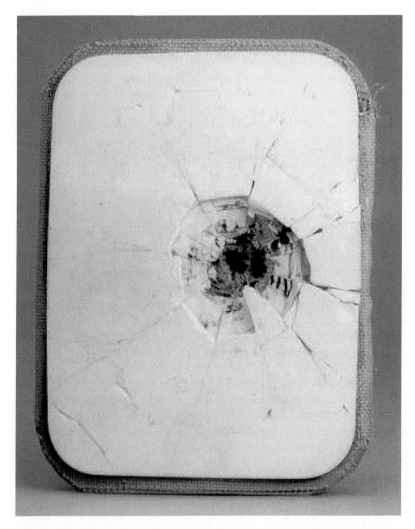

FIGURE 4-2. Alumina ceramic plate backed by a composite designed to defeat high-energy bullets.

energy acts over a very small impact area and enables the projectile to perforate materials. The term often used to describe the ability of a projectile to defeat its target is its *kinetic energy density*, that is, the projectile energy per unit area at the impact site. However, without consideration of projectile material, this term often is used in a misleading way. In the most general terms, an armor system defeats the projectile by absorbing this kinetic energy and spreading it over a larger area before the projectile has a chance to punch through.

Textile armors, such as those used for fragmentation or low-energy bullet defeat, usually are woven. The yarns used in woven ballistic textiles have a high specific strength and a high modulus. These properties mean that the fibers are particularly difficult to break. The high modulus allows the energy to be dissipated as a longitudinal stress wave, that is, along the yarn. Figure 4-3 shows a single cross-over in a woven textile. As the projectile impacts a certain point on one of the yarns, the energy imparted will travel along the yarn. When it meets the cross-over, it divides via a number of possible mechanisms. It can continue along the yarn (transmission), it can be reflected back along the yarn, or it can travel along the crossing yarn (diversion). This is a single cross-over on a single layer. For example, in a one centimeter by one centimeter square, there could be well over 100 of these cross-overs. No body armor will consist of a single layer; most will use more than 15 layers, and some even more than 40 layers. Not all the energy is dissipated in the first layer, and hence the same mechanism continues through the consecutive layers until the projectile does not have sufficient energy to continue. This continual process means that the first layer has been defeated by shearing (cutting) of the yarns. This shearing is a second mechanism of energy absorption and probably absorbs more of the energy than the longitudinal dissipation.

If a high-velocity bullet is fired from almost any range except the most extreme, it is unlikely to be defeated by a textile armor alone. For the defeat of these bullets, a hard strike face is necessary. The armor uses the hardness of the strike face to break up or distort the projectile before the composite backing spreads the energy over a greater area. Figure 4-4 shows the cross-sectional view of a ceramic-faced, composite-backed armor plate. As

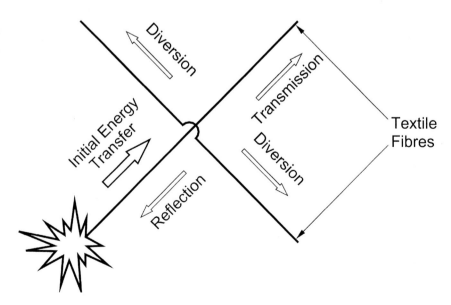

FIGURE 4-3. Distribution of the bullet's energy in textile fibers.

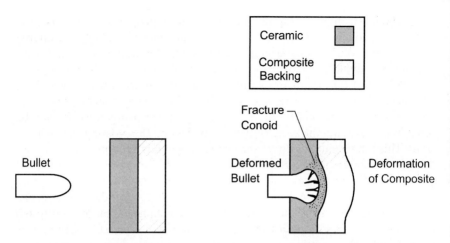

FIGURE 4-4. Defeat of a high-energy projectile by ceramic and composite.

the bullet impacts the armor, which usually is harder than the bullet, the nose of the bullet distorts. The shock pressure of the impact also fractures the ceramic. In some ceramics, such as alumina, the fracture pattern takes the form of a conoid (conical fracture), thus imparting the residual energy over a much larger area of the composite backing. Additionally, as the bullet passes through the ceramic, it is initially mushroomed, thus increasing the surface area and reducing the kinetic energy density. It then is broken up by the ceramic as it continues its path to the backing. By the time the bullet residue reaches the backing, it is accompanied by the fragments of ceramic, and these fragments are defeated by the composite backing using a mechanism similar to that of the woven textile described above.

Types of Personal Armor

The ballistic protective T-shirt does not exist. Materials must be tailored into clothing items that have minimal impact on the performance of the wearer (while still maintaining adequate coverage), and they must be compatible with other equipment the wearer is carrying.

The military ballistic helmet presents the greatest challenges; it needs to be compatible with weapon sights, communications sets, respirators, ocular protection, etc.

Body armor on the thorax must enable to wearer to lose heat, aim weapons, sit in a vehicle, crouch, wear load-carrying equipment, etc. If the armor is not comfortable, if it excessively degrades performance, or if the wearer has no confidence in its performance, it will not be worn.

Combat Helmets

Within NATO countries, combat helmets are constructed of textile-based composites. The helmet can be constructed of ballistic nylon, para-aramid, UHMWPE, or PBO. Figure 4-5.1 is the UK GS Mk6 Combat Helmet. In this configuration it has the anti-riot (public order) equipment fitted: a polycarbonate visor, with a seal at the top to stop burning fluids pouring down the face, and a blunt impact-resistant and fire-retardant nape protector.

Most combat helmets will be of a similar generic design. The differences that are seen in geometry are due to the requirement for compatibility with other equipment. Figure 4-5.2 is that of crew members of armored fighting vehicles. The shape around the ears is to enable communications equipment to be worn.

Figure 4-5.3 is a representative low-energy bullet protective helmet, which also has a high level of fragmentation protection.

All UK helmets have a high level of nonballistic impact or "bump" protection. This is achieved using a liner within the helmet shell made of an impact-absorbing material such as closed-cell polymeric foam.

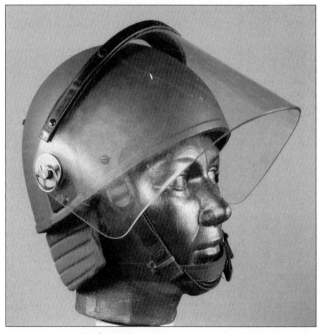

4-5.1

FIGURE 4-5.1, 4-5.2, and 4-5.3. Patterns of military helmets. 1. General combat helmet with antiriot (public order) equipment attached; 2. helmet for a crew of armored fighting vehicles; 3. a ballistic helmet designed to defeat low-energy bullets.

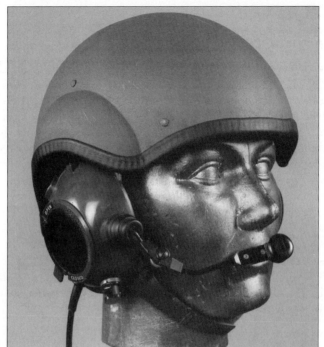

4-5.2

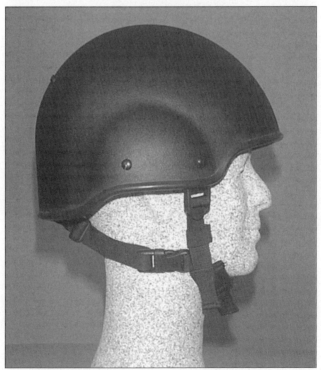

4-5.3

FIGURE 4-5.1, 4-5.2, and 4-5.3. *Continued*

Torso Armor—Ballistic

These items are designed to protect the torso from antipersonnel fragments and low- or high-energy bullets. The textile garment alone provides protection from the fragments and/or low-energy bullets. To increase the level of protection to include that from high-energy bullets, a rigid insert plate is added.

Figure 4-6 is the UK's Combat Body Armor (CBA). The rectangular pocket on the front is the location of the rigid ceramic plate.

Figure 4-7 is a police body armor that includes low-energy bullet protection in the garment and larger high-energy bullet protective plates. Most bullet-resistant plates will be of the larger size. The small plate in the UK

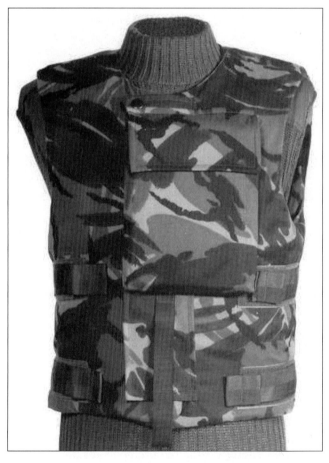

FIGURE 4-6. UK Combat Body Armor principally designed to stop antipersonnel fragments. Note the pocket for inclusion of a plate to defeat high-energy rifle bullets.

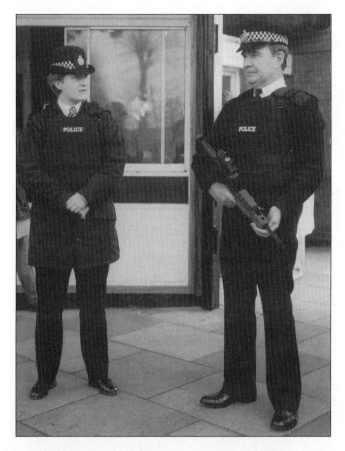

FIGURE 4-7. Police armor—a combination of aramid to defeat low-energy bullets and large plates for high-energy projectiles.

CBA (shown in Figure 4-6) is an exception; it was introduced to keep the weight to an absolute minimum in a theater where rapid medical assistance was available. There are a number of differences between Police and Military Body Armors; these are summarized in Table 4-3.

EOD (Bomb Disposal) Suits

The most extensive ensemble of personal armor is that used by personnel involved in EOD. These operators spend a significant proportion of their time close to large explosive devices that are designed to kill or injure those much further away. Therefore, the requirements for protection are greater than for any other type of user of personal armor. For most users of armor designed to defeat fragment threats, it is assumed that they will not be close

TABLE 4-3. Comparison of military and police requirements for body armors

Criteria	Military	Police
Main threats	Fragmentation	Stab
	High-energy bullets	Low-energy bullets
Weight	Low	May be slightly higher
Protection level	Usually a compromise due to other factors	Often has to be complete protection for a specified low-energy bullet threat
Specifications	Often designed to meet specific requirements of the user	Usually to a national or international standard
Wear time	Could be a very long time	Usually for a standard working shift, or less

enough to the device for any of the associated blast to be an issue (the lethal area for fragments usually considerably exceeds that for blast waves). This is not the case for the EOD operator; he/she is very close to the device and blast overpressure levels will be severe. For this reason, an EOD suit should provide protection from both fragmentation and blast. In Figure 4-8, the area covered by the two-part rigid plate system (being removed in the picture) has blast-protective materials and construction, as well as a very high level of fragmentation protection. The fragmentation protection of the rigid plate may be up to three times that of a CBA. The helmet will be of similar construction to a combat helmet, but of higher performance. The visor should have as high a ballistic performance as the helmet, but it also requires good optical properties.

Torso Armor—Knives

Contrary to expectation, armor that defeats bullets or fragmentation is not necessarily very good at stopping knives or other sharp weapons. Most current knife armors comprise a metallic mesh or chain mail backed by aramid (Figure 4-9). Textile armors are now being developed that combine knife and bullet protection, obviating the need for a metallic or ceramic outer layer.

The test standards for knife protection are different to those developed for bullets. Most standards refer to defeating a specific geometry of blade that possesses a specific energy upon impact.

In UK, there are three protection levels dependent upon the risk; an officer on routine patrol will not need the same degree of protection as an officer entering the premises where there is a known knife threat. Reflecting the various threats, standards refer to energies of 24, 33 and 43 Joules, with maximum allowable penetrations of 7 millimeters. Manufacturers can determine compliance by firing "knife missiles" from an air cannon or dropping from a drop tower.

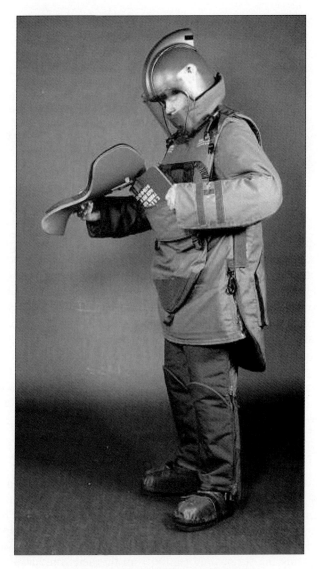

FIGURE 4-8. The UK Mk4 EOD suit.

The UK law-enforcement view on stab armors is that the purpose of the armor is to prevent the officer sustaining "serious or permanent injury"; trauma may occur, particularly if a low-specification armor is attacked by an energetic stab. Clinicians need to be aware that penetrating trauma still may occur behind knife armors, although the depth of penetration will be reduced significantly compared to the unprotected thorax.

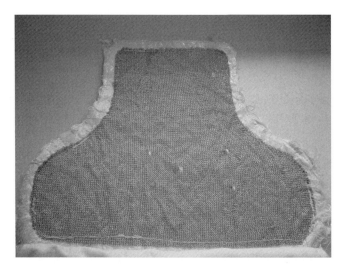

FIGURE 4-9. A representative knife armor—chain mail backed with aramid.

Medical Issues Associated with Armor Use

Evidence for Reduction in Casualty Numbers

For law-enforcement officers attacked with specific bullets, it is self-evident whether an armor has performed effectively. There is no doubt that thoracic armors save lives.

Gathering evidence that the military use of armor has made a significant benefit in terms of the frequency of KIA; DOW and the Wounded is less clear cut because of confounding factors when comparing casualty rates in different conflicts. The frequency of casualties in these three groups is not determined solely by the threat, the tactical environment, and the armor systems deployed. The standard and timeliness of medical care has a significant impact on casualty rates.

In comparing the surgical mortality from thoracic trauma in conflicts in which thoracic armors were not deployed (37% for the US Army in World War I) to those in which they were (10% mortality in Korea), differences can probably be ascribed to developments in cardiovascular trauma management and the use of antibiotics[2] as well as the provision of personal armors. It could also be argued that armors reduce the tempo tactically, and this indirectly may affect the ballistic threat to personnel.

Notwithstanding the caveats raised above, there is evidence that armors make a difference. The percentage wounds (fatal and nonfatal) to the thorax for the US Army in World War II were 13%; thoracic armor was not worn commonly in this war. In Korea, where thoracic armor was worn reasonably routinely, the incidence of thoracic wounds was less—eight percent had fatal or nonfatal thoracic wounds. Carey ascribed the lower-than-predicted incidence of brain wounds sustained by soldiers in a Corps Hospital in Desert Storm to the effectiveness of modern aramid-based helmets and troop discipline in wearing armor.[3] He also noted that brain-injured Iraqi casualties who either wore no helmets or helmets of inferior design and coverage usually were injured over the superior aspect of the cranial vault. The two US casualties suffered wounds to the inferior aspect, the projectiles entering the head below the helmet.

In their retrospective review of 125 combat casualties from an urban battle in Somalia, Mabry et al. commented that an important contribution to medical management was the prevention of small fragment wounds to the abdomen, where any evidence of penetrating injury invokes the assumption that a perforation of the abdominal wall has occurred and viscera are involved.[1] The armor reduced the requirement for diagnostic procedures and surgical exploration, thereby reducing the medical work-load. The battle was dominated by use of AK47 rifles and Rocket Propelled Grenades (RPGs). There was a relatively low rate of penetrating chest wounds, compared to the incidence in Vietnam. Two of the KIA had chest wounds and two had abdominal wounds; in these casualties, the projectiles entered the torso through the soft aramid armor (that is not designed to stop high-energy bullets/fragments). Ceramic plates were not perforated. There were at least a dozen anecdotal accounts of personnel escaping injury following impact of bullets and fragments on their torso armor.

Burkle et al.[4] undertook a prospective analysis of trauma record data in two military field trauma centers in the Persian Gulf War (1991). The 402 cases were a mixture of US personnel, allies, and prisoners of war. Pene-trating "shrapnel" (sic) wounds to the chest were observed in 2% of coali-tion forces but in 15% of "enemy" forces. The disparity in the provision and use of thoracic armor undoubtedly contributed in part to this difference.

Behind Armor Blunt Trauma

Behind-armor blunt trauma (BABT) is the spectrum of nonpenetrating injuries to the torso resulting from the impact of projectiles on personal armors. Although the armor may stop the actual penetration of the projec-tile through the armor, the energy deposited in the armor by the retarded projectile may be transferred through the armor backing and body wall. It may produce serious injury to the thoracic and abdominal contents behind the plate. With very available high-energy bullet impacts (such as a 12.7-millimeter bullet striking a boron carbide plate), the nonpenetrating thoracic injuries may result in death.

The existence of BABT as a clinical entity was reported first in the late 1970s amongst police officers wearing flexible body armor struck with handgun bullets. Behind-armor blunt trauma may occur behind flexible textile-based armors and also behind rigid armors principally constructed from ceramic materials.

Behind-armor blunt trauma has been identified as an emerging problem that has implications for the designers of personal armor systems, the operational performance of soldiers and law-enforcement officers, and for the medical management of casualties. There are two principal reasons for its growing prominence:

1. An increase in the caliber and available energy of bullets that may be used in peace-keeping, urban-violence, and other operational scenarios;
2. The desire of the designers of personal armor systems to reduce the weight and thickness of soft armors and armor plates—a strategy that plainly will buy benefit in terms of the burden on personnel, but will exacerbate the problem of dissipating the energy in the armor system. Armors are designed to absorb energy, but the rapid deformations of the armors may result in a greater proportion of the energy of the retarded projectile being propagated into the body.

The earliest case report of the lethal indirect effect of a high-energy round was described in 1969—the case of a US Army sergeant shot accidentally with an M-16 bullet at close range during the Vietnam War. There was no description of "rigid" body armor or other retardation, but the round did not penetrate the pleural cavity. After a short period of respiratory and haemodynamic stability, the soldier rapidly deteriorated and died within 45 minutes of admission. Massive pulmonary contusions alone were seen at post-mortem.

In a civilian setting, Carroll and Soderstrom[5] described five cases of BABT in police officers wearing Kevlar soft-body armor struck by handgun bullets. All survived with no significant cardio-respiratory sequelae.

One of the few accurately documented examples of severe but survivable BABT was presented as recently as 1995.[6] A humanitarian aid worker working in Sarajevo was struck by a Soviet 14.5-millimeter bullet (at unknown range) while wearing "complete" body armor. Apart from skin and muscle damage, his cardio-respiratory status was stable. A chest radiograph revealed no rib fractures and a small haemothorax only, which was managed with a chest drain. A subsequent radiograph on the same day revealed a developing pulmonary contusion corresponding to the site of impact. The patient made an uneventful recovery.

The important issue with BABT is that historically it has been associated largely with the defeat of low-energy bullets (such as from handguns) by flexible textile armor systems. Many armor manufacturers offer "trauma attenuating backings" (TABs) to reduce these injuries behind soft armors. However, it now is emerging as a significant military problem, particularly behind rigid armor plates designed to defeat high-energy bullets. It also is plain that the higher-energy threats used in modern times in urban law enforcement also render it a problem in the civilian medical scenario.

Behind-armor blunt trauma is caused by the deformation of the rear surface of the armor (plate or textile) occurring as a result of the dissipation of the energy of the retarded bullet. This deformation has a number of biophysical sequelae that are dependent upon its rate (peak velocity) and gross dynamic deformation:

- The strike of a bullet on the armor plate generates a short duration stress (pressure) wave that is coupled into the body;
- The rear of the plate then deforms locally at high velocity towards the body and accelerates the body wall—this also generates a stress wave;
- The deflection of the body wall under the armor applies local shear to the wall (e.g., rib) and shear is transferred to underlying tissues—thoracic and abdominal viscera;
- The plate as a whole moves and results in a distributed load to the body, leading to additional torso wall displacement.

Thus, the pathology observed is a combination of stress-wave–induced trauma and shear resulting in local damage to the body wall and viscera. The incidence and severity is dependent upon the energy of the impact and the characteristics of the armor (and TAB, if present); these factors determine the peak velocity and maximum gross deflection of the body wall. The pathology is the commonly observed pattern of non penetrating trauma from high-energy localized impacts: rib fracture, pulmonary contusion, pulmonary laceration, cardiac contusion, hepatic trauma, and bowel contusion.

Trauma generally is localized to the contact area and underlying tissues, but the generation of stress waves in the retardation process of high-energy bullets against plates may lead to more widespread pulmonary trauma, similar to that observed in casualties exposed to blast waves— "blast lung."

Law-enforcement agencies publish standards for body armor that are designed to limit the severity of BABT. Manufacturers of armor systems have to demonstrate compliance of their products with these standards. Test procedures are a compromise between fidelity to the biophysical processes of BABT and a test regimen that does not require enormous investment and specialized knowledge from manufacturers. Current standards in the UK are based on the maximum back-face deformation of armor, determined by indentation of Roma Plastilina®. Police armor is assigned to five threat groups ranging from lightweight flexible armor intended for use by unarmed officers in very low-risk patrolling duties (HG1/A—this armor may be used covertly or overtly) to armor designed to stop soft-core rifle ammunition and shotguns at close range. The maximum deformation permitted in the Plastilina backing material is 44 millimeters for the HG1/A group and 25 millimeters for the more severe threat groups. Similar standards are used in the US.

The North Atlantic Treaty Organization has reviewed the threat from BABT in military operations and concluded from the available knowledge that for military rifle bullets:

- the BABT injury potential of defeated very high-energy bullets (i.e., 12.7-millimeter caliber) is significant;
- that of 7.62-millimeter bullets is largely dependent on the armor design;
- there is no evidence of significant BABT injury from 5.56-millimeter military bullets.

The energy transferred from armor may be absorbed, dissipated, or redistributed using the TABs placed between the armor system and the body. These TABs vary in design depending on the threat to be countered—in the most extreme example of attenuating the energy transfer of a retarded 12.7-millimeter bullet, the TABs are constructed from a stiff-foamed polymer of substantial thickness. On the basis of the NATO assessment, the focus for attenuating BABT has been for the 12.7-millimeter and more severe 7.62-millimeter threats. For low-energy handgun bullets striking textile armors and 5.56-millimeter bullets striking ceramic plates, the risk of life-threatening injury is very low. Nevertheless, BABT may be present and the physician is advised to recognize the potential for pulmonary, cardiac, and hepatic trauma (dependent upon impact site), even in the absence of a defect on the skin.

Removal of Armor

The removal of clothing for the survey of a casualty is compounded by the presence of body armor and the supine posture. Aramids such as Kevlar cannot be cut with the type of implements normally found in medical facilities. Most thoracic armors open at the front or at the side (or both) and are sleeveless; in practice, they can be removed with relative ease, if the removal is planned.

Medical teams should develop drills to remove armor systems; the particular pattern of armor worn by the law-enforcement or military population they serve will be defined and teams need to familiarize themselves with the nature of the protective equipment issued operationally.[6]

Removal of EOD suits is very problematic, as there may be no frontal and side openings (to maintain integrity of the suit when subjected to severe blast, the opening may be at the rear) and the legs and arms will be heavily armored with aramid. The lower-limb armor may be in the form of a salopette, which may be removed relatively easily, but the presence of bulky, relatively tight-fitting sleeves on the upper jacket will make removal with spinal immobilization very difficult. Some suits, such as the UK Mk4, have the aramid seams marked to facilitate emergency removal.

It is difficult to offer specific advice on removal because the designs of suits vary, but the general principles are:

- it is futile and a waste of time to try and cut the aramid (unless cutters specifically designed to cut aramid are available);
- there is little point in searching for *covert* seams—the designers try to ensure that there are not any—so utilize marked seams (if any);
- if time permits, the manufacturers should be able to advise on the removal;
- undertake a rapid survey of the design of the armor (seeking "Velcro" straps and zips that most likely are to be out of sight for EOD suits) and develop a strategy for its removal. Rolling of the casualty during the primary survey may be inevitable in order to gain access to initiate resuscitation and to effect removal of the arms from sleeves for the secondary survey.

There may be either clinical or tactical requirements in the military to assess casualties who still are wearing body armor. Harcke et al.[7] used plain film and computed tomography of simulated casualties clothed with aramid helmet, torso armor (plate and aramid textile), and de-mining suit sleeve. Helmets may contain metal components. They concluded that if conditions so dictate, patients wearing military-pattern personal armor can be satisfactorily examined radiographically through the armor systems. This conclusion also is undoubtedly applicable to civilian medical staff dealing with armor systems used by law-enforcement officers.

Perforation of Armor by Bullets

Textile armors will not stop high-energy bullets. If the textile armor is defeated by a bullet, will the presence of the armor exacerbate the trauma? The ballistic basis for this potential problem is that as a result of its passage through the textile, the bullet may be influenced thus:

- deformation or break-up;
- induction of yaw (the deviation of the axis of the body of the bullet from its line of flight);
- instability arising from a reduction in the balance of angular velocity (spin) and longitudinal velocity.

Each of these factors could lead to an increase in the total energy transferred to a target and changes in the distribution of energy along the track.

The scientific evidence is limited and equivocal. The characteristics of the bullet range, strike angle, armor construction, and thickness all will influence the effect that the armor has on the bullet during its passage and it is inappropriate to offer generalized statements. Knudsen[8] demonstrated instability of 7.62-millimeter AK-47 bullets (demonstrated by an increase in yaw) after passage through soft aramid comprising 28 plies. The yaw induction also was dependent upon strike angle. The consequences of the yaw induction upon a tissue-simulant target behind the armor were not investigated, but intuitively the temporary cavity in tissue would be more proximal and energy transfer would be greater. It is difficult to judge the overall clinical consequences. More recently, experiments in the UK have indicated *increased* stability of 5.45-millimeter and 5.56-millimeter bullets after passage through aramid—the temporary cavity volumes were reduced in soap behind the armor when compared to shots into soap with no armor.[9]

This issue requires more research to determine clinical impact, but it is unlikely that torso wounds will be unequivocally significantly increased in *clinical* severity by the passage of a high-energy bullet through textile armor.

If a high-energy bullet defeats ceramic armor, the effects on a soft target behind the plate will be dependent upon how overmatched the bullet is to the armor. If only just overmatched, the steel core of the bullet may emerge from the back face of the armor and enter the body with relatively low energy—the jacket and lead components may be captured in the plate. At the other extreme, multiple bullet fragments arising from erosion of the bullet by the ceramic and pieces of the ceramic armor may perforate the composite backing of the plate to result in gross, but relatively superficial high-energy transfer wounds.

Acknowledgements. Graham Smith and John Croft of the Police Scientific Development Branch, Sandridge, UK provided information on knife armors.

References

1. Mabry RL, Holcomb JB, Baker AM, Cloonan CC, Uhorchak JM, Perkins DE, Canfield AJ, Hagmann JH. United States Army Rangers in Somalia: An analysis of combat casualties on an urban battlefield. *J Trauma*. 2000;49:515–528.
2. Carey ME. An analysis of US Army combat mortality and morbidity data. *J Trauma*. 1988;28(suppl):S515–S528.
3. Carey ME. Analysis of wounds incurred by US Army Seventh Corps personnel treated in Corps hospitals during Operation Desert Storm, February 20 to March 10, 1991. *J Trauma*. 1996;40(suppl):S165–S169.
4. Burkle FM, Newland C, Meister SJ, Blood CG. Emergency medicine in the Persian Gulf War—Part 3: Battlefield casualties. *Ann Emerg Med*. 1994; 23:755–760.
5. Carroll AW, Soderstrom CA. A new non-penetrating ballistic injury. *Ann Surg*. 1978;188:735–737.
6. Ryan JM, Bailie R, Diack G, Kierle J, Williams T. Safe removal of combat body armor lightweight following battlefield wounding—a timely reminder. *J R Army Med Corps*. 1994;140:26–28.
7. Harcke T, Schauer DA, Harris RM, Campman SC, Lonergan G. Imaging body armor. *Mil Med*. 2002;167:267–271.

8. Knudsen PJT, Sorensen OH. The destabilising effect of body armour on military rifle bullets. *Int J Legal Med*. 1997;110:82–87.
9. Lanthier J-M. The effects of soft textile body armour on the wound ballistics of high velocity military bullets. MSC Thesis, Cranfield University College of Defence Technology, Shrivenham, Wiltshire, UK; 2003.

Further Reading

Abbott TA, Shephard RG. Protection against penetrating injury. In: Cooper GJ, Dudley HAF, Gann S, Gann DS, Little RA, Maynard RL. (eds). Scientific Foundations of Trauma. Oxford: Butterworth Heinemann; 1997:83–100.
Cannon L. Behind armour blunt trauma—an emerging problem. J R Army Med Corps. 2001;147:87–96.

5
Forensic Aspects of Ballistic Injury

JEANINE VELLEMA and HENDRIK JOHANNES SCHOLTZ

The Clinician's Role

Clinical forensic medicine is best defined as the application of forensic medical knowledge and techniques to the solution of law in the investigation of trauma involving living victims.[1-5] In the setting of emergency departments, these techniques include the correct forensic evaluation, documentation, and photography of traumatic injuries, as well as the recognition and proper handling of evidentiary material for future use in legal proceedings.[1-8]

While the tasks of documenting, gathering, and preserving evidence traditionally have been considered to be the responsibility of the forensic pathologist or the police, the roles of the trauma physician and forensic investigators actually have several areas of complementary interest. These arise from the dual purposes of providing immediate care for the individual victim or patient and the longer-term reduction and prevention of injury and violence in the community as a whole.[6,9]

Appropriate documentation and handling of evidence by trauma personnel assist the forensic pathologist in evaluating cases of initially non-fatal traumatic deaths and assist the police and legal authorities responsible for investigating both civil and criminal cases in deceased and surviving injured patients.[6]

In addition, emergency physicians could play an important role in informing police about patients presenting to them with non-fatal forensic-related problems such as gunshot wounds. In these instances, consent to report must be obtained from the patient so as not to breach physician–patient confidentiality. Patients should be advised that it is in their interest, as well as the interest of the wider community, to report offences, but it remains the patients' decision whether such offences are reported.[9,10]

In September 2003, the General Medical Council (GMC) in the UK published "Reporting Gun Shot Wounds. Guidance for Doctors in Accident and Emergency Departments." The guidelines were developed with the Association of Chief Police Officers and supported by the British Association of

A&E Medicine. In essence, the guidance is that the police should be informed whenever a person has arrived at a hospital with a gunshot wound, but initially identifying details such as the patient's name and address usually should not be disclosed. The treatment and care of the patient remains the doctor's first concern. If the patient's treatment and condition allow them to speak to the police, then they should be asked if they are willing to do so. If they refuse or cannot consent, then information still may be disclosed if it is believed this is in the public interest or is required by law. The patient should be informed of the disclosure and an appropriate record made in their notes. Copies of the guidelines can be obtained from the GMC.

Thus, while the main priority of trauma physicians always will be to provide timeous and optimal care for the individual living patient that cannot be compromised, they also could serve society in general by applying some forensic principles in their approach to patients who are victims of violence.[5–8]

The Forensic Evaluation

In a firearm-related injury, the direction that a bullet travels through a body may have little relevance in a patient's clinical management, but it usually has profound medico-legal implications. The appearance of a gunshot wound may not only indicate the bullet's direction and trajectory, but also the type of ammunition and weapon used and the range of gunfire. Additionally, it may assist with the manner of gunshot injury or death with respect to it being accidental, homicidal, or suicidal in nature.[2,11]

Proper forensic evaluation of patients in the clinical environment is often neglected in the hurried setting of a resuscitation.[6,12] Such an evaluation should be documented comprehensively and should include a history and physical examination with accurate descriptions of wound characteristics supplemented by diagrams or line drawings.[3–8,13] Use of a proforma, which includes a simple diagram, has been shown to improve the quality of documentation.[14–17]

Ideally, photographs should be taken whenever possible. However, consent must be obtained first from patients for photography, unless they are unconscious. The consent form must become a permanent part of the patient's medical records. In unconscious patients, "implied consent" is the legal construct used to secure consent when the photographs may aid in the subsequent conviction of those individuals who perpetrated a crime. If implied consent was used, the physician later must obtain consent from either the patient or next of kin.[3]

In addition to the above documentation, recognizing, collecting, and preserving physical evidence while maintaining a "chain of custody" is another important responsibility of trauma personnel; this will be dealt with comprehensively later in this chapter.[1-8,12-16]

Documentation of Gunshot Wounds

Emergency physicians are ideally positioned to describe and document gunshot-wound appearances before such wounds are altered by surgical intervention or the healing process.[3,17]

The interpretation of gunshot wounds with respect to "entrance and exit," direction of fire, or type of firearm or ammunition used need not be commented on. Clinicians should confine themselves to recording accurately the location, size, and shape of all wounds, as well as any unusual marks or coloration associated with these wounds. Surgical procedures such as drain sites must also be recorded to prevent subsequent interpretive difficulties for the forensic pathologist, should the patient die.[17-20]

Differentiation between entrance and exit wounds can be difficult, and information from patients or witnesses may be false or inaccurate. In a study of 271 gunshot-wound fatalities, it was found that trauma specialists had misclassified 37% of single exiting gunshot wounds with respect to entrance or exit wounds and 73.6% of multiple gunshot wounds had been misinterpreted with respect to total number of wounds, as well as erroneous identification of entrance or exit wounds.[17]

If descriptive documentation is accurate, acknowledged experts in forensic wound ballistics can use these descriptions to make the necessary forensic interpretations pertaining to direction and range of gunfire, as well as type of weapon and ammunition used.[17-22]

An emergency physician may be called upon by the courts to give evidence regarding injuries sustained by a gunshot victim and, in nonfatal gunshot victims, may be the only person who can testify as a witness of fact to the original appearances of the gunshot wounds.

An expert witness is someone who, because of training and depth of experience, may be asked to give an opinion based on the observation of others, as opposed to merely testifying as to the facts of the case.[12]

Thus, an emergency physician may be called as a "factual" witness regarding the wound(s) appearances, but may also be called as an expert witness regarding the severity or lethality of a wound. The expert forensic ballistics witnesses may be asked to interpret the documented factual findings in a gunshot-wound victim and define the wound descriptions as entrance or exit, as well as give an expert opinion as to range and direction of fire, type of firearm, and ammunition used.[12]

The quality of both factual and expert testimony will depend on the accuracy of the original clinical documentation, which in turn may influence the outcome of the court case.[1-8,15-22]

Forensic Concepts

Accurate descriptions of gunshot wounds require a basic understanding of firearms, ammunition and wound ballistics, as well as the relevant forensic terminology.[2,3] Ballistics is defined as the science of motion of projectiles and can be divided into interior ballistics, the study of the projectile in the gun; external ballistics, the study of the projectile moving through the air; and terminal ballistics, the study of the effects the projectile causes when hitting a target, as well as the counter effects produced on the projectile.

Wound ballistics is considered a subdivision of terminal ballistics, which concerns itself with the motions and effects of a projectile in tissue.[23–25]

Chapter 2 dealt with firearms and ammunition and Chapter 9 deals with clinical ballistics and surgical wound management. Only a brief summary of some pertinent forensic issues pertaining to the above will be given here.

Forensic Aspects of Firearms and Ammunition

When a firearm is discharged, the primer is crushed and ignited by the firing pin producing an intense flame, which ignites the propellant gunpowder in the cartridge case. The rapidly burning gunpowder results in the formation of relatively large volumes of very hot gas within the cartridge case, and the pressure of these gases on the base of the projectile result in the projectile being forced out of the cartridge and propelled through the barrel of the firearm.

As a consequence of these events, the ejected projectile is accompanied by a jet of flame, hot compressed carbon monoxide-rich gases, soot, propellant particles, primer residue, metallic particles stripped from the projectile, and vaporized metal from the projectile and cartridge case.[23–32]

In revolvers, similar substances may emerge from the cylinder-barrel gap, the amount of which will depend on the manufacture, quality, and age of the weapon.[23] These residues are most commonly referred to as gunshot residue (GSR), but the terms cartridge-discharge residue (CDR) or firearm-discharge residue (FDR) also are used.[32]

Additional components that may be expelled and deposited on a bullet when a firearm is discharged are the elements fouling the barrel of a firearm. These could include rust particles, lubricating oil, dirt, and even biological material resulting from blowback of blood and tissue into the barrel of the weapon, as sometimes happens in hard-contact entrance wounds.[23,24,27–31]

This has forensic relevance in that:

1. in addition to the ejected bullet, the residual materials resulting from the discharge of a firearm may impart specific characteristics to the appearances of gunshot entrance wounds depending on the range and angle of discharge of a firearm, the type of firearm and type of ammunition used;[23–31]

2. the description, detection, and identification of expelled residual materials may provide valuable investigative information, allowing for scientific range estimates, identification of the ammunition or firearm(s) used, and thus identification of the assailant(s).[23,24,32]

It is of major clinico-forensic importance for trauma personnel to recognize that in addition to the bullet and its cartridge case, all of the above barrel emissions constitute potential evidentiary material that may be deposited in and on the clothing, hair, body, and wounds of a gunshot-wound victim, or even an assailant. By being aware of the presence and value of gunshot-related evidence, such evidence may be identified, collected and preserved rather than inadvertently being destroyed.[1-8,13-16]

Forensic Aspects of Wound Ballistics

Penetrating projectiles can be classified broadly into two major groups, namely fragments and bullets. Fragments from military munitions are the most common wounding agents in war, although fragmentation injuries also may occur following civilian terrorist bombings. Bullets are the predominant penetrating missiles in civilian clinical practice.[36]

Weapons originally designed for military use also are used frequently in civilian settings, leading to blurring of the distinction between military wounds arising from high-velocity rifles and fragments and civilian wounds arising from handguns with lower muzzle velocities.[37]

There are three mechanisms whereby a projectile can cause tissue injury:

1. in a low-energy transfer wound, the projectile crushes and lacerates tissue along the track of the projectile, causing a *permanent cavity*. In addition, bullet and bone fragments can act as secondary missiles, increasing the volume of tissue crushed.[15,23-35,36-42]
2. In a high-energy transfer wound, the projectile may impel the walls of the wound track radially outwards, causing a *temporary cavity* lasting 5 to 10 milliseconds before its collapse, in addition to the permanent mechanical disruption directly produced in (1) (Figure 5-1).[23-31,36-42]
3. In wounds where the firearm's muzzle is in contact with the skin at the time of firing, tissues are forced aside by the gases expelled from the barrel of the firearm, causing a localized *blast injury* (Figure 5-2).[15,38]

Several misconceptions exist about the wounding effects of high-velocity projectiles, particularly when their kinetic energy (as determined by muzzle or impact velocity alone) is presumed to be the sole determinant in size of temporary cavity formation.[36-43]

The severity and size of a gunshot wound is related directly to the total amount of *kinetic energy transfer* to the tissues, not merely the total amount of kinetic energy possessed by the projectile. Kinetic energy transfer is proportional to the degree of retardation of the projectile in the tissue, which in turn is determined by four main factors[23,36-43]:

Temporary cavitation effects on exit wounds

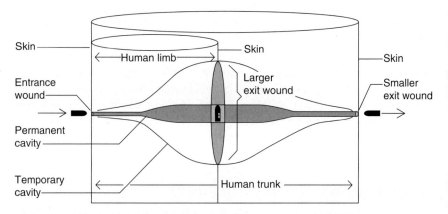

FIGURE 5-1. Schematic profile of the variable sizes of exit wounds caused by the same projectile, as influenced by the diameter of the temporary cavity at the point of exit. The narrow column represents the diameter of a limb and the wider column, the diameter of a trunk.

1. The amount of kinetic energy (KE) possessed by the bullet at the time of the impact, which is dependent on the velocity and mass of the bullet $(KE = \frac{1}{2}mv^2)$.[23–25,36]

2. The angle of yaw of a bullet at the time of impact, which in turn is dependent on the physical characteristics of the bullet (its length, diameter, and density), the rate of twist imparted by the barrel, and the density of the air. The greater the angle of yaw when a bullet strikes a body, the

Contact gunshot wound of the head

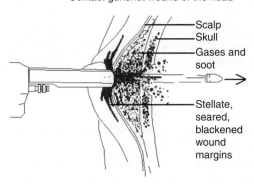

FIGURE 5-2. Contact gunshot wound of the head showing compressed gases expanding between the scalp and the outer table of the skull, with soot deposition in the subcutaneous tissues and on the bone.

greater the retardation of the bullet and consequently the greater the amount of kinetic energy transfer. This explains why unstable projectiles in flight cause larger entrance wounds on impact with the body. Once the bullet enters the denser medium of tissue, its yaw angle increases progressively until the bullet becomes completely unstable, tumbles and rotates by 180 degrees, and ends up travelling base forward. Tumbling of the bullet in tissue increases the presented cross-sectional area of the bullet, resulting in more direct tissue destruction and increased retarding (drag) forces, with consequently greater kinetic energy transfer and larger temporary cavity formation. The sudden increase of the drag force also puts strain on the bullet, which may lead to the break up of the bullet and more tissue destruction.[23]

3. The caliber, construction, and configuration of a bullet also influence the amount of kinetic energy transfer to tissue[23]:

- Blunt-nose bullets and expanding bullets designed to mushroom in tissues are retarded more than streamlined bullets, resulting in more kinetic energy transfer to the tissue.
- The caliber and shape (bluntness of the nose) of a bullet determine the initial presented cross-sectional area of the bullet and thus the drag of the bullet, but are of less importance when bullet deformity occurs.
- Deformation of a bullet depends on both the construction of the bullet and the bullet velocity.
- Construction of a bullet refers to the jacket, the length, thickness, and hardness of the jacket material, the hardness of the lead in the bullet core, and the presence or absence of special features, such as a hollow point.
- Soft- and hollow-point rifle bullets expand and may shed lead fragments from the core, irrespective of whether they strike bone, resulting in a lead snowstorm image as visualized on X-ray. This fragmenting phenomenon appears to be related to velocity and does not happen with handgun bullets unless they strike bone. The lead fragments in turn act as secondary missiles increasing the size of the wound cavity.
- A full metal-jacketed rifle bullet also may break up in the body without striking bone because of its velocity and tendency to yaw radically. As stated earlier, the significant yaw results in a sudden increase in the drag force, straining the structure of the bullet and resulting in break up of the bullet.

4. The fourth factor influencing kinetic energy transfer is the density, strength, and elasticity of the tissue penetrated by the bullet and the length of the wound track. The denser the tissue, the greater the angle of yaw and consequently the greater the degree of retardation and kinetic energy transfer.[23]

Thus, while the *capacity* of a projectile to cause tissue damage is defined traditionally by its available kinetic energy, the muzzle velocity of a firearm and the impact velocity of a projectile can be misleading indicators of their potential for injury when the *kinetic energy transfer variables* are ignored.[3,36,43]

Temporary cavitation is merely a transient displacement or stretching of tissue where the size of the cavity is determined by the characteristics of the tissue and the amount of energy transferred. The damage and external wound appearances caused by a temporary cavity can vary greatly depending on its size and anatomic location (Figure 5-1). Tissues containing a large amount of elastic fibers, such as lung, muscle, or bowel, can withstand some mechanical displacement without significant damage, but denser tissues with few elastic fibers, such as liver and spleen, and encased tissues, such as the brain, may be lacerated severely.

While considered rare, temporary cavitation may cause vascular disruption and bone fractures distant to the permanent wound track.[36,39,40]

Forensic Terminology and Gunshot Wound Appearances

Gunshot wounds may be either *penetrating* or *perforating*. The term *penetrating* wound is used when a bullet enters the body or a structure, but does not exit. The term *perforating* wound is used when a bullet passes completely through the body or a structure.[23]

Entrance Wounds

Range of fire is the distance from the muzzle to the victim and can be divided into four broad categories: contact, near-contact or close-range, intermediate-range, and distant-range. Each category has specific identifying features that are imparted both by the bullet and the various emissions accompanying the bullet from the muzzle of a firearm.[3,23,24]

The presence of clothing or hair acting as intermediary barriers may obscure the typical wound characteristics of contact, close-range, and intermediate-range wounds. It is of great forensic importance that the integrity of such intermediary barriers be maintained and such items preserved as evidentiary material.

Other intermediary targets such as doors or windows also may influence the appearances of entrance wounds as discussed under the heading, "Atypical Entrance Wounds."[23,24]

It must be noted that the size of an entrance wound is a poor indicator of the caliber of the wounding bullet because of variations in anatomic anchoring and elasticity of skin.[23]

Contact Wounds

In contact wounds, the muzzle of the firearm is held in contact with the victim's body or clothing at the time of discharge. Contact wounds may be subdivided further into hard-contact, loose-contact, and incomplete- or angled-contact wounds. In the latter, the complete circumference of the muzzle is not in contact with the body.[3,23,24]

In hard-contact wounds, the muzzle is pressed firmly against the body. All the muzzle emissions accompanying the bullet—the flame, the hot gases, the soot, the propellant particles, the primer residue, and metal particles— are forced into the wound (Figure 5-2). The wound appearance can vary from a small perforation with searing and blackening of the wound edges caused by the hot gases and flame, to a large, gaping stellate wound, with soot visible within and around the wound and searing of the wound edges from hot gases and flame.[23,24]

The large wounds occur over areas where only a thin layer of skin overlies bone, such as the head. On discharge of the firearm, the compressed gases injected between the skin and the skull expand to such an extent that the skin stretches and tears. These tears radiate from the center, resulting in a large stellate or cruciform entrance wound with blackened, seared wound tissues and margins[3,23] (Figure 5-3A,B). The inner wound tissues may appear cherry pink due to the carbon monoxide in the gases.[23]

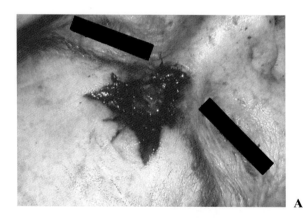

A

Contact entrance wound over bony area

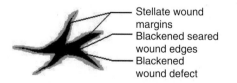

Stellate wound margins
Blackened seared wound edges
Blackened wound defect

B

FIGURE 5-3 (A, B). Contact gunshot wound of the forehead showing a large, stellate, lacerated wound with soot blackening visible within the wound and on the wound margins.

Stellate lacerated wound appearances are not only found in hard-contact entrance wounds, but also may be found in tangential, ricochet, or tumbling bullet entrance wounds, as well as some exit wounds. However, in these wounds, soot and propellant will not be present within and around the wound, and the wound margins will not be seared.[3,23,24]

In some hard-contact wounds, the gases expanding in the subcutaneous tissues may slam the stretched skin against the muzzle of the firearm with enough force to leave behind a muzzle-imprint abrasion or contusion on the skin (Figure 5-4). Patterns like these may be helpful in determining the type of firearm used and should be described, documented, and ideally photographed before wound alteration by debridement, surgery, or healing.[3,23,24]

In both loose-contact and incomplete- or angled-contact wounds, soot and other gunshot residues are present within and around the wound. Soot, which is carbon, is produced by the combustion of propellant and imparts a black color to the areas where it is deposited. In addition, flame and hot gas emissions result in searing of the skin around the wound. Scattered grains of propellant may accompany the jet of gas and be deposited in the seared and blackened zones of skin. The angle between the muzzle and the skin will determine the soot and searing pattern.[3,23]

In a perpendicular loose- or incomplete-contact wound, the distance between the muzzle and the skin is too small for propellant particles to

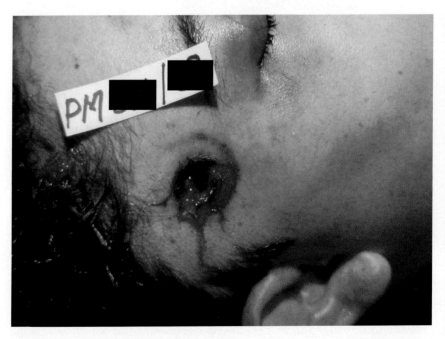

FIGURE 5-4. Hard-contact gunshot wound of the temple, with a partial muzzle-imprint abrasion around the soot-blackened wound.

disperse and mark the skin; the resultant wound appearance is that of a round central defect surrounded by a zone of soot overlying seared skin.[23,24] In an angled loose- or incomplete-contact wound, the zone of searing and soot deposition around the wound is elongated in shape. A fan-shaped pattern of powder tattooing resulting from propellant grains skimming over the seared skin may be observed at the distal end of the entrance wound. This pattern can indicate the direction in which the gun was angled.[23]

Close-Range or Near-Contact Wounds

There is considerable overlap between the appearance of close-range and loose-contact wounds, making it difficult to differentiate the two. Both have an entrance defect with a surrounding zone of seared, soot-blackened skin. Close-range can be defined as the maximum range at which soot is deposited on the wound or the clothing, usually with a muzzle-to-target distance of up to 30 centimeters in handguns.

Because some of the soot can be washed away, its presence and configuration should be described accurately and documented, and photographed if possible, prior to cleansing or surgical debridement (Figure 5-5). Clean-

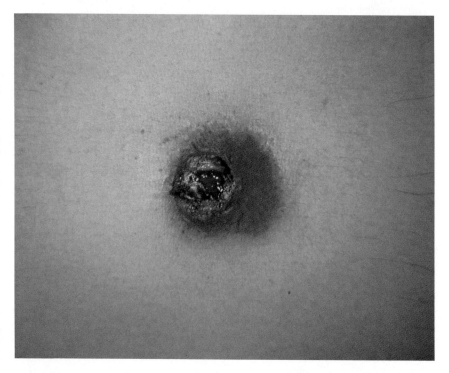

FIGURE 5-5. Slightly angled near-contact wound with the wider zone of soot-blackened skin on the same side as the muzzle of the weapon, i.e., pointing towards the weapon.

ing a wound with a spray of hot water or pouring hydrogen peroxide on wounds caked with clotted blood should wash away or dissolve the blood but preserve the soot pattern. Propellant particles may be deposited in the seared zone surrounding the wound defect, but tattooing from the dispersal of propellant generally is not seen.[23]

Intermediate Range Wounds

The hallmark of intermediate-range wounds is the phenomenon of so-called powder tattooing. This tattooing consists of numerous reddish-brown punctate abrasions surrounding the entrance wound, caused by unburned and partially burned propellant particles impacting against the skin (Figure 5-6). Tattooing may be observed in wound-to-muzzle distances between one centimeter and one meter, but generally is found at distances of less than 60 centimeters in handguns. The lesions of tattooing are actual small abrasions and thus cannot be washed off.[3,23,24,28,29]

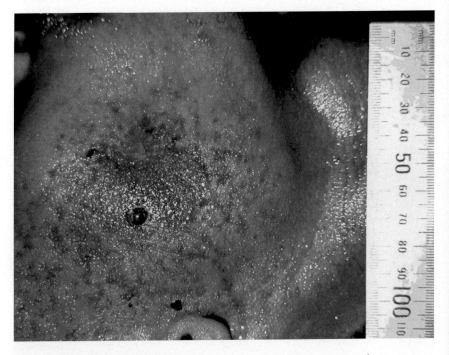

FIGURE 5-6. Powder tattooing around an intermediate-range gunshot entrance wound.

With respect to searing, soot deposition, and powder tattooing, the following must be noted[23]:

- The zone size, concentration, and pattern of both soot deposition and powder tattooing depend on the muzzle-to-target distance and angle, the type of propellant powder and ammunition, the barrel length, and the caliber and type of weapon.
- Accurate documentation and photography of patterns of skin searing, soot deposition, and powder tattooing accompanied by simple line drawings will allow for comparative test-firing studies to give more accurate range-of-fire estimates.
- Test firing is conducted at forensic ballistic laboratories where the offending weapon is fired at a target from different ranges using similar ammunition to that which caused the wound. The target appearances then are compared with those of the wound and the range determined.
- Intermediary barriers such as hair or clothing may obscure or prevent skin searing, soot deposition, or powder tattooing from occurring (Figure 5-7). At close and intermediate ranges, ball powder may perforate one to two layers of cloth to produce powder tattooing, but flake powder usually does not even perforate one layer of cloth. Clothing also may result in

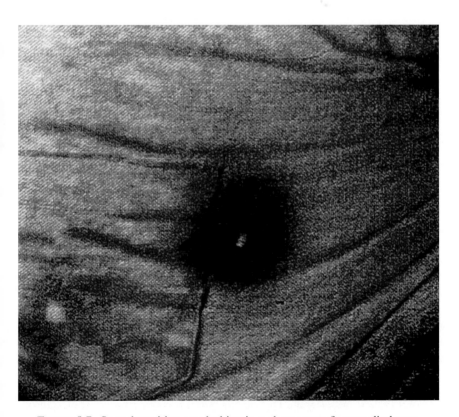

FIGURE 5-7. Soot deposition on clothing in a close-range firearm discharge.

redistribution of soot and powder patterns among the layers of clothing or on the skin in a hard-contact wound, altering the wound appearance to that of a loose-contact wound. It also may absorb completely the soot of a close-range wound, altering its appearance to mimic that of a distant-range wound.

– The correct handling of the clothing of gunshot-wound victims as evidentiary material will allow for further forensic investigations pertaining to range, direction, and firearm or ammunition identification to be conducted on such items.

– Microscopic examination and elemental analyses could be performed on excised gunshot wounds to assist with range, as well as entrance versus exit wound determinations.[23,30,35]

Distant-Range Wounds

In distant-range entrance wounds, the only marks left on the body are produced by the mechanical action of the bullet perforating the skin. There is no searing, soot deposition, or tattooing associated with the skin defect.[23]

Regardless of range, most entrance wounds have a zone of abraded epidermis surrounding the entrance hole, which is called an "abrasion ring" or "abrasion collar." This abrasion ring traditionally is considered to be caused by friction between the bullet and the epithelium, which occurrs as the bullet indents and perforates the skin.[23,24,27–31] In a recent study utilizing high-speed photography and the "skin–skull–brain model," it was postulated that the abrasion ring is due to the massive temporary overstretching of the skin adjacent to the bullet perforation.[33] The abrasion ring is due neither to the bullet's rotational movement nor to thermal effects of the bullet on the skin. The width of an abrasion ring varies with the caliber of the firearm, the angle of bullet entry, and the anatomic location. The abrasion ring may be concentric or eccentric, depending on the angle between the bullet and the skin (Figure 5-8A).

Distant-range entrance wounds of the palms, soles, and elbows do not have abrasion rings and appear stellate or slit-like due to the thickness and rigidity of the skin in those regions. Some high-velocity distant entrance wounds may have no abrasion ring and may show small "micro-tears" radiating outwards from the edges of the perforation, which may be visualized with a dissecting microscope.[23]

Most distant-range entrance wounds are oval to circular with a punched-out, clean appearance to the margins, totally unlike those of exit wounds.[23] A contusion ring may also be present around the wound defect due to damaged blood vessels in the dermis.[33] However, distant entrance wounds over bony surfaces may have stellate or irregular appearances.[23,24]

Distant-range wounds may have a gray coloration to the abrasion ring, which is called bullet wipe. This occurs when powder residue, soot, gun oil, or dirt deposited on the bullet surface as it moves down the barrel is rubbed

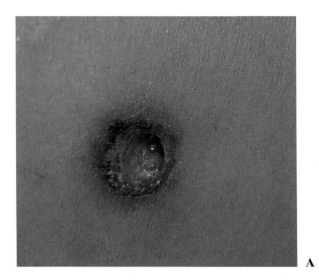

A

Distant-range gunshot entrance wound

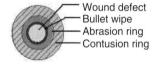

Wound defect
Bullet wipe
Abrasion ring
Contusion ring

B

FIGURE 5-8 (A, B). Slightly angled distant-range gunshot entrance wound with punched-out neat wound margins. A slightly eccentric abrasion ring and narrow contusion ring are present around the wound defect.

off the bullet by the skin as the bullet penetrates the body. Bullet wipe is commonly observed in clothing overlying entrance wounds and is also referred to as a grease ring[23,24,27,28,33] (Figure 5-8B).

It is not possible to determine an exact range of fire in distant-range entrance wounds. Here, only the ring of bullet wipe may be of value in linking a wound to a weapon because metallic elements from the primer, cartridge case, and bullet may be present in the bullet wipe.[23] However, it must be re-emphasized that soot and propellant from close- and intermediate-range wounds may be deposited on the clothing overlying the wound, resulting in a skin wound that *appears* to be of distant-range.[3,23,24,26–31]

Exit Wounds

Most exit wounds have similar characteristics irrespective of whether they result from contact, intermediate, or distant ranges of firing. An exit wound typically is larger and more irregular than an entrance wound. This is mainly due to two factors[23,24]:

i. increasing projectile instability as it travels through the tissue, resulting in accentuated yaw, eventual tumbling, and the bullet exiting base first if the wound track is long enough;

ii. projectile deformation in its passage through the tissues as seen in the mushrooming of a bullet.

Both factors result in a larger area of projectile presented at the exit site, with a resultant larger, more irregular exit wound. Exit wounds result from the stretching force of the bullet overcoming the resistance of the skin. The skin is perforated from the inside out, causing eversion of the wound margins and protrusion of tissue tags through the wound defect[23,24] (Figure 5-9).

Exit wounds can be difficult to interpret because they vary in size and shape and are not necessarily consistently larger than their preceding entrance wounds. Factors other than projectile deformation and projectile instability affecting the size and appearance of an exit wound include[23,24]:

i. velocity and temporary cavitation effects of a bullet at the point of exit; (Figure 5-1)

ii. fragmentation of the bullet;

iii. secondary missile formation, such as bone or jacket fragments accompanying the bullet through the exit wound;

iv. bone under the skin in the area of exit;

v. objects pressing against the skin in the area of exit.

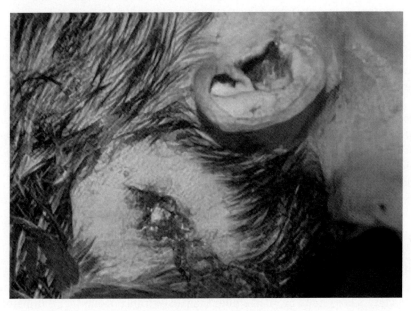

FIGURE 5-9. Irregular exit wound with eversion of the wound margins.

Atypical Entrance Wounds

Atypical gunshot entrance wounds occur when bullets become unstable and nonaxial in their flight before striking the body. Unstable nonaxial flight may be caused by intermediary objects, ricochet, inappropriate weapon–ammunition combinations, poor weapon construction, or use of silencers, muzzle brakes, and flash suppressors. Of significance in these instances is that distant-range gunshot entrance wounds may be confused with contact, close-, or intermediate-range entrance wounds, and even exit wounds, particularly when intermediary objects or ricochet bullets are encountered.[23,44]

If a bullet passes through an intermediary object, before penetrating a body, fragments of glass and even bullet fragments may strike the skin, producing stippling around the entrance wound, mimicking an intermediate-range gunshot entrance wound.[23,44,45,46] Di Maio[23] defines the term "stippling" as multiple punctate abrasions of the skin due to the impact of small fragments of foreign material. If the material is propellant, it is called powder tattooing, but if the stippling is produced by material other than propellant, it is called pseudo-powder tattooing.

Pseudo-powder tattoo marks generally are larger, more irregular, and more sparse than true powder tattoo marks, and fragments of foreign material from the intermediary object, such as glass, may be found embedded in the marks[23] (Figure 5-10).

Pseudo-soot blackening effects may occur in ricochet off material such as black asphalt, with deposition of fine black asphalt powder on a victim. Likewise, the lead core of a bullet may disintegrate following ricochet or intermediary object perforation, with powdered or vaporized lead deposition on a victim simulating soot blackening.[23,45,46,47]

The entrance wound of an unstable or deformed bullet may have a large stellate configuration. In the absence of any stippling or pseudo-soot, it may mimic a contact entrance wound or mimic an exit wound.[23] Bullets recovered from a body following ricochet or intermediate object impaction may be markedly altered in appearance, or even fragmented. If the recovered bullet is handled correctly, forensic scientific examination of such a bullet could reveal the type of material the bullet impacted prior to penetrating the body. This may facilitate the subsequent scene reconstruction and legal proceedings.[13,23,24]

Contact gunshot wounds from firearms fired with silencers, muzzle brakes, or flash suppressors may leave unusual patterns of seared, blackened zones around their entrance wounds (Figure 5-11). These result from the diversion of muzzle gases by such devices. A silencer may even filter out all the soot and powder emerging from the barrel.[23]

A graze wound resulting from tangential contact with a passing bullet may reveal the direction of fire. Careful hand-lens examination of such a wound may reveal skin tags on the lateral wound margins of the

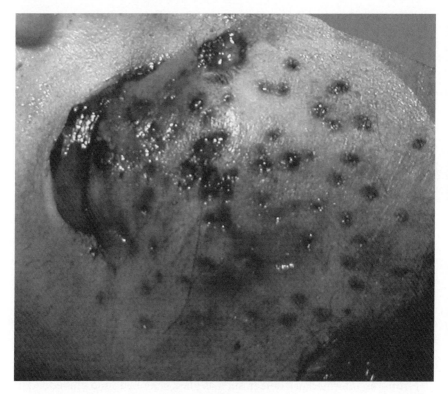

FIGURE 5-10. Larger, more irregular stippling or pseudo-powder tattooing due to fragments of glass.

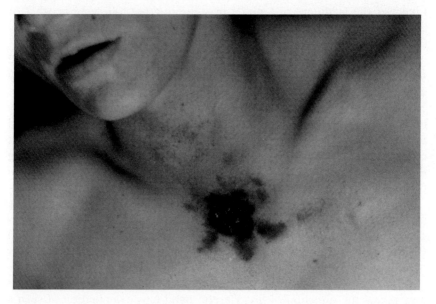

FIGURE 5-11. "Petal" pattern of soot and searing around a contact entrance wound. A flash suppressor was attached to the muzzle of the military rifle used to inflict this wound.

graze-wound trough pointing towards the weapon. The lacerations along the wound-trough margins point in the direction the bullet moved.[23,48] Piling up of tissue may occur at the exit end.[23]

A pseudo-gunshot wound may be defined as an external wound with features resembling those of a gunshot wound, which on further examination is shown to be non-gunshot in origin, such as a stab wound caused by a pointed instrument like a screwdriver[24,49] (Figure 5-12).

Atypical Exit Wounds

Exit wounds may have abraded margins resembling the abrasion collars of distant entrance wounds. This occurs when the skin is reinforced or supported by a firm object at the instant the bullet exits. The exiting bullet everts the skin, impacting and abrading it against the firm object, such as a floor, a wall, or even tight garments like belts or brassieres. These wounds are called shored exit wounds.[3,23,24] Occasionally, the pattern of the material may be imprinted on the edges of the wound.[23] Elemental analysis of excised shored exit wounds by scanning electron microscope–energy dispersive X-ray spectrometry (SEM-EDX) may reveal the nature of the shoring material.[23,50]

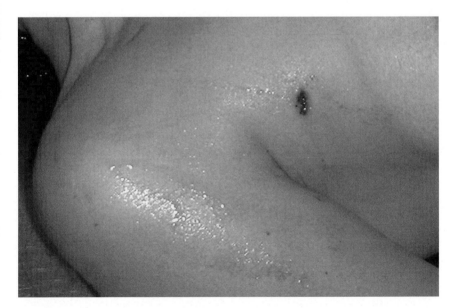

FIGURE 5-12. Oval pseudo-gunshot entrance wound with an "abrasion ring" around the wound defect. This penetrating wound was inflicted with a screwdriver.

Shotgun Wounds

Shotgun wounds are also classified on the basis of range of fire into contact, close-range, intermediate-range, and distant-range wounds.

The components of a shotgun discharge giving rise to differing wound appearances include the propellant, flame, soot, carbon-monoxide–rich gases, pellets, wads, detonator constituents, and cartridge-case fragments.[23,24,27] The terms used to describe the effects of these shotgun components are the same as for rifled weapons.[24]

The characteristics of shotgun entrance wounds vary with the caliber (gauge) of the weapon, degree of choke, size and number of pellets, as well as the range of fire. Searing, soot deposition, and powder tattooing may be present in close-range and intermediate-range shotgun wounds. The precise range of discharge for a given shotgun can be accurately assessed only by test firing that shotgun with the same brand of ammunition and then comparing the findings with the description of the shotgun wound.[23,24,27]

The wound description should include[23,24,31]:

i. The presence of a wad in the wound and the measurements of the wound defect, as well as the searing, blackening, and powder tattooing patterns around the wound. (Close-range: <30 cm).

ii. The presence of a wad in the wound and measurements of the wound defect, noting the presence or absence of crenated or scalloped wound edges and surrounding powder tattooing. (Intermediate-range: 30–120 cm).

iii. Measurement of the diameter of the spread of "satellite" pellet wounds around the measured central defect and the presence or absence of an adjacent wad impact abrasion. (Distant-range: >120 cm) (Figure 5-13A and 5-13B).

iv. The absence of a central wound defect with measurement of the diameter of the spread of pellet wounds. (Distant-range: >600–1000 cm)

v. The presence of a wad or pellets in the clothing.

The range estimates given in brackets above are only a rough guide.

Perforating wounds of the trunk from shotgun pellets are uncommon, but when they do occur, the exit wounds vary from large, irregular, gaping wounds caused by a mass of pellets exiting, to single, slitlike exit wounds produced by single pellets.[23,27]

When found, shotgun pellets and wads should be removed and handled as evidence, as examination of the wad could indicate the gauge of the shotgun and make of the ammunition, whereas the pellets will give the pellet size and shot category.[23]

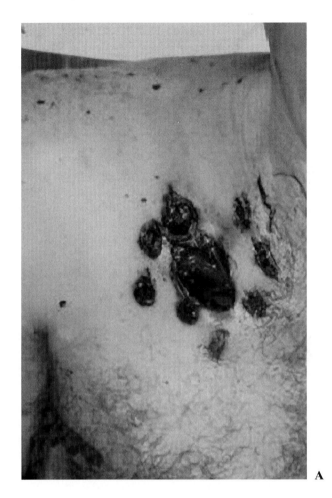

A

Distant-range shotgun entrance wound

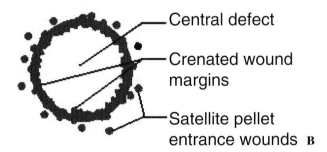

Central defect

Crenated wound margins

Satellite pellet entrance wounds **B**

FIGURE 5-13 (A, B). Distant-range shotgun entrance wound with surrounding satellite pellet entrance wounds. Range is estimated at 1.5 to 2 meters.

Forensic Evidence

The value of forensic evidence in gunshot cases in determining ranges of fire, entrance versus exit wounds, types of ammunition and firearms, manners of injury, and even identification of the assailant cannot be over-emphasized. Therefore the collection, handling, and documentation of evidence during the initial evaluation of a gunshot victim should be standard practice in the emergency setting.[1,3–8] Hospitals should have written protocols that incorporate proper procedures for the collection and retaining of forensic evidence.[6,7,51] A clear understanding of what constitutes evidence is necessary for the successful implementation of such protocols.[4,52]

The term *evidence* is used to describe the nature by which information is presented to the courts; it may be either *informational*, by way of documents and orally, or *physical*, by way of objects such as bullets.[4,52] All physical evidence must be collected carefully, packaged, sealed, and labelled, and it should include the patient's name and hospital number, as well as date and time of specimen collection, specimen type, site of collection, and collector's name and signature.[4,7,13,51,53]

Informational Evidence

In the context of gunshot victims, informational evidence should include a history, examination, and accurate documentation of the gunshot injuries on admission, supplemented with line diagrams, X-rays, and, where possible, photographs. Objective descriptive terminology stating location, size, and shape of wounds and any unusual marks or coloration should be used to describe the wounds, rather than making potentially inaccurate ballistic interpretations.[1–8,11–22] All iatrogenic interventions must also be recorded to prevent subsequent interpretive difficulties by the forensic pathologist.

X-ray studies indicating the location and the number of bullets in the body must be included. The path and fragmenting nature of a bullet may be revealed, but opinions regarding the type of ammunition used are best left to ballistics experts.[8,11–24] When bone is traversed in the path of a bullet, an X-ray may provide valuable information as to the direction of fire, as the bullet displaces the bone fragments in the direction it travels.[23,24]

Physical Evidence

Physical evidence is real, tangible, or latent matter that can be visualized, measured, or analyzed.[4] Any belongings, body fluids or tissues, or foreign objects found in or on the patient constitute potential evidence. If physical evidence is very small or microscopic, it is referred to as "trace evidence."

In gunshot victims, physical evidence would include:

  i. trace evidence such as:
   – gunshot residue (GSR) or blood-spatter on the victim's hands, hair, and clothing[23,32,54–59]
   – hairs, debris, or fibers on the victim's body or clothing[4,7,53,60]
   – blood or tissue under the victim's fingernails[3,23,54]
 ii. blood, urine, or tissue samples
iii. clothing with or without bullet holes
 iv. bullets and cartridge cases in the victim's body or clothing.[4–7,13,51,53]

Trace Evidence

The individual collection of trace evidence by "tape lift" or "swabbing" ideally should be performed by trained forensic personnel and falls outside the scope of the emergency trauma surgeon.[4,32] However, by merely collecting and preserving the clothing of a gunshot victim in totality, trace evidence collection and analyses of GSR, fibers, hairs, debris, or blood on the clothing can be performed at forensic laboratories.[4,7,23,32,53–60]

If a physical altercation occurred prior to the shooting incident, fingernail scrapings could be used for comparative DNA analyses. Special crime kits for the collection of such samples are available in most centers, but ideally staff with appropriate forensic training should collect these samples.[1–8,16]

Once the patient is stable, GSR testing on the hands of victims could be performed by forensic investigators, as particles may be detectable for up to 12 hours following the shooting incident, using SEM-EDX techniques. A GSR test may determine whether a person has fired a firearm by testing for primer-residue constituents containing barium nitrate, antimony sulfide, and lead peroxide.[23,32,55–59]

If GSR or DNA testing is to be performed on the patient's hands, the hands should not be cleaned with soap or alcohol. Paper bags should be placed over the hands and secured with elastic bands. Plastic bags should not be used as condensation or moisture in the plastic bags may wash away primer residue or cause fungal degradation of biological evidence.[3,4,7,13,23,53]

Laboratory Samples

Admission blood samples for alcohol or drug analyses taken prior to dilution by volume expanders or transfusions will yield the most accurate results. Urine specimens also may be used, but they are less valuable for quantification of results.[7] The victim's blood could be used for comparative DNA analysis with blood spatter found at a scene, on a suspect, or on a firearm, as well as with tissue particles found on a spent bullet recovered at a scene.[23,54]

Surgical debridement of a gunshot wound will permanently alter the wound appearance. If not properly documented, photographed, or retained for microscopic evaluation, this may result in misinterpretation by subsequent examiners.[1–8,51] Excised wound margins could allow for microscopic and SEM-EDX evaluation in cases where it is important to[23,30,35,51,55–58]:

- confirm the range of an entrance wound
- establish whether one is dealing with the pseudo-effects of soot blackening or powder tattooing
- establish which of two gunshot wounds is the entrance wound
- ascertain the type of weapon or ammunition used.

For SEM-EDX GSR trace analysis, the excised skin specimen should be placed outer surface upwards on a layer of dry gauze, on top of a piece of cotton wool dampened (not soaked) with formalin, then placed inside a specimen bottle. The skin sample must be secured in this position by placing another piece of dry gauze over it before closing and sealing the bottle. Suspension of the specimen in liquid formalin should be avoided to prevent particles from being washed off prior to analysis (B. A. Kloppers, personal communication).

Clothing

The clothing of victims often contains valuable clues, including trace evidence and macroscopic bullet holes.[13] Examination of clothing may reveal information as to range and direction of fire, type of ammunition and firearm used, and allow for confirmatory trace evidence analysis. Therefore, all clothing of gunshot victims should be preserved and retained.[3–8,13,23,24,32,54–60,61]

Emergency personnel should not cut through the convenient starting point of the bullet holes for purposes of removing clothing because disruption of the bullet defect site may destroy evidence. Clothing should be searched for pieces of spent bullets such as bullet jackets.[13,53] It also should be noted whether any garments on the victim were "inside out," as clothing fibers bend in the direction of the path of the bullet, and the true orientation of the fabric may be important to forensic investigators in confirming the circumstances surrounding the incident.[13,23]

Propellant residue and soot will deposit on clothing in contact, close-, and intermediate-range discharges, as they would on skin (Figure 5-7). Contact wounds in synthetic material may even cause "burn holes." Bullet-wipe residue also may be observed as a gray to black rim around an entrance hole in clothing. Trace evidence on retained clothing, including fibers, debris, blood spatter and GSR, may be detected and analyzed to corroborate or complement macroscopic findings with respect to circumstances, range, and direction of fire and type of firearm or ammunition used.[3,23,32,54–60]

Bloody garments should be air dried before being packaged in correctly labelled paper bags to prevent degradation of evidence by fungal or bacterial elements.[4,7,13,23,53]

Bullets and Cartridge Cases

When bullets or projectile fragments are found or surgically removed from the patient, their integrity must be maintained as much as possible for subsequent ballistic investigations.[23,24,53] A bullet's unique markings are called *class characteristics*, which result from its contact with the rifling in the gun's barrel when the firearm is discharged. They may indicate the make and model of a firearm using comparative analytical techniques.[23,24] Standard metal instruments such as forceps can scratch the jacket or lead of the bullet, producing marks that could hamper or prevent analysis of bullet striations, and thus firearm identification.[23,62] Russel et al.[62] suggested using a "bullet extractor" to accomplish the dual purpose of safe handling (as in the case of bullets with pointed ends, jagged projections, and sharp edges, for example the Black Talon Bullet) and evidence preservation. The bullet extractor is a standard curved Kelly forceps fitted with two-centimeter lengths of standard-gauge rubber urinary catheter as protective tips.[62]

The retrieved projectile should be examined for macroscopic trace evidence such as fibers and glass. If none is found, the projectile may be rinsed gently to remove excess blood or body fluids.[62] If the surgeon chooses to mark the bullet with his initials, such marks should be put on the base of the bullet so as not obliterate the rifling marks on the side of the bullet.[23]

Deformed sharp-edged bullets or bullet fragments should be placed in hard plastic containers rather than traditional bullet envelopes to prevent accidental puncture through the envelopes and subsequent loss or injury.[62,63] The bullet container or envelope should be annotated with the date, time, anatomical location of the bullet, the name and hospital number of the gunshot victim, and the collector's name. Tamper-proof seals should be used whenever possible.[23,53,62]

Cartridge cases that may be found in the victim's clothing also have unique microscopic marks on their bottoms or sides, imparted by contact with the firing pin, the breechlock, the magazine of semiautomatic weapons, and extractor and ejector mechanisms. These may be used to identify the type, make, and model of the firearm used. Therefore they should be handled and preserved in the same careful way as described above for bullets.[23]

The Deceased Gunshot Victim

When a gunshot victim dies in the hospital, the clinical documents forwarded to the forensic pathologist must indicate clearly whether any bullets or projectiles were retrieved from the body of the patient. The location of the bullet before retrieval must be noted. The documents must also include a summary history and examination of the victim at the time of admission, accurate admission wound descriptions, and subsequent iatrogenic procedures performed. If the death is delayed for a period of time, a summary of the patient's management, clinical progress, and any complications must also be recorded. If X-rays were taken, the exact location of any remaining projectiles must be documented clearly.[1–8,13,61]

If a gunshot wound victim dies soon after arrival at the hospital, it is recommended that the deceased's hands be encased in paper bags. If the clothing is still on the body, it should not be removed before placing the body in a body bag for transfer to the mortuary.[4] To facilitate the comparison of clothing defects with wounds on the victim's body, all removed clothing still in the custody of the hospital should accompany the body to the mortuary.[53] All intravenous lines, catheters, tubes, sutures, and drains should be left in situ to minimize possible confusion of gunshot wounds with surgical wounds.[4]

The Chain of Custody

The chain of custody is the pathway that physical evidence follows from the time it is collected until it has served its purpose in the legal investigation of an incident. A record of the chain of custody will reflect the number of times a piece of evidence has changed hands or location prior to its final destination.[4] Minimizing the times that evidentiary items change hands will assist in protecting the integrity and credibility of such evidence.[53] Failure to protect the chain of custody may cause evidence to be inadmissible in court, even though it is physically present, as defense attorneys often attempt to cast doubt on the integrity of the evidence by attacking the chain of custody.[4,53]

All potential evidentiary items should be placed in appropriate containers that can be sealed with tape and labelled appropriately.[4,53] A standard chain-of-custody form attached to the container could be used to document all transfers of the evidence, with the dates, details, and signatures of all the individuals who handled the evidence recorded on it. A copy of this chain-of-custody form should be kept in the patient's hospital record. If the chain is properly recorded, hospital personnel may not be required to testify in subsequent court proceedings, especially when testimony is needed simply to establish the chain of custody.[4,51,53]

Written protocols incorporating the proper handling of forensic evidence, together with standard chain-of-custody forms should be implemented at all hospitals.[6,7,51] A hospital "property custodian" should be appointed to safeguard all evidentiary items until their collection by law-enforcement officials.[4,7]

Explosions and Evidence

With the dramatic increase in the incidence of domestic bombings and mass-casualty incidents worldwide, all hospitals must have mass-casualty plans in place in order to optimize medical care for victims.[64,65] In addition, emergency departments must recognize that criminal prosecution or civil litigation against parties responsible for injurious explosions may follow such events. While it may be very difficult in mass-casualty situations, the forensic aspects of documentation and evidence collection must remain in place.[37,65]

A variety of explosive devices exist, including many which are home-made. Emergency health-care workers must protect themselves and their patients from further injury by ensuring that contaminated clothing and potential flammable material is removed from the patient, keeping in mind that all material removed is potential forensic evidence and should be treated as such.[64] Clothing and hair of victims may contain macroscopic and trace evidence that may reflect the type of explosive used, confirm the chemical composition of incendiary devices, indicate the presence or absence of fire or smoke, and may provide clues as to the location of a patient in relation to the blast.[27–29,64]

The patterns of injuries and shrapnel retained in patients may also provide valuable information as to all of the above. Careful descriptions and documentation of all injuries, total-body X-ray investigations, and retrieval of foreign materials during surgery that may include bomb fragments, must be performed.[27,28,37] Small metal objects forming part of the bomb mechanism may be invaluable in allowing experts to recognize the handiwork of a particular bomb maker or terrorist group.[27–29]

Conclusion

When clinicians are remiss in the adequate forensic evaluation of gunshot patients, it could have far-reaching medico-legal implications in the increasingly litigious construct of society and could result in obstruction of the ends of justice with respect to the forensic and legal needs of individual patients, as well as society in general.[1–8,16,20,52]

Three separate retrospective analyses have shown that clinical records in gunshot cases routinely lack adequate wound descriptions.[14,18–22] In addition, the correct handling of potentially short-lived evidentiary material and the preservation of a chain of custody is frequently neglected in clinical settings.[5–8]

If a gunshot victim is killed outright and examined by a competent forensic pathologist, precise descriptions of the wounds will be obtained and forensic evidence will be handled correctly. However, if the patient initially survives and remains in hospital for a period of time, then wound healing or sepsis and surgical interventions can cause considerable difficulty in interpretation for the forensic pathologist if the documentation of gunshot wounds and iatrogenic procedures and the collection of forensic evidence have been neglected.[13,15,17–20]

In summary, the comprehensive forensic evaluation of a gunshot victim should include the following:

i. recording of the patient's and clinician's names, date and time of admission, full history and examination, and date and time of death (when applicable)
ii. recording of anatomical location, size, shape, and characteristics of the gunshot wound(s), including associated marks or coloration
iii. recording of surgical resuscitative procedures, as these may obscure or alter gunshot wound appearances, or result in "additional wounds"
iv. augmentation of narrative descriptions with X-rays, diagrams, and photographs where possible
v. use of a proforma, including a simple line drawing, to improve the quality of documentation
vi. refraining from "forensic interpretations" of gunshot wound appearances with respect to entrance, exit, direction, or range of fire
vii. recording of the patient's clinical management, progress, or complications, as well as special investigations and further surgical interventions
viii. recording and correct handling of all evidence collected and proper maintenance of the chain of custody.

Lastly, a succinct observation by William S. Smock[3] that reflects the merits of clinical forensic training and the consequent appreciation of the value of forensic evidence in the emergency department, bears iteration:

"What was once considered confounding clutter that gets in the way of patient care (such as clothing and surface dirt) takes on a whole new significance when recognised for what it really is - evidence."[3]

Acknowledgments. With special thanks to Fiona Bester, the Deputy Librarian of the University of the Witwatersrand Health Sciences Library, and her members of staff, Senior Superintendent B.A. Kloppers, the Operational Commander of the Ballistics Unit at the Forensic Science Laboratory in Pretoria, and Raymond Cherry, our Departmental Research Assistant, for their invaluable assistance in the preparation of this chapter.

References

1. Eckert WG, Bell JS, Stein RJ, Tabakman MB, Taff ML, Tedeschi LG. Clinical forensic medicine. *Am J Forensic Med Pathol.* 1986;7:182–185.
2. Smock WS. Forensic emergency medicine. In: Marx JA, ed. *Rosen's Emergency Medicine*, 5th ed. St Louis, MO: Mosby; 2002:828–841.
3. Olshaker JS, Jackson CM, Smock WS. *Forensic Emergency Medicine.* Philadelphia: Lippincott Williams and Wilkins; 2001.
4. Muro GA, Easter CR. Clinical forensics for perioperative nurses. *AORN J.* 1994;60:585–591, 593.

5. Smock WS, Nichols GR, Fuller PM. Development and implementation of the first clinical forensic medicine training program. *J Forensic Sci*. 1993;38:835–839.
6. Carmona R, Prince K. Trauma and forensic medicine. *J Trauma*. 1989; 29:1222–1225.
7. Mittleman RE, Goldberg HS, Waksman DM. Preserving evidence in the emergency department. *Am J Nurs*. 1983;83:1652–1654.
8. Smialek JE. Forensic medicine in the emergency department. *Emerg Med Clin North Am*. 1983;1:693–704.
9. Hargarten SW, Waeckerle JF. Docs and cops: a collaborating or colliding partnership? *Ann Emerg Med*. 2001;38:438–440.
10. Shepherd JP. Emergency medicine and police collaboration to prevent community violence. *Ann Emerg Med*. 2001;38:430–437.
11. Randall T. Clinicians' forensic interpretations of fatal gunshot wounds often miss the mark. *JAMA*. 1993;269:2058, 2061.
12. Apfelbaum JD, Shockley LW, Wahe JW, Moore EE. Entrance and exit gunshot wounds: incorrect terms for the emergency department? *J Emerg Med*. 1998;16:741–745.
13. Godley DR, Smith TK. Some medicolegal aspects of gunshot wounds. *J Trauma*. 1977;17:866–871.
14. Ross RT, Hammen PF, Frantz EI, Pare LE, Boyd CR. Gunshot wounds: evaluating the adequacy of documentation at a Level I trauma center. *J Trauma*. 1998;45:151–152.
15. Bowley DM, Vellema J. Wound ballistics—An update. *Care of the Critically Ill*. 2002;18:133–138.
16. Ryan MT. Clinical forensic medicine. *Ann Emerg Med*. 2000;36:271–273.
17. Collins KA, Lantz PE. Interpretation of fatal, multiple, and exiting gunshot wounds by trauma specialists. *J Forensic Sci*. 1994;39:94–99.
18. Fackler ML, Mason RT. Gunshot wounds: Evaluating the adequacy of documentation at a level I trauma center. *J Trauma*. 1999;46:741–742.
19. Fackler ML. How to describe bullet holes. *Ann Emerg Med*. 1994;23:386–387.
20. Fackler ML, Riddick L. Clinicians' inadequate descriptions of gunshot wounds obstruct justice: Clinical journals refuse to expose the problem. *Proceedings of the American Academy of Forensic Sciences*. 1996;149.
21. Voelker R. New program targets death investigator training. *JAMA*. 1996;275:826.
22. Shuman M, Wright RK. Evaluation of clinician accuracy in describing gunshot wound injuries. *J Forensic Sci*. 1999;44:339–342.
23. Di Maio VJM. *Gunshot Wounds*, 2nd ed. Boca Raton, FL: CRC Press; 1999.
24. Fatteh A. *Medicolegal Investigation of Gunshot wounds*. Philadelphia: JB Lippincott; 1976.
25. Sellier KG, Kneubuehl BP. *Wound Ballistics and the Scientific Background*. Amsterdam: Elsevier Science; 1994.
26. Gordon I, Shapiro HA, Berson SD. *Forensic Medicine*, 3rd ed. Edinburgh: Churchill Livingstone; 1997.
27. Knight B. *Forensic Pathology*, 2nd ed. New York: Oxford University Press; 1996.
28. Spitz WU, Fischer RS. *Medicolegal Investigation of Death*. Springfield: Charles C Thomas; 1993.
29. Mason JK. *Forensic Medicine*. London: Chapman Hall Medical; 1993.

30. Adelson L. *The Pathology of Homicide*. Springfield: Charles C Thomas; 1974.
31. Knight B. *Simpson's Forensic Medicine*, 10th ed. London: Edward Arnold; 1991.
32. Romolo FS, Margot P. Identification of gunshot residue: a critical review. *Forensic Sci Int*. 2001;119:195–211.
33. Thali MJ, Kneubuehl BP, Zollinger U, Dirnhofer R. A study of the morphology of gunshot entrance wounds, in connection with their dynamic creation, utilizing the "skin-skull-brain model". *Forensic Sci Int*. 2002;125:190–194.
34. Mason JK, Purdue BN. *The Pathology of Trauma*, 3rd ed. New York: Oxford University Press—Arnold; 2000.
35. Adelson L. A microscopic study of dermal gunshot wounds. *Am J Clin Pathol*. 1961;35:393–402.
36. Cooper GJ, Ryan JM. Interaction of penetrating missiles with tissues: Some common misapprehensions and implications for wound management. *Br J Surg*. 1990;77:606–610.
37. Ryan JM, Rich NM, Dale RF, Morgans BT, Cooper GJ. *Ballistic Trauma*. London: Arnold; 1997.
38. Fackler ML. Civilian gunshot wounds and ballistics: Dispelling the myths. *Emerg Med Clin North Am*. 1998;16:17–28.
39. Fackler ML. Wound ballistics. A review of common misconceptions. *JAMA*. 1988;259:2730–2736.
40. Fackler ML. Gunshot wound review. *Ann Emerg Med*. 1996;28:194–203.
41. Hollerman JJ, Fackler ML, Coldwell DM, Ben-Menachem Y. Gunshot wounds: 1. Bullets, ballistics, and mechanisms of injury. *AJR Am J Roentgenol*. 1990;155:685–690.
42. Mendelson JA. The relationship between mechanisms of wounding and principles of treatment of missile wounds. *J Trauma*. 1991;31:1181–1202.
43. Lindsey D. The idolatry of velocity, or lies, damn lies, and ballistics. *J Trauma*. 1980;20:1068–1069.
44. Donoghue ER, Kalelkar MB, Richmond JM, Teass SS. Atypical gunshot wounds of entrance: An empirical study. *J Forensic Sci*. 1984;29:379–388.
45. Dixon DS. Tempered plate glass as an intermediate target and its effects on gunshot wound characteristics. *J Forensic Sci*. 1982;27:205–208.
46. Stahl CJ, Jones SR, Johnson FB, Luke JL. The effect of glass as an intermediate target on bullets: Experimental studies and report of a case. *J Forensic Sci*. 1979;24:6–17.
47. Sellier K. *Forensic Science Progress, Volume 6, Shot Range Determination*. Berlin: Springer-Verlag; 1991.
48. Dixon DS. Determination of direction of fire from graze gunshot wounds. *J Forensic Sci*. 1980;25:272–279.
49. Prahlow JA, McClain JL. Lesions that simulate gunshot wounds—further examples II. *J Clin Forensic Med*. 2001;8:206–213.
50. Dixon DS. Characteristics of shored exit wounds. *J Forensic Sci*. 1981; 26:691–698.
51. Murphy GK. The study of gunshot wounds in surgical pathology. *Am J Forensic Med Pathol*. 1980;1:123–130.
52. Mc Lay WDS. *Clinical Forensic Medicine*, 2nd ed. London: Greenwich Medical Media; 1996.
53. Schramm CA. Forensic medicine. What the perioperative nurse needs to know. *AORN J*. 1991;53:669–683, 686–692.

54. Karger B, Nüsse R, Bajanowski T. Backspatter on the firearm and hand in experimental close-range gunshots to the head. *Am J Forensic Med Pathol.* 2002;23:211–213.
55. Zeichner A, Levin N. Casework experience of GSR detection in Israel, on samples from hands, hair, and clothing using an autosearch SEM/EDX system. *J Forensic Sci.* 1995;40:1082–1085.
56. Wolten GM, Nesbitt RS, Calloway AR, Loper GL, Jones PF. Particle analysis for the detection of gunshot residue I: scanning electron microscopy/energy dispersive x-ray characterization of hand deposits from firing. *J Forensic Sci.* 1979;24:409–422.
57. Wolten GM, Nesbitt RS, Calloway AR. Particle analysis for the detection of gunshot residue III: The case record. *J Forensic Sci.* 1979;24:864–869.
58. Tillman WL. Automated gunshot residue particle search and characterization. *J Forensic Sci.* 1987;32:62–71.
59. Fojtášek L, Vacínová J, Kolá P, Kotrlý M. Distribution of GSR particles in the surroundings of shooting pistol. *Forensic Sci Int.* 2003;132:99–105.
60. Laing DK, Hartshorne AW, Cook R, Robinson G. A fiber data collection for forensic scientists: collection and examination methods. *J Forensic Sci.* 1987; 32:364–369.
61. Finck PA. Ballistic and forensic pathologic aspects of missile wounds. Conversion between Anglo-American and metric-system units. *Mil Med.* 1965; 130:545–563.
62. Russell MA, Atkinson RD, Klatt EC, Noguchi TT. Safety in bullet recovery procedures: A study of the Black Talon bullet. *Am J Forensic Med Pathol.* 1995;16:120–123.
63. McCormick GM, Young DB, Stewart JC. Wounding effects of the Winchester Black Talon bullet. *Am J Forensic Med Pathol.* 1996;17:124–129.
64. Maxson TR. Management of pediatric trauma: Blast victims in a mass casualty incident. *Clin Ped Emerg Med.* 2002;3:256–261.
65. Wightman JM, Gladish SL. Explosions and blast injuries. *Ann Emerg Med.* 2001;37:664–678.

Further Readings

1. Olshaker JS, Jackson CM, Smock WS. *Forensic Emergency Medicine.* Philadelphia: Lippincott Williams and Wilkins; 2001.
2. Di Maio VJM. *Gunshot wounds,* 2nd ed. Boca Raton, FL: CRC Press; 1999.
3. Fatteh A. *Medicolegal Investigation of Gunshot wounds.* Philadelphia: JB Lippincott; 1976.
4. Knight B. *Forensic Pathology,* 2nd ed. New York: Oxford University Press; 1996.
5. Sellier K. *Forensic Science Progress, Volume 6, Shot Range Determination.* Berlin: Springer-Verlag; 1991.

6
Ballistic Trauma, Armed Violence, and International Law

ROBIN M. COUPLAND*

Ballistic trauma is perceived, quite reasonably, as being the domain of emergency-department personnel, military doctors and nurses, and trauma surgeons. They are expected to treat the people suffering ballistic trauma. The other medical domain that feeds off an understanding of ballistic trauma is forensic medicine; reconstruction of an event in which use of a weapon resulted in ballistic trauma can provide evidence for the process of justice. Between these two medical applications of understanding ballistic trauma sits the physical subject of wound ballistics, which is the study of the interaction of missiles and tissue and can really only be studied in a laboratory using tissue simulants such as gelatine or soap.[1]

A nonmedical subject to which an understanding of ballistic trauma applies is that part of international humanitarian law pertaining to means and methods of warfare.[2,3] There exist certain treaty-based instruments of international law that were drawn up, in part, to prevent injury and suffering of soldiers on the battlefield excessive to that necessary to put them out of action. Examples are: prohibitions on explosive or expanding bullets (agreed upon in the 1868 St Petersburg Declaration and the 1899 Hague Declaration respectively); weapons that injure by fragments that cannot be detected by X-rays;[4,5] blinding lasers;[4,6] and antipersonnel mines.[7] There also is a general prohibition on any weapon "of a nature to cause superfluous injury or unnecessary suffering."[8]

In relation to small-caliber bullets, debate has raged for more than one hundred years around the question of how much ballistic trauma is necessary to put the soldier out of action and how much would be excessive to this objective.[9] This debate is unresolved despite greater understanding of the differences between the ballistic trauma caused by prohibited bullets and that caused by nonprohibited bullets.[3,10] It is made no clearer by the

---

* R.M. Coupland is the medical adviser on armed violence and the effects of weapons to the legal division of the International Committee of the Red Cross. The opinions expressed are the author's own and do not represent the views or policy of the International Committee of the Red Cross.

fact that police can and do use ammunition in handguns that, if used in armed conflict, would contravene the 1899 Hague Declaration.[11] While this debate ultimately hinges on a health issue, many doctors have an ethical problem with entering into it; first, they do not wish to be involved in studies ascertaining how much injury can or should be inflicted to the human body in war because this acknowledges that some degree of injury is acceptable and therefore somehow legitimizes war; second, they see a simpler preventive health solution, that is, to stop the use of weapons.[12] Nevertheless, it seems that nation states continue to settle their differences by resorting to armed conflict; the origins and application of international *humanitarian* law start with this assumption, uncomfortable though it is, and the aim of this body of law is to limit the degree of suffering involved.

However, health professionals cannot ignore the interface of other bodies of international law and the injury and suffering brought by weapons solely because, for some, examining the nature of the effects of certain weapons in relation to instruments of international humanitarian law raises an ethical dilemma. What is clear from every-day news is that injury and suffering in every corner of the world results from the use of weapons, which inflict injury by ballistic trauma, but which are not specifically prohibited or regulated; namely, artillery, mortars, aerial bombs, grenades, assault rifles, and handguns. It is not only the technical features of these weapons such as rate of fire, bullet velocity, or area covered by explosive force that are responsible for these effects, but also their widespread availability[13,14] and, above all, how they are used.[15,16] The people who suffer are not only combatants, but also prisoners of war and, above all, civilians. In attempting to limit the absolute worst excesses of armed violence, the International Criminal Court recently has become a reality. The court has jurisdiction over the crime of aggression, the crime of genocide, crimes against humanity, and war crimes. It is highly pertinent that the crimes have been defined precisely in legal terms, and virtually every crime listed represents, not surprisingly, a health issue resulting from some form of ballistic trauma or threat of it.[17] In brief, ballistic trauma is much more than a health-care or surgical issue; it is a massive global health issue that demands prevention. Furthermore, a whole range of other health and legal issues follow if one includes fear of ballistic trauma; migration, infectious disease, lack of clean drinking water, malnutrition, and lack of access to health care; these are but a few of the follow-on effects that result from people's insecurity because of the fear of being shot. This means that virtually all the data pertaining to the health impact of conflict can be interpreted as data about the effects of armed violence using weapons that inflict ballistic trauma. It also means that the legal instruments that are vehicles for prevention are not only international humanitarian law, but also the Charter of the United Nations, the international laws of arms control and disarmament, and human-rights law.

The above provides justification for why a broader approach to prevention of ballistic trauma warrants inclusion in a book such as this. This chapter does not continue further with the debate of why or how certain weapons themselves might be prohibited based on their purported excessive effects on the individual soldier. It provides a generic approach—albeit an unconventional public health approach—to many important issues at the core of which lies ballistic trauma or threat of ballistic trauma. There are two contemporary, recurrent, and critically important issues that are ultimately issues of ballistic trauma. These are first, unintended civilian deaths and injuries when explosive weapons are used against military objectives in populated areas, and second, massacres and enforced disappearances. In relation to both these phenomena, the presented analytical framework may provide a decision-making tool for policy makers, diplomats, armed-forces personnel, and lawyers working in different areas of international law.

A Public Health Approach to Armed Violence Resulting in Ballistic Trauma

Analysis of any war, rebellion, or massacre tends to focus on political motives, who is the guilty party, and sometimes on the weapons used if they are new, unusual, or spectacular. However, when the story extends to the victims (those who have suffered ballistic trauma), somehow rational argument gets lost to sentiment, emotion, or outrage. Responsibility for surviving victims is left to health professionals who themselves are struggling under multiple constraints that often includes fear for their own security. A rational overview of the context is difficult because this health issue arises in precisely those contexts in which rational thinking is suppressed and data collection may be perceived as pointless, or even unethical. Another consideration is that there is something so profoundly shocking or, dare it be said, exciting about armed violence that it defies objective analysis. It is also a health subject in which, for some inexplicable reason, figures are cited to emphasize the horrible nature of it all and in an authoritative manner, but without evidence or citation; the universally cited, but untrue statistic that "90% of casualties of modern wars are civilian" is an example.[18,19] It is of fundamental importance that violence and above all, collective violence, is at last being approached as a global health issue.[20]

To take the first steps in a more rational approach, the following series of simple and logically connected assertions should be considered:

- Ballistic trauma is an effect of use of weapons. (The Oxford English Dictionary defines a weapon as a "material thing designed or used or usable as an instrument for inflicting bodily harm").
- The use of a weapon is an act of violence. (The World Health Organization's definition of violence is "the intentional use of physical force or power, threatened or actual, against oneself, another person, or against a

group or community, that either results in or has a likelihood to result in injury, death, psychological harm, maldevelopment or deprivation.")
- An act of armed violence results in a health problem for the victim. (The World Health Organization's definition of health is "a state of complete physical, mental and social well-being and not merely the absence of disease.")
- Threat of use of a weapon is also an act of armed violence and also can exert an effect on health (according to the above definitions of violence and health).
- If the determinants of the health effects of armed violence can be identified, preventive strategies could be identified.

It follows that identifying the determinants of ballistic trauma or fear of ballistic trauma in any given context provides the elements of a preventive framework.

An analytical framework of armed violence is offered here that can be applied to any effects of any act of armed violence committed with any weapon. In most cases, this framework does little more than underscore the obvious. Where it may prove useful is in the analysis of complex situations and as a tool for dialogue about a variety of issues relating to assistance and protection of victims of war and international law. It could help us to talk common sense about something that is difficult to approach in common-sense terms.

An analytical framework is a tool for sorting and prioritizing a variety of information about a given subject or context. Incoming information is categorized appropriately and the relationship between the categories is established. In the field of health, such an analytical framework brought new understanding to global child mortality.[21] Obviously, in an analytical framework of armed violence, the *effects* of an act of armed violence, which can be measured in many and varied ways, make up one of the categories; the other categories are made up of the determinants of these effects.[22]

How can the determinants of the effects of armed violence be categorized? Another series of assumptions helps us:

- Before the victim or victims can suffer any effects of the use of a weapon in a given context, they must in some way be vulnerable (increasing vulnerability simply means increasing potential to suffer the effects);
- Before a particular weapon is used, at some previous time the weapon has to be transferred into the hands of the user;
- Before transfer, the weapon has to be produced;
- Before production, the weapon has to be designed.[23,24]

Thus, important potential determinants of the effects of armed violence are found in the vulnerability of the potential victims and along the continuum of "design-to-production-to-transfer-to-use." It follows that whatever the nature of armed violence, and whatever effects are being considered, the key determinants of the effects are:

- the vulnerability of the victim (the potential to suffer the effect);
- the psychological potential for violence (intentional *use* of physical force);
- the potential number of weapons in use (corresponding to *production* and *transfer*);
- the potential of the weapon to cause the effect (corresponding to *design*).

Thus, five categories of information are identified: the effects of armed violence and the four categories given by the determinants of these effects.

An essential part of this analytical framework is understanding the interaction of these determinants. There are two core concepts: first, effects of armed violence are produced only as long as the potential of each determinant is above zero—each is a necessary but not sufficient cause of the effects in question; second, the potential for violence using weapons must be influenced by the user's perceptions of the effects and of the other three determinants—the complex relationship between weapons and violence is played out in the psychology of the user or users. By extrapolation, the nature of the weapons themselves and their availability are major determinants of the nature, timing, and extent of armed violence.

In analyzing any act of armed violence, the first step is to identify the effects of concern. The next step is to identify the determinants of these effects. Although one of the determinants may weigh more heavily in the interaction than others, no single determinant stands alone; determinants from the other three categories also must come into play. Addressing only one determinant may be ineffective in preventing or limiting any given effect of armed violence unless that determinant is eliminated completely. Analyzing or reporting any act of armed violence involves asking:

1. What is the effect or effects that could be reduced or eliminated?

Bearing in mind that all four determinants must be present in some way, four other questions follow:

2. In what way were the victims vulnerable?
3. How many potential users of the weapon or weapons were so armed or how many weapons were put into use?
4. What was the potential of the weapon or weapons to cause the effect or effects?

Given the answers to questions 1 through 4:

5. What conclusions can be drawn or further questions asked about:
   - preventing or limiting the effects
   - the context in which the weapon or weapons are, were, or would be used
   - the intent of the user or users of the weapon
   - what law might apply

Application of the Framework for Use of Explosive Weapons in a Populated Area

Civilian injuries in a populated area under bombardment always generate headline news. The hospital images usually are heart rending, especially as the context may have rendered the hospital nonfunctional. Media analysis revolves around whether the act of bombardment intentionally targeted civilians or whether the target was a legitimate military objective. The bombardment may be described as "heavy" and the area covered by explosive force seems to be an issue only if cluster bombs are used. Targeting errors are "regrettable." The fact that there is an emotional and "moral" distance brought by these weapons forces recognition of an important nexus between the technology, intent, and law.[16,25–28] How these factors interact to generate civilian deaths and injuries is never reported. In brief, one never sees or hears a public health expert on the news explaining this particular "epidemic" of ballistic trauma; this is in stark contrast to infectious diseases.

If we apply the above analytical framework, the effect we are concerned about (and should not lose sight of) is the number of civilians killed or injured. This framework, by placing reduction or prevention of a particular effect foremost, forces us to think beyond the political or strategic situation and beyond whether the combatants have violated international humanitarian law or whether the wounded receive adequate surgical care in hospital.

It is not necessary to go through the steps formally answering questions 1 to 5 above before identifying preventive measures. However, specific questions become obvious.

What contributes to the civilians' vulnerability?
Do they have access to shelters? (If not, could they have such access?)
How vulnerable are they if they stay in their homes given the weapons being used?
Are they injured by flying glass as the windows in their homes are shattered? (If so, distribution of adhesive plastic sheeting may reduce injuries while resolution of the conflict is negotiated.)
Are they injured in bread queues or at water-distribution points? (If so, the distribution of these vital commodities could be changed in time or space so as to reduce the number people waiting in an exposed location.)

Two legal questions relate to the interaction of law and vulnerability.

Has the civilian population been warned of the likelihood of an attack?[29] (If so, they may be instructed about where to go during a bombardment.)
Have military objectives been placed in close proximity to civilians?[30] (If so, they should be removed.)

Legal questions relating to the interaction of the psychological aspects of violence, the kind of weapons used, and the number of weapons used also become apparent. In terms of choice of weapon or the number with which they are delivered, does the attack represent an "indiscriminate attack"[31] and have "all feasible precautions" been taken to avoid civilian deaths and injuries?[32]

Asking questions such as these has led the International Committee of the Red Cross (ICRC) to call for a prohibition of use of cluster bombs in populated areas beause of the difficulty of using these weapons in a manner that can discriminate between military target and civilians and civilian infrastructure.[33]

Have the inaccuracies in the use of weapons been taken into account? Any weapon that delivers explosive force has some degree of inaccuracy, whether due to user factors or the inherent technology of the weapon; obviously, the more weapons are used, the greater the number that will miss their target. When explosive force is used against military targets in populated areas, the number delivered is a strong predictor of unintended civilian deaths and injuries. Is using large numbers compatible with taking "all feasible precautions"?

When this form of armed violence is reported, these questions are not asked routinely in this way, and so responsibilities are not identified clearly and routinely. The same considerations of preventive factors might be a useful part of dialogue between a commander working under a United Nations mandate and two belligerent parties. Negotiating withdrawal of military objectives from a populated area may be linked to withdrawal of artillery to a certain distance, but withdrawal of artillery may *increase* the potential for civilian deaths and injuries if the bombardment restarts from the new positions; inaccuracies are simply multiplied by distance. Likewise, moving a vulnerable population out of an area may only elevate their vulnerability in the short term; in order to avoid further civilian deaths and injuries, determinants of other categories must be reduced simultaneously, e.g., there must be a simultaneous cease fire.

The analytical framwork has thrown light on some of the determinants of unintended civilian deaths and injuries. They are: use of explosive weapons in large numbers against military objectives and in populated areas where civilians have limited means to reduce their vulnerability. Preventive measures have been revealed by considering how these determinants interact. Logic tells us that these determinants, if quantified, could also serve as predictors.

Massacres, Enforced Disappearances, and Missing People

Reports of massacres or discoveries of mass graves are all too common. There are no reports of weapons that, when used in combat, produce the effect of total or near-total mortality among those wounded.[34,35] Therefore, when there is a situation of a certain number killed by firearms and no wounded (and the world's attention is focused on who is going to point the finger of blame at the presumed perpetrators of the massacre), reference to the above framework immediately reveals that the victims must have been brought to an exceptionally high degree of vulnerability. They must have been disarmed, wounded, arrested, tied up, or confined in some way.[35] The explanation usually given is that the victims were soldiers "killed in a battle" or civilians "caught in the crossfire." Political dialogue or media reporting simply could include an observation that such a number of dead people with comparatively few wounded or no wounded at all simply is not compatible with the explanation given.

However shocking the news of yet another massacre may be, when the bodies are hidden or cannot be identified, another layer of misery is superimposed; families may live in the agony of uncertainty for years. The issue of people who are reported missing as a result of armed conflict and internal violence is one of the world's most disturbing problems. The necessity of a multidisciplinary approach to people missing as a result of armed conflict or internal violence only became apparent in early 2003 at an international conference, where it was acknowledged that the problem required three tracks.[36]

First, ascertaining the fate of those who had been taken prisoner, abducted, tortured, or murdered in large numbers or who eventually vanished without trace. These investigations fall to the United Nations, human-rights groups, international criminal lawyers, and forensic specialists because the authorities who should conduct the investigation are often the perpetrators.

Second, assisting the families who suffered the mental torture of uncertainty about the fate of their relatives fell to family associations, health professionals, psychologists, social workers, nongovernmental organizations, and the Red Cross. Forensic specialists have a major part to play here through identification of the dead victims and returning their remains to the families for appropriate burial or cremation.

Third, preventing further acts that could lead to people going missing clearly involves politicians, military bodies, international lawyers, and diplomats. Prevention of this form of armed violence is of paramount importance. Health professionals have roles and responsibilites in relation to all three tracks.[37]

An unresolved or disputed issue of missing people can be a major obstruction to any peace process, a major political issue following a conflict, fuel for the next conflict, and a major constraint to transitional justice and the return to democracy. When information is manipulated for political reasons, as is frequently the case, it serves only to inflame the anxieties and indignation of the families and affected commnities.

In relation to this chapter, those who are missing or who disappear and who suffer in ways that defy imagination ultimately have ballistic trauma inflicted upon them or have been coerced, abducted, or arrested by threat of ballistic trauma. The litmus test of the potential usefulness of the presented analytical framework is examining whether in applying it to the missing and disappeared, it indicates useful preventive measures. It is the litmus test because the people most likely responsible are those authorities who are least likely to listen to a preventive argument; consequently, they are unlikely to change their policies or admit that those under their command are responsible for violations of international humanitarian law or human-rights law.

A first step involves understanding the phenomenon. The analytical framework can be applied to the act or acts necessary to make people disappear systematically—that is, to arrest them, to interrogate and torture them, and then to kill them in a way and in a place that makes finding their bodies difficult or impossible. The potentially measurable effects of armed violence that could be considered are multiple. Some examples are the number of arbitrary arrests in a given time or given area; the number of families deprived of the male of the household; number of prisoners executed; and, obviously, the number of people arrested and who subsequently have not been seen or heard of.

The victims' vulnerability comes from being a civilian, unarmed, arrested, bound, or blindfolded. The physical potential to cause these effects come from the wounding potential of firearms and the fact that authorities can muster large number of armed people. Obviously, the physical potential is much greater if assault rifles are used as opposed to handguns. Considering the interaction of the physical potential for this form of armed violence and the vulnerabilities is the key to understanding how the violence can be planned only at a high level. To arrest a number of people, a certain number of armed people are needed. To execute the same number once they are confined or tied up requires many fewer because the arrested already are extremely vulnerable. Then to move and dispose of the bodies in a way that the chances of their being found are minimized must, by necessity, involve as few as people as possible. Therefore the arrested have to enter a system whereby their vulnerability is elevated systematically in a series of steps so permitting at each step the involvement of fewer and fewer people until the person is killed and the body disposed of. The stepwise escalation of vulnerability and the simultaneous stepwise reduction of people must be planned together to minimize the chances of the bodies being found at a later date.

None of this is astonishing, nor does it obviously throw up realistic preventive strategies. Those responsible usually are immune to or are supposedly enforcers of the domestic laws of the country concerned. But analyzing the armed violence required to make people disappear in large numbers shows that organization is a prerequisite and refutes in a generic way and without direct accusation that such disappearances cannot be due only to excessive use of force by a few police or members of armed forces; it shows that a system is required that must involve people highly placed in the military and most likely the government as well. A leader or commander cannot easily claim ignorance given this analysis. Preventing such disappearances by changing the behavior of the authorities should therefore be achievable by diplomatic pressure and sanctions. If the situation is extreme, use of force may be necessary to change the authorities.[38]

Data in relation to massacres, extrajudicial killings, and disappearances have been published and could be brought to bear in a way that generates accountability.[35,39,40] As with unintended civilian injuries, this raises the question of whether there are predictors to which other agencies or governments could be sensitive to justify stronger diplomatic demarches or political actions at an earlier stage. Identifying predictors might enable international actors to break at an early stage or even preclude the cycle of atrocity, resentment, hatred, and revenge attacks, thereby lessening the need for intervention with military force at a later stage. The predictors might include news reports of a certain number of arbitrary arrests per month, training of police in military tactics, equipping regular police with military assault rifles, military rule, and a large proportion of the population living in poverty. Common sense tells us these are all ingredients, but there is, as yet, no indication of their relative importance in relation to the recipe for a high-risk situation.

Ballistic Trauma and Humanity

Most international news reports refer to acts of armed violence, threats of armed violence, effects of armed violence, agreements that restrain the capacity for armed violence, or means of inflicting armed violence. Most of the armed violence reported employs weapons that inflict ballistic trauma on their victims. It is obvious that armed violence and the trauma that results from it are very much in our collective conscience and determine how international affairs are played out.

Anthropologists and historians argue that human cultures and a world built on the notion of the nation state are born of acts of armed violence, the capacity to inflict armed violence, and agreements that restrain this capacity.[41,42] In other words, armed violence resulting in ballistic trauma has always carried a fundamental importance for human existence because the basis of group defence or law enforcement is ultimately about how individuals or groups apply force to or threaten each other. This is why most societies recognize that certain members should carry weapons legitimately. While this baseline view of militarism and law enforcement by police may appear simplistic, it is safe to say that ballistic trauma and its prevention are somehow profoundly implicated in how all humans live and interact.

When the term "humanity" is used, it is used interchangeably between two meanings. One refers to the collective existence of all humans; the other implies an attitude, morality, or sentiment of good will towards fellow humans.[43,44] The links between the management of ballistic trauma and humanity would at first glance appear to confined to assisting victims of war in the spirit of humanity (the first principle of the International Red Cross and Red Crescent Movement). Looking beyond this may appear the equivalent of asking how many angels can dance on the head of a pin; however, it is worth considering both meanings of humanity in terms of the title of both this book and this chapter for three reasons. First, the importance in human existence of armed violence that results or would result in ballistic trauma has been alluded to above; this importance pertains to humanity in the first sense, that is, of collective existence of all humans. Second, humanity in the second sense, that is, the sentiment, becomes more concrete if considered as the converse of inhumanity, and there are few, if any, acts of inhumanity that do not ultimately involve use of, threat of, or coercion by armed violence that results or would result in ballistic trauma. The definition of "crimes against humanity" serve as evidence.[17] Third, humanity—in both senses—is cited as a source of or even a prerequisite for international law.[45,46] In brief, notions of humanity imply not only ameliorating the effects of armed violence, but also restraining the capacity for armed violence; these notions, together with ballistic trauma and international law, are therefore profoundly linked in our collective existence.

Conclusion

Armed violence resulting in ballistic trauma should be considered for what it is—a global health issue. A public health approach to prevention is possible using an analytical framework that takes into account the determinants of the effects of armed violence. In the examples given, certain determinants of the effects of armed violence are identified and the importance of understanding how these determinants interact becomes apparent. This begs the question of whether quantification of the relative importance of the determinants could permit prediction. Prediction could lead to preventive policies in the longer term.

Our existence has been and continues to be dominated by armed violence that results in ballistic trauma, the capacity for this violence, and the means to restrain it. It seems likely that our future will continue to be likewise influenced. If the fundamental importance to humanity of armed violence resulting in ballistic trauma is recognized, referring to the presented analytical framework could have profound implications for how affairs are conducted in the international sphere and how international law, in particular, international humanitarian law, the United Nations Charter, the international law of arms control and disarmament, and human-rights law are developed and applied. Such assertions may seem far removed from the title of this book, but, at the end of the day, international law is a practical guide to the management of ballistic trauma writ large.

References

1. Sellier KG, Kneubuehl BP. *Wound Ballistics*. Amsterdam: Elsevier; 1994.
2. Kalshoven F, Zegveld L. *Constraints on the Waging of War*. Geneva: International Committee of the Red Cross; 2001.
3. Coupland R, Kneubuehl B, Rowley D, Bowyer G. Wound ballistics, surgery and the law of war. *Trauma*. 2000;2:1–10.
4. 1980 UN Convention on Prohibitions or Restrictions on the Use of Certain Conventional Weapons Which May be Deemed to be Excessively Injurious or to Have Indiscriminate Effects.
5. 1980 Protocol on Non-Detectable Fragments to the 1980 UN Convention on Conventional Weapons.
6. 1995 Protocol on Blinding Laser Weapons to the 1980 UN Convention on Conventional Weapons.
7. 1997 Ottawa Convention on the Prohibition of the Use, Stockpiling, Production and Transfer of Anti-Personnel Mines and on their Destruction.
8. Article 35.2 of 1977 Protocol I Additional to the 1949 Geneva Conventions.
9. Ogston A. Continental criticism of english rifle bullets. *Br Med J.* 1899;i:752–757.
10. Second Preparatory Committee for the Second Review Conference of the 1980 CCW. *Protocol on the Use of Small Calibre Arms Systems (Draft)*. UN Document CCW/CONF.II/PC.2/WP.2. 4 April 2001.
11. Coupland R, Loye D. The 1899 Hague Declaration concerning expanding bullets. *International Review of the Red Cross*. 2003;85:135–142.
12. World Medical Association 48th General Assembly. *Weapons and their Relation to Life and Health* [Statement]. 1996.
13. Meddings DR. Weapons injuries during and after periods of conflict: retrospective analysis. *Br Med J.* 1997;315:1417–1420.
14. International Committee of the Red Cross. *Arms Availability and the Situation of Civilians in Armed Conflict*. Geneva: International Committee of the Red Cross; 1999.
15. Meddings DR, O'Connor SM. Circumstances around weapon injury in Cambodia after departure of a peacekeeping force: Prospective cohort study. *Br Med J*. 1999;319:412–415.
16. Coupland RM, Samnegaard HO. Effect of type and transfer of conventional weapons on civilian injuries: Retrospective analysis of prospective data from Red Cross hospitals. *Br Med J.* 1999;319:410–412.
17. Articles 5–8 of the 1998 Rome Statute of the International Criminal Court.
18. Meddings DR. Are most casualties non-combatants? *Br Med J.* 1998;317:1249–1250.
19. Meddings D. Civilians and war: A review and historical overview of the involvement of non-combatant populations in conflict situations. *Med Confl Surviv.* 2001;17:6–16.
20. Krug E, Dahlberg L, Mercy J, Zwi A, Lozano R. (eds.). *World Report on Violence and Health*. Geneva: World Health Organization; 2002:213–239.

21. Moseley W, Chen L. An analytic framework for the study of child survival in developing countries. *Popul Dev Rev*. 1986;10(suppl):25–45.
22. Coupland R. Armed violence. *Med Global Surviv*. 2001;7:33–37.
23. Coupland R. The effects of weapons on health. *Lancet*. 1996;347:450–451.
24. Coupland R. The effects of weapons and the Solferino Cycle. *Br Med J*. 1999;319:864–865.
25. Grossman D. *On Killing: The Psychological Cost of Learning to Kill in War and Society*. Boston, MA: Little Brown and Co.; 1995:97–137.
26. Glover J. Humanity: A Moral History of the Twentieth Century. London: Jonathon Cape; 1999:64–88.
27. Rogers A. Zero-casualty warfare. *Int Rev Red Cross*. 2000;82:165–182.
28. Carlino M. The moral limits of strategic attack. *Parameters (US Army War Quarterly.)* Spring 2002:15–29.
29. Article 57.2c of Protocol I Additional to the 1949 Geneva Conventions.
30. Article 58 of Protocol I Additional to the 1949 Geneva Conventions.
31. Article 51.4 of Protocol I Additional to the 1949 Geneva Conventions.
32. Article 57.2a of Protocol I Additional to the 1949 Geneva Conventions.
33. International Committee of the Red Cross. *Cluster Bombs and Landmines in Kosovo*. Geneva: International Committee of the Red Cross; 2001.
34. Coupland RM. Epidemiological approach to the surgical management of the casualties of war. *Br Med J*. 1994;308:1693–1697.
35. Coupland RM, Meddings DR. Mortality associated with use of weapons in armed conflict, wartime atrocities, and civilian mass shootings: Literature review. *Br Med J*. 1999;319:407–410.
36. International Committee of the Red Cross. *The Missing*. Available at: http://www.icrc.org/eng. Accessed April 2003.
37. Coupland R, Cordner S. People missing as a result of armed conflict. *Br Med J*. 2003;326:943–944.
38. International Commission on Intervention and State Sovereignty. *The Responsibility to Protect*. Ottawa, Ontario, Canada: International Development Research Center; 2001.
39. Chevigny P. Police deadly force as social control: Jamaica, Argentina and Brazil. *Criminal Law Forum*. 1990:1;389–425.
40. Spiegel PB, Salama P. War and mortality in Kosovo, 1998–99: An epidemiological testimony. *Lancet*. 2000;355:2204–2209.
41. Keegan J. A history of warfare. London: Pimlico; 1994:386–393.
42. Chagnon NA. Life histories, blood revenge and warfare in a tribal population. *Science*. 1988;239:985–992.
43. Pictet J. *Red Cross Principles*. Geneva: The International Committee of the Red Cross; 1956:14–31.
44. Pictet J. *Development and Principles of International Humanitarian Law*. Dordrecht, Martinus Nijhoff: Henry Dunant Institute; 1983:5
45. Brownlie I. *Principles of Public International Law*. Oxford: Clarendon Press; 1998:28.
46. Coupland R. Humanity, what is it and how does it influence international law? *Int Rev Red Cross*. 2001:83;969–989.

Section 2
Clinical Care

Introduction

This section will concentrate on clinical care. Hospital-based practitioners are used to having casualties presented to them by prehospital staff. It is important that they understand what has gone on in the prehospital arena and how this has influenced the care the casualty has received.

The initial chapters on resuscitation, anesthesia, and clinical ballistics give general outlines for clinical care of the ballistic casualty.

Specific issues are then addressed in more detail in the chapters looking at particular body regions.

Finally, there is a review of how to train surgeons to manage ballistic trauma—a pressing problem where medical training is geared towards producing specialists rather than generalists.

7
Prehospital Care

MARK BYERS and PETER F. MAHONEY

Introduction

Prehospital care of the ballistic casualty should be considered as two intertwined areas:

1. Management of the situation.
2. Management of the casualty.

Managing the situation involves understanding what is happening at the ballistic incident, who is in charge, the medic's role within this situation, and what medical advice and actions are appropriate.

Managing the injured casualty consists of first aid and advanced care *appropriate to the situation.*

The Situation: Three Environments of Care

Medics who attend ballistic trauma will find themselves providing care in one of three environments: non-permissive, semipermissive, and permissive. This also has been described as Care Under Fire, Tactical Field Care, and Combat Casualty Evacuation Care.[1,2]

The Non-Permissive Environment: Care Under Fire

This may occur when a tactically trained medic or medically trained member of an assault team is providing care. A non-permissive environment implies that either the medic or the casualty is under a direct threat. The risks may range from being inside a dangerous structure to being present during a shooting and under fire. It is not a place in which to deliver medical care. The aim is to extract the casualty in any way practicable without the medic becoming a casualty.

The Semi-permissive Environment: Tactical Field Care

This environment is not safe, but the direct threat is removed (albeit probably temporarily). Casualty and rescuer might be behind cover, but there is no guarantee the potential assailant or threat will not move and threaten them again.

The Permissive Environment: Combat Casualty Evacuation Care

A permissive environment is a safe environment. In this area the medic should be highly visible and have access to the full range of equipment and resources carried by any prehospital-care practitioner. This does not mean that the medic should delay the casualty's move to hospital.

All three environments will exist around an incident and also can be related to areas of operational control (see Figure 7-1).

Care in these environments is considered later in the chapter.

Unprotected and untrained staff should not enter the inner cordon, which should be controlled by the police or military.

The Prehospital Environment

Preparation

Preparing for the prehospital environment begins long before the call out.

Prehospital medical practitioners require proper training, the correct clothing and equipment, and an understanding of the environment in which they are working.

Training

The type and level of training required depends on where you are working, for whom you are working, and why you are working there. An individual responding as part of civilian Emergency Medical Service (EMS) has different requirements to the medic working with a military group or police firearms team. A progressive training path is given in Appendix 7-3.

Clothing

Dress with safety in mind—either to be seen or not to be seen, depending on the setting. Prehospital-care practitioners providing care in a permissive location should wear high-visibility clothing, jackets or tabards, trousers or

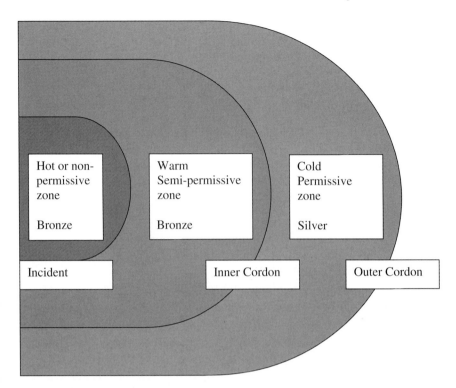

| Hot or non-permissive zone | Warm Semi-permissive zone | Cold Permissive zone |
| Bronze | Bronze | Silver |

| Incident | Inner Cordon | Outer Cordon |

FIGURE 7-1. Zones of care. The non-permissive, semi-permissive, and permissive environments respectively translate to the so called Hot, Warm, and Cold zones around an incident. There is an approximate correlation with the command zones described in the Major Incident Medical Management and Support (MIMMS) course and manual (see ref. 3 and Appendix 7.3). Bronze describes tactical command at an incident and silver describes operational command. Gold or strategic command is some way distant to the incident. Bronze of MIMMS equates approximately to the Hot (non permissive) and Warm (semi permissive) zones, the areas inside the inner cordon. Silver of MIMMS equates to the Cold (permissive) zone between the inner and outer cordons. The permissive zone beyond the outer cordon is within the Gold area.

coveralls, and a helmet that is sufficiently robust and meets the safety specification for the job. The clothing also should conform to the dress codes of the organization being represented. Clothing should be marked clearly with the name and position/specialty of the practitioner, and at night, they should have reflectors and a torch, preferably a head torch. Guidance for BASICS (British Association for Immediate Care) Doctors on prehospital clothing can be found on the BASICS website (http://www.basics.org.uk).

Practitioners in the tactical environment should wear the same protective clothing as the tactical team. This should include, as a minimum, ballistic body armor and a ballistic helmet. This equipment is heavy and unwieldy, and practice is required to operate efficiently in it. Ballistic protection is considered in Chapter 4.

Medical Equipment

This should be adequate for the task, but this needs to be balanced against the necessity to carry it. The practitioner working in a safe area has far more latitude than the practitioner working within a safety cordon. The tactical medic must balance utility with load and should carry as little as possible packed as small as possible. Suggested packing lists can be found in Appendix 7.2.

The Prehospital Environment

Practice

The ballistic incident may range from an accident at a rural shooting ground to a siege and hostage situation. Each situation presents its own problems. What follows is a generic approach that can be adapted to circumstances.

Arriving at the Scene

On receipt of a request to attend an incident involving firearms, it is important to consider:

- *who* has made the request;
- who is in charge of the situation (usually police) If there is no police presence at the scene, it is prudent to confirm they will be attending.
- *where* you are to report [the incident control point (ICP)];
- the *type* of incident;
- routes in and out;
- the numbers of casualties involved;
- who else is attending.

The acronym METHANE (see Table 7-1) developed and taught by the Advanced Life Support Group (ALSG) in their Major Incident Medical Management and Support course[3] can be adapted to help remember the information that is required and provides a format for sending a situation report or reporting an incident. Major Incident Medical Management and Support is used by the UK military and is also being taught by a number of North Atlantic Treaty Organization (NATO) armies (T.J. Hodgetts, personal communication, November 2003).

Table 7-1. METHANE report.

From MIMMS Manual BMJ Books 2002.
With permission of BMJ and Prof TJ Hodgetts

M—My name or name of person requesting assistance
E—Exact location of the incident
T—Type of incident
H—Hazards affecting the incident
A—Access routes to the Incident Control Point
N—Numbers of casualties and severity
E—Emergency services involved or required.

For a simple accident, it may just be a case of being taken to the casualty, ensuring scene safety (such as confirming where the weapon involved is), giving appropriate care, and arranging evacuation to hospital.

A more complex situation may require:

- a clear statement of your tasks;
- the commander's concept of how the operation will progress;
- current intelligence and any information on the numbers and locations of the threat;
- numbers of casualties, locations, and routes to and from them;
- other agencies present, such as police, fire, ambulance, and military;
- clothing and equipment required;
- who is escorting you around the incident;
- the location of support services in the event of a long operation (such as catering);
- signal commands being employed.

Finally, watches should be synchronized to the same time as the commanders (see Appendix 7.1).

Scene Assessment

The first rule of any prehospital-care incident is safety. This includes safety of the medic, other members of the emergency services, of the public, of the casualty, and of the scene. Every year, prehospital-care providers are injured or killed in both the civilian and military environments because of failing to follow this rule.

Prior to voluntarily entering the scene, the practitioner should understand the level of risk. If a casualty is seen to be lying on the ground, is it safe to approach? If the environment is non-permissive, then a value judgement should be made. The situation will not improve if the rescuer becomes a casualty. A casualty who has suffered a high-velocity head wound is unlikely to survive regardless of the level of care provided, and if the perpetrator were still at large, it would be foolhardy to enter the area. It may be possible to assess the casualty from a safe place, construct a secure approach, and ensure a successful outcome. Do not rush into an incident until after a proper assessment of risk has been made and heed advice from the experts.

Non-permissive Environment

Treatment

This should be rapid and simple:

A. consider turning the casualty to a recovery position or similar to prevent airway obstruction. Cervical spine (C spine) control is not going to be achieved in these circumstances.
C. hemorrhage control by direct pressure or tourniquets.

Extract the casualty by whatever means is possible. This may mean physically dragging the casualty to cover.

ABC or CAB?

ABC is "airway, breathing, and circulation", the accepted Advanced Trauma Life Support/Battlefield Advanced Trauma Life Support (ATLS/BATLS) approach to trauma management.[4,5] CAB stands for "Catastrophic hemorrhage, Airway, and Breathing."

Potential survivors are most at risk of bleeding to death. "Catastrophic hemorrhage, Airway, and Breathing" requires one to deal rapidly with catastrophic or massive hemorrhage by applying pressure to the bleeding point (by kneeling on the wound or the application of a tourniquet) and then move onto airway care. A casualty with non-compressible hemorrhage needs surgical intervention and only the management of *life-threatening* airway and breathing problems should delay their transfer to surgery.

Semi-permissive Environment

Treatment

Within tactical medical care, this is likely to be working within the police cordon. If the medic has to go forward into this area, an escort should be provided. The medic should be protected at all times while within the cordon by a suitably trained member of the incident team. This is most likely to be a police officer trained in the use of firearms. The officers' role is not to act as a drip stand or extra pair of hands, but to provide security.

The focus remains on getting the medic and casualty to safety, but if time is available, further care can be carried out:

A. management of the airway using simple maneuvers and adjuncts such as nasopharyngeal airways. C spine control may be appropriate in a blunt injury, but not in a penetrating injury (see below);

B. Asherman Chest Seals™ if access to a sucking chest wound is possible; Possibly needle decompression of a tension pneumothorax (very difficult to assess in this location)

C. continued hemorrhage control (dressings and tourniquets).
Extracting the casualty: depends on potential threat. If the situation is volatile, then rapid extraction is needed.

Cervical Spine Control?

Cervical spine immobilization is employed in the management of the blunt trauma casualty where clinical signs, symptoms, or the mechanism of injury lead one to suspect biomechanical instability in the cervical spine. The concern is that further movement will cause or aggravate a spinal cord injury.

In penetrating trauma, this approach has been reviewed for a number of reasons:

- Ballistic injury to the cervical spine has a very high fatality rate. Much of this is due to adjacent vascular structures being disrupted. Such wounds may or may not involve the spinal cord.[6]
- In the survivor, these wounds generally are accepted to be stable (see Chapter 16) and moving the casualty is unlikely to cause neurological injury.
- Placing collars and other immobilization devices in a non-permissive environment will have minimal benefit, cause evacuation delays, and the delays may endanger both casualty and rescuer.[5,7]
- A cervical collar may obscure developing life-threatening injuries such as a developing hematoma in the neck that can compromise the airway.[8]

In the military environment, c spine immobilization for penetrating injury to the neck is not advocated.

Where a penetrating injury has occurred along side a blunt injury (e.g., casualty shot in neck and falls off a roof), then immobilization is carried out for the blunt injury unless to do so would endanger both the casualty and the rescuer.

Permissive Environment

The practitioner can perform the assessments and treatments *appropriate to the casualty's condition*, as will be discussed below. The aim is not to delay definitive hospital treatment.

The decisions that need to be made are how quickly can the patient be transferred safely and by what means can this be achieved?

– *Do nothing at the scene that cannot be carried out safely in transit, and*
– *do nothing in transit that would not be better carried out in a hospital.*

Ballistic trauma is still relatively uncommon in most parts of the UK so it is important to guard against becoming overawed by the injury or the situation.

Do Not Forget the ABCs

ASSESS

A. Is the airway clear? If not, what must be done to secure it? Will a simple adjunct be sufficient, or must the patient have a definitive airway (surgical or endotracheal) to allow transfer?

B. What is required to improve respiration? Can any defect be closed with an Asherman Chest Seal™? Does the patient now need chest drainage, or will a needle thoracostomy do? How much oxygen is available? Is evacuation by helicopter or other aircraft? Does this influence my decision on chest drainage?

C. Has all compressible hemorrhage been secured? Is there uncompressible hemorrhage that needs the attention of a surgeon? Does the patient now need intravenous (IV) access, or can it be secured in transit? Does the patient need fluids, and if so, is hypovolemic or normotensive resuscitation appropriate? (Fluid resuscitation is considered further in Chapter 8)

D. What neurological assessment of the patient is required? Does the patient need a Glasgow Coma Score (GCS) or is an AVPU Score sufficient? AVPU means "is the casualty **A**lert or responding to **V**oice or only responding **P**ain or **U**nresponsive? Is the patient's airway at risk because of neurological trauma and a decreased consciousness level?

E. Does the patient have any extremity trauma? Does the casualty need limb splintage or pelvic compression straps to improve survival? Can the patient be stabilized on the stretcher and evacuated, or is a traction splint needed first?

A secondary survey rarely is required in prehospital care unless time and location dictate it and it usually is achieved better in hospital.

Multiple Casualties

Triage of multiple casualties is considered in Chapter 26.

Evacuation and The Chain of Care

The prehospital practitioner should not see him or herself as acting in isolation, but as part of a team whose aim is to return the casualty to health. The aim is to do what is appropriate at each level to ensure safe movement onto the next, but not to perform procedures that are better done further down the chain of care.

Within the UK military environment this is described as "roles." Role 1 is care under the direction of a doctor (such as a Regimental Aid Post), Role 3 provides hospital-level care, and Role 4 is definitive care, usually provided away from the conflict, (e.g., the NHS and associated military facilities). Role 2 provides the link between Roles 1 and 3. A Role 2 facility with surgical teams attached is described as "Role 2+".[9]

Monitoring should be employed prior to or during evacuation. The minimal level of monitoring is a fully trained medic looking after the patient and who is capable of dealing with any unexpected emergencies that may occur.

The use of electronic monitors for pulse oximetry, electrocardiogram (ECG), and blood pressure will be dictated by availability and the situation. Prehospital monitoring used by London Helicopter Emergency Medical Service (HEMS) has been described by Morley.[10]

Packaging and Transfer

The default transport is a properly equipped and crewed emergency ambulance providing a rapid move to a suitable hospital.

At shooting incidents, military, police, and medical helicopters may be in attendance. When used correctly, helicopters can provide a rapid move to hospital, but a number of factors need to be considered.

An Emergency Air Ambulance or a police helicopter with dual police and ambulance tasking should be suitably crewed and equipped to care for and transport casualties. A police helicopter operating only in the police role or military helicopter not configured for casevac are unlikely to have the appropriate crew and equipment. That is not to say they cannot be used effectively if crew and equipment can be carried by them.

Not all hospitals have a helicopter landing site (HLS). Of those that do, few are suitable for night operations in the UK. A significant number are some distance away from the emergency department, and an additional ambulance journey may be required from the HLS to the hospital.

The Crime Scene

It is nearly always inevitable that, unless at war, a ballistic incident will be a crime scene. This will often apply in peace support and "post conflict" military operations. This has implications for the medic.

If the incident is to be investigated, it is incumbent on all involved to contaminate the scene as little as possible. The practitioner should not interfere with the scene unless it is an unavoidable part of the treatment of a casualty. The dead should not be moved unless it is to gain access to the living. If they are moved, this must be recorded. Artifacts, weapons, and shell casings should not be moved. The death should be confirmed by a doctor in the presence of a police officer. The medical practitioner's movements and role within the incident need to be documented. At the end of the incident, nobody should leave the scene without the permission of the incident commander. Forensics is considered further in Chapter 5.

Summary

Ballistic trauma produces many problems for the prehospital practitioner. These are not just related to the injuries, but also to the hazards of the situation. Proper training, equipment, and clothing, coupled with an awareness of the dangers encountered and knowledge of how to act and react to the particular circumstances, should lead to the best possible outcome for the casualty and team. Understand the command structure of the incident, the roles and responsibilities of all involved, and the need of the police to investigate the scene. It is not a situation for the amateur, but for a committed and experienced individual who is properly trained. If such an incident is encountered unexpectedly then remember safety, situational awareness and risk assessment. Clinically do simple procedures well followed by timely transfer of the casualty to an appropriate hospital. Above all else remember individual safety.

Aide Memoire

Be prepared.
Be familiar with equipment. Keep equipment up to date.
Train regularly with supported service.
Receive METHANE report.
Arrive Safely.
Receive orders.
Non-permissive care: Clear airway. Control Hemorrhage. CAB.
Semi-permissive care: Minimal care consistent with safety. Transfer as soon as possible.
Permissive care: All you need to, nothing you do not.
Rapid package and transfer by the most appropriate means.

References

1. Butler FK, Hagmann J, Butler E. Tactical combat casualty care in special operations. *Mil Med*. 1996;161(suppl 3):3–16.
2. De Lorenzo RA, Porter RS. *Tactical Emergency Care: Military and Operational Out of Hospital Medicine*. Upper Saddle River, NJ: Brady Prentice Hall; 1999.

3. Advanced Life Support Group. *Major Incident Medical Management and Support*. 2nd ed. London: BMJ Books: 2002.
4. American College of Surgeons Committee on Trauma. Advanced Trauma Life Support Student Course Manual. 6th ed. Chicago, IL; 1997.
5. Battlefield Advanced Trauma Life Support. 2nd ed. 2000. D/AMD/113/23. AC No 63726. Available from: Defense Storage and Distribution Center, Mwrwg Road, Llangennech, Llanelli, Carmathenshire SA14 8YP.
6. Bellamy RF. The nature of combat injuries and the role of ATLS in their management. In: *Combat Casualty Care Guidelines: Operation Desert Storm*. Washington DC: Office of the Surgeon General, Center of Excellence, Walter Reed Army Medical Center; February 1991.
7. Holcolmb J, Mabry R. Trauma: Primary and secondary survey. In: Whitlock WL, (chief ed.) *Special Operations Forces Medical Handbook*. Jackson, Wyoming: Teton NewMedia; 2001:7-1–7-5.
8. Barkana Y, Stein M, Scope A, Major R, Abramovich Y, Friedman Z, Knoller N. Prehospital stabilisation of the cervical spine for penetrating injuries of the neck- is it necessary? *Injury*. 2000;31:305–309.
9. *The Organisation of Medical Support in Army Medical Services Core Doctrine. Principles*. 2000, Crown Copyright.
10. Morley AP. Prehospital monitoring of trauma patients: Experience of a helicopter emergency medical service. *Br J Anaesthesia*. 1996;76:726–730.

Further Reading

Prehospital Care
1. Greaves I, Porter K, eds. *Pre-hospital medicine. The principles and practice of immediate care*. London: Arnold; 1999. ISBN 0340676566.

Field and Tactical Medical Care
2. McDevitt I. *Tactical Medicine: An Introduction to Law Enforcement Emergency Care*. Boulder, CO: Paladin Press; 2001. ISBN 1 581602553.
3. *Care in the Field for Victims of Weapons of War*. ICRC 2001. Available at: http://www.icrc.org.
4. Husum H, Gilbert M, Wisborg T. Save Lives, Save Limbs. Life Support for Victims of Mines, Wars and Accidents. Penang: Third World Network: 2000. ISBN 983 9747428.

Appendix 7.1. Orders Process

The orders process: Information required by you or those working for you.

Ground Brief—a short description of the ground/terrain/environment in which you will be working.
Situation Report—Up-to-date information on what is happening, including the threat, casualties, and supporting assets.
Task—Your task specifically.
Execution of the Task—The commanders' concept of the operation, his intentions and plan, and your role within it. In addition, details of all the tasks delegated to individuals in the team and their place in the overall

plan. Finally, coordinating instructions, including timings, movement, and routes to be used.

Support Information—Dress and equipment. The location and arrangements of facilities available for feeding, washing, sleeping, and personal hygiene during the task.

Signals and Commands—Pre-arranged signals, their meanings, and the command structure.

The Time—Synchronize your watch with the commanders.

Appendix 7.2. Suggested Packing Lists

Tactical Care Provider: All you need and nothing you don't	Pre-hospital Care Provider: All you need (if you can carry and work with it).
Rucksack (small) Tactical Medical Vest (a waistcoat with multiple equipment pouches)	Rucksack (large)
Airway 1. Oro/naso-pharyngeal airway 2. Surgical airway kit	**Airway** (with C spine control if needed 1. Oro/naso-pharyngeal airways 2. Surgical airway kit 3. Self Inflating Bag-Valve-Mask set 4. Advanced airway equipment eg: *Laryngeal Mask, Laryngoscope, Endo-Tracheal Tubes, End-tidal CO2 detector.* 5. Cervical Collars
Breathing: 1. Asherman Chest Seals™ 2. Large bore cannulae	**Breathing:** 1. Asherman Chest Seals™, 2. Large bore cannulae 3. Field Chest Drainage sets.
Circulation: 1. Tourniquets 2. Dressings-Roller bandages, Field Dressings	**Circulation:** 1. Tourniquets 2. Dressings: Roller bandages, Field Dressings 3. Triangular bandages 4. Tape 5. Intravenous cannulae

	6. Intravenous fluids and giving sets 7. pressure infuser 8. Interosseus access and infusion kits
Drugs 1. Opiate analgesic 2. Antiemetic	**Drugs** 1. Opiate analgesic 2. Antiemetic 3. Benzodiazepine 4. Primary care medications **Diagnostic**: 1. Stethoscope, 2. sphygmomanometer, 3. Torch, 4. Blood sugar testing set, 5. Ophthalmoscope, 6. Auroscope.
Dress: tactical: as per group being supported **Torch if tactically appropriate**	**Dress**: Helmet, High Visibility Jacket, over trousers, Safety Boots, Torch
	Paed Kit: Paediatric aidememoires, triage tapes and trauma kit
Packaging: straps, splints and stretchers to assist drag and rapid removal of casualty	**Packaging** (depending on nature of injury-blunt or penetrating) Spinal boards Head blocks Splints Extrication kit
Administration: Triage Cards Chem. lights (Multiple colours)	**Administration**: Triage cards, paperwork, reference manuals

Appendix 7.3. Training

a. *Basic first aid*. Basic first aid as taught by British Red Cross, St. John Ambulance, and the Military gives the tools for initial casualty care with minimal resources. Basic first-aid courses can be accessed from local Red Cross and St. John training organizations.

b. *Specific prehospital training*. Progressive training and qualification in prehospital care is offered and overseen in the UK by the Faculty of Prehospital Care at the Royal College of Surgeons (RCS) of Edinburgh.

Training is delivered by organizations such as BASICS Education Ltd. An initial qualification is the RCS's Pre-Hospital Emergency Care Certificate. After this comes the Diploma in Immediate Medical Care (Dip IMC) and the Fellowship in Immediate Medical Care (FIMC). *Contact:* Faculty of Pre-Hospital Care, The Royal College of Surgeons of Edinburgh, Nicolson Street, Edinburgh EH8 9DW; e-mail: prehosp@rcsed.ac.uk; BASICS Education Ltd., Turret House, Turret Lane, Ipswich IP4 1DL; e-mail: educ@basics.org.uk.

c. For Major Incident Management Training: Major Incident Medical Management and Support Course (MIMMS). *Details from:* Advanced Life Support Group, http://www.alsg.org.

d. For working within the military environment, clinical courses such as Battlefield Advanced Trauma Life Support (BATLS) and Battlefield Advanced Resuscitation Training (BARTS) have been developed. These usually are offered only to the military, but the training manual *Battlefield Advanced Trauma Life Support* (2nd Edn 2000), D/AMD/113/23. AC No 63726 can be obtained from: Defense Storage and Distribution Center, Mwrwg Road, Llangennech, Llanelli, Carmathenshire SA14 8YP.

e. *Additional Training.* Additional tactical and field training is needed for individuals providing close medical support to police and military organizations. This needs to be geared around the likely operating environments of these organizations.

8
Resuscitation and Anesthesia for the Ballistic Casualty

PAUL R. WOOD, ADAM J. BROOKS, and PETER F. MAHONEY

Introduction

The first part of this chapter focuses on the assessment and resuscitation of the ballistic casualty. The second part discusses the anesthetic considerations required for these patients.

Resuscitation

Preparation

Medical facilities in all locations—urban, rural, or austere—need to prepare to receive casualties well before they arrive. In a civilian hospital, this is likely to involve activating the trauma team and notifying other key personnel. In a military field hospital, this preparation will include putting a system in place to remove safely the casualty's weapons and ammunition (Figure 8-1).

Casualties exposed to chemicals or other noxious agents will need decontamination before entering the hospital.

Trauma Teams

The trauma team needs to be briefed with any prehospital information that is available. The objectives of the trauma team are to identify, assess, and treat life-threatening injuries. The running of the team is aided by an effective and organized team leader and clear allocation of tasks and roles to the team members in advance of the casualty arriving.

Driscoll[1,2] demonstrated the advantage of a trauma team approach with horizontal organization. These works showed that there is improved efficiency of the resuscitation and a reduction in the time taken for the casualty to receive definitive care when tasks are carried out simultaneously by the team members.

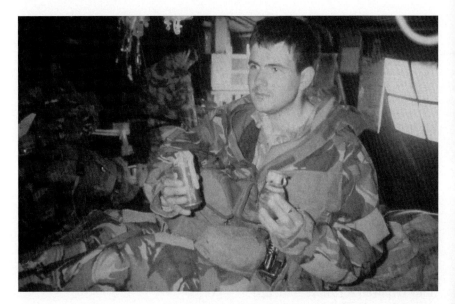

FIGURE 8-1. During one of many training exercises in the 1990–1991 Gulf War, troops were used as exercise casualties to test the hospital. This soldier had arrived in the resuscitation department with his hand grenades still on his person.

The ideal size of the team has not been defined, but is probably between 6 and 10 team members, including doctors, nursing staff, and a radiographer.

Team Activation

A hospital receiving trauma needs to define what criteria will initiate trauma team activation. These can be based on a combination of history, vital signs, or injuries. Many systems build a substantial overtriage into the system to prevent serious injuries being missed (Table 8-1).

Most systems include any gunshot wound as an activation criteria. In field hospitals, this may be augmented to include blast- and mine-related injuries.

Clinical

The principles that guide resuscitation of the ballistic casualty are essentially those described in the Advanced Trauma Life Support/Battlefield Advanced Trauma Life Support (ATLS/BATLS) Courses. The following section will highlight the differences and peculiarities associated with resuscitation of ballistic injury.

TABLE 8-1. Trauma activation criteria

Airway compromise
Signs of pneumothorax
Saturations <90%
Pulse >120 or systolic blood pressure (BP) 90-millimeters
  mercury (Hg)
Unconscious > five minutes
An incident with five or more casualties
An incident involving fatality
High-speed motor-vehicle crash
Patient ejected from the vehicle
Knife wound to the groin and above
Any gunshot wound or blast or mine injury
Significant burns (Chapter 21)
Fall from >8 meters
Child with altered consciousness, capillary refill >3 secs, pulse
  >130
Child pedestrian or cyclist hit by a vehicle

Adapted from *Better Care for the Severely Injured*, Royal
College of Surgeons of England and British Orthopedic
Association, 2000.

Airway & Cervical Spine Control

Simple First

It is easy to become fixated on advanced airway procedures and forget
about simple ones. The primary issue is ensuring oxygenation of the casualty. The method will depend on the casualty's injuries, the skill of the caregiver, and the resources available (Figure 8-2).

There are a number of other airway issues that are associated with
ballistic trauma, especially where it involves the head and neck.

Collars

The issue of cervical spine immobilization for ballistic injury is considered
in Chapters 7 and 16.

In the ballistic casualty, the pragmatic approach is that cervical spine
immobilization should be undertaken in the presence of blunt injury and
combined blunt and penetrating injury, but not in penetrating ballistic
injury alone.

In the presence of a cervical collar, laryngoscopy becomes more difficult.
Criswell et al.[3] described a successful management plan:

i. An assistant provides manual in-line immobilization of the cervical
    spine.
ii. The equipment stabilizing the cervical spine is removed (in the case of
    collars, this may mean unfastened and opened rather than completely
    removed).

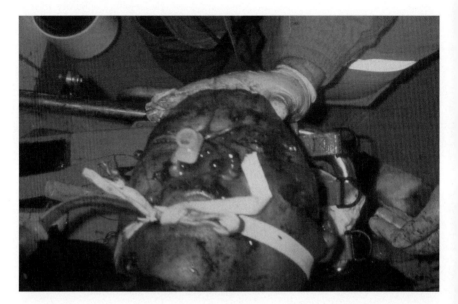

FIGURE 8-2. Gunshot Wound (GSW) face. This casualty had multiple GSW to the face and head (fired from both a 9-millimeter pistol and 7.62-millimeter AK 47). He was very agitated, with a decreased conscious level. The paramedic used a jaw thrust to attain an airway, then a nasopharyngeal tube to help maintain it. The hospital the paramedic went to refused the patient for economic and political reasons. A helicopter team was called, but they had to finish another job first. When they arrived, they anesthetized the casualty and performed endotracheal intubation. This was difficult, as the casualty had facial swelling and other damage from the bullets. The paramedic had successfully managed the casualty's airway for 2 hours using simple methods.

iii. The patient is preoxygenated (ideally 2 to 3 minutes, but this depends on their condition).
iv. A separate assistant applies cricoid pressure.
v. The patient receives anesthetic drugs and rapid-acting neuromuscular-blocking drugs.
vi. The patient's trachea is intubated, the endotracheal tube position is checked, and the tube is secured.
vii. The stabilizing devices are reapplied.

In this situation, management must include appropriate equipment and a rehearsed plan for dealing with a grade 2–3 laryngoscopy and failed intubation. A gum-elastic bougie and a small-diameter (uncut) endotracheal tube should be available.

Compression

Survivors of penetrating trauma to the neck are at risk of tracheal compression from hemorrhage. If this is suspected, and particularly if the patient is to be moved for computerized tomography (CT) or other imaging, the trachea should be intubated early under controlled conditions rather than as an emergency when the airway is compromised, narrowed, or displaced.

Partial severance of the trachea (Figures 8-3 and 8-4) is a rare but potentially disastrous situation, and attempted endotracheal intubation may complete the disruption. Extreme care must be exercised with positioning the head and neck, and subsequent successful management will depend upon the availability of expertise in fiberoptic bronchoscopy and/or tracheostomy.[4,5]

Burns

Burns of the head and neck represent a potential major airway hazard. If there is any doubt over the possibility of developing airway compromise, then early endotracheal intubation is required, especially if patient transfer is anticipated.

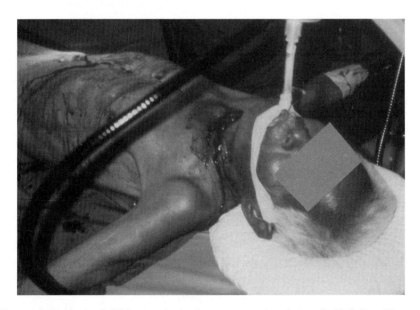

FIGURE 8-3. Cut neck. This casualty had an open trachea from a knife injury. He was managed at a resource-limited field hospital by anesthesia, gentle endotracheal intubation, and a tracheostomy. An alternative would have been a tracheostomy as the first procedure.

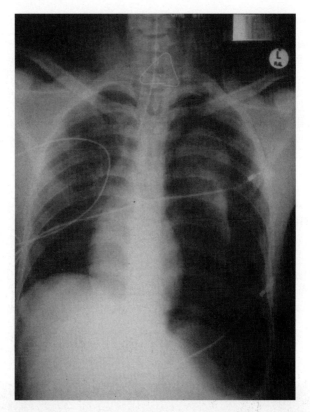

FIGURE 8-4. Shot neck. This casualty arrived *in extremis* with a gunshot wound to the front of the neck. Air was bubbling from the wound. He presented a similar dilemma to the patient in Figure 8-3. He was intubated with a 7.0 endotracheal tube. Attending surgeons indicated they would have done a rapid percutaneous tracheostomy. An X ray taken immediately after intubation demonstrated the tension pneumothorax. Everyone had been concentrating so much on "A" that "B" had deteriorated. The triangle in the front of the neck is a bullet marker. The bullet had clipped the top of the left pleura. Following chest drainage and formal tracheostomy, the casualty made a good recovery.

In the absence of anesthetic training, drugs, and equipment to achieve this, or in other situations where endotracheal intubation is not possible or has failed, an urgent surgical airway is required.

In most situations, this means a surgical cricothyridotomy. The aim is to secure the airway with a cuffed tracheostomy tube of 6.0-millimeter internal diameter or greater. This provides a definitive airway through which the patient can breathe or receive intermittent positive-pressure ventilation.

On very rare occasions in the prehospital environment, it may be necessary to perform a cricothyroidotomy in an awake patient with progressive airway obstruction. This will require local anesthesia of the area either by careful infiltration or by bilateral superficial cervical plexus blocks. The latter approach has the advantage of not distorting the cricothyroid membrane, and it also avoids the risk of causing coughing by inadvertent puncture of the membrane.

Breathing

The exact diagnosis of chest injury in patients with major trauma can be difficult. This is especially so in the noisy field environment or during transport in an ambulance or helicopter. The main concerns are recognizing and appropriately treating the immediately life-threatening thoracic injuries and detecting pneumothorax and hemothorax.

Approximately 15% of low-energy transfer ballistic injuries to the chest will require emergency surgery; the remainder can be managed by the placement of a chest drain. The mortality associated with high-energy transfer wounds is significantly greater, and those that survive to reach a medical facility may have significant tissue destruction and loss. The elastic composition of the lung makes it relatively resistant to the effect of high-energy transfer and cavitation, unlike the solid abdominal organs. Plain X ray is the mainstay of thoracic imaging in trauma, although CT of the thorax has been shown to delineate well the track of a missile through the lungs.[6]

Penetrating chest trauma may result in an open or sucking chest wound. These can be managed by the application of an Asherman chest seal™ (Rusch, Duluth, USA) applied over the defect; this provides a seal around the injury and one-way valve for drainage of air. Following this, a chest drain should be inserted.

Circulation/Hemorrhage Control

Recognition

The detection of the clinical signs of hemorrhagic shock is essential in assessing the injured patient. These include visible bleeding, tachycardia, poor peripheral perfusion, and, in later stages, decreased conscious level. Visible bleeding needs to be controlled quickly by direct pressure, elevation, and/or tourniquets. The history and clinical signs should produce a high index of suspicion for nonvisible bleeding.

Clinical examination for intra-abdominal and thoracic bleeding at the medical facility may be augmented with lightweight portable, hand-held ultrasound machines during the circulation assessment of the primary survey. These have been validated in the diagnosis of hemoperitoneum[7] using the Focused Assessment with Sonography for Trauma (FAST) technique.[8]

Broadly, then, hemorrhage can be differentiated into:

i. *Compressible* hemorrhage that can be controlled by direct pressure or limb splinting. When this bleeding is controlled (i.e., the "tap" turned off) (Figure 8-5), the casualty can receive fluid resuscitation with near-normal blood pressure as the goal.

ii. *Noncompressible* hemorrhage (for example, bleeding into the abdomen or chest) that requires urgent surgical intervention. (i.e., the "tap" cannot be turned off in the resuscitation department). Current views are that management of this situation may involve hypotensive resuscitation.

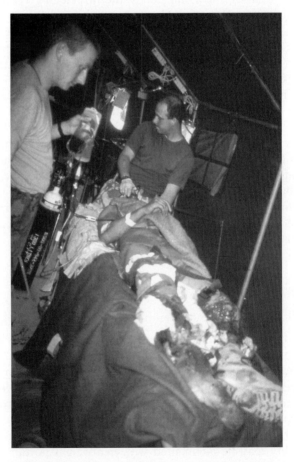

FIGURE 8-5. 1991 Gulf War. This casualty had severe leg injuries from a mine blast. The medics on the scene had controlled the bleeding using tourniquets.

Hypotensive Resuscitation

Hypotensive or minimal-volume resuscitation to a systolic blood pressure of *around* 80 to 90-millimeters Hg is increasingly being advocated in trauma resuscitation. This is not a new approach, as vascular surgeons have been advocating a minimal-fluid resuscitation approach for ruptured aneurysms for a number of years. The approach is based on the belief that giving excess fluid may raise the blood pressure, disrupt clots, cause rebleeding, and increase blood loss.[9] Clinical data from Houston (where 598 consecutive patients were allocated into either a standard, high-volume fluid resuscitation group or a minimal preoperative fluids group) has been quoted as supporting this approach.[10] The study showed a trend towards reduced blood loss and a statistically significant reduction in mortality in the minimal resuscitation group.

Dutton et al. have since challenged this work in a randomized study of patients in hemorrhagic shock.[11] There was no difference in mortality between patients resuscitated to a blood pressure of 70-millimeters Hg or greater than 100-millimeters Hg.

Certainly this technique is not appropriate in all trauma patients[12] and is not recommended in patients with prolonged entrapped or with head injury where it is vital to maintain an adequate cerebral perfusion pressure to ensure the best outcome from the cerebral injury.[13,14]

Consensus guidelines for prehospital trauma care state that fluid should not be given to trauma patients before hemorrhage control if a radial pulse can be felt. In the absence of a radial pulse, 250-milliliter aliquots of normal saline may be given, but stopped temporarily once the pulse returns.[9] The patient should be monitored for subsequent deterioration. In penetrating torso trauma, the presence of a central pulse may be considered adequate.[9]

This strategy requires rapid definitive surgical control of hemorrhage, and it may be the timing of surgery rather than the volume of fluid transfused that is the defining issue.

Fluids

The choice of intravenous resuscitation fluid remains contentious. In fixed civilian establishments, the choice of fluid (crystalloid, colloid, blood, or hypertonic hyperosmotic solutions) will be influenced by both its clinical effect and unwanted effects. In the military factors such as weight, ease of transport and storage characteristics must be considered.

Different scientific models of hemorrhage have been developed in an attempt to analyze this complex issue. Various studies have been performed comparing the effects of different fluid regimes.[15,16] Definitive evidence for the use of hypertonic saline dextran (HSD) is limited; however, HSD may have an advantage in traumatic head injury.[17]

Massive Transfusion Protocols

The massively bleeding patient poses acute problems. Massive transfusion, defined as greater than twice the circulating blood volume, is associated with severe physiological and metabolic disturbances. Substantial blood loss and replacement result in severe coagulation disturbances that are complicated by hypothermia and acidosis. Expedient blood and blood component therapy is required.

Massive transfusion policies have been developed for exsanguinating patients in many units (Table 8-2). These provide rapid standardized component therapy in proportion to the blood used, and they can be automatically repeated until discontinued. In addition, efforts must be made to minimize the physiological disturbances associated with transfusion. All infused fluids and blood should be warmed to reduce core hypothermia. Consideration should be given to recovery of noncontaminated blood and autotransfusion.

Damage Control Ground Zero

Damage control surgery (DCS) has become the accepted approach for the trauma patient *in extremis*.[18] The prehospital/resuscitation phase is where the patient who will benefit from DCS is recognized and efforts are made to expedite their passage to the operating room.[18] This approach has been termed "Damage Control Ground Zero". Damage control is an integral part of the casualty's resuscitation in the circulation/hemorrhage stage of the primary survey. The surgical goal is rapid hemorrhage control and limitation of contamination. Resuscitation continues (following the surgery) in the intensive-care unit, before definitive surgery is undertaken at 24–48 hours, once acidosis, hypothermia, and coagulopathy have been corrected.

Disability

The majority of casualties who sustain a high-energy transfer wound to the head do not survive to medical care.[19,20] In head-injured survivors, the primary head injury can be compounded by secondary injury as a result of hypoxia and hypotension. The fundamental principle of resuscitation for central nervous system injury is prevention of secondary brain insult through avoidance of hypoxia, hypercapnia, and hypotension.

TABLE 8-2. From the trauma center at Penn, Hospital University of Pennsylvannia, USA

Massive transfusion pack
10 units group O noncross-matched–packed red blood cells
6 units of platelets
4 units of thawed fresh frozen plasma

There is an obvious conflict between the need to maintain blood pressure and cerebral perfusion pressure and the need to avoid uncontrolled bleeding from the abdomen and chest.

Military penetrating brain injuries frequently arise from fragments, rather than bullets. In this situation, casualties who *survive* to reach medical care are a preselected group who generally have received low energy transfer fragment injuries; the outcome for both survival and rehabilitation in this group is good.[20,21] (Exceptions can occur when very rapid evacuation systems bring live casualties with unsurvivable brain injuries to the medical facility within minutes of injury).

Environment

Ballistic casualties, especially those that received their injuries in an austere location or on a battlefield, may be markedly hypothermic on arrival at the medical facility. Climatic conditions, transport times, and the severity of injury will affect this. Hypothermia compounds coagulopathy and is associated with increased mortality. During resuscitation and in the operating room, active measures including warm air blankets and environment control, and warmed fluids should be employed routinely.

Summary—Resuscitation

Resuscitation of the ballistic casualty requires an organized approach that addresses the basics of trauma resuscitation through ATLS/ BATLS guidelines and recognizes the unique characteristics of these devastating injuries.

The following section concentrates on practical guidance for the anesthetic management of the casualty with ballistic injury.

Anaesthesia

Patients are likely to present for anesthesia in two broad phases;

Early:
1. as part of the patient's resuscitation, including anesthesia for surgical control of hemorrhage and "damage control" surgery (Chapter 10),
2. anesthesia for early wound debridement and major fracture stabilization.

These "acute" interventions usually will take place in a casualty who is shocked, cold, and likely to be at risk of pulmonary aspiration. The anesthetic management here follows the general principles of emergency anesthesia. Successful management depends not only on technical skills, but also on the ability to continually reassess patients whose clinical condition may be subject to rapid and unexpected deterioration. The areas of particular concern in the ballistic casualty will be discussed below.

Late:
This includes anesthesia for re-look and delayed procedures. Anesthesia in this situation will depend on the patient's overall condition. A "re-look" for continued bleeding is likely to be similar to the acute interventions outlined above and not uncommonly will involve intensive-care patients where the surgery will be a necessary part of their ongoing management.

In contrast, an anesthetic for delayed primary suture in a single-limb injury in a well resuscitated and prepared patient several days post injury is more likely to be similar to a routine anesthetic.

Planning Anesthesia

Casualties injured by modern munitions containing preformed fragments are likely to have multiple penetrating injuries to different body areas[22] and may need frequent repositioning during surgery (Figure 8-6).[23] Fragments and bullets cross body cavities and regions; therefore, the theater team must be prepared for the surgeon having to convert an abdominal operation into a thoracic one and vice versa.

A suggested plan of management is:

1. Preoxygenation and rapid sequence induction with endotracheal intubation. The appropriate range of equipment to manage a potentially

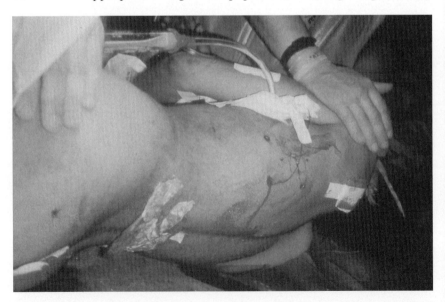

FIGURE 8-6. A casualty from the first Gulf War being treated at 32 Field Hospital. The casualty had multiple-fragment injuries involving both abdominal and thoracic cavities. The majority of these injuries were in the casualty's back and not seen until the casualty was rolled during resuscitation. The casualty had a left pneumothorax. This had been detected by clinical examination early in the resuscitation and treated with a chest drain.

difficult airway must be readily available. This includes a range of endotracheal tubes, gum-elastic bougie, and a surgical airway kit.

2. Which induction agent? This depends on what drugs you are familiar with and what you would normally use in a shocked, hypovolemic patient.

In the author's view, Ketamine[24] [1 to 2 milligrams per kilogram (mg/kg), depending on the level of hemorrhagic shock in the casualty) is an excellent induction agent. Following initial rapid muscle relaxation with suxamethonium (1 to 1.5 mg/kg) and endotracheal intubation, muscle relaxation can be maintained with Vecuronium, pancuronium, or an equivalent.

3. How to maintain anesthesia? Again, this depends on what techniques you are familiar with and your normal practice for the unstable, shocked casualty. In very resource-limited environments, one of the authors (P.F.M.) tends to use Ketamine boluses or infusions until hemostasis is achieved, then gradually introduces a volatile anaesthetic agent.

4. What intravenous access? The aim is to be able to give a number of different drugs (induction agents, muscle relaxants, antibiotics, analgesics, inotropes) and fluids at the time and in the quantities that are required.

The issue is that a balance has to be achieved between time taken for anesthetic preparation (siting lines for access and monitoring) and the need to start surgery to achieve hemostasis.

It is reassuring to start a difficult anesthetic with central venous monitoring, direct arterial monitoring, and several sites for fluid and drug administration. This is rarely achievable or practical with a patient in extremis.

A practical plan is:

Ask the surgeon, "How much time do we have?"
Site lines according to your skill:
- an individual skilled at getting central access will achieve this while someone else is struggling with a peripheral line (in this case, "central access" means a large-bore rapid-infusion device, not a multilumen monitoring line).
- Cervical collars and injuries will restrict the sites available for central access
- If, however, you have sufficient peripheral access for drug administration and rapid fluid replacement once hemostasis is obtained go with this.

Hypotensive resuscitation should be maintained until surgical hemostasis is achieved. Although a systolic blood pressure of 90-millimeters Hg is often quoted, in practice, a pressure that produces at least 0.5 milliliters of urine per kg per hour is satisfactory (assuming there is not a head injury). Noninvasive blood pressure (NIBP), electrocardiograph (ECG), pulse oximetry, capnography, and urine output are sufficient monitoring during resuscitation and anaesthetic induction.

If red cells are needed urgently, then O Rh negative or group-specific blood is used until a definitive cross-match is available. Fluids must be warmed and must be capable of being infused under pressure; all other measures should be taken to prevent hypothermia, such as covering the patients head with dressings or blankets and the use of warm air blowers. As surgery progresses, additional monitoring is added to evaluate the effectiveness of surgery and fluid resuscitation. This requires central venous pressure (CVP) and direct arterial pressure measurement.

As the patient's condition stabilizes, arterial blood gas analysis, coagulation screens, and platelet count should be used to adjust ventilation and fluid management. Near patient monitoring of coagulation using the thromboelastogram (TEG) is established in liver transplantation and cardiac surgery and has potential in trauma patients.[25]

Resuscitative Endpoints

A hypothetical trauma patient well resuscitated from hypovolemia involving massive transfusion ideally would have minimal evidence of the physiological consequences of cellular hypoxia. An elevated blood lactate or failure to clear a high lactate concentration predicts a poor outcome.[26]

The figures in Table 8-3 are acceptable endpoints, but again it is stressed that investigations are supplementary to clinical acumen and trends are often more significant than isolated numbers.

Problems in the Operating Theater

If the patient's condition unexpectedly deteriorates, the original diagnosis must be reviewed in light of the mechanism of injury and the possible anatomical and physiological consequences. The following differential diagnoses must be considered (some, of course, are fundamental to any general anaesthetic).

Airway and Ventilation

One of the concerns for the anesthetist is that intermittent positive-pressure ventilation (IPPV) following endotracheal intubation can cause

TABLE 8-3. Endpoints of resuscitation

1. pH 7.35–7.45
2. Base deficit −3.0 or higher with a lactate concentration of 1.0 mmol per liter or less
3. Core temperature >35.5 degrees centigrade
4. International normalized ratio (INR) <1.5 PT* <16 seconds PTT** <42 seconds
5. Hemoglobin (Hb) 80 grams per liter or greater
6. Platelets >50 × 10^9 per liter
7. Fibrinogen >1 gram per liter

* PT = prothrombin time.
** PTT = partial thromboplastin time.

tension in an existing pneumothorax and, in addition, may reduce cardiac output in the hypovolemic patient.

If the patient cannot be adequately ventilated, or oxygenation is inadequate, the following issues should be considered.

a. Has the endotracheal tube slipped into a main stem bronchus?
b. Is there an undiagnosed chest injury?
c. If present, is the chest drain performing as intended?
d. If a blast injury has occurred, is the patient already developing ventilation perfusion mismatch due to a developing lung injury?

When there is progressive difficulty in ventilating the patient associated with an increase in the airway pressures, always assume an obstructed airway until proved otherwise. This is particularly so if the airway was established with difficulty and has now become obstructed due to bleeding, soiling, endotracheal tube kinking, etc.

Difficulty ventilating due to intrinsically stiff lungs may be associated with unacceptably high airway pressures. In this situation, the recognized intensive-care ventilation strategy of permissive hypercapnia, using small tidal volumes and rapid respiratory rates, may be necessary to avoid further barotraumas. If the theater ventilator is capable, then pressure-controlled modes of ventilation may be appropriate.

Circulation

The differential diagnosis of unexplained hypotension includes: bleeding from a missed injury, a missed high spinal cord lesion, undiagnosed tension pneumothorax, cardiac contusion, infarction, or tamponade.

Less commonly, anaphylaxis from colloids, drugs, or a transfusion reaction may be responsible. Cardiac ischemia on the ECG of a previously fit young adult may be associated with profoundly low hemoglobin, particularly in the presence of ischemic limb injuries.

Poor urine output following restoration of a normal CVP in crush injuries is an ominous marker of impaired renal function due to myoglobinuria and the development of renal tubular necrosis. A forced mannitol diuresis is necessary to save renal tubular function; a renal output of at least 100 milliliters per hour is required.

Deterioration of the patient at a later stage associated with persistent bleeding or massive transfusion may reflect a dilutional coagulopathy or the onset of disseminated intravascular coagulation (DIC). Treatment of this complication will require expert hematological advice and treatment with fresh frozen plasma, platelets, and cryoprecipitate, depending on the results of hematological and clotting studies. These investigations will need to be repeated on a regular basis. The use of antifibrinolytic drugs as an attempt to reduce transfusion volumes continues to attract interest. A variety of different drugs have been used, but there are few studies to support their

166 P.R. Wood et al.

routine use. Aprotinin is used in liver resection surgery and may be of benefit in liver trauma.[27] The use of Factor VIIa is considered in the chapter on abdominal and pelvic trauma.

Critical Care

Intensive care of the ballistic trauma patient is discussed in Chapter 22.

Conclusion

Anesthesia for ballistic trauma can be challenging and will frequently test both the technical and diagnostic abilities of the anesthetist.

Practical management needs to follow a logical sequence of assessment and treatment and should be kept as simple as possible.

Frequent discussion between the anesthetist and surgeon and reassessment of treatment priorities is vital to maximize the chance of a successful outcome.

References

1. Driscoll PA, Vincent C. Variation in trauma resuscitation and its effect on outcome. *Injury*. 1992;23:110–115.
2. Driscoll PA, Vincent C. Organising an efficient trauma team. *Injury*. 1992;23:107–110.
3. Criswell JC, Parr MJA, Nolan JP. Emergency airway management in patients with cervical spine injury. *Anaesthesia*. 1994;49:900–903.
4. Huh J, Milliken JC, Chen JC. Management of tracheobronchial injuries following blunt and penetrating trauma. *Am Surg*. 1997;63:896–899.
5. Mussi A, Ambrogi MC, Ribechini A, Lucchi M, Menoni F, Angeletti CA. Acute major airway injuries: Clinical features and management. *Eur J Cardiothoracic Surg*. 2001;20:46–51.
6. Hanpeter DE, Demetriades D, Asensio J, Berne TV, Velmahos, Murray J. Helical computed tomographic scan in the evaluation of mediastinal trauma. *J Trauma*. 2000;49:689–694.
7. Brooks A, Davies Br, Connolly J. Prospective evaluation of handheld ultrasound in the diagnosis of blunt abdominal trauma. *J R Army Med Corps*. 2002;148:19–21.
8. Rozycki GS, Oschner G, Schmidt JA, et al. A prospective study of surgeon-performed ultrasound as the primary adjuvant modality for injured patient assessment. *J Trauma*. 1995;9:492–500.
9. Greaves I, Porter K, Revell MP. Fluid resuscitation in Pre-hospital trauma care: A consensus view. *J R Coll Surg Edinb*. 2002;47:451–457.
10. Bickell WH, Wall MJ Jr, Pepe PE, Martin RR, Allen MK, Mattox KL. Immediate versus delayed fluid resuscitation for hypotensive patients with penetrating torso injuries. *N Engl J Med*. 1994;331:1105–1109.
11. Dutton RP, Mackenzie CF, Scalea TM. Hypotensive resuscitation during active hemorrhage: impact on in-hospital mortality. *J Trauma*. 2002;52:1141–1146.
12. Pepe PE. Shock in polytrauma. *BMJ*. 2003;327:1119–1120.

13. Bickell WH, Bruttig SP, Millnamow GA, O'Benar J, Wade CE. Use of hypertonic saline/dextran versus lactated Ringer's solution as a resuscitation fluid after uncontrolled aortic hemorrhage in anesthetized swine. *Ann Emerg Med.* 1992;21:1077–1085.
14. Martin RR, Bickell WH, Pepe PE, Burch JM, Mattox KL. Prospective evaluation of preoperative fluid resuscitation in hypotensive patients with penetrating truncal injury: A preliminary report. *J Trauma-Inj Infect Crit Care.* 1992;33:354–361, discussion 361–362.
15. Wiggers CJ. *Physiology of Shock.* New York: Common Wealth Fund; 1950:121–146.
16. Myers C. Fluid resuscitation. *Eur J Emerg Med.* 1997;4:224–232.
17. Wade CE, Grady JJ, Kramer GC, Younes RN, Gehlsen K, Holcroft JW. Individual patient cohort analysis of the efficacy of hypertonic saline / dextran in patients with traumatic head injury and hypotension. *J Trauma.* 1997;42:s61–s65.
18. Johnson JW, Gracias VH, Schwab CW, Reilly PM, Kauder DR, Shapiro MB, Dabrowski GP, Rotondo MF. Evolution in damage control for exsanguinating penetrating abdominal injury. *J Trauma.* 2001;51:261–269.
19. Surgical management of penetrating brain injury. *J Trauma.* 2001;51:S16–S25.
20. Prognosis in penetrating brain injury. *J Trauma.* 2001;51:S44–S49.
21. Coupland RM, Pesonen PE. Craniocerebral war wounds: non specialist management. *Injury.* 1992;23:21–24.
22. Spalding TJW, Stewart MPM, Tulloch DN, Stephens KM. Penetrating missile injuries in the Gulf war 1991. *Br J Surg.* 1991;78:1102–1104.
23. Adley R, Evans DHC, Mahoney PF, Riley B, Rodgers CR, Shanks T, Skinner TA, Swinhoe CF, Yoganathan S. The Gulf war: Anaesthetic experience at 32 Field Hospital Department of Anaesthesia and Resuscitation. *Anaesthesia* 1992;42:996–999.
24. Wood PR. Ketamine: Pre-hospital and in hospital use. *Trauma.* 2003;5:137–140.
25. Kaufmann CR, Dwyer KM, Crews JD, Dols SJ, Trask AL. Usefulness of thromboelastography in assessment of trauma patient coagulation. *J Trauma.* 1997;42:716–720, discussion 720–722.
26. Abramson D, Scalea T, Hitchcock R, Trooskin SZ, Henry SM, Greenspan J. Lactate clearance and survival following injury. *J Trauma.* 1993;35:588–589.
27. Kovesi T, Royston D. Pharmacological approaches to reducing allogeneic blood exposure. *Vox Sang.* 2003;84:2–10.

Further Reading

Resuscitation
Fluid resuscitation of combat casualties. *J Trauma.* 2003;54(suppl 5s).
Rhee P, Alam HB, Ling GSF. Hemorrhagic shock and resuscitation. In: Tsokos GC, Atkins JL, eds. *Combat Medicine: Basic and Clinical Research in Military, Trauma and Emergency Medicine.* Totowa, NJ: Humana Press Inc.; 2003:177–218. ISBN 1 58829 070 0

Anesthesia
Gwinnutt C, Bethelmy L, Nolan J. Anaesthesia in trauma. *Trauma.* 2003;5:51–60.
Cantelo R, Mahoney PF. An introduction to field anaesthesia. *Curr Anaesth Critical Care.* 2003;14:126–130.

9
Clinical Ballistics: Surgical Management of Soft-Tissue Injuries—General Principles*

DONALD JENKINS, PAUL DOUGHERTY, and JAMES M. RYAN

The goal in treatment of soft tissue wounds is to save lives and limbs, preserve function, minimize morbidity, and prevent infections through early and aggressive surgical wound care far forward on the battlefield.

Treat the wound, not the weapon.

All war wounds are contaminated and should not be closed primarily

Presurgical care is aimed primarily at prevention of infection. Typically, a sterile dressing should be placed in the field as soon as possible, and this dressing should be left undisturbed until surgery. A one-look soft tissue exam may be performed upon initial presentation to the definitive treatment facility because the infection rate increases with multiple examinations prior to surgery. Initial wound cultures are unnecessary and a waste of valuable resources. Antibiotics should be administered for all penetrating wounds as soon as practical, preferably even in the tactical field scenario, if possible. In these war wounds, antibiotics are therapeutic, not prophylactic, but keep in mind that antibiotics are not a replacement for surgical treatment.

Surgical wound-management priorities involve understanding that life-saving procedures should be done before limb and soft tissue wound care. In order to save limbs, vascular repair and compartment release must be undertaken expeditiously, even simultaneously, if possible. In order to best

---

* The opinions expressed herein are the private views of the authors and are not to be construed as official or reflecting the views of the US Department of the Army, or the US Department of the Air Force, or the US Department of Defense.

minimize or prevent infection in war wounds, wound surgery needs to be accomplished within 6 hours of wounding, sterile dressings must be applied properly and maintained, antibiotics need to be well utilized, and fractures must be immobilized.

Superficial penetrating fragment (single or multiple) injuries usually do not require surgical exploration. Simply cleanse the wounds with antiseptic and scrub brush. Nonetheless, depending upon location and clinical presentation, maintain high suspicion for vascular injury or intra-abdominal penetration. Avoid "swiss cheese" surgery (in an attempt to excise all wounds and retrieve fragments).

Primary Surgical Wound Care

The techniques important to master in primary surgical wound management include the proper use of limited longitudinal incisions, the excision of all foreign material and devitalized tissue, copious wound irrigation, splinting extremities for transport to improve pain control, leave wounds open (no primary closure of war wounds), and proper use of antibiotics (Figure 9-1).

As seen in the accompanying graphics, the mainstay of surgical technique is the use of limited longitudinal incisions as originally described by Larrey for the purpose of debridement (see box).

Débridement (unbridling or unleashing)
The term was introduced by Baron Dominique Jean Larrey (1766–1842), Surgeon to Napoleon's Imperial Guard. He used it to describe the process of laying a wound open to facilitate removal of bullets, bits of loose cloth, detached pieces of bone, and soft tissue. He and his contemporaries did not excise tissue in the modern sense, and his procedure was much less extensive than the formal wound excision practiced today.

Wounds are extended with incisions parallel to the long axis of the extremity to expose the entire deep zone of injury. At the flexion side of joints, the incisions are made obliquely to the long axis in order to prevent the development of flexion contractures. The use of longitudinal incisions, rather than transverse ones, allows for proximal and distal extension, as needed, for more thorough visualization and debridement.

In the current day, we have extended the technique to include wound excision of nonviable tissue. For skin, a conservative excision of 1 to 2 millimeters of damaged skin edges is performed. Excessive skin excision is

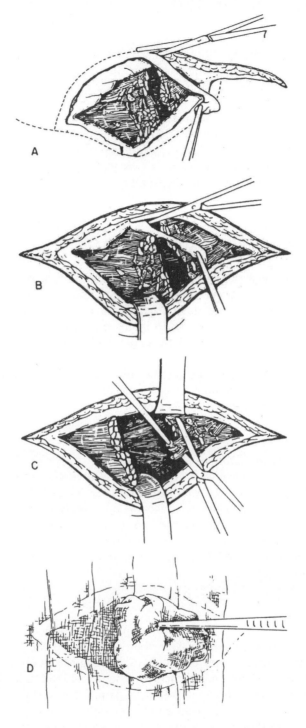

FIGURE 9-1. Technique of debridement in soft-tissue wounds. (A) Line of incision and excision of traumatized skin. (B) Excision of traumatized fascia. (C) Excision of devitalized muscle. (D) Technique of wound dressing. (From Emergency War Surgery, 2nd US revision. NATO Handbook 1988. US Government printing office, Washington, DC).

avoided; questionable areas can be assessed at the next debridement. For fat, damaged contaminated fat should be generously excised. For fascia, one must bear in mind that the damage to the fascia is often minimal relative to the magnitude of destruction beneath it. Shredded, torn portions of fascia are excised, and the fascia is opened widely through longitudinal incisions to expose the entire zone of injury beneath. Complete fasciotomy is often required.

Wound Excision

Removal of dead muscle is important to prevent infection (Figure 9-2 shows wound excision of a high-energy gunshot wound of thigh). Accurate initial assessment of muscle viability is difficult. Tissue-sparing debridement is acceptable if follow-on wound surgery will occur within 24 hours. More aggressive debridement is required if subsequent surgery will be delayed for more than 24 hours. Sharply excise all nonviable, severely damaged, avascular muscle. Color, contractility, consistency, and capillary bleeding (circulation)—the "4 Cs"—may be unreliable for initial assessment of

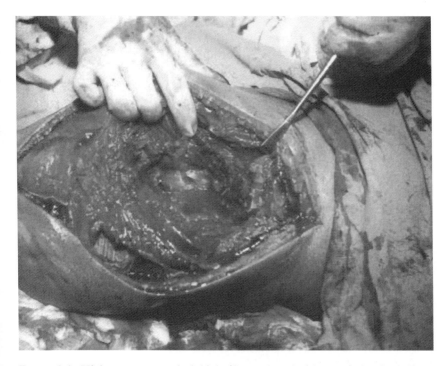

FIGURE 9-2. High-energy wound of thigh. (Reproduced with permission from Ryan JM, *Ballistic Trauma: Clinical Relevance in Peace and War*. London: Arnold; 1997:113).

muscle viability. Color is the least reliable sign of muscle injury. Surface muscle may be discolored due to blood, contusion, or local vasoconstriction. Contraction is assessed by observing the retraction of the muscle with the gentle pinch of a forceps. Consistency of the muscle may be the best predictor of viability. In general, viable muscle will rebound to its original shape when grasped by a forceps, whereas muscle that retains the mark has questionable viability. Circulation is assessed via bleeding tissue from a fresh wound. Transient vasospasm, common with war wounds, may not allow for otherwise healthy tissue to bleed.

Bones, Nerves, and Tendons

For bone, fragments with soft-tissue attachments and large free articular fragments are preserved. Remove all devitalized avascular pieces of bone smaller than thumbnail size that have no soft-tissue attachment. Deliver each of the bone ends of any fracture independently, clean the surface, and clean out the ends of the medullary canal. Nerves and tendons do not require debridement, except for trimming frayed edges and grossly destroyed portions. Primary repair is not performed at the initial debridement. To prevent desiccation, use soft tissue or moist dressings for coverage. Only minimal debridement of a vessel is required for a successful repair and limiting infection.

Management of Vascular Injury

Major artery and vein damage can pose special difficulty. Smaller vessels may be ligated, but major vessels should be repaired (for closer examination, see Chapter 18). Where possible, the ends should be trimmed and sutured. If any tension is likely to develop, a reversed vein graft may be inserted to bridge the gap and the repair, then covered by healthy muscle. The rest of the wound should be left open for delayed primary closure. Synthetic grafts are best avoided in the field surgical environment—the risk of graft failure due to sepsis is an ever-present threat. However, a temporary plastic shunt may be employed to revitalize tissue distal to the site of injury prior to definitive repair. In combined arterial and venous injury, concomitant shunting of both vessels may be necessary. Temporary shunting has an important place where major vascular injury is associated with complex fractures of long bones. Here, blood flow is re-established via the shunt(s), and the fracture is reduced and immobilized using an external fixator, after which definitive vascular repair is undertaken.

Irrigation and Wound Dressing

Irrigation serves to remove small particulate matter, clots, bacteria, debris, and other foreign matter. Following surgical removal of debris and nonviable tissue, irrigation is performed until clean. Several liters of fluid are required and varies based on degree of contamination, age of wound, and surgeon experience. While sterile physiologic fluid is preferred, do not deplete resuscitation fluid resources: one may use potable water as an alternative. According to preference, there may be additional efficacy if the last liter of irrigant contains antibiotics.

In the civilian setting, local soft-tissue coverage is often required in complex wounds with extensive tissue loss. The development and rotation of flaps for this purpose should not be done during primary surgical wound care in the field environment. Local soft-tissue coverage through the gentle mobilization of adjacent healthy tissue in order to prevent drying, necrosis, and infection is recommended. Saline-soaked gauze is an alternative.

NO PRIMARY CLOSURE OF WAR WOUNDS

When dressing a wound, take care not to plug the wound with packing material, as this prevents proper wound drainage. Leaving the wound open allows the egress of fluids, avoids ischemia, allows for unrestricted edema, and avoids the creation of an anaerobic environment. Lastly, place a nonconstricting, nonocclusive dry dressing over the wound.

Wound Management After Initial Surgery

Ideally, the wound should undergo a planned second debridement and irrigation in 24 to 72 hours and subsequent procedures until a clean wound is achieved. It is likely that this serial wound debridement will occur at different facilities by different surgeons as the patient traverses the echelons of care. Timing and duration of transport becomes an important planning factor for the surgeon to consider: if a casualty were to depart the surgical facility at the 23-hour point on a 48-hour trip, one should consider a second debridement prior to departure. Between procedures there may be better demarcation of nonviable tissue or the development of local infection. Early soft-tissue coverage is desirable within 3 to 5 days, when the wound is clean, in order to prevent secondary infection. Delayed closure (3–5 days) requires a clean wound that can be closed without undo tension. This state may be difficult to achieve in war wounds and should not be performed if the casualty will not be under direct surgical observation. Soft-tissue war wounds heal well through secondary intention without significant loss of function. This is especially is true of simple soft-tissue wounds. Definitive closure with skin grafts and muscle flaps should not be done in the conflict area.

Crush Syndrome

When a victim is crushed or trapped with compression on the extremities for a prolonged time, there is the possibility for the crush syndrome (CS), characterized by ischemia and muscle damage or death (rhabdomyolysis). In rhabdomyolysis, there is an efflux of potassium, nephrotoxic metabolites, myoglobin, purines, and phosphorous into the circulation, resulting in cardiac and renal dysfunction. Reperfusion injury can cause up to 10 liters of third-space fluid loss per limb, which can precipitate hypovolemic shock. Acute renal failure (ARF) can result from the combination of nephrotoxic substances from muscle death (myoglobin, uric acid) and hypovolemia, resulting in renal low-flow state. The recognition of crush syndrome relies on proper history and physical exam. Suspect CS in patients in whom there is a history of being trapped (urban operations, mountain operations, earthquakes, or bombings) for a prolonged period (from hours to days). Note that a clear history is not always available in combat, and the syndrome may appear insidiously in patients that initially appear well. A thorough exam must be done with attention to extremities, trunk, and buttocks. The physical findings depend on the duration of entrapment, treatment rendered, and time since the victim's release. Extremities initially may appear normal just after extrication. Edema develops rapidly with resuscitation and the extremity becomes swollen, cool, and tense. The patient often may have severe pain out of proportion to exam. Anesthesia and paralysis of the extremities can mimic a spinal cord injury with flaccid paralysis, but there will be normal bowel and bladder function in the CS patient. Again, in the trunk/buttocks, the patient may have severe pain out of proportion to exam in tense compartments.

Laboratory findings in CS are predictable and diagnostic. Creatinine phosphokinase (CK) is elevated with values usually >10 000 international units per milliliter. The urine initially may appear concentrated and later change color to a typical reddish-brown color, so called "port-wine" or "iced-tea" colored urine. The urine output decreases in volume over time. Due to myoglobin, the urine dipstick is positive for blood, but microscopy will not demonstrate red blood cells (RBCs). The urine may be sent to check for a myoglobin, but results take days and should not delay therapy. Hematocrit/hemoglobin (H/H) can vary depending on blood loss, but in isolated crush syndrome H/H is elevated due to hemoconcentration from third-spacing fluid losses. With progression of the CS, serum potassium and CK increase further with a worsening metabolic acidosis. Creatinine and blood urea nitrogen (BUN) will rise as renal failure ensues. Hyperkalemia is typically the ultimate cause of death from cardiac arrhythmia.

The primary goal of therapy is to prevent acute renal failure in crush syndrome. Again, the key is to suspect, recognize, and treat rhabdomyolysis early in victims of entrapment. Therapy should be initiated as soon as possible, preferably in the field, while the casualty still is trapped. Ideally, it is recommended to establish intravenous (IV) access in a free arm or leg vein. Avoid potassium- and lactate-containing IV solutions. At least one liter should be given prior to extrication and up to one liter per hour (for short extrication times) to a maximum of six to ten liters per day in prolonged entrapments. As a last resort, amputation may be necessary for rescue of entrapped casualties (ketamine 2 mg/kg IV for anesthesia and use of proximal tourniquet).

Hospital care continues that begun in the field, with attention to the other injuries and electrolyte anomalies, which must be treated while continuing fluid resuscitation to protect renal function. To monitor urine output, a Foley catheter is placed. The goal is to establish and maintain urine output >100 cubic centimeters per hour until pigments have cleared from the urine. If necessary, also add sodium bicarbonate to the IV fluid (1 amp/liter D5W) to alkalinize the urine above a pH of 6.5. If unable to monitor urine pH, put one amp in every other IV liter. Additionally, consider the administration of mannitol: 20% solution, one to two grams per kilogram over four hours (up to 200 grams per day) in addition to the IV fluids. Central venous monitoring may be needed with the larger volumes (may exceed 12 liters per day to achieve necessary urine output) of fluid given.

Electrolyte abnormalities to be monitored and addressed include: hyperkalemia, hyperphosphatemia, hypocalcemia, and hyperuricemia. Acute renal failure requiring dialysis occurs in many of those with severe rhabdomyolysis. Rapid evacuation to an appropriate capable facility is necessary for casualty survival from CS in such cases. The surgical management centers on diagnosis and treatment of Compartment Syndrome (see below)—remember to check torso and buttocks as well. Amputation should be considered in casualties with irreversible muscle necrosis/necrotic extremity.

Compartment Syndrome

Compartment syndrome may occur with an injury to any fascial compartment. The fascial defect caused by the injury is not adequate to fully decompress the compartment, and compartment syndrome still may occur. Mechanisms of injuries associated with compartment syndrome include any injury resulting in open or closed fractures, penetrating wounds, crush injuries, vascular injuries, and reperfusion following vascular repairs. The early clinical diagnosis of compartment syndrome includes: pain out of proportion; pain with passive stretch; and tense, swollen compartments. Late clinical diagnosis includes findings of paresthesia, pulselessness, pallor, and paralysis. In the field setting, the diagnosis of compartment pressures is best made on clinical grounds. Measurement of compartment pressures is not recommended in the combat zone: if the surgeon suspects it, just do the fasciotomy. In fact, prophylactic fasciotomy should be considered in several circumstances outlined below.

- High-energy wounds
- Intubated, comatose, sedated
- Closed head injuries
- Circumferential dressings or casts
- Vascular repair
- Prolonged transport
- High index of suspicion.

The technique of fasciotomy is well described in any surgical text or atlas. Every war surgeon should familiarize themselves with this anatomy and these techniques prior to deployment. Some key points in fasciotomy of the arm include: open both compartments [anterior flexors (biceps, brachialis) and posterior extensors (triceps)]; the lateral skin incision runs from the deltoid insertion to the lateral epicondyle; attempt to spare the larger cutaneous nerves; release the intermuscular septum between the anterior and posterior compartments; protect the radial nerve as it passes through the intermuscular septum from the posterior compartment to the anterior compartment just below the fascia; and release the fascia overlying each compartment with longitudinal incisions.

For thigh fasciotomies, all three compartments [the anterior (quadriceps), the medial compartment (adductors), and the posterior compartment (hamstrings)] must be released. The key points in technique include: the lateral incision is made from greater trochanter to lateral condyle of the femur; the iliotibial band is incised and the vastus lateralis is reflected off the intermuscular septum bluntly, releasing the anterior compartment; and the intermuscular septum then is incised the length of the incision, releasing the posterior compartment. This release of the intermuscular septum should not be made close to the femur, as there are a series of perforating arteries passing through the septum from posterior to anterior near the bone. The medial adductor compartment is released through a separate antero-medial incision.

For calf fasciotomies, all four compartments [lateral compartment (containing peroneal brevis and longus), anterior compartment (containing extensor hallucis longus, extensor digitorum communis, tibialis anterior, and peroneus tertius), superficial posterior compartment (containing gastrocnemius and soleus) and deep posterior compartment (containing the flexor hallucis longus, flexor digitorum longus, and the tibialis posterior)]. A two-incision technique is recommended. These incisions must extend the entire length of the calf in order to release all of the compressing fascia and skin. The lateral incision is made centered between the fibula and anterior tibial crest. The lateral intermuscular septum and superficial peroneal nerve are identified, and the anterior compartment is released in line with tibialis anterior muscle proximally toward the tibial tubercle and distally toward anterior ankle. The lateral compartment then is released through this incision in line with the fibular shaft, proximally toward the fibular head and distally toward the lateral malleolus. A second incision is made medially at least two centimeters medial to the medial-posterior palpable edge of the tibia, not over or near the subcutaneous surface of the tibia in order to prevent exposure of the tibia when the tissues retract. The saphenous vein and nerve are retracted anteriorly and the superficial compartment is released through its length, and then deep posterior compartment over the FDL is released. Then identify the tibialis posterior and release its fascia.

In the foot, there are five compartments to consider: the interosseous compartment (bounded by lateral 1st metatarsal medially, metatarsals and dorsal interosseous fascia dorsally, and the plantar interosseous fascia plantarly); the lateral compartment (bounded by 5th metatarsal shaft dorsally, the plantar aponeurosis laterally, and the intermuscular septum medially); the central compartment (bounded by the intermuscular septum laterally and medially, the interosseous fascia dorsally, and the plantar aponeurosis plantarly); the medial compartment (bounded by the inferior surface of the 1st metatarsal dorsally, the plantar aponeurosis extension medially, and the intermuscular septum laterally); and the calcaneal compartment (containing the quadratus plantae muscle). The foot may be released through a double dorsal incision technique. One incision placed slightly medial to 2nd metatarsal, reaching between 1st and 2nd metatarsals into medial compartment and between 2nd and 3rd metatarsals into the central compartment. A second dorsal incision is made just lateral to 4th metatarsal, reaching between 3rd and 4th metatarsals into central compartment and between 4th and 5th metatarsals into the lateral compartment. In order to spare the dorsal soft tissues, a single-incision medial fasciotomy may be used. A medial approach to the foot is made through the medial compartment, reaching across central compartment into interosseous compartments dorsally and lateral compartment releasing all the way across the foot.

Fasciotomy wound management should include the same open-wound guidelines outlined earlier in this chapter. Following the fasciotomy, the fasciotomy wound undergoes primary surgical wound management, removing all devitalized tissue, as discussed above. As with all war wounds, the fasciotomy is left open and covered with sterile dressings.

Shotgun Injuries

Shotguns are used increasingly in war and conflict. Injury is typically inflicted at close range, posing special problems. It is never possible to remove all the shot, and indeed, to do so would result in unacceptable damage to uninjured soft tissues. Wound excision should be carried out on the majority in the manner already described, particularly looking for indriven wadding and visible plugs of clothing. The retention of lead shot within the wound can result in dangerously high lead concentrations, which should be monitored. With time, lead levels fall as a result of encapsulation of the lead pellets by fibrous tissue.

Summary

Ballistic injury in the military environment poses unique difficulties. The lesson of history is that you cannot take the experience of an urban hospital onto the battlefield. What may be feasible for a single victim managed in peacetime could lead to disaster if transposed to a field hospital in wartime. Military concepts such as wide exposure, debridement, extensive would excision of devitalized soft tissue, delayed primary closure of wounds, and avoidance of prosthetic devices (vascular grafts and internal fixation devices for fractures are examples) were hard learnt on past battlefields and should not be discarded easily into the dustbin (trashcan in the USA) of history.

In conclusion, we list some helpful "Dos and Do Nots"

Do:
– Incise skin generously
– Incise fascia widely
– Indentify neurovascular bundles
– Excise all devitalized tissue
– Remove indriven clothing
– Leave the wound open on completion of surgery
– Dress wounds lightly with fluffed up gauze
– Record all injuries on field medical cards

Do Not:
– Excise too much skin
– Practice keyhole surgery
– Repair tendons or nerves at first surgery
– Remove attached pieces of bone
– Close the deep fascia
– Insert synthetic materials
– Pack the wound
– Close the skin

Further Reading

Coupland RM. *War Wounds of Limbs—Surgical Management*. Oxford: Butterworth-Heinmann; 1993.
Dufour D, Kroman Jensen S, Owen-Smith M, Salmela J, Stening GF, Zetter Ström B. *Surgery for the Victims of War*. Geneva: International Committee of the Red Cross: 1998.

Husum H, Chai SC, Fosse E. *War Surgery—Field Manual*. Malaysia: Third World Network; 1995.

Husum H, Gilbert M, Wisborg T. *Save Lives Save Limbs—Life Support for Victims of Mines, Wars and Accidents*. Malaysia: Third World Network; 2000.

Molde Å, Naevin J, Coupland R. *Care in the Field for Victims of Weapons of War*. Geneva: International Committee of the Red Cross; 2001.

Ryan JM. Warfare injuries. In: Russell RCG, Williams NS, Bulstrode CJK, eds. *Bailey and Love's Short Practice of Surgery*. 23rd ed.. London: Arnold; 2000:281–290.

10
Damage Control

BENJAMIN BRASLOW, ADAM J. BROOKS, and C. WILLIAM SCHWAB

Introduction

Massive hemorrhage is a major cause of trauma-related mortality and is the second most common cause of death after central nervous system injuries in the prehospital setting.[1] Moreover, uncontrolled bleeding is the most common cause of early in-hospital mortality (first 48 hours) due to major trauma.[2] During the last two decades, advances in prehospital care and trauma bay efficiency (especially in busy urban trauma centers) has led to more severely injured trauma patients surviving to the point of operative intervention. Regarding penetrating-trauma patients, the increasing use of powerful semiautomatic firearms by the civilian population has manifested in patients arriving with multiple penetrations and more severe tissue destruction. These patients often are wounded in multiple body cavities, suffering massive hemorrhage and both physiological and metabolic exhaustion.

A combination of profound acidosis, hypothermia, and coagulopathy, also known as the "lethal triad", is commonly noted in these patients. The "traditional surgical approach" to such patients, in which surgeons would repair all identified injuries at the initial operation, often led to patient demise despite control of anatomic bleeding.

During the peak of American gun violence in the late 1980s and early 1990s, urban trauma centers accumulated a wealth of experience in treating these severely injured patients and the concept of "Damage Control" surgery was born.

Damage control is a traditional Navy term[3] that refers to keeping a badly damaged ship afloat after major penetrating injury to the hull so as to maintain mission integrity. Typical procedures for temporary righting and stabilizing the vessel classically involved stuffing mattresses into gaping holes in the ship's hull, extinguishing local fires, and "dogging down" watertight doors to limit flooding and spread of damage.[4] These measures, which keep the ship afloat, allow for the assessment of other damage and afford time to establish a feasible plan for definitive repair. The analogy to the care of the seriously injured is obvious.

For the trauma surgeon, damage control describes the technique of abbreviated laparotomy, with rapid and precise containment of hemorrhage and contamination and temporary intra-abdominal packing for initial injury control. Following this, the patient is transferred to the surgical intensive care unit (ICU) for physiologic resuscitation. Subsequently, the patient returns to the operating room for definitive repair of all injuries and, if possible at that time, abdominal wall closure. This approach must not be deemed as surgical failure or an abandonment of proper surgical technique. Instead, it has proven to be an aggressive, deliberate strategy to combat the pattern of physiologic failure that accompanies major blunt and penetrating trauma.

History

The history of present-day damage control surgery is grounded in the early successes realized with hepatic packing for uncontrolled hemorrhage.[5]

Pringle, in 1908, first described the concept of hepatic packing in patients with portal-venous hemorrhage.[6] In 1913, Halstead went on to modify this technique by suggesting that rubber sheets be placed between the packs and the liver to protect the parenchyma.[7]

As surgical techniques, instruments, and materials improved, packing for control of hepatic hemorrhage fell from favor, and by the end of the second World War (WW II), primary repair re-emerged as the preferred approach. This continued through the era of the Viet Nam war.

The technique started to re-emerge when, in 1976, Lucas and Ledgerwood described a prospective 5-year evaluation of 637 patients treated for severe liver injury at the Detroit General Hospital. Three patients underwent perihepatic packing, and all three survived.[8]

In 1979, Calne and colleagues reported four patients in whom massive hemorrhage from severe hepatic trauma was managed initially by conservative surgery and packing. The patients then were transferred by ambulance for definitive surgery. All of these patients survived.[9] Two years later, at the Ben Taub General Hospital, Feliciano and colleagues reported a 90% survival in ten patients in whom intra-abdominal packing for control of exsanguinating hepatic hemorrhage was used. These authors noted that this technique appeared to be lifesaving in highly selected patients in whom coagulopathy, hypothermia, and acidosis made further surgical efforts likely to increase hemorrhage.[10]

In 1983, Stone and colleagues described a stepwise approach to the exsanguinating, hypothermic and coagulopathic trauma patient that included abbreviated laparotomy and extensive intra-abdominal packing (beyond the scope of just hepatic injuries). They made suggestions for temporizing maneuvers for other injured organs, such as the intestines and urinary tract. Once hemodynamic stability was achieved and the coagulopathy corrected, the patient was returned to the operating room (OR) for definitive surgical repairs and abdominal closure. Eleven of 17 patients, deemed to have a lethal coagulopathy, survived as a result of this strategy.[11] In this landmark study, the three phases of present-day damage control were defined.

Over the next decade, the concept and its application continued to evolve. In 1993, Rotondo and Schwab coined the term "Damage Control" and detailed a standardized three-phase approach that yielded a 58% survival rate.[12] When applied to select cohorts of patients, that is, a maximum injury subset with major vascular injury and two or more visceral injuries, survival increased further to 77%.

As outlined in their paper:

- part one (DC I) consists of immediate exploratory laparotomy with rapid control of bleeding and contamination, abdominal packing, and abbreviated wound closure.
- Part two (DC II) is the ICU resuscitative phase where physiologic and biochemical stabilization is achieved and a thorough tertiary examination is performed to identify all injuries.
- In part three (DC III), re-exploration in the OR is undertaken and definitive repair of all injuries is performed.

In 2001, Johnson and Schwab introduced a fourth component to the damage control sequence, "Damage Control Ground Zero" (DC 0)[13] (Figure 10-1). This represents the earliest phase of the damage control process that occurs in the prehospital setting and continues into the trauma bay. Here the emphasis is on injury-pattern recognition for potential damage control beneficiaries. This manifests in truncated scene times for emergency medical service (EMS) and abbreviated emergency department resuscitation by the trauma team. Rapid-sequence intubation, early rewarming maneuvers, immediate blood product resuscitation, and expedient transport to the OR are the key elements of "DC 0" in the trauma bay.

As reported survival rates in this maximally injured subset of patients has continued to rise, so has the popularity of the damage control approach. A recent collective review by Shapiro and colleagues of over 1000 damage control patients revealed an overall 50% survival.[14] The high morbidity rates (overall morbidity 40%) are not surprising and include wound infection (5–100%), intra-abdominal abscess (0–80%), dehiscence (9–25%), bile leak (8–33%), enterocutaneous fistula (2–25%), abdominal compartment syndrome (2–25%), and multisystem organ failure (20–33%). Other common morbidities in damage controlled patients include hepatic necrosis, intestinal obstruction or prolonged ileus, anastomatic leak, and pancreatic fistula.

The damage control philosophy stresses survival as the ultimate goal. Means to achieve this goal in this unique patient population are aggressive and prolonged ICU stays and multiple operations, which are often unavoidable.[15]

The Four Phases of Damage Control - Current

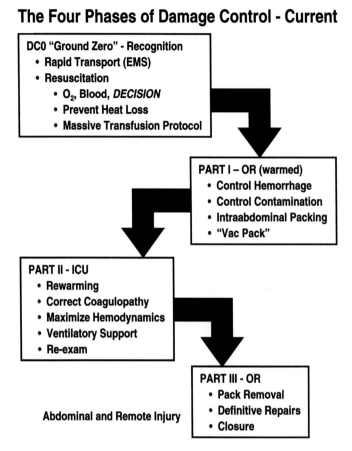

DC0 "Ground Zero" - Recognition
• Rapid Transport (EMS)
• Resuscitation
  • O$_2$, Blood, *DECISION*
  • Prevent Heat Loss
  • Massive Transfusion Protocol

PART I – OR (warmed)
• Control Hemorrhage
• Control Contamination
• Intraabdominal Packing
• "Vac Pack"

PART II - ICU
• Rewarming
• Correct Coagulopathy
• Maximize Hemodynamics
• Ventilatory Support
• Re-exam

Abdominal and Remote Injury

PART III - OR
• Pack Removal
• Definitive Repairs
• Closure

FIGURE 10-1. The four components of the Damage Control Sequence. [Johnson JW, Gracias VH, Schwab CW, et al. Evolution in damage control for exsanguinating penetrating abdominal injury. *J Trauma*. 2001; 51(2): 261–271] (Hoey BA, Schwab CW. Damage control surgery. *Scand J Surg*. 2002;91;92–103).

Indications for Damage Control

Although major liver injury and progressive coagulopathy remain the most frequent indications for damage control, the list has continued to expand. Because of the associated morbidity that often accompanies the process, patient selection and proper timing is crucial.

Early identification of patients who require damage control promotes optimal results. Inappropriate use of this strategy on more stable patients subjects them to associated morbidities.

Rotondo and colleagues defined a "maximal injury subset" of patients suffering penetrating injuries that clearly benefit from the damage control procedure.[10] These are patients with a major vascular injury, two or more hollow viscus injuries, and profound shock. In their initial damage control series, patients with this complex of injuries who underwent definitive laparotomy had an 11% survival rate compared with 77% for those in whom damage control was employed. Later, Rotondo and Zonies[16] expanded upon and organized the "key" factors in patient selection for damage control (Table 10-1).

Moore and colleagues[17] have also published their major indications for abbreviated laparotomy/damage control. In their estimation, the decision to proceed with damage control usually is based on a combination of these factors and may be influenced additionally by the resources available (e.g., inadequate blood products, limited surgical expertise, multiple casualties).

Table 10-2 is a comprehensive list of damage control triggers used at the University of Pennsylvania for initiating the damage control pathway. In general, the decision to proceed with damage control ultimately must be made when the surgeon recognizes a trend towards physiologic exhaustion.

Since this is often an intraoperative decision based on the severity of injuries identified at exploration, constant communication between the anesthesiologist and the surgeon regarding the patient's response to ongoing resuscitation is essential.

Damage Control—Pathophysiology

In the late 1970s and early 1980s, an epidemic of penetrating injuries was encountered in many urban trauma centers across the United States. Blood banks in these institutions developed the capability of delivering massive

TABLE 10-1. Key factors in patient selection for damage control (Rotondo & Zonies The damage control sequence and underlying logic. Surg Clin North Am. 1997; 77:761–777)

Conditions
  High energy blunt torso trauma
  Multiple torso penetrations
  Hemodynamic instability
  Presenting coagulopathy and/or hypothermia
Complexes
  Major abdominal vascular injury with multiple visceral injuries
  Multifocal or multicavitary exsanguination with concomitant visceral injuries
  Multiregional injury with competing priorities
Critical Factors
  Severe metabolic acidosis (pH < 7.30)
  Hypothermia (temperature <35°C)
  Resuscitation and operative time >90 minutes
  Coagulopathy as evidenced by development of nonmechanical bleeding
  Massive transfusion (>10 units packed red blood cells)

Source: With permission from Hoey BA, Schwab CW. Damage control surgery. Scan. J Surg. 2002;91;92–103.

TABLE 10-2. Triggers used at the University of Pennsylvania for initiating the damage control pathway

Severe shock with:
- Hypothermia (<95°F or 35°C), acidosis, coagulopathy
- Suboptimal response to resuscitation
- Inability to perform definitive repair: physiologic, equipment*, judgement*
- Inaccessible major anatomic injury (IVC, intrahepatic, retroperitoneal, pelvis) and demand for nonoperative control* (vascular control best accomplished by angiographic embolization)
- Need for time consuming procedure(s)* (Whipple, etc.)
- Indeterminate serious injury* (pancreatic head/duct)
- Need to reevaluate abdominal contents (intestinal ischemia)

* Shock may be absent.

quantities of blood products to keep pace with the transfusion requirements of all but the most severely injured patients.[18] Consequently, trauma surgeons were able to continue operating on such patients until a common constellation of metabolic derangements developed. These were characterized by the triad of a clinically obvious coagulopathy, profound hypothermia, and metabolic acidosis. Each entity seemed to reinforce both of the other derangements, resulting in an apparently irreversible metabolic downward spiral towards death.

Damage control was developed to reverse this "bloody vicious cycle," as Kashuk and colleagues[19] coined it. Each component is discussed in more detail below.

Hypothermia

Hypothermia is defined as a core temperature of less than 35°C. The adverse consequences of hypothermia first were studied extensively during WW II in experiments performed to determine the tolerance of and rescue logistics for downed pilots in the North Atlantic.[16]

In 1987, Jurkovich and colleagues reported that 66% of severely injured patients admitted to a Level I trauma center were hypothermic.[20] They noted a 60% increase in mortality when patients with core temperatures of 34°C were compared to patients with core temperatures of 32°C or less.

Cushman and colleagues,[21] in their review of iliac vascular injuries in 1997, reported a four times greater risk of dying for the hypothermic patient (initial core temperature of less than or equal to 34°C). They also found that if the patient's last body temperature in the operating room was less than 35°C, the risk of death was nearly 40 times greater than that for euthermic patients. Practically impaired myocardial contractibility, cardiac irritability, a left shift in the oxygen–hemoglobin saturation curve, and impaired coagulation capability are the most important complications of hypothermia.[15]

There are many causes of hypothermia in severely injured trauma patients. Hypovolemic shock adversely affects oxygen delivery and consumption, which ultimately decreases the body's ability to produce heat.[22] This is exacerbated further by the frequent intoxication of trauma patients, which causes vasodilatation. Trauma patients often are not only exposed to severe low temperatures in the field prior to transport, but despite efforts to maintain warm temperatures in the trauma bay and operating rooms, hypothermia often is exacerbated early in the patients hospitalization. On arrival to the bay, the patient is unclothed and fully exposed to allow for complete injury identification. A patient to room temperature gradient of 15°C is common and will result in heat loss from the body by convection.[23]

Suggested maneuvers to prevent or reverse hypothermia during the damage control process include:

1. Use of heat lamps and warmed blankets in the trauma bay
2. Infusion of crystalloid solution and blood products through a warming device such as the Level I fluid warmer
3. Increasing OR room temperature to more than 30°C
4. Covering body parts out of the operative field with a warming device such as the Bair Hugger or warmed towels
5. Warmed ventilator circuit
6. Irrigating Foley catheter, nasogastric tube, and thoracostomy tubes with warmed saline during laparotomy
7. Irrigation of other opened body cavities during the operative procedure.

Acidosis

Prolonged hypovolemic shock is associated with tissue ischemia and a shift from aerobic to anaerobic metabolism. Lactic acid is produced, resulting in profound metabolic acidosis, which further exacerbates the coagulopathic state.[24] In addition, acidosis causes the uncoupling of beta-adrenergic receptors, which reduces the patient's response to endogenous and exogenous catecholamines. This lowers cardiac output, induces hypotension, and increases susceptibility to ventricular arrhythmias. Lactate clearance has been correlated closely with the degree of oxygen delivery and oxygen consumption as endpoints of resuscitation.

In 1993, Abramson and colleagues showed that the rate of lactate clearance predicts survival in severely injured trauma patients. Whereas 100% of patients survived when lactate levels normalized within 24 hours, only 14% survived when clearance occurred at 48 hours.[25]

During damage control, aggressive measures must be instituted immediately to limit the degree of acidosis and promote lactate clearance with return to aerobic metabolism. These include rapid control of hemorrhage and optimization of oxygen delivery via aggressive resuscitation with blood products. Placement of a pulmonary artery catheter (PAC) and an arterial line are of great assistance in guiding therapy. Oxymetric PACs allow for continuous mixed venous oxygen saturation monitoring, which is helpful when titrating medications and fluids to optimize oxygen delivery.

Coagulopathy

The observed coagulopathic state of the exsanguinating trauma patient is multifactorial. Dilution and consumption of clotting factors, hypothermia, and acidosis are all contributory effects.

Dilutional thrombocytopenia is the most common coagulation abnormality occurring in trauma patients who receive transfusion volumes greater than 1.5 times their blood volume. After replacement of one blood volume, only about 35 to 40% of platelets remain in circulation. Moreover, dilution of procoagulant factors is a recognized complication of massive crystalloid and colloid resuscitation.[26]

The clotting cascade involves a series of temperature-sensitive serine-dependent esterase reactions that become relatively inhibited during hypothermia.[27]

In 1990, Reed and colleagues reported clotting abnormalities equal to profound factor deficiencies during hypothermia.[28]

Rohrer and Natale showed a dramatic increase in mean prothrombin time (PT) and partial thromboplastin time (PTT) with a decreasing assay temperature in pooled plasma from normal volunteers.[29] However, these standard assays of clotting function all are performed at a standardized temperature of 37°C, thus underestimating the degree of coagulopathy in the hypothermic patient.

Platelet function also is affected by hypothermia. Research in this area has shown links between hypothermia and decreased thromboxane B2 production. Furthermore, a number of in vitro studies describe the temperature-sensitive nature of the inositol triphosphate messenger system at the GPIIb-IIIa platelet–thrombin receptor site, which ultimately is responsible for the activation of protein kinase C and the initiation of platelet adherence, aggregation, and release.[30] This may explain the frequent clinical observation of platelet dysfunction in the hypothermic patient despite a normal quantitative platelet level.

Massive tissue damage, shock, and hypothermia cause severe malfunction within the fibrinolytic system. Under normal circumstances, fibrinolysis serves to clear thrombi from the microvasculature and to limit excessive thombus formation. In the trauma patient, massive clotting factor activation resulting from multiple injuries may lead to uncontrolled activation of the fibrinolytic system.[31] This particularly is true in selected injury complexes such as severe head and lung injury. Severe pulmonary contusions or the breakdown of the blood–brain barrier have been shown to release tissue thromboplastin into the systemic circulation.[32] This in turn causes extensive intravascular activation of the coagulation cascade and the formation of thrombin and subsequent fibrin clots. Consequently, coagulation factors and fibrinogen are depleted and disseminated intravascular coagulation (DIC) develops.

In 1992, Kearney and colleagues demonstrated that head injury is associated with elevation of D-dimer levels (fibrinogen degradation products), prolongation of the PT, and reduction of both antithrombin III and fibrinogen levels.[33]

Obviously, the multifactorial interactions leading to coagulopathy in the exsanguinating trauma patient are extremely complex and, to date, not completely understood. Early aggressive resuscitation with appropriate blood products and rewarming maneuvers is necessary to correct the coagulopathy and prevent further physiologic and metabolic deterioration.

The Damage Control Sequence

Damage Control—Ground Zero

Damage Control Ground Zero is the earliest phase of the damage control process and occurs in the prehospital setting and continues into the trauma bay. The emphasis is on injury pattern recognition for patients likely to benefit from damage control.

– For the EMS providers, this manifests in truncated scene times and early notification of the trauma response team.
– For the trauma team, abbreviated emergency-department resuscitation is the goal. Gaining large-bore intravenous (IV) access, rapid-sequence intubation, chest tube placement if indicated, early rewarming maneuvers, immediate blood product resuscitation, and expedient transport to the OR are the key elements of DC 0 in the trauma bay. For the rapid workup of penetrating trauma in the unstable patient, minimal diagnostic X-rays are required. A chest X-ray following intubation is imperative to confirm tube placement and identify hemo- and/or pneumothorax that might compromise the patient during transport to the OR. If blunt trauma also is suspected, spinal precautions must be observed, including the placement and/or continuation of a cervical collar. A pelvic X-ray is required to rule out pelvic ring instability and the need for a temporary stabilization device to reduce the pelvic volume and tamponade bleeding. The blood bank needs to be made aware that there is the potential for massive transfusion requirement. Additionally, a cell-saver device should be mobilized to the OR for the collection and reinfusion of shed blood intraoperatively. It is in this phase of the damage control sequence that broad-spectrum intravenous antibiotics and tetanus prophylaxis should be administered.

Damage Control Part I—The Initial Laparotomy

The primary objectives of the initial laparotomy are control of hemorrhage, limiting contamination and the secondary inflammatory response, and temporary abdominal wall closure to protect viscera and limit heat loss. All of this is done by the most expedient means possible.

Preparation

The operating room should be warmed to approximately 27°C before the patient's arrival, and the anesthesiologists should prepare their circuit to deliver warmed oxygen and anesthetic agents. As the patient is transferred onto the operating room table, the nursing team prepares the instrument trays, which should consist of a standard laparotomy set and vascular and chest instruments, including a sternal saw. A large supply of laparotomy pads must be immediately available for the initial packing. It is useful to have a cart stocked with damage control equipment (Table 10-3) available in the room, thus reducing the time OR personnel are away.

The patient is placed in a supine position on the table with upper extremities abducted at right angles on arm boards. Positioning of the electrocardiogram (ECG) leads and monitoring equipment must not limit the options for surgical exposure. In anticipation of the need for a median sternotomy, resuscitative left thoracotomy, or bilateral tube thoracostomy, no leads or tubing should be present on the anterior or lateral chest wall. The patient is prepped from chin to mid thighs, extending down to the table laterally should thoracotomy be necessary. A urinary catheter and nasogastric tube are inserted during the prep if not already performed in the trauma bay.

Surgery should not be delayed while waiting for the insertion of invasive monitoring devices, that is, arterial lines or central venous lines. These can be placed during the procedure, either by the anesthesiologists or members of the surgical team if in the prepped region.

TABLE 10-3. Damage control essential equipment

Basic:
- Abdominal, vascular, and chest instruments (including sternal saw)

Damage control essentials:
- Packs
- Shunts (sterile plastic conduits)
- Balloon catheters (large Foley of various sizes with 30 cc balloons)
- Sterile silastic bags
- Adhesive plastic
- Hemostatic agents
- Benzoine
- Suction drains

Incisions

The most expeditious incision for abdominal exploration is the vertical midline extending from the xiphoid process to the pubic symphysis. In the setting of a suspected severe pelvic fracture, the inferior limit of this incision initially might be curtailed to just below the umbilicus, allowing for continued tamponade of a potential large pelvic hematoma.

If the patient has had a previous midline incision, a bilateral subcostal incision can be employed. This allows for rapid access to the peritoneal cavity away from the expected midline adhesions involving bowel and omentum. These adhesions then can be divided rapidly under direct vision.

Hemorrhage Control

Once the peritoneum is entered, the next steps need to be performed in a rapid but orderly fashion. Large clots are removed manually. A large hand-held abdominal wall retractor is used sequentially around the periphery of the abdomen to provide space for the packing of all four quadrants. Surgeons on opposite sides of the table trade retraction and packing as appropriate. The falciform ligament is divided to prevent iatrogenic injury to the liver during pack placement in the right upper quadrant. The cell-saver suction should be in place to maximize autologous blood capture and return. While packing the abdomen, the surgeon is assessing the degree and location of the most significant injuries.

Knowledge of the trajectory of the projectiles may aid in assessing potential sites of major bleeding or organ injury. Next, a large self-retaining abdominal retractor is placed to free up the surgeons and provide maximal exposure.

Once the peritoneum is opened, any tamponade effect that had been provided by the abdominal wall is lost immediately. This may induce abrupt and severe hypotension. If the patient remains profoundly hypotensive after packing, control of aortic inflow should be obtained. Manual occlusion of the aorta at the diaphragmatic hiatus can be performed quickly to control abdominal exsanguination and give the anesthesia team some time to catch up with volume replacement. This maneuver also has been shown to augment cerebral and myocardial perfusion.[34] It is performed by passing the hand anterior to the stomach and posterior to the left hepatic lobe. In this position, the abdominal aorta can be palpated immediately to the right and posterior to the esophagus. Control is obtained by compressing it between the thumb and the index finger or by compression against the vertebral column with the hand or an aortic occlusion device.

If prolonged occlusion is necessary, or if surgical hands need to be freed up, a vascular clamp can be placed on the aorta after minimal dissection is performed. First, the diaphragmatic attachments of the left hepatic lobe are divided and the lobe is retracted to the right. Next, a longitudinal incision is made in the hepatogastric ligament approximately one centimeter medial to the esophagus. The muscle fibers of the right crus of the diaphragm then can be split longitudinally by blunt finger dissection to fully expose the aorta and allow for the placement of a large, curved vascular clamp (Figure 10-2).

Between occlusion of the aorta and intra-abdominal packing, the majority of significant bleeding should be controlled temporarily. Next, packs are removed in a sequential fashion, beginning in the areas least likely to harbor the source of major hemorrhage. This will provide space to pack the bowel away from the areas of hemorrhage and create maximal exposure.

Initial control of major vascular hemorrhage is performed rapidly using a variety of techniques. If an injury is amenable to rapid arteriorraphy or venorrhaphy, this is the treatment of choice. Simple lateral repairs are performed immediately utilizing appropriate vascular clamps for proximal and distal control.

Definitive reconstruction of complex arterial injuries, however, should be delayed unless the surgeon is confident that placing a prosthetic interposi-

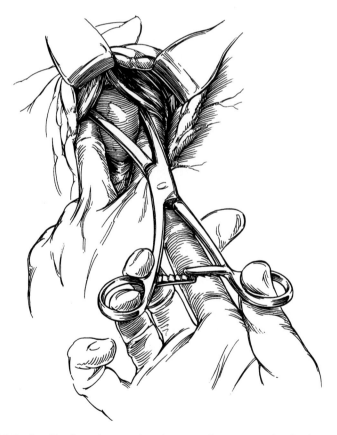

FIGURE 10-2. Application of a vascular clamp on the aorta at the diaphragm. (Hoey BA, Schwab CW. Damage control surgery. *Scand J Surg*. 2002;91:92–103).

tion graft [i.e., woven Dacron or polytetrafluoroethylene (PTFE)] can be done rapidly and there is not significant contamination present from concomitant bowel injury.

The placement of temporary intravascular shunts (i.e., thoracostomy tubes, silastic catheters, or commercially available heparin-bonded devices) in the more critical vessels [abdominal aorta, superior mesenteric artery (SMA), iliac and common femoral arteries, etc.] has been well described.[35,36] This technique is an excellent rapid alternative to arterial ligation, which often can put end organ and limb viability in jeopardy.

Experience with prolonged use of intravascular shunts in humans is limited. Johansen and colleagues reported three patients with lower-extremity intravascular shunts in place that underwent air transfer to a Level I trauma center for definitive care. Shunt times ranging from 12 to 17 hours were well tolerated and extremity ischemia minimized. No anticoagulation was used and no evidence of shunt thrombosis or distal emboli was observed.[37]

Experimentally, Aldridge and colleagues found that heparin-bonded polyvinylchloride intravascular shunts remained patent in the arterial circulation for a 24-hour period without evidence of distal embolization and no increase in coagulation factor or platelet consumption or red blood cell destruction. In that same model, venous shunts often were noted to be partially lined with mural thrombus. One of ten venous shunts thrombosed within 24 hours.[34] The value of major abdominal and pelvic vein shunting in critically injured patients is controversial, as published patency rates are low. However, it has been proposed that temporary shunting may help control short-term edema during acute high-volume resuscitation.

If no significant intra-abdominal bleeding has been identified, a retroperitoneal source should be considered and explored. This begins with the evisceration of the small bowel to inspect the aorta, iliac arteries and veins, and inferior vena cava. Next, retroperitoneal viscera (i.e., colon, kidneys, and duodenum) are mobilized.

Prolonged repair for bleeding from solid organ injuries must be avoided. Splenic and renal hemorrhage is managed best with resection. Bleeding from liver parenchyma is dealt with by manually displacing the liver inferiorly, followed by packing over the dome with multiple laparotomy pads. The space between the diaphragm and the liver is obliterated. Here the initial ligation of the falciform ligament helps prevent iatrogenic injury as the liver is mobilized. Next, the inferior surface of the liver is also tightly packed.

Ongoing bleeding from deep parenchymal injury then is controlled by the Pringle maneuver (temporary hepatic vascular inflow occlusion by compression of the Porta Hepatis within the lateral edge of the gastrohepatic ligament) followed by finger fracture to expose deep intraparenchymal bleeding vessels for suture ligation or clip application.[38]

More complex injuries (such as transhepatic gunshot wounds with long narrow columns of shredded hepatic parenchyma and active bleeding) require more innovative techniques. Insertion and inflation of a Foley catheter balloon or the use of an inflated Penrose drain over a red rubber catheter is a useful technique.[39,40]

Other strategies can be employed to deal with larger, actively bleeding liver parenchymal disruptions. Placement of hemostatic agents, such as microfibrillar collagen, cellulose sheets, or even fibrin glue within the liver wound itself, may provide additional hemostatic support.[41]

We have had great anecdotal success with the "liver tampon." This consists of a sausage-sized piece of absorbable gelatin sponge (Gelfoam™) cut into two centimeter by eight centimeter strips, soaked in thrombin solution, stacked to appropriate width, and wrapped in a sheet of oxidized cellulose (Surgicell™). It is stuffed into the parenchymal defect, followed by additional packing to effectively tamponade the bleeding and provide a hemostatic milieu.

In all cases of complex hepatic injury, we immediately follow the completion of DC I with angiography. Even in those cases where hemostasis seemingly is achieved, we have been surprised at the high incidence of intrahepatic arterial bleeding or arterio-venous fistula revealed by angiogram, which require therapeutic embolization. The care of the patient while in interventional radiology (IR) will be discussed in the DC II section.

Controlling Contamination

The second priority in a damage control laparotomy, following hemorrhage control, is to control the spillage of intestinal contents or urine from hollow viscus injuries.

Simple bowel perforations that are limited in size and number are repaired using a single-layer continuous suture and then tagged for later reinspection. More extensively injured bowel segments can be either isolated (using cotton umbilical tapes passed through the mesentery) or stapled across (using a linear stapler) on both sides of the wound. To save time, formal resection and reconstruction are avoided, as is stoma creation and feeding tube placement.

With high-velocity penetrating wounds, the extent of bowel wall edema and blast injury effects often are under appreciated at the initial operation; this can cause delayed bowel ischemia and threaten anastamoses and stomas. Therefore, bowel continuity is deferred until DC III following reevaluation of bowel viability.

Biliary tract and pancreatic injuries can be controlled temporarily by intra- or extraluminal tube drainage. This is important because of the damaging effects of the pancreatic enzymes and bile on surrounding tissues. Definitive repair or resection is delayed until physiologic restoration is achieved. Drains are brought out laterally through the flank at the mid-axillary line and intra-abdominal packs are carefully placed so as not to cause kinking of these tubes. Adjunctive studies, including endoscopic retrograde cholangiopancreatography (ERCP) or intraoperative distal pancreatography can be obtained prior to definitive repair if pancreatic and/or bile duct anatomy remains in question.[42]

Once all vascular and bowel injuries have been controlled, intra-abdominal packing is performed. This technique is especially important when coagulopathy is recognized and extensive retroperitoneal or pelvic dissection has been performed.[43,44] Folded laparotomy pads are placed over any solid organ injury and all dissected areas. Packing should be tight enough to provide adequate tamponade without impeding venous return or arterial blood supply.

Abdominal Closure

Abdominal closure is the final step prior to transport to the ICU. In all damage control cases, fascial closure is not recommended at the initial laparotomy. Secondary to reperfusion injury and ongoing capillary leakage during resuscitation, intestinal and abdominal wall edema will continue and potentially cause intra-abdominal hypertension, abdominal compartment syndrome, and fascial necrosis if there is not adequate provision for volume expansion. Skin-only closures allow for considerable expansion of the abdominal contents and wall while maintaining an insulating protective environment.

One of the most rapid methods of closing the abdomen is to place towel clips in the skin. Alternatively, a simple running nonabsorbable suture placed in the skin is adequate and has the added advantage of allowing ancillary studies (i.e., arteriogram) without radiopaque clamps obstructing the view.

At times, even skin closure is not possible because of massive bowel edema (i.e., bowel protrudes above the abdominal wall when viewed horizontally across the abdomen). In this situation, our practice has evolved from temporary silo-type devices (i.e., the Bogotá bag) to the placement of a vacuum pack (vac-pac) dressing (Figures 10-3–10-6). This dressing allows rapid temporary abdominal coverage and considerable increase in abdominal volume. Controlled egress of fluid from the abdomen is permitted and a sterile barrier is maintained while providing a durable dressing for possible prone-position ventilation.

First, the omentum, if present, should be used to drape the small bowel. Then a large Ioban™ (3M, St. Paul, MN) sheet is held adherent-side up as a sterile blue surgical towel is placed on top. The edges then are folded in and the completed pack is placed over the intestines and tucked beneath the fascia with the Ioban™ side in contact with the bowel to create a non-adherent surface. Two flat Jackson Pratt drains are laid alongside the pack and their ends brought out through separate skin stab wounds cephalad to the upper apex of the incision. A second large Ioban™ sheet then is placed adherent-side down over the abdomen and the intra-abdominal pack. To ensure that the Ioban™ sticks securely to the skin, all abdominal hair,

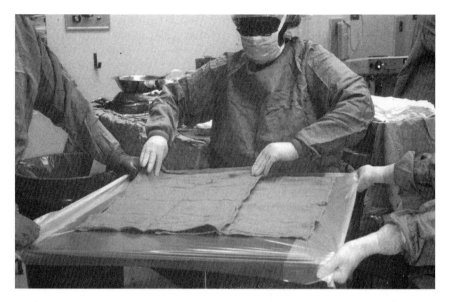

FIGURE 10-3. A sterile towel is covered on one side with adhesive plastic dressing and placed over the intestines and tucked under the fascial edges. (Hoey BA, Schwab CW. Damage control surgery. *Scand J Surg*. 2002;91;92–103).

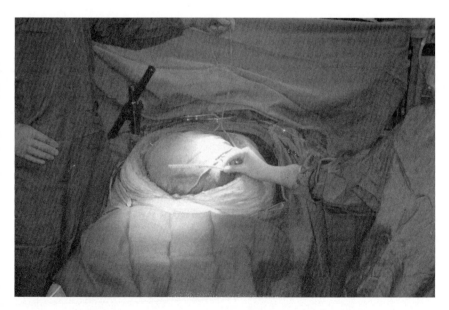

FIGURE 10-4. Closed suction drains are placed above the towel in the subcutaneous gutters and brought out superiorly through long subcutaneous tunnels. (Hoey BA, Schwab CW. Damage control surgery. *Scand J Surg*. 2002;91;92–103).

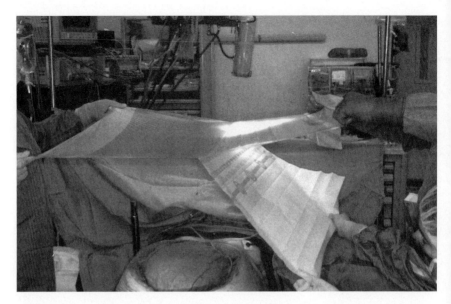

Figure 10-5. A second large adhesive drape is placed over the entire abdomen. (Hoey BA, Schwab CW. Damage control surgery. *Scand J Surg.* 2002;91;92–103).

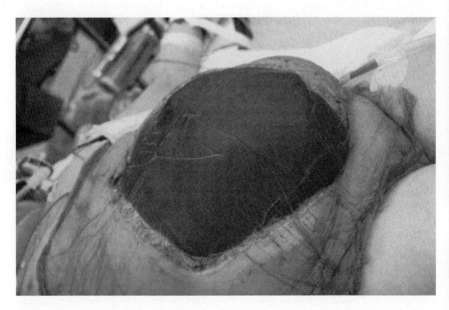

Figure 10-6. The drains are placed on continuous low suction, creating a vacuum effect; the wound is sealed. (Hoey BA, Schwab CW. Damage control surgery. *Scand J Surg.* 2002;91;92–103).

especially in the groin and the suprapubic areas, is shaved and the skin is painted with a thin layer of benzoin. No effort is made to approximate skin edges or force the abdominal wall edges together. The drains are placed on low-pressure, continuous wall suction, creating a vacuum. The drains allow controlled egress of fluid and blood, and the layered plastic dressing maintains a sterile, waterproof barrier.

Further Procedures

Damage Control Part I cannot be considered complete until all surgical bleeding is arrested, and occasionally a patient will require an interventional radiology procedure to achieve or prolong hemodynamic stability.

Uncontrolled surgical bleeding may not respond to packing alone, and often interventional radiology techniques are necessary to halt bleeding that could not be addressed adequately in the OR. This is particularly true for complex hepatic, retroperitoneal, pelvic, or deep muscle injuries that, because of location, are not amenable to surgical control or would require lengthy surgical exploration, often in the setting of coagulopathy.

Aberrant hepatic arterial anatomy is fairly common and branches arising from the SMA or celiac trunk are difficult to identify intraoperatively, but readily are seen on angiography. This also is true of bleeding lumbar arteries, as well as deep pelvic arterial bleeds.[45]

It is essential that DC II strategies be initiated and maintained during the time the patient spends in the interventional suite. Appropriate monitors, suction devices, respiratory support, patient and fluid warming devices, as well as capable nursing personnel must be available as the IR suite is transformed into an extension of the surgical ICU.

Damage Control Part II—ICU Resuscitation

The goal of DC II is to reverse the sequelae of shock-related metabolic failure and support physiologic and biochemical restoration. Here, simultaneous treatment of all physiologic abnormalities is essential. Preparations for this phase should begin prior to the completion of the initial laparotomy: warming the room, setting up appropriate hemodynamic monitoring devices, ventilator placement, preparing patient and IV fluid warming devices, communication with the blood bank, and assuring adequate nursing availability. The first several hours in the ICU are extremely labor intensive and often require the collaborative efforts of multiple nurses and ancillary staff.

One of the keys to physiologic restoration is the establishment of adequate oxygen delivery to body tissues. Invasive monitoring devices are used to direct this maximization of hemodynamics. In our practice, femoral artery catheters are preferred, as Dorman and colleagues showed that they provided more accurate measures of systolic and mean arterial pressures than radial artery catheter measurements if a patient required high vasopressor support during volume resuscitation.[46]

The use of the pulmonary artery catheter remains controversial. Although it has never been proven to enhance patient outcome in the critically ill, in the damage control subset of injured patients, the volumetric oximetry pulmonary artery catheter is a useful tool to assist in guiding resuscitation based on parameters of preload[47] and oxygen delivery.[48]

To date, the exact hemodynamic endpoints that patients must attain following severe injury in order to reliably survive remain controversial. Moreover, resuscitating patients to arbitrary endpoints of normal or supranormal hemodynamic and oxygen transport variables has not been shown to predict survival. Abramson and colleagues, however, did show that serum lactate clearance correlates well with patient survival and that the ability to clear lactate to normal levels within 24 hours was paramount to ensuing patient survival.[49]

Immediate and aggressive core rewarming not only improves perfusion, but also helps reverse coagulopathy. All of the warming maneuvers initiated in the trauma bay and operating room are duplicated in the ICU. These include increasing ambient room temperature, use of a turban or heating device on the patient's head, the application of a convective warm-air blanket or fluid-circulating heat blanket over the trunk and extremities, use of a heating cascade on the ventilator, administration of all resuscitative fluids and blood products through a high-flow warming system, and pleural, gastric, or bladder lavage with warmed fluids.

Occasionally, extracorporeal circulation devices such as veno–venous bypass and arterial–venous bypass via femoral vessel cannulation are necessary for rapid correction of severe hypothermia (core temperature 28–32°C). Rewarming rates of 2°C to 3°C per hour can be achieved with these devices. The limitations of veno–venous bypass include the need for systemic anticoagulation while arterial–venous bypass can be maintained with a heparin-bonded system.[50] However, this requires a normal systolic blood pressure to drive the flow. Gentilello and colleagues showed that failure to correct a patient's hypothermia after a damage control operation is a marker of inadequate resuscitation or irreversible shock.[51]

An aggressive approach to correction of coagulopathy is paramount in DC II. Standard therapy to correct coagulopathy includes reversal of hypothermia and administration of fresh frozen plasma (FFP), which is rich in factors V and VIII. Repletion of clotting factors with FFP continues until laboratory values of the PTT and international normalized ratio (INR) are normalized. Platelet levels also should be followed and corrected accordingly. Likewise, fibrinogen levels should be assessed and, if necessary, cryoprecipitate infused. All blood products should be warmed prior to infusion.

Factor VIIa

Recently, a new adjunct to the treatment of coagulopathy has been reported. Recombinant activated factor VII (rFVIIa) was developed as a prohemostatic agent for the treatment of bleeding episodes in patients with hemophilia A or B with inhibitors to factor VIII or IX, respectively. Recombinant activated factor VII is almost identical in structure and activity to human factor VII. It becomes active after forming a complex with tissue factor, which is located in the subendothelial media, and thus only is exposed to circulating blood after vessel injury. Formation of the tissue factor–rFVIIa complex initiates activation of factors IX and X, inducing a thrombin burst and faster formation of the fibrin clots at the site of vascular injury.[52]

A case report described the first successful use of rFVIIa in an exsanguinating penetrating trauma patient:[53]

A 19 year old soldier sustained a high-velocity rifle injury to the inferior vena cava and continued to bleed despite conventional surgical and medical attempts to restore hemostasis. Administration of rFVIIa 60 µg/kg corrected the coagulopathy and a second dose 1 hour later resulted in immediate cessation of bleeding.

Following this, the compassionate use of rFVIIa for patients suffering massive life-threatening bleeding as a result of surgery or trauma was approved by the Ethical Committee of the Israeli Ministry of Health. A subsequent series of seven critically ill coagulopathic multitransfused trauma patients, in whom conventional medical and surgical hemostatic techniques had failed, were treated with rFVIIa 40 to 120 µg/kg. The diffuse bleeding decreased within five minutes of the administration of 1 to 3 doses of rFVIIa, allowing identification of the vessels requiring surgical intervention. Blood requirements, PT, and activated PTT (aPTT) all were significantly decreased compared with pretreatment values after rFVIIa administration. Three of the seven patients died from causes other than bleeding or thrombotic events, and no thromboembolic complications were reported in any patient.[54]

Throughout DC II, the patient should remain sedated and receive complete ventilatory support. Arterial blood gases are used to guide ventilator adjustments.

Tertiary Survey

During this phase, a complete physical examination or "tertiary survey" of the patient should occur. Appropriate radiographs should be obtained to evaluate for additional skeletal injuries based on physical findings.

Immobilization and/or traction devices are applied when indicated. In the case of associated blunt mechanism, completion of the spine survey is imperative. Peripheral wounds are addressed and vascular integrity of all injured limbs is assessed frequently.

Adjunctive studies such as computed tomography (CT) scanning should be obtained at this time unless the patient is too unstable for travel.

Recruitment of consultants for all definitive repairs should occur early in this phase, and both the extent and priority of repairs must be established.

Unplanned Reoperation

Two subgroups of patients emerge who require "unplanned" reoperation during DC II prior to achieving physiologic restoration.

The first is the group of patients who continue to require packed red blood cell transfusions despite a corrected coagulopathy and normalized core temperature. These patients usually are found to have ongoing surgical bleeding from a vascular site that was not treated adequately during the initial damage control operation. Once recognized, immediate operative re-exploration to localize and stop the bleeding must occur. These patients have a very high mortality rate.[12,15]

The second group requiring unplanned return to the operating room have developed abdominal compartment syndrome (ACS). This syndrome, first suggested in 1863 by Marey, is a term used to describe a constellation of physiologic sequelae of increased intra-abdominal pressure (IAP) or intra-abdominal hypertension (IAH). It is characterized clinically by a tensely distended abdomen, elevated intra-abdominal pressure and peak airway pressure, impaired ventilation associated with hypoxia and hypercarbia, decreased urine output, increased systemic vascular resistance (SVR), and decreased cardiac output.[55]

Abdominal compartment syndrome has a reported incidence of 6% in patients with severe abdominal and/or pelvic trauma undergoing emergency damage control laparotomy.[56]

These patients are at high risk for the development of IAH from several causes: the use of bulky abdominal packs, continued bleeding into the abdominal cavity from uncorrected coagulopathy; bowel distension and edema from extensive resuscitation volumes (>10 liters), or mesenteric vascular injuries and abdominal wall edema.

Management of the open abdomen with the vacuum pack closure technique does not obviate the development of ACS.[57] This may be due to the efficiency with which the vac-pac dressing is able to contain the abdominal volume and allow subsequent intra-abdominal pressure increases to continue.

Vigilant monitoring of intra-abdominal pressure is mandatory in this patient population to recognize IAH and treat it expediently before ACS develops. This is done by intermittently transducing a urinary bladder pressure through the urinary catheter as described by Kron and colleagues.[58]

The technique consists of instilling 50 milliliters of saline into the urinary bladder via the Foley catheter. The tubing of the collecting bag is clamped and a needle is inserted into the specimen-collecting port of the tubing proximal to the clamp. This needle is attached to tubing that leads to a monitoring device (i.e., a central venous pressure monitor). Bladder pressures above 25 mm Hg signify intra-abdominal hypertension. Patients who develop intra-abdominal hypertension must be treated immediately to prevent ACS and its associated extreme mortality.[59]

Treatment consists of opening the patient's abdomen to relieve the pressure. If ongoing blood loss is suspected as the cause of the increased intra-abdominal pressure, this best is performed in the operating room, where lighting and equipment availability is maximized as long as the patient can tolerate the necessary transport. The alternative is to open the abdomen at the bedside in the ICU under sterile conditions. Occasionally, adequate decompression can be achieved without extensive operative intervention by incising the external Ioban™ drape of the vacuum pack to allow for further expansion of the neoabdominal wall prior to placement of a new sterile Ioban™ cover.

Damage Control Part III—Definitive Reconstruction

The primary objectives of DC III are definitive organ repair and fascial closure. Timing for this stage is critical to successful outcome. The decision to proceed is made on the belief that all physiologic and biochemical deficits have been corrected. The patient should be normothermic and should have normal coagulation studies and a normal pH and lactate. This state usually takes 24 to 36 hours to achieve following aggressive ICU management.

Occasionally, the timing of definitive repair is influenced by other clinical circumstances:

- One pressing concern that often leads to early planned reoperation is salvage of an ischemic limb due to shunt occlusion or suboptimal vascular repair following restoration of a normal coagulation profile.
- Other situations in which early planned reoperation is advisable include bowel that has been interrupted at several sites, resulting in a closed-loop obstruction that threatens bowel viability, and suboptimal control of spillage at the initial laparotomy from packed or drained duodenal, kidney, or bladder disruption.

Once in the operating room, the patient is prepped appropriately and draped for the definitive repairs ahead. The temporary abdominal dressing is prepped into the field prior to removal and subsequent exposure of the abdominal contents.

All packs are irrigated copiously and removed carefully; teasing them slowly away from all surfaces to avoid clot disruption. The surgeon must be prepared to accept failure if bleeding is encountered on pack removal that does not originate from an accessible vascular injury.

When repeated attempts to control the bleeding using local hemostatic measures fail, immediate repacking is the safest course of action to prevent massive blood loss and recurrent physiologic deterioration.

Following successful pack removal, a complete re-examination of the abdominal contents should occur, with particular attention paid to any previous repairs made during DC I.

Significant injuries often are overlooked, or only partially defined, during the rapidly performed initial laparotomy in an exsanguinating unstable patient.

Additional sites of bleeding are controlled, vascular repairs are performed, and intestinal continuity is restored using standard anastomatic techniques. Any bowel anastamoses should be covered with omentum and/or tucked-under mesentery to provide protection.

If fascial closure is not possible, percutaneous feeding tubes and stomas should be avoided, as they are associated with a high leak rate and make subsequent mobilization and separation of abdominal wall components difficult when closure eventually is performed. Instead, primary anastamoses should be created for gastrointestinal continuity, and both nasogastric tubes and nasoduodenal tubes should be placed and directed into position intraoperatively for proximal decompression and feeding, respectively.

If creation of a stoma becomes necessary, it should be placed laterally (lateral to the rectus muscles) through the obliques. Ideally, an ostomy should lie between the anterior and mid-axillary line of the abdominal wall.

Abdominal Closure

Once all of the repairs are completed, formal abdominal closure without tension is the final step in the planned reoperation sequence. Maneuvers to temporarily approximate the fascial edges should be performed with clamps. If gentle adduction allows the fascial edges to approximate, a standard fascial closure should be possible. However, persistent edema within the retroperitoneum, bowel wall, and abdominal wall often renders primary closure impossible at this time.

In general, if, when the abdomen is viewed from across the operating table, the bowels are above the level of the skin, then a low-tension primary closure is unlikely. A good rule to follow is that if the peak airway pressure rises more than 10 centimeters H_2O during temporary fascial approximation, then the fascia should be left open and the vac-pac closure replaced.

The patient then is returned to the ICU and aggressive diuresis is implemented over the next few days to decrease bowel and body wall edema if hemodynamically tolerated. During this period, the patient undergoes a daily abdominal washout, reinspection, and meticulous replacement of the vac-pac dressing so as not to promote fistula formation. This can occur at the bedside if personnel and resources are readily available. The majority of damage controlled open abdomens can be closed primarily within one week, especially if there is no sign of intra-abdominal infection.

The Whitman Patch^{TM} is used occasionally to assist in stepwise fascial closure during the period of diuresis. This device consists of two thin sheets of semi-rigid material comprised of a nonadherent undersurface with a Velcro-like material on the outer surface. Tiny perforations are present over the sheets to allow for the egress of third-space fluids. These sheets are sutured to the fascia on both sides of the abdominal wound, and when over-lapped with slight tension, allow for partial fascial approximation without threat of loss of domain. In effect, the fascia is trained under minimal tension and the gap between its edges can be reduced slowly with each sub-sequent daily abdominal washout. The nonadherent smooth undersurface prevents fistula formation, as the bowel wall is not irritated by contact. The patch is removed prior to definitive fascial closure. A limiting factor in the decision to use this device is its relatively high cost ($1000–$1200 per device). Alternatively, a stepwise silo-type closure can be performed with a durable nonadherent material (i.e., an opened three-liter intravenous bag sewn to the fascial edges) in a manner similar to that described in the pediatric surgical literature for neonates with an omphalocele or gastrochisis.[59] Gradual reduction in the size of the silo, and hence the wound, is achieved as the bag is incised, trimmed, and sutured closed during abdominal washout procedures.

Delayed Fascial Closure

If fascial closure still is not achieved after 7 to 10 days, the surgeon faces a number of alternatives that will cover the abdominal defect, but will leave the patient with a large ventral hernia. The first of these involves closing the skin with no attempt at fascial reapproximation. The patient then would undergo repair of the abdominal wall defect several months later. This often is not possible, as the gap is too wide, and despite skin flap mobilization, the edges cannot be approximated.

Alternatively, a vicryl (polyglycolic acid) mesh is placed over the entire abdominal wall defect and sutured to the fascial edges with the omentum, if available, first draped over the bowel so that frequent dressing changes do not promote formation of enteric fistulae.

Careful daily dressings with saline-soaked gauze are performed over this mesh, and the wound is allowed to granulate through the material. Once a smooth bed of granulation tissue is established (2–3 weeks), a split-thickness skin graft is applied to the granular bed.

Over the next 6 to 12 months, this skin graft will mature, separate, and develop a thin layer of connective tissue or fat between the underlying viscera. At this point, the patient is ready for excision of the skin graft and definitive reconstruction.

Many reconstructive techniques have been described in the literature, including the use of preoperative tissue expanders[60] and abdominal wall component separation with bilateral rectus release to achieve primary com-ponent closure with extra-fascial mesh support.[61] The involvement of a plastic surgeon at this step is advisable.

Damage Control—Beyond the Abdomen

More and more case reports are being generated describing the adaptation of damage control principals to severely injured patients with single or multiple injuries to regions of the body other than the abdominal cavity.

Damage control orthopedics describes caring for the patient with severe extremity injury in "extremis." The goal is hemorrhage control and maintenance of flow to distal tissues of the affected limb(s). External fixation of long bone and pelvic ring fractures is performed as an emergency procedure. Formal vascular repair occurs only if simple, otherwise temporary shunts are utilized. Rapid debridement and dressing placement then is performed and the patient is resuscitated in the ICU. This approach has been shown to minimize the duration of initial surgery, hypothermia, and additional blood loss. Formal internal fixation is delayed until the patient's physiology is restored.[62–64]

Damage control surgery principles have been applied selectively in the chest. In the physiologically exhausted patient, the definitive operation is abandoned in favor of an abbreviated thoracotomy.

In an unstable patient with a penetrating lung injury, stapled, non-anatomic wedge resection or pulmonary tractotomy with direct suture ligation of bleeding vessels can be performed. The latter technique works well when the site of hemorrhage is secondary to a deep through and through stab wound or gunshot wound. Here, the pulmonary parenchyma bridging the wound tract is divided using a linear stapling/cutting device. This permits direct inspection of the tract, with selective ligation of bleeding points and control of air leaks.[65]

Although packing of the pleural cavity is an option to temporarily control bleeding, it has obvious physiological consequences related to compression of the heart, great vessels, and viable lung tissue.

A recent case report out of Ben Taub General Hospital describes the "pulmonary hilum twist" as a thoracic damage control technique to control hemorrhage for severe lung trauma when a suitable hilar clamp is unavailable or if hilar control is particularly difficult with instrumentation. This procedure involves division of the inferior pulmonary ligament, then anterior rotation of the lower lobe over the upper lobe, achieving vascular occlusion. This occlusion can be maintained during resuscitation, and definitive resection can follow once physiologic parameters have improved.[66]

A report from Los Angeles described extending damage control principals to the neck.[67] In this report, bleeding in an unstable patient who had sustained a gunshot wound to zone II of the neck initially was controlled by insertion of two Foley catheters into the wound tract and inflation of the balloons. Uncontrollable hemorrhage from the vertebral vessels was encountered intraoperatively during exploration. Standard operative techniques to control bleeding only led to more hemorrhage as the patient became acidotic, hypothermic, and coagulopathic. The decision to damage control was made and the wound was packed tightly and the patient taken to the ICU for resuscitation, followed by the interventional radiology suite for embolization.

Damage Control—Trauma System Applications

The damage control approach can be applied in any operating room by general surgeons. Therefore, DC I principles are ideal for smaller hospitals where experience with these complex injuries may be limited and the resources necessary for resuscitation may be unavailable. Once DC I is completed and hemorrhage control is assured, the patient can be transferred to a regional trauma center for definitive repair.

References

1. MacKenzie EJ, Fowler CJ. Epidemiology. In: Mattox KL, Feliciano DV, Moore EE, eds. *Trauma*. 4th ed. New York: McGraw-Hill; 2000:21–39.
2. Sauaia A, Moore FA, Moore EE, et al. Epidemiology of trauma deaths: A reassessment. *J Trauma*. 1995;38:185–193.
3. Gaynor F. *The New Military and Naval Dictionary*. New York, NY: Philosophical Library Publishers; 1951.
4. Department of Defense. *Surface Ship Survivability*. Washington, DC: Department of Defense; 1996. Naval War Publication 3-20.31.
5. Richardson JD, Franklin GA, Lukan JK, et al. Evolution in the management of hepatic trauma: A 25-year perspective. *Ann Surg*. 2000;232:324–330.
6. Pringle J. Notes on the arrest of hepatic hemorrhage due to trauma. *Ann Surg*. 1908;48:541–549.
7. Halsted W. Ligature and suture material: the employment of fine silk in preference to catgut and the advantages of transfixing tissues and vessels in controlling hemorrhage—also an account of the introduction of gloves, gutta-percha tissue and silver foil. *JAMA*. 1913;LX:1119–1126.
8. Lucas C, Ledgerwood A. Prospective evaluation of hemostatic techniques for liver injuries. *J Trauma*. 1976;16:442–451.
9. Caln R, McMaster P, Pentlow B. The treatment of major liver trauma by primary packing with transfer of the patient for definitive treatment. *Br J Trauma*. 1978;66:338–339.
10. Feliciano D, Mattox K, Jordan G. Intra-abdominal packing for control of hepatic hemorrhage: A reappraisal. *J Trauma*. 1981;21:285–290.
11. Stone H, Strom P, Mullins R. Management of the major coagulopathy with onset during laparotomy. *Ann Surg*. 1983;197:532–535.
12. Rotondo M, Schwab CW, McGonigal, et al. Damage control: An approach for improved survival in exsanguinating penetrating abdominal injury. *J Trauma*. 1993;35:373–383.

13. Johnson JW, Gracias VH, Schwab CW, et al. Evolution in damage control for exsanguinating penetrating abdominal injury. *J Trauma*. 2001;51(2):261–271.
14. Shapiro MB, Jenkins DH, Schwab CW, et al. Damage control: Collective review. *J Trauma*. 2000;49:969–978.
15. Morris J, Eddy V, Blinman T, et al. The staged celiotomy for trauma: Issues in unpacking and reconstruction. *Ann Surg*. 1993;217:576–584.
16. Rotondo MF, Zonies DH. The damage control sequence and underlying logic. *Surg Clin North Am*. 1997;77:761–777.
17. Moore EE, Burch JM, Franciose RJ, et al. Staged physiologic restoration and damage control surgery. *World J Surg*. 1998;22(12):1184–1190.
18. Burch JM, Denton JR, Noble RD. Physiologic rational for abbreviated laparotomy. *Surg Clin North Am*. 1997;77:779–782.
19. Kashuk JL, Moore EE, Millikan JS, et al. Major abdominal vascular trauma: A unified approach. *J Trauma*. 198222:672–679.
20. Jurkovich GJ, Greiser WB, Luterman A, et al. Hypothermia in trauma victims: An ominous predictor of survival. *J Trauma*. 1987;27:1019–1024.
21. Cushman JG, Feliciano DV, Renz BM, et al. Iliac vessel injury: Operative physiology related to outcome. *J Trauma*. 1997;42:1033–1040.
22. Weg JG. Oxygen transport in adult respiratory distress syndrome and other acute circulatory problems: Relationship of oxygen delivery and oxygen consumption. *Crit Care Med*. 1991;19:650–657.
23. Gregory J, Flancbaum L, Townsend M, et al. Incidence and timing of hypothermia in trauma patients undergoing operations. *J Trauma*. 1991:31:795–800.
24. Ferrara A, MacArthur J, Wright H, et al. Hypothermia and acidosis worsen coagulopathy in the patient requiring massive transfusion. *Am J Surg*. 1990;169:515–518.
25. Abramson D, Scalea T, Hitchcock R, et al. Lactate clearance and survival following injury. *J Trauma*. 1993;35:584–588.
26. Lynn M, Jeroukhimov I, Klein Y, et al. Updates in the management of severe coagulopathy in trauma patients. *Intensive Care Med*. 2002;28:s241–s247.
27. Patt A, McCroskey B, Moore E. Hypothermia-induced coagulopathies in trauma. *Surg Clin North Am*. 1988;68:775–785.
28. Reed R, Bracey A, Hudson J. Hypothermia and blood coagulation: Dissociation between enzyme activity and clotting levels. *Circ Shock*. 1990;32:141–152.
29. Rohrer M, Natale A. Effect of hypothermia on the coagulation cascade. *Crit Care Med*. 1992;20:1402–1405.
30. McGowan E, Detwiler T. Modified platelet responses to thrombin. Evidence for two types of receptor or coupling mechanisms. *J Biol Chem*. 1986;261:739–746.
31. Gentilello LM, Pierson DJ. Trauma critical care. *Am J Respir Crit Care Med*. 2001;163:604–607.
32. Goodnight SH, Kenoyer G, Rapaport SI, et al. Defibrination after brain tissue destruction: A serious complication of head injury. *N Engl J Med*. 1974;290: 1043–1047.
33. Kearney T, Bentt L, Grode M, et al. Coagulopathy and catecholamines in severe head injury. *J Trauma*. 1992;32:608–611.
34. Garcia-Rinaldi R, et al. Unimpaired renal, myocardial, and neurologic function after cross clamping of the thoracic aorta. *Surg Gyn Obstetr*. 1976;143:249–252.
35. Reilly PM, Rotondo MF, Carpenter JP, et al. Temporary vascular continuity during damage control: Intraluminal shunting for proximal superior mesenteric artery injury. *J Trauma*. 1995;39:757–760.

36. Aldridge SD, Badellino MM, Malaspina PJ, et al. Extended intravascular shunting in an experimental model of vascular injury. *J Cardiovasc Surg.* 1997; 38(2):183–186.
37. Johansen KH, Hedges G. Successful limb reperfusion by temporary arterial shunt during a 950-mile air transfer. *J Trauma.* 1989;29:1289–1291.
38. Pachter HL, Spencer FC, Hofstetter SR, et al. Significant trends in the treatment of hepatic trauma. Experience with 411 injuries. *Ann Surg.* 1992; 215:492–502.
39. Poggetti RS, Moore EE, Moore FA, et al. Balloon tamponade for bilobar transfixing hepatic gunshot wounds. *J Trauma.* 1992;33:694–697.
40. Demetriades D. Balloon tamponade for bleeding control in penetrating liver injuries. *J Trauma.* 1998;44:538–539.
41. Shen GK, Rappaport W. Control of nonhepatic intra-abdominal hemorrhage with temporary packing. *SGO.* 1992;174:411–413.
42. Carrillo C, Folger RJ, Shaftan GW. Delayed gastrointestinal reconstruction following massive abdominal trauma. *J Trauma.* 1993;34:233–235.
43. Feliciano DV, Mattox KL, Burch JM, et al. Packing for control of hepatic hemorrhage. *J Trauma.* 1986;26:738–743.
44. Saifi J, Fortune JB, Graca L, et al. Benefits of intra-abdominal pack placement for the management of nonmechanical hemorrhage. *Arch Surg.* 1990;125:119–122.
45. Kushimoto S, Arai M, Aiboshi J, et al. The role of interventional radiology in patients requiring damage control laparotomy. *J Trauma.* 2003;54:171–176.
46. Dorman T, Breslow MJ, Lipsett PA, et al. Radial artery pressure monitoring underestimates central arterial pressure during vasopressor therapy in critically ill surgical patients. *Crit Care Med.* 1998;26:1646–1649.
47. Cheatham ML, Safcsak K, Block EF, et al. Preload assessment in patients with an open abdomen. *J Trauma.* 1999;46:16–22.
48. Bishop MH, Shoemaker WC, Appel PL, et al. Prospective, randomized trial of survivor values of cardiac index, oxygen delivery, and oxygen consumption as resuscitation endpoints in severe trauma. *J Trauma.* 1995;38:780–787.
49. Abramson D, Scalea TM, Hitchcock R, et al. Lactate clearance and survival following injury. *J Trauma.* 1993;35:584–589.
50. Gentilello LM, Cobean RA, Offner PJ, et al. Continuous arteriovenous rewarming: Rapid reversal of hypothermia in critically ill patients. *J Trauma.* 1992; 32:316–325.
51. Gentilello LM. Practical approaches to hypothermia. In: Maull KI, Cleveland HC, Feliciano DV, Rice LL, Trunkey DD, Wolfoth CC, eds. *Advances in Trauma and Critical Care.* Vol 9. St. Louis, MO: Mosby; 1994:9.
52. Lynn M, Jeroukhimov I, Klein Y, et al. Updates in the management of severe coagulopathy in trauma patients. *Intensive Care Med.* 2002;28:s241–s247.
53. Kenet G, Walden R, Eldad A, et al. Treatment of traumatic bleeding with recombinant factor VIIa. *Lancet.* 1999;354:1879.
54. Martinowitz U, Kenet G, Segal E, et al. Recombinant activated factor VII for adjunctive hemorrhage control in trauma. *J Trauma.* 2001;51:431–439.
55. Ivatury RR, Sugerman HJ. Abdominal compartment syndrome: A century later, isn't it time to pay attention? *Crit Care Med.* 2000;28:2137–2138.
56. Ertel W, Oberholzer A, Platz A, et al. Incidence and clinical pattern of the abdominal compartment syndrome after "damage control" laparotomy in 311

208   B. Braslow et al.

patients with severe abdominal and/or pelvic trauma. *Crit Care Med.* 2000;28:
1747–1753.
57. Gracias VH, Braslow B, Johnson J, et al. Abdominal compartment syndrome in
the open abdomen. *Arch Surg.* 2002;137:1298–1300.
58. Kron IL, Harman PK, Nolan SP. The measurement of intra-abdominal pressure
as a criterion for exploration. *Ann Surg.* 1984;199:28–30.
59. Rowlands BJ, Flynn TC, Fischer RP. Temporary abdominal wound closure with
a silastic "chimney". *Contemp Surg.* 1984;24:17–20.
60. Livingston DH, Sharma PK, Glantz AI. Tissue expanders for abdominal wall
reconstruction following severe trauma: Technical note and case reports.
J Trauma. 1002;32:82–86.
61. Fabian TC, Croce MA, Pritchard E, et al. Planned ventral hernia. Staged management for acute abdominal wall defects. *Ann Surg.* 1994;219:643–650.
62. Przkora R, Ulrich B, Zelle B, et al. Damage control orthopedics: A case report.
J Trauma. 2002;53:765–769.
63. Nowotarski PJ, Turen CH, Brumback RJ, et al. Conversion of external fixation
to intramedullary nailing for fractures of the shaft of the femur in multiply
injured patients. *J Bone Joint Surg Am.* 2000;82:781–788.
64. Scalea TM, Boswell SA, Scott JD, et al. External fixation as a bridge to
intramedullary nailing for patients with multiple injuries and femur fractures:
Damage control orthopedics. *J Trauma.* 2000;48:613–621.
65. Wall MJ, Villavicencio RT, Miller CC, et al. Pulmonary tractotomy as an
abbreviated thoracotomy technique. *J Trauma.* 1998;45:1015–1023.
66. Wilson A, Wall MJ, Maxson R, et al. The pulmonary hilum twist as a thoracic
damage control procedure. *Am J Surg.* 2003;186:49–52.
67. Firoozmand E, Velmahos G. Extending damage-control principals to the neck.
J Trauma. 2000;48:541–543.

11
Neck Injury

John P. Pryor and Bryan Cotton

Introduction

Colloquialisms such as "Go for the throat," and "He went straight for the jugular," demonstrate the layperson's appreciation for the vulnerability of the neck. Although the first recorded case of penetrating neck injury was found in the Edwin Smith papyrus[1] in 1800 BC, it was not until 1552 that Ambroise Paré performed the first surgical control of a cervical vascular injury.[2]

To this day, penetrating neck injuries continue to challenge the surgeon's knowledge of anatomy and technical ability. The management of a firearm injury involving the neck, more so than in any other area, requires the surgeon to make quick and accurate decisions about operative timing and approaches.[3] In no other region are problems with airway and hemorrhage control so dire and immediate. Thus, injury patterns and treatment algorithms must be clearly defined and understood before being faced with a patient with a penetrating wound to the neck.

With so many vital anatomic structures in a relatively small space, the majority of gunshot wounds (GSW) to the neck will demand immediate surgery. However, some injuries will be amendable to selective, nonoperative care. Success with nonoperative management has changed the algorithms for penetrating neck injuries over the last two decades. Prior to this time, mandatory exploration for all penetrating neck injuries was deemed standard of care.[4]

In the early 1980s, high-volume institutions with considerable experience in firearm injuries began reporting the selective, nonoperative management of patients with Zone II wounds presenting without physical exam evidence of vascular or aerodigestive injuries.[5,6] Concurrently, improvements in diagnostic technology such as helical computed tomography (CT) and interventional radiology augmented the sensitivity and specificity of the physical exam in detecting injuries. Several studies over the last decade supported the nonoperative approach of selected patients after an appropriate diagnostic evaluation had excluded injury.[7–9]

Despite these advances in selective nonoperative care, all surgeons who care for victims of gunshot injuries must be confident with operating in the neck and superior mediastinum. These skills are developed by refining anatomical knowledge, understanding diagnostic techniques, and mastering surgical options for a variety of injuries.

Anatomy

A surgeon who ventures into this area, whether electively or in a crisis, should have a solid, thorough knowledge of head, neck, and chest anatomy. The neck is bounded by the skull base superiorly, the thoracic inlet inferiorly, and contains numerous vital structures in a relatively small area.

Posteriorly, the central nervous system passes through the neck along the protected course of the spinal column, whereas the sympathetic chain, several cranial nerves, and the vagus nerve remain relatively unprotected in the accompanying soft tissue.

The hypopharynx and esophagus are situated ventral to the spinal column, separated by potential space lined by the prevertebral fascia. This prevertebral space communicates with the superior mediastinum and can be a potential area for spread of blood, air, or pus from the neck into the chest.

The course of the arterial vessels begins at the base of the neck with the aortic arch and its branches (Figure 11-1). As the common carotid arteries (CCA) near the thyroid and the hypopharynx, they divide into the internal and external carotid arteries. The internal carotid artery (ICA) is found lateral to the external carotid artery (ECA) and easily can be identified operatively by its lack of branches in the neck.

The internal jugular vein (IJV) is located anterior and lateral to the CCA, just underneath the sternocleidomastiod muscle (SCM). During the standard anterior SCM approach to the CCA, the vein is identified and retracted laterally with the muscle to gain access to the artery. Often a large facial vein is found crossing from the jugular vein laterally to the face. The facial vein often is ligated to free the SCM and IJV dissection. There is a thin investing layer of tissue, the carotid sheath that contains the CCA, the IJV, and the vagus nerve lying posterior and lateral to the CCA. Care should be taken to identify and avoid injury to the vagus during control of the CCA.

The aerodigestive structures are medial to the vessels (Figure 11-2). The thyroid cartilage is an easily identified surface marker for the larynx, with the cricrothyroid cartilage positioned just below and attached by the cricrothyroid membrane. The trachea begins just below the epiglottis at the level of the fifth cervical vertebra and is intimately related posteriorly to

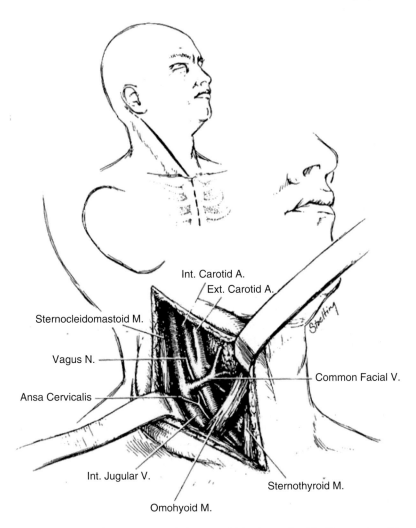

Int. Carotid A.

Ext. Carotid A.

Sternocleidomastoid M.

Vagus N.

Common Facial V.

Ansa Cervicalis

Int. Jugular V.

Sternothyroid M.

Omohyoid M.

FIGURE 11-1. Operative anatomy of the carotid is shown in this illustration. (From Ward RE. Injury to the cervical cerebral vessels. In: Blaisdell FW, Trunkey DD, eds. *Trauma Management: Cervicothoracic Trauma*. New York: Thieme; 1986:273, with permission).

the esophagus. Thus, posterior tracheal wounds often are associated with concomitant anterior esophageal injury. The recurrent laryngeal nerve is located in the tracheoesophageal groove and is responsible for causing tension on the ipsilateral vocal cord. The phrenic nerve is found on the anterior surface of the anterior scalene muscle, which sits deep to the SCM. The branches of the brachial plexus pass deep to the anterior scalene muscle to enter the axilla.

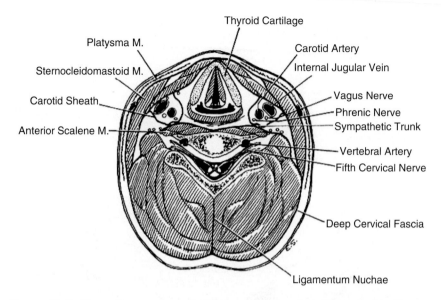

Thyroid Cartilage
Platysma M.
Sternocleidomastoid M.
Carotid Sheath
Anterior Scalene M.
Carotid Artery
Internal Jugular Vein
Vagus Nerve
Phrenic Nerve
Sympathetic Trunk
Vertebral Artery
Fifth Cervical Nerve
Deep Cervical Fascia
Ligamentum Nuchae

FIGURE 11-2. Operative anatomy of the deep neck space is shown in this illustration. (From Ward RE. Injury to the cervical cerebral vessels. In: Blaisdell FW, Trunkey DD, eds. *Trauma Management: Cervicothoracic Trauma*. New York: Thieme; 1986:273, with permission).

A system of dividing the neck into zones is useful to define anatomic regions of injury that correlate with diagnostic and therapeutic algorithms specific to those areas. The most common classification system divides the neck into three zones anterior to the lateral border of the sternocleidomastoid muscle (Figure 11-3):

- Zone I is bounded by the thoracic outlet at the clavicles and the cricoid cartilage;
- Zone II encompasses the area between the cricoid and the angle of the mandible;
- Zone III contains structures from the angle of the mandible to the base of the skull.

Each zone presents different challenges for the surgeon. Proximal vascular control of Zone I injuries is difficult and often involves an approach through a sternotomy or thoracotomy. Zone III injuries pose problems with distal control and special techniques such as mandibular subluxation may be needed. The approach to each zone of injury is discussed in length below.

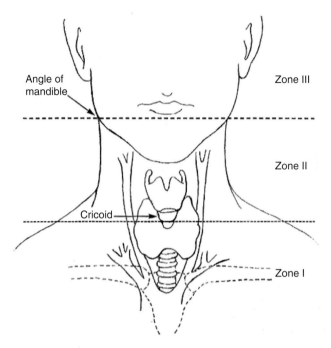

FIGURE 11-3. The neck typically is divided into three zones of injury. Each zone has preferred diagnostic and therapeutic approaches (From Maxwell, RA. Penetrating Neck Injury. In: Peitzman AB, Rhodes M, Schwab CW, Yealy DM, Fabian TC, eds. *The Trauma Manual.* Philadelphia: Lippincott Williams & Wilkins; 2002:192, with permission) (See also Figure 23.2).

Initial Assessment

Patients often arrive unstable with obvious active bleeding, an expanding hematoma, or airway compromise. Priorities include digital control of bleeding while all attention is focused on establishing a secure airway.

Airway

Since many patients with penetrating neck injuries will require an emergent airway procedure, rapid assessment is paramount. Since expanding hematomas and soft tissue swelling make endotracheal intubation more difficult as minutes go by after an injury, an experienced provider should attempt airway control as soon as possible.

A rapid sequence technique should be employed that uses cricoid pressure, liberal suctioning, sedatives, and paralytics to afford the best opportunity of success on the first pass. A trained individual should be at the head of the bed ready for a rescue technique, such as cricrothyroidotomy if endotracheal intubation fails.

In some cases, an endotracheal tube will not pass secondary to laryngeal and tracheal deviation from a neck hematoma and a surgical airway will be necessary and should be performed without hesitation.

On occasion, a neck incision performed as part of an emergency surgical airway will relieve the pressure on the airway, allowing the endotracheal tube to pass. Endotracheal tube or trachestomy tube placement should be confirmed with an end tidal CO_2 device.

Hemorrhage Control

Once the airway is secure, other maneuvers can be performed, including hemorrhage control and assessment for other injuries.

Control of external bleeding is accomplished best with direct digital control by a provider taking proper universal precautions.

Pressure should be applied in the area of the vessel injury, which may be far from the surface wound, allowing blood to exit. Simply plugging the surface wound will not slow bleeding and will cause an expansion of the hematoma over the area of vessel injury.

The exact area of vessel bleeding is not always obvious, and the practitioner should attempt pressure in different areas until the bleeding seems to minimize. Clamping of exposed vessels should only be done if the vessel is identified clearly and a vascular clamp is available. Blind clamping in an open wound often leads to associated nerve damage, increased vessel wall damage, and ineffectual hemorrhage control. Practitioners who have obtained digital control can be scrubbed into the operative field, continuing to hold pressure until operative control is obtained.

Breathing

Every neck wound should be thought of as a possible chest wound. The chest is examined and an early chest radiograph (CXR) is obtained to rule out hemopneumothoraces. Pleural capping seen on CXR may indicate injury to the great vessels and hemorrhage into the superior mediastinum (Figure 11-4). A completely normal CXR has been shown to be sensitive for ruling out great vessel injury.[10]

A full secondary examination should follow, including inspection of the back, axilla, and groin areas, to look for additional surface wounds. Blood should be available, and, if shock is already present, transfusion should not be delayed.

Deficit

The neurologic examination is very important in patients with potential carotid injury. A hemiplegia may herald inadequate collateral cerebral blood flow from a damaged carotid system and may greatly influence the

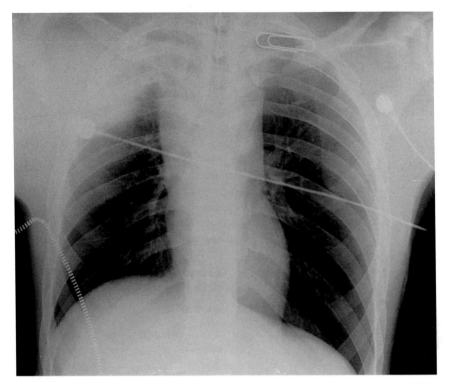

FIGURE 11-4. A chest radiograph in a patient with a gunshot wound to the base of the neck. The paperclip marks the surface wound on the anterior chest. Notice the large pleural cap on the right side as a result of hemorrhage from a proximal right common carotid injury.

operative decision-making. Thus, it is important to obtain and document a gross neurologic examination before the patient is sedated for intubation.

As opposed to patients injured by blunt trauma, firearm injuries are more likely to be associated with spinal cord injury. In addition to being a younger population, these patients are more likely to suffer complete spinal cord injury with subsequent paraplegia or tetraplegia than their blunt counterparts.[11]

Penetrating Injury and Cervical Spine Immobilization

Numerous authors have challenged the existence of cervical spine instability from a firearm injury in a patient who is neurologically intact. Apfelbaum and colleagues considered[12] cervical spine immobilization to be standard care in a blunt trauma patient.[12,13] This standard for blunt injury has been extrapolated to the patient with penetrating injury to the neck.[13]

The disadvantage of having a collar in place is that life-threatening injuries such as expanding neck hematomas may be overlooked.

Large studies dealing with combat casualties have shown that the incidence of unstable cervical spine injuries is less than 2%,[14] whereas the rate of missed life-threatening injuries by having a hard collar applied may be as high as 22%.[15]

Authors from these studies concluded that cervical spine immobilization in penetrating neck trauma is "neither prudent nor practical."

Investigation

Patients who arrive stable, without impending airway compromise or active bleeding, can be managed with appropriate trajectory-guided diagnostic studies. Patients with so-called soft signs, including hematemesis, hemoptysis, hoarseness or change in voice, dysphagia, or odynophagia, mandate further diagnostic evaluation.

Prior to considering nonoperative or selective management on a patient with penetrating neck trauma, one must consider the diagnostic modalities that are available and what degree of reliability can be placed on each of them.

The initial management of this group of patients should proceed in a similar fashion to that of the unstable patient. Although the sense of urgency may not appear as obvious, these patients have the potential for rapid deterioration; thus, early assessment of the airway, breathing, and circulation is essential. Some centers rely solely on the physical exam to guide their decisions for operative or nonoperative management, whereas others will employ a cadre of diagnostic tests to definitively exclude injuries to the structures within the neck.[4,16]

Trajectory Determination

As early as 1987, Pass and colleagues noted that findings on plain radiographs (prevertebral soft tissue swelling, missile fragmentation, missiles adjacent to major vessels) could be useful in predicting anatomic injury.[17] Identifying and marking all wounds (with radio-opaque markers such as a paper clip) and assessing possible trajectories with radiographs and or CT can help define likely anatomic injuries and guide diagnostic evaluations.[18] Nemzek and colleagues noted in clinical findings that plain radiographs lack the specificity necessary to exclude injuries to the neck structures. They concluded that a high index of suspicion, based on the bullet trajectory, is essential for early diagnosis of aerodigestive injuries.[18]

Compared to missiles that do not cross the midline, transcervical GSWs are twice as likely to injure vital structures in the neck. This has led some authors to suggest that these wounds be considered as a separate category of neck trauma, and even advocate mandatory exploration in this special population.[19] Demetriades and colleagues also noted a high incidence of injuries in transcervical GSWs, but found that less than one-fourth of patients required exploration.[9] They concluded that a careful clinical examination combined with the appropriate diagnostic tests could safely select the appropriate treatment.

Over the last decade, numerous authors have examined the role of CT scan in the trajectory determination of penetrating torso injuries.[20–22] Recently, several institutions have examined the use of CT scan in accurately determining the missile trajectory and, therefore, defining the anatomic injuries in penetrating neck trauma.[23] Gracias and colleagues retrospectively evaluated helical CT scan in firearm injuries to the neck.[24] Approximately 60% of patients had "trajectory consistent with injury" excluded by CT scan (Figure 11-5). Forty percent underwent angiography

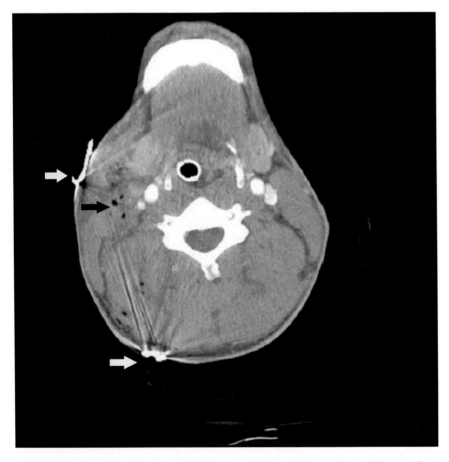

FIGURE 11-5. A computed tomography image of the neck in a patient with a gunshot wound. In select cases, CT can be used to determine trajectory and screen for possible injuries. White arrows indicate clips used to mark entrance and exit wounds; black arrow indicates air in tissue along the bullet path (see also Figure 23-3).

because of proximity, and less than ten percent required endoscopy. They concluded that, in stable patients with penetrating neck injuries, CT scan can safely and accurately determine trajectory consistent with injury. A prospective study from Mazolewski and colleagues noted sensitivity of CT scan for significant injury was 100%, with a specificity over 90%.[23] They concluded that CT scan could help to eliminate the need for mandatory exploration and limit the need for further diagnostic testing.

Vascular Evaluation

In the neck, evaluation of the vascular system begins with a rapid search for the "hard signs" of vascular injury, which include pulsatile bleeding, expanding hematomas, and bruits. Patients with these hard signs require immediate operative care, as discussed below.

Once hard signs have been excluded, vascular assessment proceeds with an examination for any neurologic deficits. Neurological deficits such as hemiplegia or unilateral cranial nerve deficit are soft signs of carotid injury and also may need exploration.

Early in the evaluation of these stable patients is the decision whether or not to use angiography to identify vascular injury. The decision involves understanding the utility of the procedure and the indications based on physical examination.

Angiography

In patients who are hemodynamically stable, without hard signs of injury, angiography remains the gold standard for evaluating and excluding arterial injury.[25] When an injury is found, angiography can provide invaluable anatomical information that may aid in planning the operative approach, especially when more than one zone is involved. In addition, angiography may have a therapeutic role in selected cases where embolization or endovascular stenting is possible.

The procedure most often is performed in the radiology department, although some centers have angiography capabilities in the operating room. A typical exam will visualize the innominate, common, internal, and external carotid arteries, the subclavian arteries, and both vertebral arteries.[26]

Angiography has its greatest utility in Zone I and Zone III injuries. Because these areas have a greater difficulty of operative exposure relative to Zone II, precise anatomical information on the location and extent of injury is paramount.[27] Angiography for Zone III injuries has been shown to facilitate triage decisions, and many injuries, with the use of various interventional techniques, can be managed without surgical exploration.[28]

Until recently, the majority of trauma centers recommend a policy of routine angiography to screen for vascular injury and to minimize non-therapeutic neck explorations.[29-30] The procedure, however, is an invasive and costly procedure with a yield in most centers of less than two percent.[11] Thus, a more modern approach is to use angiography in selected patients with soft signs of injury or a concerning trajectory determined by other diagnostic tests (CT scans).

Physical Examination

Several studies over the past decade have demonstrated that, in the absence of signs of vascular injury, penetrating injuries limited to Zone II can be managed safely on physical exam alone.[5,9,11,12]

Atteberry and colleagues evaluated 28 patients with Zone II neck injuries and no signs of vascular injury.[7] They concluded that physical examination alone was safe and accurate in evaluating this patient population for vascular injury. In a follow-up study from the same institution, Sekharan and colleagues observed 91 patients with no signs of vascular injury for a 23-hour period without further diagnostic evaluation.[31] Physical examination had a false-negative rate of 0.7%. The authors concluded that physical examination is safe and accurate and much less invasive or costly than arteriography. Their follow up, however, was limited to two weeks post injury.

Supporting these findings, Biffl and Beitsch concluded that asymptomatic patients with Zone II neck injuries could be observed, in the presence of a normal physical examination, with less than a one-percent chance of a missed injury. Beitsch and colleagues retrospectively evaluated 178 patients with Zone II injuries, all of which had undergone angiography and operative exploration.[32] Biffl and colleagues extended their policy to Zone III, but continued to recommend that Zone I injuries should have an arteriogram.[33-34]

Jarvick and colleagues noted physical examination to have a sensitivity of 100% for detecting vascular injuries that required intervention.[35] In addition, they calculated the cost of using angiography as a screening tool for identifying vascular injury in patients with a normal physical examination. The authors noted the cost to be over three million dollars per central nervous system event prevented.

As for Zone I injuries, a multi-institutional study group recently published their findings on whether routine arteriography is necessary for penetrating injuries to this area of the neck. Eddy and colleagues reported the results of a study of five level-one trauma centers that examined all Zone I injuries over a ten-year period.[10] They found no arterial injuries in patients with a normal physical examination and normal chest radiograph. With some caution, the authors concluded that this subgroup of patients could be managed safely without arteriography.

Computed Tomographic Angiography

With dramatic improvements in image quality and advances in software, computed tomography is becoming the standard diagnostic tool for many traumatic injuries. Computed tomographic angiography (CTA) is performed using a high-speed helical scanner with a timed injection that results in opacification of the neck vessels during data acquisition. Images then are reconstructed with one- to three-millimeter intervals. In addition to evaluating vascular injury, it has the advantage of providing information on the soft tissue, bone, and missile trajectory all in one exam (Figure 11-6).

Munera noted CTA to be a safe alternative to conventional angiography in patients with penetrating neck injuries.[37] The authors conducted a prospective study over twenty-four months in patients with penetrating neck trauma who were referred for conventional angiography. They found CTA to have a high sensitivity and specificity for detecting major carotid and vertebral arterial injuries from penetrating trauma. Computed tomo-

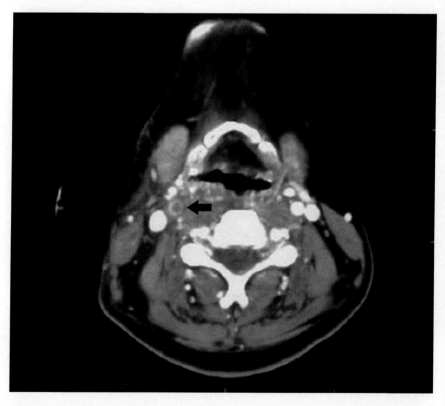

FIGURE 11-6. A CT angiogram image of the neck in a patient with a stab wound. In this case, a right carotid thrombosis (associated with a dissection) can be seen as a filling defect within the lumen of the vessel (black arrow).

graphic angiography had a 100% positive predictive value and a negative predictive value of 98% compared to conventional angiography.

In 2002, a study from the same institution found similar results and concluded that CTA could be used as the initial method of evaluation and that conventional angiography could be reserved for those patients with equivocal studies.[36]

Other authors also have investigated the role of CTA as a safe and accurate alternative to conventional angiography.[37,38] Ofer and colleagues noted that all CTA obtained were diagnostic and confirmed their findings on surgical exploration. The authors concluded that CTA of the carotid arteries might be used as an accurate decision tool for surgical intervention.

Color Flow Doppler

In the early 1990s, Color-flow Doppler (CFD) began augmenting angiography in the evaluation of arteriosclerotic carotid artery disease. Shortly thereafter, Fry and colleagues reported their results on the application of CFD to traumatic carotid injuries.[39] Their prospective study of 100 patients found no false positives or false negatives compared to angiography as the gold standard. Although the study only included eight injuries, they concluded that CFD was as accurate as conventional angiography in diagnosing cervical vascular injuries.

Corr reported similar findings and made recommendations for utilizing CFD to screen for injury.[40] After evaluating fifty-two patients prospectively with CFD, Montalvo and colleagues were more cautious in their recommendations of CFD replacing angiography in penetrating neck injuries.[41]

Demetriades and colleagues evaluated several diagnostic modalities among a group of 223 patients.[42] After excluding patients with injuries that did not require intervention, CFD had a sensitivity and specificity of 100%. They estimated the financial impact of developing an algorithm based on their findings and noted the cost of evaluating penetrating neck injuries would decrease from 450000 to 30000 US dollars.

Although CFD is inexpensive and noninvasive, most authors are quick to point out that this test is extremely operator dependent and that physicians specializing in sonography interpreted their studies.

Magnetic Resonance Angiography

The use of magnetic resonance angiography (MRA) has been shown to be accurate in diagnosis of blunt cerebrovascular injury (BCVI).[43-45] Magnetic resonance angiography allows direct visualization of mural thrombus and determination of the length of the dissection. Dissections are characterized by eccentric hyperintense signaling on T1-weighted and T2-weighted images.[46] However, Biffl and colleagues have noted the limitations of MRA in detecting lower-grade injuries, which are the type of carotid injuries noted in most series of angiograms for penetrating neck injuries.[47–50] Other authors have published similar conclusions regarding the role of MRA in the evaluation of penetrating neck injuries.[21,51,52] Currently, there is insufficient data to suggest that MRA be used as the definitive evaluation of penetrating neck injuries.

Esophageal and Pharyngeal Evaluation

Digestive tract injuries are difficult to diagnose preoperatively when other life-threatening injuries obscure the subtle signs of hypopharyngeal or esophageal trauma. Clinical findings suggestive of hypopharyngeal or esophageal penetration include:

– dysphagia
– odynophagia
– hemoptysis
– hematemesis
– subcutaneous emphysema.

Major injuries often are accompanied by pneumomediastinum on CXR or CT scan. Missed injuries can cause severe irritation and eventual infection of the soft tissue in the neck, and potentially the chest. Thus, early diagnosis and treatment is important to avoid major morbidity.

Physical Examination

Mandatory exploration for patients with penetrating neck injuries has been advocated, in part, to avoid a missed (and potentially fatal) injury to the hypopharynx and esophagus.[34,53] Proponents of selective management, however, have argued that the high incidence of negative explorations and the associated morbidity outweighed the small chance of missing a digestive tract injury.[54] Several recent studies have examined the ability of clinical examination to detect injury in these patients.[9,34,45,46]

Investigators at the University of Southern California (USC) have published several articles regarding the accuracy of clinical examination and other diagnostic modalities in detecting esophageal injuries from penetrating trauma.[8,26] They found signs or symptoms suggestive of esophageal injury in over twenty percent of patients presenting with penetrating neck injuries, but confirmed injuries in less than three percent. However, of the 152 patients without clinical signs or symptoms, none had an injury requiring an operation (negative predictive value of 100%).

To determine safe criteria for the management of patients with crepitance of the neck, Goudy and colleagues reviewed the charts of 236 patients with the diagnosis of aerodigestive tract injury or subcutaneous emphysema.[55] Nineteen patients were identified with cervical emphysema and/or crepitance. Of these, twenty percent complained of dysphagia and two-thirds had hoarseness or stridor. Diagnostic laryngoscopy identified injuries to the hypopharynx or larynx in 80% of patients.

Other investigators, however, have shown the inaccuracy of clinical findings in predicting penetrating injury to the aerodigestive tract. Noyes noted that the more common and sensitive physical findings (shock, expanding hematoma, hemorrhage, and subcutaneous crepitance) are not specific for the organ injured and often occur in the absence of serious injury.[56] These authors reported an overall accuracy of 72% when clinical findings were used to predict injuries in penetrating neck wounds.

An evaluation of physical examination performed by Back and colleagues was even less promising.[57] Clinical signs or symptoms suspicious for digestive tract injury were present in only three of the eight patients with documented injury. Most of these clinical findings were nonspecific and could be attributed to laryngotracheal injuries. Studies by other authors also have stressed the unreliability of using clinical findings alone.[58]

Despite the promising results from USC investigators, physical examination does not appear reliable in excluding injuries to the esophagus following gunshot wounds.

Esophagography Versus Esophagoscopy

Controversy remains in the literature as to the optimal methods of evaluating the aerodigestive tract after firearm injury.

Diagnostic options range from mandatory surgical exploration to various combinations of radiographic and endoscopic inspection to close clinical observation. Much of the ongoing disagreement created by proposed management algorithms is derived from the difficulty in detecting aerodigestive tract injuries relative to vascular injuries caused by penetrating wounds.[50]

A retrospective review of 23 cervical esophageal injuries showed that contrast esophagography had only a 62% success rate in identification of cervical esophageal violations compared to 100% for rigid esophagoscopy.[59] However, rigid esophagoscopy is associated with serious complications such as dental injuries, bleeding, and aspiration. Critics of rigid evaluation also have noted the need for general anesthesia and less image quality as reasons to utilize flexible esophagoscopy.[55,56,57]

Flexible endoscopy is being used more often by young surgeons who completed their training with little to no experience with rigid esophagoscopy. Srinivasan and colleagues evaluated fifty-five patients who underwent emergent flexible endoscopy for the evaluation of penetrating neck injuries in an attempt to determine if flexible endoscopy was safe and what impact it had on the management of the patient with penetrating neck injury.[60] Flexible endoscopy was performed safely in all patients with a sensitivity of 100% and specificity of 92% for detecting an esophageal injury. The authors concluded that flexible endoscopic examination of the esophagus is safe in the early evaluation of penetrating neck injuries. Their findings are similar to that of Flowers and colleagues, who noted 100%

sensitivity and 96% specificity for flexible endoscopy. Critics, however, have noted that the "blind passage" of the flexible scope through the hypopharynx increases the risk of missing mucosal defects in the upper cervical esophagus.[59]

Contrast studies require a stable, cooperative patient and are difficult to obtain in agitated or intubated patients. The sensitivity of contrast esophagography in patients with esophageal trauma varies from 48 to 100%.[61] The contrast agent and technique employed for esophageal evaluation both have a significant effect on the sensitivity and accuracy of this modality.[59] Water-soluble agents are less viscous and dense and therefore are less likely to coat the mucosa adequately. Up to fifty percent of esophageal perforations will be missed if a water-soluble agent is used alone.[62] To slow contrast transit time, and therefore provide a more adequate study, the patient should be placed in the decubitus position. Patients unable to safely swallow should have the contrast agent instilled through a nasogastric tube under pressure.[59] A thorough and properly performed swallow study should detect eighty to ninety percent of esophageal injuries.[59,63]

Combined Modalities

When used alone, esophagoscopy and esophagography have sensitivities of sixty to eighty percent. Combining the two, however, increases the sensitivity of detecting esophageal injury following penetrating trauma to well over ninety percent.

Demetriades and colleagues noted that physical examination combined with both endoscopy and esophagography detected 100% of penetrating esophageal injuries.[39] Weigelt and colleagues evaluated 118 patients with penetrating neck injuries and no evidence of hard signs. The combination of esophagography with esophagoscopy identified all esophageal injuries. The authors concluded that patients with penetrating neck trauma and minimal clinical findings should be evaluated initially with arteriography and esophagography.[64]

Glatterer and colleagues evaluated twenty-one injuries to the cervical esophagus, all of which underwent surgical exploration. Esophagography was positive in seventy-five percent of patients, esophagoscopy was positive in eighty-three percent.[65] A combination of the two modalities would have detected all esophageal injuries.

Laryngotracheal Evaluation

Injuries to the larynx and trachea are uncommon, but are associated with significant morbidity and mortality. The risk of death and complications associated with these injuries can be minimized by aggressive airway control and an expedient search for occult injuries, respectively.

The endotracheal approach to intubation has been shown to be safe in selected patients with laryngotracheal injuries.[66] This approach allows for controlled placement of the endotracheal tube, as well as the evaluation of the hypopharynx, larynx, and proximal trachea through direct laryngoscopy. Once the airway is controlled, a careful evaluation of the laryngotracheal tree should be undertaken.

Physical Examination

Patients with laryngotracheal injury often present with obvious signs of airway injury, such as stridor, dyspnea, or subcutaneous crepitance.[54] As with the digestive tract, physical examination findings are sensitive for detecting airway injury, but they lack specificity.

Some authors have suggested that asymptomatic patients could be observed safely regarding potential airway involvement.[22,35]

Others, however, have suggested patients at risk receive endoscopic evaluation in the form of diagnostic laryngoscopy, tracheobronchoscopy, or both.

Diagnostic Laryngoscopy (DL) and Tracheobronchoscopy

Diagnostic laryngoscopy is utilized to evaluate the hypophayrnx following Zone III injuries, whereas tracheobronchoscopy is suited better for examination of Zones I and II. Demetriades and colleagues noted that DL detected all major injuries to the laryngotracheal region, as well as mild injuries such as pharyngeal edema and submucosal hemorrhage.[67]

Other authors have noted that DL detects over ninety percent of laryngotracheal injuries, and when combined with tracheobronchoscopy, sensitivity approaches one hundred percent.[13,58]

More recently, investigators at the University of Southern California prospectively evaluated 149 patients with penetrating neck injuries using flexible endoscopy.[67] They noted abnormalities in approximately sixteen percent of endoscopies and no missed injuries. They concurred with previous authors that flexible fiberoptic bronchoscopy is the diagnostic modality of choice in detecting laryngotracheal injuries.

Operative Approaches

In general, patients should be positioned in the supine position with the arms abducted to ninety degrees to allow access to the neck, chest, and proximal arm. Positioning with the patient's arms tucked and at their sides is a reasonable option if the patient's trajectory is determined to be one in which proximal control can be obtained without the need for thoracotomy.

Unless a cervical spine injury is suspected, the neck should be extended and rotated to the opposite side (15–20 degrees) (see Figure 11-1). To allow for full neck extension, the shoulders should have a bolster placed under them (pillow, rolled sheet(s)).

Skin preparation should extend from the ears to the middle of the abdomen, with at least one groin prepped out for the possibility of saphenous vein harvest.

The scrub team should have a full vascular and thoracic set available, including a sternal saw, vascular shunts, and Fogarty balloon catheters. A blood recycling system, such as a cell saver, should be immediately available. The exact incision depends on the anticipated injury and the neck zone that needs to be explored.

Zone I Injury

Injuries involving the superior mediastinum and Zone I of the neck are very challenging and require the most forethought on how to approach them. Patients with injuries in this area almost always present with unstable vital signs or in extremis, and thus there is often little time for extensive preoperative planning. A median sternotomy with a sternocleidomastoid extension is the most versatile approach, allowing exposure of the great vessels and carotid system on the side of the extension.[24,68] The only limitation of this approach is difficulty controlling the proximal left subclavian artery, which exits the aorta in a very posterior position in the left chest.

If there is a suspicion of a proximal left subclavian artery injury, the best incision for proximal control is a posterior, high (3–4 interspace) thoracotomy.

Utilization of a supraclavicular incision can provide exposure and allow for vascular control of injuries to the right subclavian and distal two-thirds of the left subclavian artery.[25]

Extension into a "trap-door" sternotomy is rarely necessary to approach or repair any neck injury.[24] A median sternotomy provides ample exposure for injuries involving the innominate or common carotid arteries at the takeoff of the aorta. Early division of the innominate vein will allow full exposure to the base of these great vessels and can be done with minimal morbidity.

Dissection of the mediastinal fat and thymus remnant can be accomplished quickly by dividing all tissue above the vessels with an endovascular stapling device.

Zone II Injury

An anterior sternocleidomastoid (SCM) incision is the standard for adequate exposure of unilateral neck injuries.

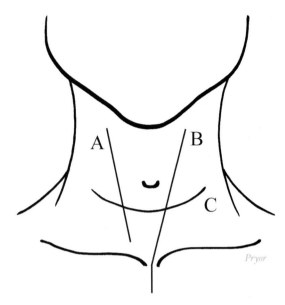

FIGURE 11-7. Operative approaches to the neck include (A) the sternocleidomastoid incision, (B) the sternocleidomastoid incision with sternotomy extension, and (C) the collar incision.

Bilateral SCM incisions joined inferiorly or in the mid-portion (H-shaped incision) can be used for bilateral injuries (Figure 11-7). The incision should be planned in such a way that a tracheostomy, if needed, can be performed through a separate incision.

Alternatively, for bilateral exploration, a transverse (collar) incision can provide adequate exposure for the majority of Zone II injuries. Both the collar and the SCM incisions can be extended quickly into the chest should a sternotomy be required.[69] Carotid injuries in Zone II can be visualized adequately through either incision. If the extent of injury extends into either Zone I, a sternotomy may be used if more proximal exposure is necessary. For those extending distally (or into Zone III), division of the omohyoid and/or digastric muscle will increase exposure. Care should be taken to avoid injury to the hypogastric and glossopharyngeal nerve that pass medial to lateral, superficial to the internal carotid in this area. If necessary, anterior subluxation of the mandible may be utilized for those injuries requiring extreme distal exposure.[70]

After making the skin and subcutaneous incision along the lateral border of the SCM, the facial vein will be encountered crossing lateral to medial into the internal jugular. The internal jugular vein (IJV), which lies just deep to the SCM, is retracted laterally, exposing the carotid sheath. If hematoma is seen within the sheath, proximal control of the common carotid artery should be obtained. After vascular control, full exposure of the injury is necessary, including inspection of the posterior wall of the vessel. The trachea and esophagus lie medial to the vessels and can be explored fully through the standard SCM incision.

Zone III Injury

Due to the inherent difficulty in evaluating and obtaining vascular control in this area, selective management of injuries to Zone III has arisen out of necessity. Management of vessel injury high in Zone III is approached best by interventional angiography, where selective embolization can be used to arrest hemorrhage (Figure 11-8). If proximal control can be obtained, distal control of Zone III (and even some Zone II) injuries can be obtained through the placement and inflation of a Fogarty balloon catheter. This allows for the surgeon to further expose necessary vessels for vascular control or provides control of distal bleeding until interventional radiology or endovascular treatments can be employed.

If distal control of a high Zone II injury is necessary in the operating room, there are several techniques that can be used to access the distal internal and external carotid vessels. Division of the posterior belly of the digastric muscle will begin to free more length on the carotid distally. Anterior subluxation of the mandible can be performed by traction on the jaw, pulling the jaw forward out of the temporomandibular joint. Some maneuver will be needed to hold the jaw in this prognathic position. Alternatively, resection of the angle of the mandible or styloid process has been described, although these are more complex procedures to perform.[71]

Associated injury involving the hypogastric and glossopharyngeal nerve increases as the exposure proceeds towards the base of the skull.

Difficult Management Decisions

Should Carotid Artery Injuries be Repaired?

Carotid artery injuries account for ten to twenty percent of life-threatening injuries that occur in patients with penetrating neck trauma, and the literature evaluating the management of these injuries is controversial.[72–74]

The primary objective during operative management is to restore antegrade flow to the carotid and preserve neurological function.

Carotid injuries should be repaired unless the surgeons is faced with:

1. uncontrollable hemorrhage,
2. ongoing hemodynamic instability,
3. a comatose patient presenting with no evidence of antegrade flow, or
4. a devastating vessel injury technically impossible to temporize with a vascular shunt.[75]

In these circumstances, ligation can and should be employed.[70,71]

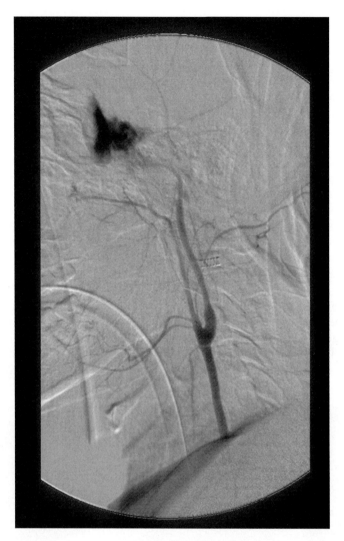

FIGURE 11-8. This cerebral angiogram in a patient with a Zone III neck gunshot wound shows active exsanguination from a very distal carotid injury. The only approach to this injury is by endovascular embolization.

Some authors also have advocated ligation if there is little to no "back bleeding" from the carotid artery, citing the likelihood of worsening an established ischemic infarct or risk of embolizing a distal clot with attempts at restoring blood flow.[72,73]

Injuries involving the external carotid exclusively can be ligated with minimal morbidity.

How Should Carotid Injuries be Repaired?

Some authors have advocated the routine use of shunts during the repair, while others argue that they should only be employed if "back" pressures are less than 60 millimeters Hg.[74] A shunt should be used if there will be a significant delay in the arterial repair, such as in cases where multiple other injuries need immediate attention. Commercially available carotid shunts are preferable; however, any suitable conduit may substitute is needed (Figure 11-9).

If available, heparin-bonded shunts may help to prevent small thrombus formation with embolization during the shunting procedure. Long-term shunts should only be considered in dire circumstances on account of the risk of embolization.

Vessels damaged by gunshot injury typically have intimal damage beyond the lacerated ends of the artery. Adequate dedridement is necessary back to normal looking vessel free of intimal dissection or mural hematoma before repair should be attempted.

Primary repair is not often possible in gunshot injury because adequate debridement of nonviable tissue often leaves a significant gap in vascular continuity. Likewise, a vein or Dacron patch is only rarely an option because the tissue around even a small defect often is damaged and should be debrided. The best option for repair is a formal bypass graft (Figure 11-10) Options for homogenous conduit include saphenous vein from the groin,

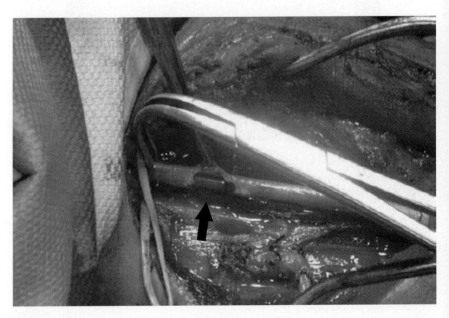

FIGURE 11-9. A gunshot wound to the right common carotid artery with an intraluminal shunt in place (black arrow).

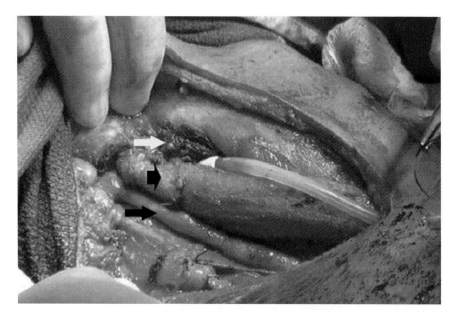

FIGURE 11-10. This patient had both a carotid transection and a pharyngeal injury. Note that the sternocleidomastoid muscle (thick black arrow) has been rotated to protect the vascular anastamosis (thin black arrow) from the drain exiting superiorly (white arrow).

ipsilateral facial vein, or contralateral external jugular vein. The ipsilateral internal and external jugular should be preserved to help with venous outflow on the side of arterial repair.[75]

Polytetrafluoroethylene (PTFE) grafts have been employed with increased frequency when primary repair is not possible. Recently, Thompson and colleagues advocated the use of PTFE as the conduit of choice, even in settings where a saphenous vein is available.[74] They noted the comparable patency and infection rates with PTFE versus saphenous graft. The majority of studies supporting the use of PTFE, however, have evaluated patency rates following lower-extremity revascularizations.

Consideration should be given to associated injuries, especially to the aerodigestive tract. If an esophageal injury is repaired or drained near the vascular repair, some would advocate using vein instead of foreign material to reduce the risk of graft failure. Any vascular repair that is associated with an esophageal or pharyngeal wound should be protected with a muscle flap, using SCM or strap muscles. The muscles are rotated to cover the vascular anastamosis and protect it from any saliva leak from the digestive tract injury. Vascular principles such as those used in elective procedures— "flushing out" the artery prior to completion of the anastomosis, completion angiography, and systemic heparinization—should be employed.[70]

Repair of the innominate and subclavian arteries can be accomplished using similar principles as those applied to the carotid arteries. Dacron grafts may be used for proximal injuries, especially when an end-to-side anatamosis must be made on the aorta. Over thirty percent of patients with these injuries traditionally have had associated brachial plexus injuries. Some authors suggest that clavicular resection may have as much to do with this phenomenon as the injuries themselves. Should a supraclavicular approach be chosen and an interposition graft be necessary, the conduit can be tunneled beneath the clavicle without having to resect the clavicle.[76] This usually can be accomplished after "stripping off" the attachments of the pectoralis major and SCM muscle. This avoids the functional difficulties that often are encountered postoperatively following clavicular resection. This also obviates the need for reconstructive surgery in the future.

How Can Bleeding from a Vertebral Artery be Controlled?

Control of the vertebral artery is among the most difficult vascular exposures in the entire human body. The majority of the vessel is contained within the vertebral foramina of the spine. In addition, the soft tissue surrounding the anterior spine includes a venous plexus, the brachial plexus, phrenic nerve, and scalene muscles. Moreover, simple proximal ligation rarely stops bleeding on account of the rich back bleeding often present in the vertebral system. Thus, without question, the most successful way to control bleeding from a vertebral artery is by angiography and embolization. If a penetrating trajectory is highly suspicious of a vertebral injury, angiography should be performed if at all possible before operative exploration. If this is not possible on account of exsanguination from that or an associated injury, operative control may be necessary. If true proximal and distal control is not possible, other options include balloon tamponade or packing of the injury. Balloon tamponade can include a Foley urinary catheter that is placed into the gunshot tract and inflated. Alternatively, a Fogarty type intraluminal catheter can be placed anterograde through an arterotomy in the proximal vertebral artery and inflated in the area of injury. Both of these maneuvers are temporary control measures until definitive control is obtained with angiography.

Packing is also an option, either with hemostatic material such as surgicell or bone wax, which works well between the bone fragments of the spine.

Operative exposure of the vertebral artery is best obtained through a supraclavicular incision extending from the insertion of the sternoclavicular head to the lateral third of the clavicle. The carotid sheath is identified and retracted laterally and the supraclavicular fat pad separated, exposing the thyrocervical trunk and scalene muscles. Exposure is maximized by ligation of the thyrocervical vessels and division of the anterior scalene. Care should be taken to avoid and protect the phrenic nerve. The vertebral artery will be noted as the deepest structure lying within the fossa.

What is the Role of Endovascular Stents in Neck Trauma?

Following successful use of endovascular stents in patients with carotid artery disease, Coldwell and colleagues reported on the use of endovascular stents to treat complications following carotid artery injury.[77] Since their report of stent treatment of a carotid pseudoaneurysm after trauma, numerous authors have utilized successfully the endovascular approach to address penetrating cervical vascular injuries.[78–81] Duane and colleagues noted the viable option of endovascular techniques in managing difficult, often inaccessible, vascular injuries of the neck. Stent deployment in their patients allowed nonoperative management of Zone III vascular injuries.

Strauss and colleagues reported the successful management of subclavian artery injuries through an endovascular approach.[83] The vessels were occluded at the time of evaluation, but underwent thrombectomy and stent deployment without difficulty. Both patients had patency confirmed on one-year follow up. Other authors have noted these and additional advantages to the endovascular approach. These include the ability to embolize those vessels not amenable to stenting, treating traumatic AVFs, and addressing occluded vessels in a delayed fashion. The role of endovascular stents in managing cervical vascular injuries continues to evolve.

How Should Esophageal Injuries be Managed?

The repair of an injury to the cervical esophagus is approached best through an anterior SCM incision. Should there be an associated laryngotracheal injury, however, these combination injuries are approached best through a collar incision. Maximal exposure of the esophagus is achieved through retraction of the trachea and thyroid medially and the carotid sheath laterally. An indwelling nasogastric tube can facilitate not only the localization of the esophagus, but the identification of the esophageal injury (through the instillation of air or methylene blue).[82] Nonviable edges should be debrided sharply prior to primary repair, which then is carried out in one of two methods.

The two-layered repair is performed with an interrupted submucosal (absorbable suture) and a muscular layer (nonabsorbable suture). Alternatively, a single-layered repair can be performed in an interrupted fashion (nonabsorbable suture). Whether a single- or two-layered repair is chosen, good mucosal and muscular approximation is necessary to prevent delayed leakage. The area around the repair should be drained with a closed drainage system.

Associated tracheal injuries and hemodynamic instability place the patient at increased risk of tracheoespohageal fistula formation. Although the majority of fistulas will heal without surgical intervention, their risk of occurrence can be minimized with a tissue flap or buttress.[82] This can be accomplished by dividing the clavicular head of the SCM muscle and mobilizing the flap between the trachea and esophagus, separating the two structures. The patient should have nothing by mouth until a barium swallow (five to seven days postoperatively) has excluded a leak.

A reduction in the number of diagnostic delays has likely accounted for the improvement in survival rates following penetrating esophageal trauma. In the patient without signs of sepsis or clinical deterioration, small injuries detected in a delayed fashion may be managed nonoperatively.[69] The majority, however, will require debridement and drainage. Although the management principles usually are centered on creation of a controlled fistula, a buttress repair of the defect should be attempted if possible. Some authors have advocated prolonged esophageal "rest" and nasopharyngeal (or T-tube) drainage to decrease the already high risk of fistula formation and anastomotic leaks. More devastating wounds may require cervical esophagostomy and parenteral nutrition.[83,84]

How is Management of Pharyngeal Wounds Different than Esophageal Wounds?

Unlike esophageal injuries, those confined to the hypopharynx frequently can be managed nonoperatively. Yugeros and colleagues evaluated fourteen patients with penetrating injuries to the hypopharynx that were managed nonoperatively.[57] They found no evidence of leaks or fistula formation, and only one patient developed a cervical abscess. Shortly thereafter, Stanley and colleagues addressed this issue in a study of seventy patients with hypopharyngeal or cervical esophageal injuries.[84] They noted a significant increase in the number of deep cervical infections and fistulas in patients with injuries below the arytenoids that were managed nonoperatively. The authors concluded that patients with injuries above the arytenoids should be managed nonoperatively, whereas those below this level should undergo primary repair. Demetriades and colleagues concurred with these authors, but stated that "major wounds" to the hypopharynx should be managed similarly to those of the cervical esophagus.[73] The role of antibiotics in these patients remains controversial.[73,82,83]

How Are Tracheolaryngeal Wounds Repaired?

Patients presenting with low-velocity GSWs to the neck will require an urgent airway in eighteen to forty-four percent of cases.[83,85] Definitive airway control prior to operative exploration may be necessary in the form of endotracheal intubation, cricothyroidotomy, or tracheostomy. In the majority of cases, however, oral endotracheal intubation will be possible. Both an anterior SCM or collar incision may be utilized to approach these injuries.

With combined esophageal injury or transcervical GSWs, however, a collar incision usually will allow improved exposure with less struggle than the standard SCM incision. Then careful dissection is carried out, retracting necessary tissues to expose the involved segment. Lateral dissection should be minimized and, if possible, avoided in order to protect the laterally based blood supply.

Most laryngeal defects from penetrating trauma can be repaired primarily. Small defects noted on endoscopy usually can be managed nonoperatively with airway protection, elevation of the head of the bed, and "voice rest." A search for the recurrent laryngeal nerve should be avoided and the dissection minimized. Proper debridement should proceed any attempt at primary repair. However, all viable tissues should be spared. Early fracture stabilization (Kirschner wires) of involved components and repair of mucosal lacerations has been associated with improved airway and voice quality.[85,86] If the cartilaginous framework has been disrupted beyond management with a primary repair, some authors have advocated "stenting" the airway with the indwelling endotracheal tube or with the placement of a silicone stent. Tracheostomy should be avoided in the area of injury, but if necessary should be placed distal to the repair to "protect" the anastomosis.

Tracheal injuries are repaired primarily in a single-layer fashion using an absorbable (3-0) suture. As with laryngeal injuries, viable tissue should be conserved and search for recurrent laryngeal nerves avoided. Large defects (>3 cm) can be repaired primarily after adequate mobilization. This can be accomplished by releasing anterior (thyroid and suprahyoid) attachments, staying clear of the lateral blood supply. Vascularized flaps (SCM muscle) should be employed to buttress the repair, decreasing the risk of fistula formation.

The role of tracheostomy in these patients remains controversial. Tracheostomy in this setting has been associated with increased risk of infection, but many have advocated its use in "protecting" the proximal repair. Most agree, however, that with very large defects (>6 cm, those requiring vascularized flaps) a tracheostomy should be placed at the time of the initial operation. Avoidance of flexion in the postoperative period (5–7 days) can be achieved with cervical collar immobilization or by suturing the chin to the presternal skin.

References

1. Breasted JH. *The Edwin Smith Papyrus*. Chicago, IL: University of Chicago Press; 1930.
2. Pare A. In: Pierre R, ed. *Oeuvres Completes*. Paris: Lyon; 1552:292.

3. DiGiacomo JC, Reilly JF. Mechanisms of injury in penetrating trauma. In: Peitzman AB, Rhodes M, Schwab CW, Yealy DM, Fabian TC, eds. *The Trauma Manual.* 2nd ed. Philadelphia: Lippincott; 2002.
4. Bishara RA, Pasch AR, Douglas DD, et al. The necessity of mandatory exploration of penetrating zone II neck injuries. *Surgery.* 1986;100(4):655–660.
5. Golueke PJ, Goldstein AS, Sclafani SJ, et al. Routine versus selective exploration of penetrating neck injuries: a randomized prospective study. *J Trauma.* 1984;24(12):1010–1014.
6. Wood J, Fabian TC, Mangiante EC. Penetrating neck injuries: Recommendations for selective management. *J Trauma.* 1989;29:602–605.
7. Atteberry LR, Dennis JW, Menawat SS, Frykberg ER. Physical examination alone is safe and accurate for evaluation of vascular injuries in penetrating zone 2 neck trauma. *J Am Coll Surg.* 1995;179:657–662.
8. Klyachkin ML, Rohmiller M, Charash WE, et al. Penetrating injuries of the neck: Selective management evolving. *Am Surg.* 1997;63:189–194.
9. Demetriades D, Theodorou D, Cornwell E, et al. Transcervical gunshot injuries: Mandatory operation is not necessary. *J Trauma.* 1996;40(5):758–760.
10. Eddy V, the Zone I Penetrating Neck Injury Study Group. Is routine arteriography mandatory for penetrating injuries to zone I of the neck? *J Trauma.* 2000;48(2):208–214.
11. McKinley WO, Johns JS, Musgrove JJ. Clinical presentations, medical complications, and functional outcomes of individuals with gunshot wound-induced spinal cord injury. *Am J Phys Med Rehab.* 1999;78(2):102–107.
12. Apfelbaum JD, Cantrill SV, Waldman N. Unstable cervical spine without spinal cord injury in penetrating neck trauma. *Am J Emergency Med.* 2000;18(1):55–57.
13. American College of Surgeons Committee on Trauma. *Advanced Trauma Life Support Student Manual.* Chicago: American College of Surgeons; 1997.
14. Barkana Y, Stein M, Scope A, et al. Prehospital stabilization of the cervical spine for penetrating injuries to the neck—is it necessary? *Injury.* 2000;31:305–309.
15. Arishita GI, Vayer JS, Bellamy RF, et al. Cervical spine immobilization of penetrating neck wounds in a hostile environment. *J Trauma.* 1989;29(3):332–337.
16. Biffl WL, Moore EE, Rehse DH, et al. Selective management of penetrating neck trauma based on cervical level of injury. *Am J Surg.* 1997;174:678–682.
17. Pass LJ, LeNarz LA, Schreiber JT, et al. Management of esophageal gunshot wounds. *Ann Thor Surg.* 1987;44(3):253–256.
18. Nemzek WR, Hecht ST, Donald PJ, et al. Prediction of major vascular injury in patients with gunshot wounds to the neck. *AJNR Am J Neuroradiol.* 1996;17(1):161–167.
19. Hirshberg A, Wall MJ, Johnston RH, et al. Transcervical gunshot injuries. *Am J Surg.* 1994;167:309–316.
20. Renz BM, Feliciano DV. Gunshot wounds to the right thoracoabdomen: A prospective study of nonoperative management. *J Trauma.* 1994;37:737–744.
21. Grossman MD, May AK, Schwab CW, et al. Determining anatomic injury with computerized tomography in selected torso gunshot wounds. *J Trauma.* 1998;45:446–456.
22. Velmahos GC, Demetriades D, Foianini E, et al. A selective approach to the management of gunshot wounds to the back. *Am J Surg.* 1997;174:342–346.

23. Mazolewski PJ, Curry JD, Browder T, Fildes J. Computed tomographic scan can be used for surgical decision making in zone II penetrating neck injuries. *J Trauma.* 2001;51:315–319.

24. Gracias VH, Reilly PM, Philpott J, et al. Computed tomography in the evaluation of penetrating neck trauma. *Arch Surg.* 2001;136:1231–1235.

25. Sclafani SJ, Cavaliere G, Atweh N, et al. Role of angiography in penetrating neck trauma. *J Trauma.* 1991;31(4):557–562.

26. Maxwell RA. Penetrating neck injury. In: Peitzman AB, Rhodes M, Schwab CW, Yealy DM, Fabian TC, eds. *The Trauma Manual.* 2nd ed. Philadelphia: Lippincott; 2002.

27. Rao PM, Ivatury RR, Sharma P, et al. Cervical vascular injuries: a trauma center experience. *Surgery.* 1993;114(3):527–531.

28. Sclafani S, Panetta T, Goldstein AS, et al. The management of arterial injuries caused by penetration of zone III of the neck. *J Trauma.* 1985;25(9):871–881.

29. Jurkovich GT, Zingarello W, Wallace J, Curreri PW. Penetrating neck trauma: Diagnostic studies in the asymptomatic patient. *J Trauma.* 1985;25:819–822.

30. Demetriades D, Theodorou D, Cornwell E III, et al. Penetrating injuries of the neck in patients in stable condition: Physical examination, angiography, or color flow doppler imaging. *Arch Surg.* 1995;130(9):971–975.

31. Sekharan J, Dennis JW, Veldenz HC, et al. Continued experience with physical examination alone for evaluation and management of penetrating zone 2 neck injuries: Results of 145 cases. *J Vasc Surg.* 2000;32(3):483–489.

32. Beitsch P, Weigelt JA, Flynn E, Easley S. Physical examination and arteriography in patients with penetrating zone II neck wounds. *Arch Surg.* 1994;129(6):577–581.

33. Biffl WL, Moore EE, Rehse DH, et al. Selective management of penetrating neck trauma based on cervical level of injury. *Am J Surg.* 1997;174:678–682.

34. Jarvick JG, Philips GR 3rd, Schwab CW, et al. Penetrating neck trauma: Sensitivity of clinical examination and cost-effectiveness of angiography. *AJNR Am J Neurorad.* 1995;16(4):647–654.

35. Munera F, Soto JA, Palacio D, et al. Diagnosis of arterial injuries caused by penetrating trauma to the neck: Comparison of helical CT angiography and conventional angiography. *Radiology.* 2000;216(2):356–362.

36. Munera F, Soto JA, Palacio DM, et al. Penetrating neck injuries: Helical CT angiography for initial evaluation. *Radiology.* 2002;224(2):366–372.

37. Ofer A, Nitecki SS, Braun J, et al. CT angiography of the carotid arteries in trauma to the neck. *Europ J Vasc Endo Surg.* 2001;21(5):401–407.

38. Wellwood J, Alcantara A, Michael DB. Neurotrauma: the role of CT angiogram. *Neuro Research.* 2002;Suppl 1:S13–S16.

39. Fry WR, Dort JA, Smith RS, et al. Duplex scanning replaces arteriography and operative exploration in the diagnosis of potential cervical vascular injury. *Am J Surg.* 1994;168(6):693–695.

40. Corr P, Abdool AT, Robbs J. Colour-flow ultrasound in the detection of penetrating vascular injuries of the neck. *S African Med J.* 1999;89(6):644–646.

41. Montalvo BM, LeBlang SD, Nunez DB Jr, et al. Color Doppler sonography in penetrating injuries of the neck. *AJNR Am J Neuroradiol.* 1996;17(5):943–951.

42. Demetriades D, Theodorou D, Cornwell E, et al. Evaluation of penetrating injuries of the neck: Prospective study of 223 patients. *World J Surg.* 1997; 21:41–48.
43. Vaccaro AR, Klein GR, Flanders AE, et al. Long term evaluation of vertebral artery injuries following cervical spine trauma using magnetic resonance angiography. *Spine.* 1998;23(7):789–794.
44. Mulloy JP, Flick PA, Gold RE. Blunt carotid injury: a review. *Radiology.* 1998;207(3):571–585.
45. Larsen DW. Traumatic vascular injuries and their management. *Neuroimag Clin N Am.* 2002;12(2):249–269.
46. Weller SJ, Rossitch E Jr, Malek AM. Detection of vertebral artery injury after cervical spine trauma using magnetic resonance angiography. *J Trauma.* 1999;46(4):660–666.
47. Miller PR, Fabian TC, Croce MA, et al. Prospective screening for blunt cerebrovascular injuries: Analysis of diagnostic modalities and outcomes. *Ann Surg.* 2002;236(3):386–393.
48. Biffl WL, Moore EE, Offner PJ, et al. Optimizing screening for blunt cerebrovascular injuries. *Am J Surg.* 1999;187:517–522.
49. Biffl WL, Moore EE, Offner PJ, et al. Blunt carotid and vertebral artery injuries. *World J Surg.* 2001;25:1036–1043.
50. Biffl WL, Ray CE Jr, Moore EE, et al. Non-invasive diagnosis of blunt cerebrovascular injury: a preliminary report. *J Trauma.* 2002;53:850–856.
51. James CA. Magnetic resonance angiography in trauma. *Clin Neurosci.* 1997;4(3):137–145.
52. Vasama JP, Ramsay H, Markkola A. Petrous internal carotid artery artery pseudoanuerysm due to gunshot injury. *Ann Otol Rhinol Laryngol.* 2001;110 (5 Pt 1):491–493.
53. Yugueros P, Sarmiento JM, Garcia AF, et al. Conservative management of penetrating hypopharyngeal wounds. *J Trauma.* 1996;40(2):267–269.
54. Ngakane H, Muckart DJJ, Luvuno FM. Penetrating visceral injuries of the neck: Results of a conservative management policy. *Br J Surg.* 1990;77:908–915.
55. Goudy SL, Miller FB, Bumpous JM. Neck crepitance: evaluation and management of suspected upper aerodigestive tract injury. *Laryngoscope.* 2002; 112(5):791–795.
56. Noyes LD, McSwain NE Jr, Markowitz IP. Panendoscopy with arteriography versus mandatory exploration of penetrating wounds of the neck. *Ann Surg.* 1986;204:21–31.
57. Back MR, Baumgartner FJ, Klein SR. Detection and evaluation of aerodigestive tract injuries caused by cervical and transmediastinal gunshot wounds. *J Trauma.* 1997;42(4):680–686.
58. Noyes LD, McSwain NE Jr, Markowitz IP. Panendoscopy with arteriography versus mandatory exploration of penetrating wounds of the neck. *Ann Surg.* 1986;204:21–31.
59. Armstrong WB, Detar TR, Stanley RB. Diagnosis and management of external penetrating cervical esophageal injuries. *Ann Otol Rhinol Laryngol.* 1994; 103(11):863–871.
60. Srinivasan R, Haywood T, Horwitz B, et al. Role of flexible endoscopy in the evaluation of possible esophageal trauma after penetrating injuries. *Am J Gastroenterol.* 2000;95(7):1725–1729.

61. Sheely CH, Mattox KL, Beall AC, et al. Penetrating wounds of the cervical esophagus. *Am J Surg.* 1975;130:707–712.
62. Leitman BS, Birnbaum BA, Naidich DP. Radiologic evaluation of thoracic trauma. In: Hood RM, Boyd AD, Culliford AT, eds. *Thoracic Trauma.* Philadelphia: WB Saunders Co; 1989:67–100.
63. Ordog GJ, Albin D, Wasserberger J, et al. 110 Bullet wounds to the neck. *J Trauma.* 1985:25:238–246.
64. Weigelt JA, Thal ER, Snyder WH 3rd, et al. Diagnosis of penetrating cervical esophageal injuries. *Am J Surg.* 1987;154(6):619–622.
65. Glatterer MS Jr, Toon RS, Ellestad C, et al. Management of blunt and penetrating external esophageal trauma. *J Trauma.* 1985;25(8):784–792.
66. Grewal H, Rao PM, Mukerji S, et al. Management of penetrating laryngotracheal injuries. *Head Neck.* 1995;17(6):494–502.
67. Demetriades D, Velmahos G, Asensio JA. Cervical pharyngoesophageal and laryngotracheal injuries. *World J Surg.* 2001;25:1044–1048.
68. Bee TK, Fabian TC. Penetrating neck trauma. In: Cameron J, ed. *Current Surgical Therapy.* St. Louis, MO: Mosby; 2001:1170–1174.
69. Britt LD, Peyser MB. Penetrating and blunt neck trauma. In: Mattox KL, Feliciano DV, Moore EE, eds. *Trauma.* New York, NY: McGraw-Hill; 2000:437–448.
70. Lickweg WG, Greenfield LJ. Management of penetrating trauma carotid arterial injury. *Ann Surg.* 1978;188:582–586.
71. Unger SW, Tucker WS, Micleza MA. Carotid arterial trauma. *Surgery.* 1980;87:477–482.
72. Wisner DH. Cervical vascular injury. In: Trunkey DD, Lewis FR, eds. *Current Therapy in Trauma.* St. Louis, MO: Mosby; 1999:190–196.
73. Wylie EJ, Hein MF, Adams JE. Intracranial hemorrhage following surgical revascularization for treatment of acute strokes. *J Neurosurg.* 1964;21:212–215.
74. Thompson EC, Porter JM, Fernandez LG. Penetrating neck trauma: An overview of management. *J Oral Maxillofac Surg.* 2002;60:918–923.
75. Old W, Oswaks R. Clavicular excision in management of vascular trauma. *Am Surg.* 1984;50:286–289.
76. Demetriades D, Chahwan S, Gomez H, et al. Penetrating injuries to the subclavian and axillary vessels. *J Am Coll Surg.* 1999;188(3):290–295.
77. Coldwell DM, Novak Z, Ryu RK, et al. Treatment of posttraumatic internal carotid arterial pseudoaneurysms with endovascular stents. *J Trauma.* 2000; 48(3):470–472.
78. Albuquerque FC, Javedan SP, McDougall CG. Endovascular management of penetrating vertebral artery injuries. *J Trauma.* 2002;53:574–580.
79. McNeil JD, Chiou AC, Gunlock MG, et al. Successful endovascular therapy of a pentrating zone III internal carotid artery injury. *J Vasc Surg.* 2002; 36(1):187–190.
80. Duane TM, Parker F, Stokes GK, et al. Endovascular carotid stenting after trauma. *J Trauma.* 2002;52:149–153.
81. Strauss DC, du Toit DF, Warren BL. Endovascular repair of occluded subclavian arteries following penetrating trauma. *J Endovasc Ther.* 2001;8(5):529–533.
82. Stanley RB, Armstrong WB, Fetterman BL, et al. Management of external penetrating injuries into the hypopharyngeal-cervical esophageal funnel. *J Trauma.* 1997;42:675–680.

83. Duplechian JK, Miller RH. Laryngeal trauma: Diagnosis and management. *J Louisiana St Med.* 1989;141(12):17–20.
84. Mathison DJ, Grillo H. Laryngotracheal trauma. *Ann Thorac Surg.* 1987;43: 254–260.
85. Borgstom D, Weigelt JA. Neck: Aerodigestive tract. In: Ivatury RR, Cayten CG, eds. *The Textbook of Penetrating Trauma.* Baltimore, MD: Williams and Wilkins; 1996:479.

12
Thoracic Injury

DOUGLAS M. BOWLEY, ELIAS DEGIANNIS, and STEPHEN WESTABY

Historical Perspective

Penetrating chest injuries have been a constant feature of man's propensity for conflict over many centuries. Of the one-hundred-thirty battle wounds documented in Homer's *Iliad*, twenty-six (20%) were to the chest.[1] Alone or in combination, spears accounted for over 80% of the thoracic injuries, and perhaps it is not surprising that 92% of these injuries were fatal, and usually immediately so.[2] Thoracic injury continued to plague armies over the years, but little progress was made in management of penetrating chest injury until the First World War (WWI). At the start of that conflict, management usually was conservative; however, problems associated with sepsis in the chest wall and pleural space meant that a conservative strategy fell from favor and an increasingly interventional approach developed. Underwater pleural drainage was not used and one-fourth of hemothoraces became septic no matter what type of missile caused the wound; of these, half died and one-third of the survivors had to be invalided out of service.[2] Immediate open operation became the accepted therapy for all but limited degrees of hemothorax, but the overall mortality of penetrating chest injury was 74%.[2] Use of drains with underwater seals had become routine by the Second World War (WWII), and other advances such as endotracheal tubes with the abilty to mechanically ventilate the lungs, blood transfusion, antibiotics, and understanding of the techniques for anatomic pulmonary resection contributed to improved management of thoracic wounds. Thoracocentesis overtook operative drainage of the chest and thoracotomy was reserved for "clear-cut" indications; nevertheless, the overall probability of succumbing to a chest wound was 61%.[2]

In a review of twelve conflicts throughout the twentieth century, the incidence of penetrating thoracic injuries has ranged between 4% and 12%.[3] In Vietnam, according to the Wound Data Munitions Effectiveness Team database, chest injury was sustained by 8% of the total number of wounded studied with an overall mortality of 71%. One quarter were evacuated alive from the battlefield, and of those, 15% underwent thoracotomy.[2] One fact is worth remembering, the probability of dying from a single assault bullet wound to the chest in Vietnam was 80%. What is apparent is the consistently high mortality of penetrating thoracic wounds in warfare; as Freud stated in his collected writings in 1924, "anatomy is destiny."[4]

In modern-day civilian practice, thoracic injury directly accounts for 20% to 25% of deaths due to trauma and thoracic injury or its complications are a contributing factor in another 25% of trauma deaths.[5] Major penetrating injury to the heart, thoracic great vessels, or pulmonary hilum usually is rapidly fatal, with few patients reaching a medical facility with chance of survival. In contrast, most patients with injuries to the pulmonary parenchyma and chest wall survive to reach help and will benefit from management without the need for thoracotomy.

The importance of rapid evacuation from the point of wounding cannot be overemphasized. In a remarkable series of 3000 war-injured patients with thoracic injury, the reported time lag from wounding to hospital for three quarters of the wounded was only four minutes; mortality for patients with injuries to the thoracic great vessels was 13% compared with a 1.2% mortality for the rest of the patients with noncardiac thoracic wounds.[6] Early provision of definitive care also leads to improved outcomes in civilian practice; it has been shown that wounded patients transported directly to hospital by private vehicles have better chance of survival than those transported who had to wait for the emergency medical services.[7] In a recent prospective, multicenter study of patients with major life-threatening injuries, the overall mortality rate of patients receiving only basic care at the scene and rapid transport was 18% compared to 29% for patients receiving scene-based advanced life support.[8]

Pathophysiology of Thoracic Wounds

Effective treatment depends on an understanding of the physiologic derangements caused by thoracic trauma. Mortality immediately after penetrating chest injuries usually occurs as a result of the following factors, either alone or in combination:

- Airway obstruction
- Tension pneumothorax
- Cardiac tamponade
- Open pneumothorax
- Exsanguination

Later causes of the high mortality and morbidity associated with thoracic injury include:

- Alterations in the mechanics of breathing: Pain after thoracic injury causes hypoventilation and failure to clear secretions. Inadequately treated hemo/pneumothorax leads to pulmonary collapse and/or clotted hemothorax, which may become infected and lead to empyema.

- Ventilation/perfusion mismatch: Mismatch between ventilation of the lung and its blood supply occurs as a direct result of pulmonary contusion/parenchymal hemorrhage. Further imbalance may occur due to bronchial occlusion through clot or secretions.

- Impairment of gas exchange: Acute respiratory distress syndrome (ARDS) is the pulmonary manifestation of both direct lung injury and indirect injury caused by the consequences of neutrophil activation with release of cytokines, complement activation, and free radical production.[9] Pulmonary edema occurs without increased hydrostatic pressure, and the associated hypoxemia can be refractory to therapeutic manipulation.[9] Acute respiratory distress syndrome is defined as PaO2/FiO2 ratio less than 200 with diffuse bilateral infiltrates on chest radiograph and no congestive heart failure. Acute respiratory distress syndrome can appear early (within 48 hours after admission) or late. Early ARDS is associated with profound hemorrhagic shock, and late ARDS frequently follows pneumonia and is associated with multiple system injury.[10]

Airway Obstruction

Many early preventable trauma deaths are due to airway obstruction. The most common cause of airway obstruction in the unconscious patient is the tongue. However, maxillofacial injuries, vomit, blood, and secretions contribute to the airway problem, and penetrating injuries can cause airway obstruction due to expansion of the hematoma in the neck or direct major airway injury. Simple measures, such as the chin lift and jaw thrust manoeuvre, or clearing and suctioning the mouth may clear the airway. In a series of patients with laryngotracheal trauma, 29% required an emergency room airway establishment because of threatened airway loss, and in 11% the airway was lost and a cricothyroidotomy became necessary.[11] The cervical spine must be protected in blunt injury and a high concentration of inspired oxygen provided; however, a definitive airway should be achieved if there is any doubt. Whenever possible, prior to attempts at endotracheal intubation, the patient should be ventilated with a bag and mask and 100% oxygen. This preoxygenation enables a period of apnea during intubation to be tolerated safely by the patient. Correct placement of the tube should be confirmed by auscultation of the epigastrium and both sides of the chest. Additional confirmation can be obtained via measurement of exhaled CO_2 by capnography. When muscle relaxants or sedatives are used the loss of muscle tone can lead to complete loss of the airway[12] prior to it being protected by an endotracheal tube or tracheostomy or cricithyroidotomy. Expert anesthetic and surgical advice is needed.

Tension Pneumothorax

Small chest wounds can act as one-way valves, allowing air to enter during inspiration, but not allowing the air to escape. Air builds up under pressure in the pleural cavity, especially if there is an associated lung injury. Patients with tension pneumothorax present in a dramatic way; they may be close to death, profoundly hypotensive or panicky, dyspnoeic, and cyanosed. Breath sounds are absent, the percussion note will be hyper resonant, and the trachea will be displaced to the opposite side (a late sign). Tension pneumothorax is a clinical diagnosis; there should be no time for X-rays (Figure 12-1). The treatment is with immediate decompression by insertion of a needle into the pleural space in the mid-clavicular line a couple of finger-breadths below the clavicle, followed by insertion of a chest drain. This is described on page 248.

Cardiac Tamponade

In trauma, cardiac tamponade results from blood in the pericardial sac restricting cardiac movement. While it is most commonly caused by penetrating injury it can occur in blunt injury. Clinical diagnosis is often difficult. Beck's triad (CS Beck, US Surgeon 1894–1971) consists of systemic

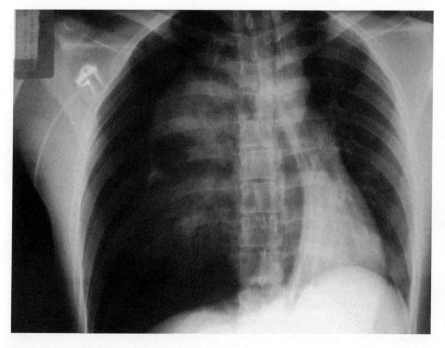

FIGURE 12-1. Right tension pneumothorax with gross mediastinal shift. An X-ray that should not have been taken.

hypotension, muffled heart sounds and distended neck veins from elevated venous pressure. Practically muffled heart sounds are difficult to assess in a noisy environment and distended neck veins may be absent in the presence of hypovolemia. Pulsus paradoxus is the physiological decrease in systolic blood pressure that occurs during spontaneous inspiration. In cardiac tamponade this may be increased to over 10 mmHg. It may also be absent or difficult to detect in a noisy environment. Tamponade may be difficult to distinguish from tension pneumothorax. The roles of pericardiocentesis and portable ultrasound in diagnosis and management are considered on page 247 and surgical management of cardiac injuries on page 252.

Open Pneumothorax

With larger penetrating wounds, air may preferentially enter the pleural cavity via the wound rather than through the trachea (Figure 12-2). If an open wound exceeds two-thirds of the cross-sectional area of the trachea in a patient breathing spontaneously, effective ventilation may cease. Complete occlusion of the wound may lead to a tension pneumothorax, and the appropriate first aid is to place an Asherman Seal™ over the wound or a dressing taped on 3 sides. (The idea is that the dressing acts as a one way valve allowing air out of the chest but not back in through the injury). Once in the hospital, a chest drain should be inserted; then the wound can be

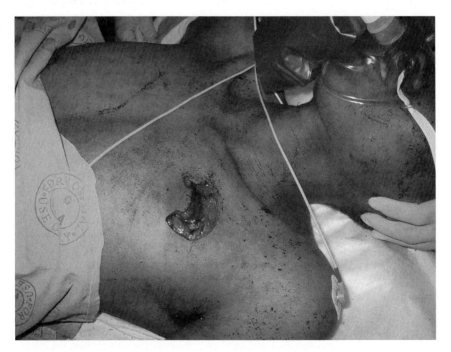

FIGURE 12-2. Open pneumothorax.

debrided and closed, as appropriate. Wartime injury can produce large defects of the chest wall; these are rare in survivors due to the nature of the injury, but reconstruction of the chest wall by prosthetic material may be required.[13]

Massive Hemothorax

With penetrating injuries to the chest, a hemothorax usually is evident on routine chest X-ray. However, if the patient is lying flat, up to a liter of blood in the chest may only cause a slightly increased haziness on the involved side. A massive hemothorax is greater than 1.5 liters of blood. The patient will be in hypovolemic shock and hypoxic. On the affected side breath sounds will be absent and the chest will be dull to percussion.

It is unusual for the blood in the chest cavity to move the mediastinum sufficiently to cause distended neck veins. Neck veins are likely to be flat due to severe hypovolemia. If there is a tension pneumothorax present in addition to the hemothorax then neck veins could be distended. Operative control of the bleeding is likely to be required.

If there is a massive hemothorax some researchers have recommended clamping the chest tube in order to allow tamponade of bleeding. In the authors' view tamponade is unlikely to happen. There is debate about the most appropriate action that should be taken in the prehospital situation.

In hospital, blood in the pleural space should be removed as completely and as rapidly as possible. If the blood is not removed it can cause empyema or fibrothorax with constriction of significant lung volumes.

Initial Assessment

Patients with thoracic trauma should be evaluated using established Advanced Trauma Life Support® (ATLS®) principles.[5] Immediate priorities are:

1. establishment of a secure airway and provision of high concentrations of oxygen,
2. establishment of adequate ventilation, and
3. control of hemorrhage.

Patients with penetrating injuries to the chest must be undressed completely and examined carefully front and back for other injuries, as it is surprisingly easy to miss a small penetrating wound to the torso. Penetrating wounds of the chest should never be probed to determine their depth or direction, as this can dislodge clots and cause severe bleeding. Attention must be paid to protection of the team of health-care workers and adequate protective measures should be taken for all patients. Potential spinal injuries must be remembered and appropriate precautions should be taken.

Diagnostic Adjuncts

Chest X-rays should be obtained as early as possible in all patients. Pneumothorax, hemothorax, subcutaneous or mediastinal emphysema, widened mediastinum, and the presence of retained missiles are all important features to be sought on the chest film (Figure 12-3). Radiopaque markers should be placed over all penetrating wounds prior to x-ray, enabling an estimation of the wounding trajectory to be made.[14]

The use of pericardiocentesis as a diagnostic and therapeutic modality in the emergency department has virtually disappeared with the introduction and widespread acceptance of portable ultrasound by the surgeon to examine the pericardial and pleural spaces for blood.[15,16] In a multicenter study of 261 patients with possible penetrating cardiac wounds, there were 225 (86.2%) true-negative, 29 (11.1%) true-positive, no false-negative, and 7 (2.7%) false-positive examinations. Patients with positive scans underwent immediate exploration and 28 of the 29 patients survived.[17]

Surgeon-performed ultrasound can detect hemothorax just as accurately and more quickly than X-ray.[18] Pneumothorax also can be diagnosed with ultrasound, although subcutaneous emphysema can make the study more difficult. In a prospective study of 382 patients, ultrasound had sensitivity

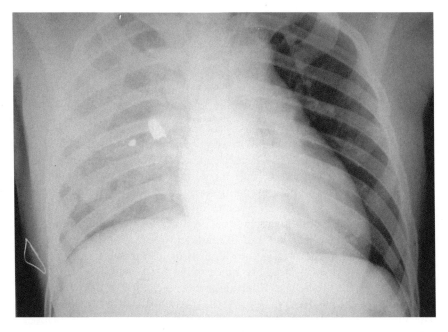

FIGURE 12-3. Gunshot wound, right chest with associated pulmonary contusion injury.

for the diagnosis of pneumothorax of 95%, the true-negative rate was 100%.[19]

Computed tomographic (CT) scanning is being used increasingly to image the trajectory of the missile and reduce the need for angiography and oesophageal investigation. Hanpeter et al.[20] reported a prospective study of 24 patients who underwent CT scan evaluation of a mediastinal gunshot wound. One patient was taken for sternotomy to remove a missile embedded in the myocardium solely on the basis of the result of the CT scan. Because of proximity of the bullet tract to mediastinal structures, 12 patients required additional evaluation with eight angiograms and nine esophageal studies. One of these patients had a positive angiogram (bullet resting against the ascending aorta) and underwent sternotomy for missile removal; all other studies were negative. The remaining 11 patients were found to have well-defined missile tracts that approached neither the aorta nor the esophagus, and no additional evaluation was required. There were no missed mediastinal injuries in this group.[20] In another prospective study of twenty-two stable patients with transmediastinal gunshot wounds,[21] CT scans demonstrated the missile trajectory was towards mediastinal structures in seven patients. Further diagnostic studies in those seven patients revealed only two patients who required operative intervention. The patients with negative CT scans were observed in a monitored setting without further evaluation and there were no missed injuries.[21] In another study[22] of fifteen patients who underwent CT solely to determine missile trajectory, a transmediastinal trajectory was excluded in nine of the fifteen (60%); of the six remaining patients who underwent investigation, two had injuries identified and subsequently repaired.[22]

Chest Tube Insertion

Insertion of a chest tube is the only procedure required for the majority of penetrating injuries to the chest. In adolescents and adults, the chest tube should be no smaller than 36 French gauge. In children, a size 28 French tube usually is appropriate. Prophylactic antibiotics have been shown to reduce the incidence of infective complications after chest drain insertion.[23] A single dose should be given prior to insertion; however, antibiotics are no substitute for scrupulous technique, even in a busy resuscitation room. The chest should be cleaned and draped, and local anaesthetic used. An incision is made in the mid axillary line, at or just above the level of the nipple. The skin incision should be made in the space below the anticipated point of entry into the chest. Blunt dissection is carried out over the superior border of the rib to avoid injuring the intercostal neurovascular bundle. The pleural space should be entered with a pair of curved artery forceps and a finger swept around the inside of the chest to ensure correct positioning inside the pleural space and to ensure that the lung is away from the chest wall. Even without previous chest surgery, up to 25% of patients will have some adhesions between the chest wall and the lung. The drain is inserted ten centimeters or so into the chest, aiming posteriorly and to the apex. The drain should be connected to an underwater drainage system; the patient is encouraged to cough vigorously while changing position to ensure re-expansion of the lung and drainage of blood. The tube must be secured with a heavy gauge suture and a chest X-ray should be taken to document correct placement of the tube. A large air leak, persistent large pneumothorax, or persistent hemothorax despite a correctly placed tube mandates a second drain and consideration for surgical intervention. Suction (up to 20 centimeters of water pressure) can be applied to the drain if required.

The timing of drain removal depends on the absence of an air leak and a reduction in the volume of chest drainage to acceptable levels (usually 50 milliliters per 24 hours). The drain should be removed with the patient either at full inspiration or full expiration. This requires teamwork between two people, one to remove the drain and temporarily occlude the wound, while the second ensures careful suture closure of the chest drain wound and places an occlusive dressing. Most authorities recommend routine chest X-ray after chest drain removal to document complete re-expansion of the lung.

The appropriate treatment of pneumothorax after penetrating injury is tube thoracostomy; however, an asymptomatic patient with a small isolated pneumothorax sometimes can be treated with observation alone. Patients with stab wounds to the chest, but a normal clinical examination and no abnormalities on chest X-ray should be re-x-rayed after a delay of around six hours, as they remain at risk for the development of a pneumothorax.

Indications for Thoracotomy

The indications for thoracotomy can be considered as immediate, early, and delayed.

Immediate Thoracotomy

Enthusiasm for emergency room thoracotomy (ERT) has waxed and waned in recent years. It is a maximally invasive procedure undertaken in an uncontrolled environment and exposes medical staff to significant risks from blood-borne pathogens (Figure 12-4). Overall survival after ERT has been as low as 4% in some series; however, ERT can be a valuable intervention in patients with penetrating chest injuries, especially cardiac tamponade.[24,25]

Emergency room thoracotomy is indicated in patients with penetrating wounds to the torso who sustained witnessed cardiac arrest or in similar patients with persistent severe hypotension (<60 millimeters Hg) with

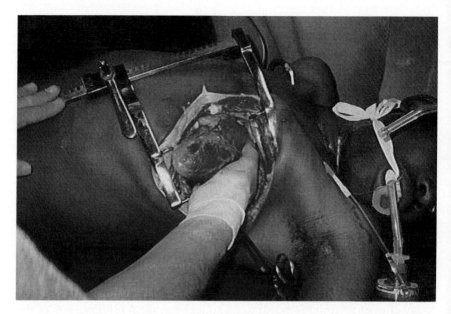

FIGURE 12-4. Emergency room thoracotomy using a left anterior approach.

suspected cardiac tamponade, exsanguinating hemorrhage, or air embolism.[26] Injury to a major airway and a pulmonary vein may allow air bubbles to enter the left side of the heart and embolization to the systemic circulation. As the air emboli migrate to the cerebral and coronary circulation, seizures and cardiac arrest may occur. In addition, air embolus may occur in the presence of a significant pulmonary parenchymal injury when the patient receives positive pressure ventilation.

If ERT is considered to be indicated, delay is fatal. A left anterolateral thoracotomy should be performed without prepping the skin at the level of the fourth or fifth interspace. The incision can be extended across the midline, but for isolated injuries to the right chest, a right thoracotomy is preferred.

Early clamping of the hilum is advisable in patients with a central lung injury or massive bleeding of undetermined origin.[26] A vascular clamp should be applied across the hilum, or alternatively, the inferior pulmonary ligament can be rapidly divided and the lung rotated forward 180 degrees.[27] Hilar control prevents air embolus and quickly controls bleeding.

If tamponade is discovered, or the bleeding is found to be cardiac in origin, the pericardium should be opened longitudinally to avoid phrenic nerve injury. Blood and clot is evacuated from around the heart and bleeding controlled using digital pressure, side-biting clamps, or by inserting a Foley catheter into the wound and blowing up the balloon.

Emergency room thoracotomy allows for direct cardiac massage to be undertaken, and large-bore intravenous lines can be inserted into the right atrium for vascular access. The descending thoracic aorta also can be cross-clamped to reduce subdiaphragmatic hemorrhage and redistribute limited blood flow to the brain and myocardium.

Patients with penetrating cardiac injury are the greatest beneficiaries of ERT, with an overall survival of approximately 10 to 19%.[28,29] When used promptly for the correct indications, ERT is an integral part of resuscitation of patients at the limit of their physiological reserve; however, indiscriminate use of ERT endangers personnel and expends vital resources with little hope of producing neurologically intact survivors.[30] Emergency room thoracotomy is the prototype "damage control" operation, where the surgical intention is to arrest hemorrhage in order to restore physiological stability prior to attempts to undertake reconstructive surgery.[31] Damage control strategies can be used during thoracotomy with immediate treatment of life-threatening injuries, and temporary closure of the incision with definitive care of injuries and formal chest closure performed when physiological characteristics were normalized. Such interventions are likely to be rare. In a study of 10787 patients admitted to a North American Trauma Center, 196 required thoracic operations and 11 of the 196 (5%) underwent a damage control thoracotomy; with all patients surviving to reach the intensive care unit (ICU).[15]

Early (<24 Hours After Injury)

The most common indication for thoracotomy after penetrating chest injury is hemorrhage, followed by airway disruption.[26,32] Indications for early thoracotomy are based on physical findings combined with information from radiological imaging of the chest. An indication for thoracotomy often is given as the drainage of 1.5 liters of blood from the chest tube. At surgery, even large-bore chest tubes are often occluded with clot, and there is usually a surprising amount of blood and clot within the chest cavity. Therefore the amount of blood loss from the tube is not always a reliable guide to the severity of intrathoracic injury. The amount of blood loss must be considered in the light of the clinical condition of the patient, but if blood loss is greater than one liter, thoracotomy should be considered. Other indications for early thoracotomy include:

1. Continued bleeding into the chest tubes of 200 milliliters per hour for 4 hours
2. Massive, continuing air leak throughout the respiratory cycle
3. Transmediastinal wounds in an unstable patient or in the absence of accurate CT imaging.
4. Large chest wall defect.

Delayed (>24 Hours After Injury)

Most patients with chest trauma are managed successfully by tube thoracostomy with careful monitoring of drainage and vital signs. Occasionally, surgical intervention may be needed, usually due to unrecognized or incompletely treated acute injuries. The most common indications for delayed thoracotomy[26] are:

1. Persistent bleeding
2. Prolonged air leak
3. Sepsis.

Although persistent, nonexsanguinating hemorrhage can be treated by thoracotomy; a reduction in severity of the surgical insult can be achieved by the use of video-assisted thoracoscopy (VATS). In a series of stable patients with ongoing thoracic bleeding, thoracoscopic control of bleeding was achieved in 82% of cases.[33] The most widespread application of VATS is in the treatment of clotted hemothorax. Many hemothoraces will liquefy and drain; however if this does not occur, then fibrothorax may occur with constriction of significant volumes of lung parenchyma. Computed tomography scans can help to define whether opacification on a plain chest X-ray is parenchymal or represents retained hemothorax.[34] Any hemothorax that persists beyond 48 hours despite adequate tube thoracostomy could be considered for VATS. If a clotted hemothorax is left, an empyema may develop. Evacuation of a purulent empyema can be achieved using VATS, but if decortication of the lung is required, then thoracotomy most often is needed. For patients with persistent air leak, VATS also allows direct visualization and stapling of the air leak zone with aspiration of associated hemothorax. This has been shown to accelerate patients' recovery.[35]

Cardiac Injuries

The two most common modes of presentation of cardiac injury are cardiac tamponade and excessive hemorrhage depending on the size of the wound in the pericardium.[36] Penetrating cardiac wounds are amongst the most lethal of all injuries; a South African review of 1198 cases of penetrating cardiac trauma showed only 6% arrived at hospital alive.[37] Nevertheless, rapid diagnosis and prompt surgical intervention can salvage patients who have signs of life at the time of presentation.[25] In addition, stable patients have a much better outcome; in a series of 296 patients with a cardiac stab wound confined to a single chamber and with no other associated extracardiac injury, the mortality rate was 8.5%.[38] Patients with penetrating cardiac wounds can be classified into five groups: lifeless, critically unstable, cardiac tamponade, thoracoabdominal injury, and those with a benign presentation.[39] Lifeless or critically unstable patients with exsanguinating hemorrhage require immediate surgical attention, but stable patients may benefit from further investigation before operation.

Much debate has centered on the significance of various factors in predicting survival after penetrating cardiac injury; there is general consensus that vital signs at presentation are a critical determinant for survival. In one study of patients with penetrating heart injury, 152 patients required ERT and only 12 (8%) survived. Of 150 patients able to be transported to the operating room for thoracotomy, 111 (74%) survived.[40] Mechanism of injury also is important, with stab wounds doing better than gunshots, and, unsurprisingly, increasing anatomical severity of injury confers worse outcomes.[40,41]

The presence or absence of cardiac tamponade may have a protective effect; in a series of 100 consecutive patients, those with tamponade had a survival of 73% (24 of 33) compared to 11% (5 of 44) in those without.[42] However, presence of tamponade does not always correlate with improved survival,[43] and it is suggested that although tamponade may protect from exsanguination, this protective effect is limited and by no means universal.

Control of cardiac bleeding may be achieved through the use of pledgeted mattress sutures; it is important to have a good look at the posterior aspect of the heart, as through-and-through penetrating injuries are common and the posterior wound tends to be smaller and may not be obvious at the time of operation. Skin staples also can be used to close a myocardial wounds with equivalent results to sutures, but less risk of needle-stick injury.[44] Penetrating injuries near the coronary arteries should be repaired with mattress sutures so that occlusion of the coronary vessels does not occur. Peripheral branches of coronary vessels damaged by penetrating injury should be ligated. If the vessel is large and the dominant vessel supplying a significant ventricular mass, an attempt can be made to repair the vessel. If repair is not possible, then ligation is recommended. If signs of progressive ischemia, cardiac failure, or uncontrolled arrhythmias develop, then formal repair with bypass is indicated.[45]

Cardiopulmonary bypass has a limited role in the management of penetrating cardiac injury; however, it also may be utilized to salvage patients with complex, multichamber injuries.[46]

All patients with penetrating cardiac injuries will require admission to an intensive care area for optimization of hemodynamic and respiratory variables. Once the immediate problems are controlled, particular attention should be paid to the development of a heart murmur, which could be suggestive of a traumatic septal defect. Ventricular septal defect (VSD) occurs in up to 4.5% of penetrating cardiac trauma, and these defects may be closed using minimally invasive (transcatheter) techniques.[47]

Missile Emboli

Bullets or missile fragments entering the chest may penetrate a blood vessel and act as emboli. The first documented case was in 1834, when a 10-year-old boy sustained a vascular injury and the fragment migrated to the right ventricle.[48] Missile emboli are rare; in the Vietnam Vascular Registry, Rich documented 22 cases of missile emboli in 7500 instances of vascular trauma, (incidence of 0.29%) of these, 19 of 22 (86%) were fragments rather than bullets.[49]

The most common presentation of missile emboli is acute arterial insufficiency;[50] however, delayed disgnosis can be common and associated with significant morbidity. Missile emboli should be suspected if:

- There is a gunshot wound without an exit wound
- Symptoms and signs do not correlate with the expected findings
- Radiological evidence of migration.

In civilian practice, approximately three quarters of missile emboli are small caliber bullets; cardiac and aortic wounds represent approximately 70% of the entry sites.[51] The majority of missile emboli follow the direction of blood flow; therefore, missiles that enter the venous circulation (or right heart) generally progress to the pulmonary circulation. Missiles that enter the aorta or left ventricle propagate into the arterial circulation and generally travel to the lower extremity (although cerebral and other sites are well described). Nearly 15% of venous emboli travel retrogradely and 10% of arterial emboli result from venous or right heart injury and have traversed a patent foramen ovale or the cardiac septum.[50]

Arterial emboli are thought to be asymptomatic in 80% of instances,[50] but the morbidity of venous emboli can be approximately one in four and some authorities have made a case for mandatory removal.[52] While it is clear that symptomatic missile emboli should be removed, asymptomatic arterial emboli in the cerebral, pulmonary, or pelvic vasculature can be safely left alone. Prior to the decision to intervene, due consideration should be given to the risk of:

- The risk of further displacement and embolism
- Propagation of clot associated with a lodged projectile
- The potential for delayed arterial insufficiency.[50]

Angiographic studies can help to plan appropriate incisions; however, intracardiac or intravascular missile emboli can be removed safely by interventional radiologists using transvascular techniques.[53]

Thoracic Great Vessel Injuries

The overall incidence of injury to the thoracic great vessels has been estimated as 5% of gunshot wounds and 2% of stab wounds to the chest.[54] Many of these patients reach the hospital dead or in severe shock due to the rapidity of the loss of a critical volume of blood and the severity of associated injuries. In one autopsy study, all patients who had sustained a penetrating injury to the ascending aorta, arch, and arch branches died before reaching the hospital.[55] Patients that arrive at the hospital with these injuries are therefore a self-selecting group, which, if treated correctly, can have good outcomes. In a series of 93 consecutive patients with penetrating injury to the aortic arch or its major branches, the overall survival was 66 of 93 (72%); of the 27 patients with aortic injury in this series, the survival was 11 of 27 (41%).[56]

In a review of forty-four consecutive patients with injuries to the intrathoracic great vessels, eighteen patients (41%) were hemodynamically stable on admission, with the remainder being unstable (46%), agonal (11%), or lifeless (2%). Forty-two patients (95%) sustained stab wounds and 2 (5%) patients had gunshot wounds. Overall mortality was 5%, and complications occurred in 7 patients (16%). The most frequent radiological abnormality was mediastinal widening in 26 patients (59%). Twenty-two patients (50%) underwent angiography with one false-negative study. A total of 48 arterial and 16 venous injuries were identified, with the innominate artery and left innominate vein the most frequently injured structures. Associated injuries to thoracic viscera occurred in 13 patients (30%). Two patients required cardiopulmonary bypass to repair their injuries.[43]

Patients with thoracic great vessel injury generally present with a wound around the thoracic inlet and can be categorized into two broad groups based on their hemodynamic status. Patients with massive or pulsatile bleeding, gross or persistent hemodynamic instability despite resuscitation should undergo immediate surgery. Patients with pulse deficits, major hematomas, widened mediastinum on plain X-ray, or a missile trajectory in proximity to a major vessel but who are not unstable should undergo angiography.

The basic principles of management have been stated by Pate et al.:[56]

– Urgent local, proximal, and distal vascular control
– Maintenance of prograde flow with shunts, if required
– Prevention of left ventricular hypertension
– Re-establishment of distal circulation by repair, grafts, or ligation and bypass.

Local control of bleeding usually can be achieved by digital occlusion or the use of tangential partially occluding clamps. Intermittent aortic occlusion, which can be partial or complete, helps to reduce blood pressure and improve exposure; however, they can lead to damaging left ventricular

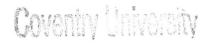
Coventry University

hypertension and should be combined with caval occlusion if possible. Intravascular shunts can be used to maintain prograde flow, and adjuncts such as Fogarty balloon catheters and autotransfusion can be useful in managing these injuries. Documentation of the preoperative neurovascular status of the patient should be performed, and ligation is always an option to save the patient's life.[57]

Penetrating wounds to the thoracic aorta are difficult to approach and control, and nonoperative treatment of small intimal injuries has been reported.[58] Sternotomy is the preferred incision, and division of the innominate vein may help the exposure. If a side-biting vascular clamp can be applied, the injury can be repaired by lateral arteriorraphy; however, cardiopulmonary bypass may be the only possible way of approaching these injuries. Injuries to the arch of the aorta can be approached via sternotomy, with extension of the incision into the neck to control the branches of the arch. Simple repairs may be undertaken without cardiopulmonary bypass. Injuries to the right brachiocephalic artery generally require division of the innominate vein for exposure; this vessel can be ligated with impunity. Simple repairs can be performed, but often a tube graft from the aortic arch to the distal innominate artery is required. This can be achieved without shunts or systemic anticoagulation.[57] The surgical approach to injuries of the left carotid artery is a mirror image of the right brachiocephalic. A median sternotomy with cervical extension is needed for exposure, and control and bypass with a tube graft may be required for complex wounds. Penetrating injuries to the descending thoracic aorta can be immediately lethal; survivors tend to have limited aortic injury, which usually can be managed by primary repair and approach should be via thoracotomy.[59] If bleeding can be controlled, outcome is often dominated by associated injury, such as spinal cord or esophageal injury.

Subclavian vascular injury can be intrathoracic, at the root of the neck or the upper extremity. Basic principles for the management of wounds at the base of the neck include use of the Trendelenberg position, if possible, to reduce the risk of air embolism and control of external bleeding with compression. If bleeding cannot be controlled by direct pressure, balloon tamponade may be attempted.[60] A Foley catheter is inserted into the wound toward the estimated source of bleeding. The balloon then is inflated until the bleeding stops or moderate resistance is felt. For supraclavicular wounds with associated hemothorax, a combination of two Foley catheters may be necessary. The first catheter is inserted as deeply as possible into the chest, the balloon is inflated, and the catheter is pulled back firmly and held in place with an artery clip. This compresses the injured subclavian vessels against the first rib or the clavicle and prevents further bleeding. If external bleeding continues, a second balloon is inserted proximally in the wound tract. Blood through the lumen of the Foley catheter suggests distal bleeding, and repositioning or further inflation of the balloon or clamping of the catheter should be considered.

In unstable patients with subclavian artery injury, sternotomy is indicated for proximal control, followed by clavicular incision regardless of the side of the injury. The "trap-door" incision does not provide good exposure; the efforts of an assistant are wasted and ribs are frequently broken in the heat of the operation. Gunshot victims are likely to be more hemodynamically compromised than stabbing victims, most probably as a result of a greater disruption of the subclavian vessels. This hypothesis is supported by the greater use of an interposition graft for the arterial repair in gunshot victims. The association of both subclavian artery injury and vein injury is also proportionately more common in patients with gunshot wounds.[61] Surgical exposure of subclavian vascular injury by a supraclavicular incision can be achieved in approximately one quarter of patients by combined supraclavicular and infraclavicular incisions in 20% and by division of the clavicle in a further 20%. The remainder require sternotomy, which then is extended as required.[62] Clavicular division generates morbidity from nonunion and sepsis, and some centers have abandoned its use. Associated injuries are common, with approximately a third of the patients sustaining an injury to the brachial plexus.[62]

Injuries to the internal mammary or intercostal arteries can cause massive hemothorax, and the presentation of these injuries can mimic great vessel or cardiac wounds. In a study of parasternal chest stabbings, injury to the internal mammary artery was associated with a mortality rate of 40%.[63] Injuries to the pulmonary arteries and veins have a very high mortality rate, and associated injuries to the heart, pulmonary arteries, aorta, and oesophagus are common. The superior vena cava can be repaired by lateral venorrhaphy, or a tube graft can be used for more complex defects. Caval injuries, either the superior or the intrathoracic inferior vena cava, are associated invariably with injuries to other organs, and the mortality rates are extremely high due to the difficulty in exposure and control of these vessels and the gravity of the associated injury.

In hemodynamically stable patients with wounds at the root of the neck, arteriography and stent-graft treatment should be considered. Stent-graft treatment can successfully treat lesions such as pseudoaneurysms and arteriovenous fistulae; however, long-term outcomes with this method of treatment are still unclear. In a series of forty-one patients with penetrating injuries to the carotid, subclavian, and proximal axillary arteries, 26 required urgent surgical exploration for active bleeding. The remaining 15 patients underwent arteriography to assess suitability for stent-graft placement, 10 patients underwent stent-graft treatment that was successful in all 10 patients, with no complications encountered during the procedure or at early review.[64]

Transmediastinal Injuries

Transmediastinal gunshot wounds (TMGSW) carry a high mortality.[13] Little controversy surrounds the treatment of hemodynamically unstable patients with TMGSW. These patients generally have cardiac or major vascular injuries and require immediate surgery. However, a proportion of patients with gunshot wounds that cross the midline will not have significant visceral injury requiring surgical intervention. In a study of 108 patients from South Africa, 51 patients (47%) were unstable at presentation and underwent immediate surgery; of these, the hemorrhage was of mediastinal origin in just over half, and one third of these patients died of intraoperative bleeding. Only 7% of the patients had aortic injury, and only one in this group survived. There were 57 (53%) stable patients who were investigated initially for injury of the aorta by angiography. It was positive in only one patient, who underwent an operation with good results. An investigation of the esophagus followed and revealed esophageal injury in 17 patients. All of them were treated operatively, 15 of them with satisfactory outcome.[59]

Debate surrounds the extent and order of the diagnostic evaluation for hemodynamically stable patients. Typically, patients undergo chest radiography and surgeon-performed ultrasound in the emergency room. Chest tubes are placed and an assessment can be made of the likely trajectory of the missile; the greatest concerns being for esophageal and aortic injury. In the "pre-CT" era, patients typically underwent contrast swallow and/or endoscopy to evaluate the esophagus and angiography to assess the aorta and great vessels. Recognizing that occult aortic injuries are very rare and that delay to diagnosis of esophageal injury contributes adversely to outcome, some authorities have recommended that the esophageal screen should be undertaken first.[58] Other experts believe that the recognition of an aortic injury is so important that angiography should take priority.[59] With the advent of helical CT scans, the first investigation for a possible mediastinal traversing injury outside of the emergency room should now be CT.[20–22]

Tracheobronchial Injuries

Half of the trachea is in the neck and half in the chest, with the bronchi originating at the level of the fourth thoracic vertebra. Because it is in contact with the esophagus along its entire length and is surrounded by vital organs, associated injuries are common and often fatal. Tracheobronchial injuries can be difficult to diagnose. The presentation of thoracic tracheobronchial injury depends on whether the injury is confined to the mediastinum or communicates with the pleural spaces. Injuries confined to the mediastinum usually present with pneumomediastinum. Injuries communicating with the pleural space usually present with a pneumothorax that persists despite adequate placement of chest tubes and a continuous air leak. Bronchoscopy is the most reliable means of achieving the diagnosis, but rigid bronchoscopy requires general anesthesia and is impossible to perform in the presence of a cervical spine injury. Flexible bronchoscopy can be undertaken without general anesthesia and allows for evaluation of the larynx and controlled insertion of an endotracheal tube, if required.[65]

Management of the airway, as with all patients, is the first priority. Blind endotracheal intubation can lead to misplacement of the tube through a transected airway, and intubation over a flexible bronchoscope is ideal. However, this usually is not available in the emergency setting. Once the airway is secure, attention can turn to the investigation and treatment of the tracheobronchial injury. The best results are obtained with early identification, debridement, and early primary repair of tracheobronchial injuries.[66] Nonoperative management is practiced for selected patients with small lesions seen on bronchoscopy. The blood supply of the trachea enters posterolaterally and care must be taken not to devascularize the trachea. As much as 4 to 5 centimeters (or half) of the thoracic trachea may be resected and primary anastomosis achieved safely. Esophageal injuries identified during repair of the trachea should be repaired simultaneously and a viable muscle flap interposed between the two repairs.

Lung Injuries

The majority of patients with penetrating injuries to the chest do not require thoracotomy. In a review of 2455 patients with chest injuries, 183 (7.4%) required thoracotomy and only 32 (1.3%) required pulmonary resection (Figure 12-5).[26] Those patients requiring thoracotomy due to injuries to the lung usually need urgent attention to stop bleeding or an air leak. When dealing with through-and-through lung injuries, simply suturing the entrance and exit wounds may not be sufficient to control bleeding from the missile track through the lung. Blood may continue to leak into the pleural space, or worse, may drain into the tracheobronchial tree and fill up the uninjured lung tissue. In these circumstances, linear gastrointestinal stapling devices may be used to open the lung parenchyma along the missile track in order to visualize and then selectively ligate bleeding vessels, this technique being known as tractotomy.[67] If it is decided that a pulmonary resection is required, it should be achieved as simply as possible. Linear staplers are a very effective means of undertaking resections of wedges of devitalized or damaged peripheral lung tissue,[26] and use of stapling devices to achieve such "lung-sparing" surgery has been shown to be associated with an improved morbidity and mortality compared with anatomical resections.[68–70] Deep hilar injuries can be very difficult to manage, and pneumonectomy with individual control of vessels prior to resection has been associated with mortality of approximately 50%.[26,70] Pneumonectomy can

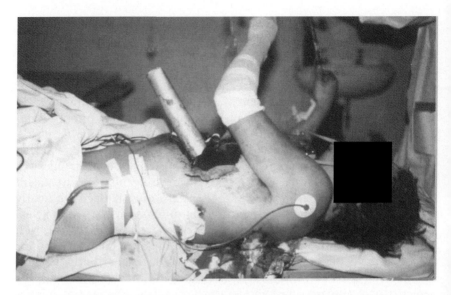

FIGURE 12-5. Impalement injury, left chest caused by a microlite boom. A formal lobectomy was required. (Reproduced with permission from Bowley DMG, Gordon M, Boffard KD. Thoracic impalement after ultralight aircraft crash. Journal Thoracic and Cardiovascular Surgery. 2003;125(4):954–955).

be achieved by en-bloc stapling of the pulmonary hilum with a proprietary stapling device; this avoids the need to formally dissect the hilum and has been associated with increased survival.[71,72] Although exsanguination is a major factor leading to death, mortality after pneumonectomy remains high, even after adequate resuscitation and is thought to be related to pulmonary edema and right heart failure. Careful attention to prevent volume overloading before and during trauma pneumonectomy and maintaining a negative fluid balance postoperatively may contribute to survival in these patients.[73]

Esophageal Injuries

Penetrating injury to the esophagus is very rare; in a series of 1961 patients with penetrating chest injuries from a busy civilian center, 0.7% of patients had intrathoracic oesophageal injuries.[58] In a retrospective review of 2500 war-injured patients from the conflict in Croatia between 1991 and 1995, 0.2% of patients sustained a penetrating injury to the thoracic oesophagus.[74] Morbidity and mortality are high; in a large contemporary series, the overall mortality was 78 of 405 (19%) and the overall complication rate was 53.5%. Diagnostic delay was associated with morbidity.[75]

Throughout its course in the chest, the esophagus is intimately related to vital organs, the trachea in the superior mediastinum, the carina and heart in the middle mediastinum, and the aorta in the lower mediastinum. Because of these intimate anatomical relationships, isolated trauma to the esophagus in the chest is almost impossible, and trauma to related vascular and airway structures confer a very high prehospital mortality. Pain on swallowing (odynophagia) is the most common symptom of esophageal injury, followed by fever, dyspnoea, and crepitus. Overall, symptoms and signs are nonspecific, and a high index of suspicion is required to achieve the diagnosis. Delay in diagnosis leads to a high incidence of mediastinitis, sepsis, and death.

Patients who require emergency surgery for the commonly associated major airway or vascular injuries should be endoscoped when they have been stabilized. Rigid or flexible esophagoscopy should be used depending on the available expertise. For the otherwise stable, cooperative patient, a simple contrast swallow study is recommended. If the patient is sitting upright, progression of contrast is rapid and so the swallow should be undertaken with the patient in the right or left lateral decubitus position. Water-soluble contrast may not show perforations in up to 10% of cases due to poor radiological density; however, barium may produce severe mediastinitis if extravasation occurs into contaminated mediastinal tissues. Gross extravasation can be ruled out using an initial water-soluble swallow, and the addition of a thin barium swallow increase the sensitivity to a small perforation overlooked on the previous study. If the diagnosis is in doubt, endoscopy should be added as well. Helical CT scans of the chest can delineate the trajectory of missiles that traverse the mediastinum. If the investigator is confident that the trajectory is well away from the oesophagus, then special investigations can be omitted.[20]

Surgical repair entails local debridement, wide drainage, primary repair of the perforation, and buttressing of the repair with a pedicle flap of viable intercostal muscle. Primary repair usually can be accomplished when the injury is operated on within 24 hours of occurrence. The blood supply to the esophagus is segmental, and excessive mobilization to achieve primary anastomosis can jeopardize the vascularity of the esophagus. In addition, the esophagus lacks a serosal coat and anastomotic leakage occurs in up to 38% of cases.[76] Approximately 50% of these leaks are asymptomatic and treatment is usually successful with wide drainage, restricted oral intake, supplemented nutrition, and antibiotics. For perforations of the lower thoracic esophagus, a gastric fundal patch can be used to close the defect. With injuries to the esophagus, distal enteral feeding is recommended and a jejunostomy should be inserted whenever possible.

If there has been a significant delay in diagnosis, mediastinal and pleural inflammation can be severe. Several techniques are possible in this setting, including esophageal diversion or exclusion. Small neglected perforations can be treated using T-tube splintage. A 24 French T-tube is used to create a controlled fistula. Mortality for esophageal injuries recognized late is often very high.

Diaphragmatic and Thoracoabdominal Injuries

The word diaphragm is derived from the Greek word meaning a partition or wall. Penetrating injuries, however, do not respect anatomical boundaries, and the diaphragm is wounded in up to 15% of all penetrating wounds to the chest. Isolated diaphragmatic injuries are uncommon; in a series of 163 patients with penetrating injuries to the diaphragm, 75% had associated intraabdominal injuries.[77] Because the diaphragm normally rises to the level of the fifth rib with expiration, it is frequently penetrated by wounds to the anterior chest below the nipple line. Gunshot wounds can injure the diaphragm from any point of entry on the torso.

Because of the intermittent negative intrathoracic pressure, abdominal viscera can herniate through diaphragmatic defects. Subsequent vascular compromise of the incarcerated viscera can lead to strangulation.[78] In a review of a series of hemodynamically stable patients with penetrating wounds to the abdomen evaluated using laparoscopy, 43% had no peritoneal penetration. Of the remaining 57% of patients with an intraperitoneal wound, one third had a diaphragmatic injury.[79] In a prospective study of 110 patients with penetrating injuries of the left thoracoabdominal area that were otherwise stable with no abdominal tenderness, 24% were found to have diaphragmatic injury. Of the patients with diaphragmatic injury, 62% had a chest X-ray reported as normal.[80] Diagnosis of an occult diaphragmatic injury after penetrating trauma depends on an initially high index of suspicion. Wounds in the diaphragm after penetrating injury are usually small, and radiological investigations such as plain X-ray, ultrasound, CT, and even MRI are likely to be of little assistance.

Minimally invasive surgical technology can be very helpful in this setting; both VATS and laparoscopy have been shown to be accurate screening tools to assess potential penetrating diaphragmatic injuries.[80] Acute diaphragmatic injuries should be approached via a laparotomy due to the high frequency of associated abdominal injuries. Diaphragmatic wounds should be sutured accurately using nonabsorbable suture material. If there is significant contamination with stomach contents, then careful toilet must be performed, extending the wound slightly to enable thorough cleansing of the hemithorax if required.

Gunshot injuries of the chest are associated with abdominal injuries in 30 to 40% of patients; however, surgical exploration of both cavities will only be required in approximately 2 to 6%, the majority of chest injuries requiring simple chest drainage.[81]

It can be difficult to decide which is the appropriate side of the diaphragm to explore first. Hirshberg and colleagues analyzed 82 consecutive patients with penetrating thoracoabdominal injuries. Nine thoracotomies (11%) and 16 laparotomies (22%) were negative, with the major causes being misleading chest tube outputs, bullet trajectories, and abdominal tenderness. Inappropriate sequencing of surgery occurred in 19 patients (23%), and 15% required reoperation within 24 hours.[82] In a study of 254 patients with thoracoabdominal injuries requiring surgical intervention, 73 (29%) underwent both thoracotomy and laparotomy. In patients undergoing a combined procedure, mortality was 43 of 73 (59%). Inappropriate surgical sequencing occurred in 32 of 73 (44%) patients. Persistent hypotension indicating that the wrong cavity had been accessed and misleading chest tube output were the leading causes of inappropriate sequencing of surgery.[83] The surgeon must be prepared to access both cavities and prepare the surgical field accordingly.

Thoracic Duct Injuries

The presence of chylous material in the chest drain after penetrating injury heralds an injury to the thoracic duct. Isolated injuries are unusual and the thoracic duct should always be considered when operating in the chest after trauma. Chylous drainage from the chest tube can be treated medically with prolonged tube thoracostomy and a diet devoid of fatty acids, but spontaneous healing rarely occurs and thoracotomy and ligation of the fistula is often required.[84] A fatty meal a few hours prior to surgery facilitates identification of the thoracic duct fistula. Repair of thoracic ductal injury using minimally invasive techniques has also been reported.[85]

Thoracic Impalements

Impalements are the most dramatic thoracic injuries; they are most commonly right sided in survivors, presumably due to the reduced risk of striking the heart or great vessels on that side.[86] A great deal of force is required to impale the thorax, and there is often extensive local tissue destruction with elements of both blunt and penetrating injury.[87] Impalement wounds are often grossly contaminated, often by soil pathogens; hence, appropriate surgical debridement and irrigation and antibiotic and tetanus prophylaxis are mandatory.[88] Patients that survive the trip to hospital are a self-selecting group; hence, the chances of survival are high because the probability is that organ injury is most probably limited to the lung and that the cardiovascular system is largely spared by the penetrating object.[86]

Cautious extrication and rapid transportation are vital, with minimal manipulation of the impaled object. The object should be left *in situ* to avoid loss of tamponade effect. Wide exposure is mandatory and the object should be extracted only after appropriate vascular control has been achieved. All necrotic tissue should be resected, but care should be taken to preserve viable lung; as an expanded lung is good protection against empyema. Complete closure of the chest should be attempted, however, delayed plastic reconstruction of the thoracic defect may be required.

Conclusion

Penetrating chest injury has been a constant challenge to medical practitioners for millennia. Our understanding of the pathophysiology of chest injury has increased, but mortality is still high. The basic principles for successful management center on the follow principles:

- Rapid evacuation to definitive care
- Appropriate first aid using ATLS® principles with rapid surgery when needed
- Use of modern diagnostic adjuncts such as ultrasound and CT
- Adequate drainage of the pleural space, which will manage the majority of survivors of penetrating thoracic injury.
- Appropriate use of thoracotomy or sternotomy.
- Optimal postoperative care with good analgesia and optimal post-injury/postsurgery physical therapy to maximize pulmonary function.

A thorough understanding of these principles, coupled with a coordinated effort from the point of wounding to the hospital and adherence to a common-sense surgical approach should lead to acceptable outcomes following penetrating thoracic injury.

References

1. Santos GH. Chest trauma during the battle of Troy: Ancient warfare and chest trauma. *Ann Thorac Surg.* 2000;69(4):1285–1287.
2. Bellamy RF. History of surgery for penetrating chest trauma. *Chest Surg Clin N Am.* 2000;10(1):55–70, viii.
3. Champion HR, Bellamy RF, Roberts CP, Leppaniemi A. A profile of combat injury. *J Trauma.* 2003;54(5 Suppl):S13–S19.
4. Freud S. Gesammelte Schriften. Vienna: Internationaler Psychoanalytische Verlag; 1924.
5. American College of Surgeons Committee on Trauma. Advanced Trauma Life Support Course. American College of Surgeons; 1997.
6. Zakharia AT. Cardiovascular and thoracic battle injuries in the Lebanon War. Analysis of 3000 personal cases. *J Thorac Cardiovasc Surg.* 1985;89(5):723–733.
7. Demetriades D, Chan L, Cornwell E, Belzberg H, Berne TV, Asensio J, et al. Paramedic vs private transportation of trauma patients. Effect on outcome. *Arch Surg.* 1996;131(2):133–138.
8. Liberman M, Mulder D, Lavoie A, Denis R, Sampalis JS. Multicenter Canadian study of prehospital trauma care. *Ann Surg.* 2003;237(2):153–160.

9. Bass TL, Miller PK, Campbell DB, Russell GB. Traumatic adult respiratory distress syndrome. *Chest Surg Clin N Am.* 1997;7(2):429–442.
10. Croce MA, Fabian TC, Davis KA, Gavin TJ. Early and late acute respiratory distress syndrome: two distinct clinical entities. *J Trauma.* 1999;46(3):361–366.
11. Vassiliu P, Baker J, Henderson S, Alo K, Velmahos G, Demetriades D. Aerodigestive injuries of the neck. *Am Surg.* 2001;67(1):75–79.
12. Demetriades D, Velmahos GG, Asensio JA. Cervical pharyngoesophageal and laryngotracheal injuries. *World J Surg.* 2001;25(8):1044–1048.
13. Flis V, Antonic J, Crnjac A, Zorko A. Air-to-surface missile wound of the thorax reconstructed with a polytetrafluoroethylene patch: Case report. *J Trauma.* 1993;35(5):810–812.
14. Brooks A, Bowley DM, Boffard KD. Bullet markers—a simple technique to assist in the evaluation of penetrating trauma. *J R Army Med Corps.* 2002; 148(3):259–261.
15. Feliciano DV, Rozycki GS. Advances in the diagnosis and treatment of thoracic trauma. *Surg Clin North Am.* 1999;79(6):1417–1429.
16. Thourani VH, Feliciano DV, Cooper WA, Brady KM, Adams AB, Rozycki GS, et al. Penetrating cardiac trauma at an urban trauma center: a 22-year perspective. *Am Surg.* 1999;65(9):811–816.
17. Rozycki GS, Feliciano DV, Ochsner MG, Knudson MM, Hoyt DB, Davis F, et al. The role of ultrasound in patients with possible penetrating cardiac wounds: A prospective multicenter study. *J Trauma.* 1999;46(4):543–551.
18. Sisley AC, Rozycki GS, Ballard RB, Namias N, Salomone JP, Feliciano DV. Rapid detection of traumatic effusion using surgeon-performed ultrasonography. *J Trauma.* 1998;44(2):291–296.
19. Dulchavsky SA, Schwarz KL, Kirkpatrick AW, Billica RD, Williams DR, Diebel LN, et al. Prospective evaluation of thoracic ultrasound in the detection of pneumothorax. *J Trauma.* 2001;50(2):201–205.
20. Hanpeter DE, Demetriades D, Asensio JA, Berne TV, Velmahos G, Murray J. Helical computed tomographic scan in the evaluation of mediastinal gunshot wounds. *J Trauma.* 2000;49(4):689–694.
21. Stassen NA, Lukan JK, Spain DA, Miller FB, Carrillo EH, Richardson JD, et al. Reevaluation of diagnostic procedures for transmediastinal gunshot wounds. *J Trauma.* 2002;53(4):635–638.
22. Grossman MD, May AK, Schwab CW, Reilly PM, McMahon DJ, Rotondo M, et al. Determining anatomic injury with computed tomography in selected torso gunshot wounds. *J Trauma.* 1998;45(3):446–456.
23. Gonzalez RP, Holevar MR. Role of prophylactic antibiotics for tube thoracostomy in chest trauma. *Am Surg.* 1998;64(7):617–620.
24. Aihara R, Millham FH, Blansfield J, Hirsch EF. Emergency room thoracotomy for penetrating chest injury: Effect of an institutional protocol. *J Trauma.* 2001;50(6):1027–1030.
25. Velmahos GC, Degiannis E, Souter I, Allwood AC, Saadia R. Outcome of a strict policy on emergency department thoracotomies. *Arch Surg.* 1995;130(7):774–777.
26. Stewart KC, Urschel JD, Nakai SS, Gelfand ET, Hamilton SM. Pulmonary resection for lung trauma. *Ann Thorac Surg.* 1997;63(6):1587–1588.
27. Wilson A, Wall MJ Jr, Maxson R, Mattox K. The pulmonary hilum twist as a thoracic damage control procedure. *Am J Surg.* 2003;186(1):49–52.

28. Asensio JA, Stewart BM, Murray J, Fox AH, Falabella A, Gomez H, et al. Penetrating cardiac injuries. *Surg Clin North Am.* 1996;76(4):685–724.
29. Rhee PM, Acosta J, Bridgeman A, Wang D, Jordan M, Rich N. Survival after emergency department thoracotomy: Review of published data from the past 25 years. *J Am Coll Surg.* 2000;190(3):288–298.
30. Ladd AP, Gomez GA, Jacobson LE, Broadie TA, Scherer LR, III, Solotkin KC. Emergency room thoracotomy: Updated guidelines for a level I trauma center. *Am Surg.* 2002;68(5):421–424.
31. Wall MJ Jr, Soltero E. Damage control for thoracic injuries. *Surg Clin North Am.* 1997;77(4):863–878.
32. Westaby S. Resuscitation in thoracic trauma. *Br J Surg.* 1994;81(7):929–931.
33. Jones JW, Kitahama A, Webb WR, McSwain N. Emergency thoracoscopy: A logical approach to chest trauma management. *J Trauma.* 1981;21(4):280–284.
34. Velmahos GC, Demetriades D, Chan L, Tatevossian R, Cornwell EE III, Yassa N, et al. Predicting the need for thoracoscopic evacuation of residual traumatic hemothorax: Chest radiograph is insufficient. *J Trauma.* 1999;46(1):65–70.
35. Lang-Lazdunski L, Mouroux J, Pons F, Grosdidier G, Martinod E, Elkaim D, et al. Role of videothoracoscopy in chest trauma. *Ann Thorac Surg.* 1997; 63(2):327–333.
36. Kulshrestha P, Das B, Iyer KS, Sampath KA, Sharma ML, Rao IM, et al. Cardiac injuries—a clinical and autopsy profile. *J Trauma.* 1990;30(2):203–207.
37. Campbell NC, Thomson SR, Muckart DJ, Meumann CM, Van M, I, Botha JB. Review of 1198 cases of penetrating cardiac trauma. *Br J Surg.* 1997;84(12): 1737–1740.
38. Velmahos GC, Degiannis E, Souter I, Saadia R. Penetrating trauma to the heart: A relatively innocent injury. *Surgery.* 1994;115(6):694–697.
39. Saadia R, Levy RD, Degiannis E, Velmahos GC. Penetrating cardiac injuries: Clinical classification and management strategy. *Br J Surg.* 1994;81(11):1572–1575.
40. Tyburski JG, Astra L, Wilson RF, Dente C, Steffes C. Factors affecting prognosis with penetrating wounds of the heart. *J Trauma.* 2000;48(4):587–590.
41. Asensio JA, Berne JD, Demetriades D, Chan L, Murray J, Falabella A, et al. One hundred five penetrating cardiac injuries: A 2-year prospective evaluation. *J Trauma.* 1998;44(6):1073–1082.
42. Moreno C, Moore EE, Majure JA, Hopeman AR. Pericardial tamponade: A critical determinant for survival following penetrating cardiac wounds. *J Trauma.* 1986;26(9):821–825.
43. Asensio JA, Murray J, Demetriades D, Berne J, Cornwell E, Velmahos G, et al. Penetrating cardiac injuries: A prospective study of variables predicting outcomes. *J Am Coll Surg.* 1998;186(1):24–34.
44. Macho JR, Markison RE, Schecter WP. Cardiac stapling in the management of penetrating injuries of the heart: Rapid control of hemorrhage and decreased risk of personal contamination. *J Trauma.* 1993;34(5):711–715.
45. Wall MJ Jr, Mattox KL, Chen CD, Baldwin JC. Acute management of complex cardiac injuries. *J Trauma.* 1997;42(5):905–912.
46. Baker JM, Battistella FD, Kraut E, Owings JT, Follette DM. Use of cardiopulmonary bypass to salvage patients with multiple-chamber heart wounds. *Arch Surg.* 1998;133(8):855–860.

47. Pesenti-Rossi D, Godart F, Dubar A, Rey C. Transcatheter closure of traumatic ventricular septal defect: An alternative to surgery. *Chest.* 2003;123(6):2144–2145.
48. Mattox KL, Beall AC Jr, Ennix CL, DeBakey ME. Intravascular migratory bullets. *Am J Surg.* 1979;137(2):192–195.
49. Rich NM, Collins GJ Jr, Andersen CA, McDonald PT, Kozloff L, Ricotta JJ. Missile emboli. *J Trauma.* 1978;18(4):236–239.
50. Michelassi F, Pietrabissa A, Ferrari M, Mosca F, Vargish T, Moosa HH. Bullet emboli to the systemic and venous circulation. *Surgery.* 1990;107(3):239–245.
51. Shannon JJ Jr, Vo NM, Stanton PE Jr, Dimler M. Peripheral arterial missile embolization: A case report and 22-year literature review. *J Vasc Surg.* 1987;5(5):773–778.
52. Shannon FL, McCroskey BL, Moore EE, Moore FA. Venous bullet embolism: Rationale for mandatory extraction. *J Trauma.* 1987;27(10):1118–1122.
53. Best IM. Transfemoral extraction of an intracardiac bullet embolus. *Am Surg.* 2001;67(4):361–363.
54. Demetriades D. Penetrating injuries to the thoracic great vessels. *J Card Surg.* 1997;12(2 Suppl):173–179.
55. Dosios TJ, Salemis N, Angouras D, Nonas E. Blunt and penetrating trauma of the thoracic aorta and aortic arch branches: An autopsy study. *J Trauma.* 2000;49(4):696–703.
56. Pate JW, Cole FH Jr, Walker WA, Fabian TC. Penetrating injuries of the aortic arch and its branches. *Ann Thorac Surg.* 1993;55(3):586–592.
57. Wall MJ Jr, Granchi T, Liscum K, Mattox KL. Penetrating thoracic vascular injuries. *Surg Clin North Am.* 1996;76(4):749–761.
58. Cornwell EE III, Kennedy F, Ayad IA, Berne TV, Velmahos G, Asensio J, et al. Transmediastinal gunshot wounds. A reconsideration of the role of aortography. *Arch Surg.* 1996;131(9):949–952.
59. Degiannis E, Benn CA, Leandros E, Goosen J, Boffard K, Saadia R. Transmediastinal gunshot injuries. *Surgery.* 2000;128(1):54–58.
60. Gilroy D, Lakhoo M, Charalambides D, Demetriades D. Control of life-threatening haemorrhage from the neck: A new indication for balloon tamponade. *Injury.* 1992;23(8):557–559.
61. Degiannis E, Velmahos G, Krawczykowski D, Levy RD, Souter I, Saadia R. Penetrating injuries of the subclavian vessels. *Br J Surg.* 1994;81(4):524–526.
62. McKinley AG, Carrim AT, Robbs JV. Management of proximal axillary and subclavian artery injuries. *Br J Surg.* 2000;87(1):79–85.
63. Ritter DC, Chang FC. Delayed hemothorax resulting from stab wounds to the internal mammary artery. *J Trauma.* 1995;39(3):586–589.
64. du Toit DF, Strauss DC, Blaszczyk M, de Villiers R, Warren BL. Endovascular treatment of penetrating thoracic outlet arterial injuries. *Eur J Vasc Endovasc Surg.* 2000;19(5):489–495.
65. Baumgartner FJ, Ayres B, Theuer C. Danger of false intubation after traumatic tracheal transection. *Ann Thorac Surg.* 1997;63(1):227–228.
66. Rossbach MM, Johnson SB, Gomez MA, Sako EY, Miller OL, Calhoon JH. Management of major tracheobronchial injuries: A 28-year experience. *Ann Thorac Surg.* 1998;65(1):182–186.

67. Asensio JA, Demetriades D, Berne JD, Velmahos G, Cornwell EE III, Murray J, et al. Stapled pulmonary tractotomy: A rapid way to control hemorrhage in penetrating pulmonary injuries. *J Am Coll Surg.* 1997;185(5):486–487.
68. Velmahos GC, Baker C, Demetriades D, Goodman J, Murray JA, Asensio JA. Lung-sparing surgery after penetrating trauma using tractotomy, partial lobectomy, and pneumonorrhaphy. *Arch Surg.* 1999;134(2):186–189.
69. Cothren C, Moore EE, Biffl WL, Franciose RJ, Offner PJ, Burch JM. Lung-sparing techniques are associated with improved outcome compared with anatomic resection for severe lung injuries. *J Trauma.* 2002;53(3):483–487.
70. Karmy-Jones R, Jurkovich GJ, Shatz DV, Brundage S, Wall MJ Jr, Engelhardt S, et al. Management of traumatic lung injury: A Western Trauma Association Multicenter review. *J Trauma.* 2001;51(6):1049–1053.
71. Tominaga GT, Waxman K, Scannell G, Annas C, Ott RA, Gazzaniga AB. Emergency thoracotomy with lung resection following trauma. *Am Surg.* 1993; 59(12):834–837.
72. Wagner JW, Obeid FN, Karmy-Jones RC, Casey GD, Sorensen VJ, Horst HM. Trauma pneumonectomy revisited: The role of simultaneously stapled pneumonectomy. *J Trauma.* 1996;40(4):590–594.
73. Baumgartner F, Omari B, Lee J, Bleiweis M, Snyder R, Robertson J, et al. Survival after trauma pneumonectomy: The pathophysiologic balance of shock resuscitation with right heart failure. *Am Surg.* 1996;62(11):967–972.
74. Ilic N, Petricevic A, Mimica Z, Tanfara S, Ilic NF. War injuries to the thoracic esophagus. *Eur J Cardiothorac Surg.* 1998;14(6):572–574.
75. Asensio JA, Chahwan S, Forno W, MacKersie R, Wall M, Lake J, et al. Penetrating esophageal injuries: Multicenter study of the American Association for the Surgery of Trauma. *J Trauma.* 2001;50(2):289–296.
76. Richardson JD, Tobin GR. Closure of esophageal defects with muscle flaps. *Arch Surg.* 1994;129(5):541–547.
77. Demetriades D, Kakoyiannis S, Parekh D, Hatzitheofilou C. Penetrating injuries of the diaphragm. *Br J Surg.* 1988;75(8):824–826.
78. Feliciano DV, Cruse PA, Mattox KL, Bitondo CG, Burch JM, Noon GP, et al. Delayed diagnosis of injuries to the diaphragm after penetrating wounds. *J Trauma.* 1988;28(8):1135–1144.
79. Ivatury RR, Simon RJ, Stahl WM. A critical evaluation of laparoscopy in penetrating abdominal trauma. *J Trauma.* 1993;34(6):822–827.
80. Murray JA, Demetriades D, Asensio JA, Cornwell EE, III, Velmahos GC, Belzberg H, et al. Occult injuries to the diaphragm: prospective evaluation of laparoscopy in penetrating injuries to the left lower chest. *J Am Coll Surg.* 1998;187(6):626–630.
81. Murray JA, Berne J, Asensio JA. Penetrating thoracoabdominal trauma. *Emerg Med Clin North Am.* 1998;16(1):107–128.
82. Hirshberg A, Wall MJ Jr, Allen MK, Mattox KL. Double jeopardy: Thoracoabdominal injuries requiring surgical intervention in both chest and abdomen. *J Trauma.* 1995;39(2):225–229.
83. Asensio JA, Arroyo H Jr, Veloz W, Forno W, Gambaro E, Roldan GA, et al. Penetrating thoracoabdominal injuries: Ongoing dilemma—which cavity and when? *World J Surg.* 2002;26(5):539–543.

84. Worthington MG, de Groot M, Gunning AJ, von Oppell UO. Isolated thoracic duct injury after penetrating chest trauma. *Ann Thorac Surg.* 1995;60(2): 272–274.
85. Buchan KG, Hosseinpour AR, Ritchie AJ. Thoracoscopic thoracic duct ligation for traumatic chylothorax. *Ann Thorac Surg.* 2001;72(4):1366–1367.
86. Robicsek F, Daugherty HK, Stansfield AV. Massive chest trauma due to impalement. *J Thorac Cardiovasc Surg.* 1984;87(4):634–636.
87. Thomson BN, Knight SR. Bilateral thoracoabdominal impalement: Avoiding pitfalls in the management of impalement injuries. *J Trauma.* 2000;49(6):1135–1137.
88. Horowitz MD, Dove DB, Eismont FJ, Green BA. Impalement injuries. *J Trauma.* 1985;25(9):914–916.

13
Penetrating Genitourinary Trauma: Management by the Nonspecialist Surgeon

Jay J. Doucet and David B. Hoyt

Introduction

The genitourinary system lies in the retroperitoneal space and shares the perineum with the rectum and major neurovascular structures. As a result, penetrating trauma to the genitourinary system usually is associated with injury to multiple organ systems and requires a multidisciplinary effort with an organized and thorough evaluation of all injuries.

Eight percent of civilian gunshot wounds include the kidney. Fifty-six percent of stab wounds and 96% of gunshot wounds to the kidney have associated injuries, most commonly the liver, small bowel, stomach, and colon.[1] In the United States, 20% of renal penetrating injury results in renal loss.

Mechanisms of Penetrating Genitourinary Trauma

Stab wounds of the genitourinary system are low-energy wounds where the injury is confined to the wound tract. Such wounds may be minor lacerations, such as a superficial parenchymal laceration as classified by the renal injury scheme shown in Table 13-1. Major lacerations into the medullary portion of the kidney may involve the collecting system and lead to urinary extravasation. About 20% of stab wounds cause vascular injuries to a main or segmental renal vein.

Gunshot wounds are more likely to cause major lacerations. The rate of deposition of energy into the tissues by the projectile's deceleration determines the wounding effect. The kinetic energy (KE) of a missile is determined by the formula $KE = \frac{1}{2} mv^2$, where m is the mass of the projectile and v is the velocity. Velocity is usually the major determinant of KE. High-velocity projectiles such as assault rifle bullets with typical muzzle velocities of 1000 meters per second may contain about 5 to 10 times more muzzle energy than low-velocity pistol bullets with typical muzzle velocities of 300 meters per second.[2] Although knowing the type of weapon used is helpful in raising suspicions of high-velocity–type injury, there are circumstances

TABLE 13-1. Kidney organ injury scoring system

Grade	Type of injury	Injury description	AIS-90
I	Contusion	Microscopic or gross hematuria, urological studies normal	2
	Hematoma	Subcapsular, nonexpanding without parenchymal laceration	2
II	Laceration	<1 cm parenchymal depth of renal cortex without urinary extravasation	2
	Hematoma	Nonexpanding perirenal hematoma confined to renal retroperitoneum	2
III	Laceration	>1 cm depth of renal cortex, without collecting system rupture or urinary extravasation	3
IV	Laceration	Parenchymal laceration extending through the renal cortex, medulla, and collecting system	4
	Vascular	Main renal artery or vein injury with contained hemorrhage	5
V	Laceration	Completely shattered kidney	5
	Vascular	Avulsion of renal hilum that devascularizes kidney	5

Advance one grade for bilateral injuries up to and including Grade III.
Source: Moore et al., 1989.[20] (With permission, Lippincott Williams and Wilkins 2003)

where wounds may not seem to match their weapons. An assault rifle bullet in the stable portion of its flight may pass through elastic tissue with minimal tissue disruption. A pistol fired against the skin, or a pistol bullet that decelerates rapidly, such as when striking bone, may cause significant tissue damage.[3]

The deposition of energy by a projectile also is determined by the viscoelastic properties of the tissues. The kidney is a relatively dense, nonelastic structure with a capsule suspended in the Gerota's fascia of elastic fat and connective tissue. Similarly, the testicle is a dense, encapsulated structure suspended in elastic aerolar tissue and skin. Missiles decelerate more rapidly and deposit energy more rapidly in denser tissue. High-velocity missiles may pass through the relatively elastic connective tissues with little effect, but can cause extensive destruction to these solid organs by the effects of cavitation and fragmentation.

Low-velocity projectiles usually cause injury only within a narrow tract defined by 1 to 5 times the bullet's caliber. High-velocity projectiles may cause cavitation and may cause disruption and lacerations of vessels and viscera outside of the actual bullet's track.[4] Some high-velocity bullets also are prone to fragmentation, causing penetrations with multiple tracts. They also may generate secondary projectiles by striking, fragmenting, and accelerating bone.[5] High-velocity injuries do not mandate excessive debridement of the genitourinary wounds, but should increase suspicions for a significant injury lateral to the expected bullet's tract.

Shotguns have special characteristics.[3] These weapons have a large caliber, smooth bore barrel with typical diameters from 1.0 centimeter (.410

caliber) to 2.0 centimeters (10 Gauge). There are a variety of projectiles that can be fired, from a single large "slug" through large buckshot (e.g., 00 Buckshot contains spheres of about .33 caliber) down to small caliber birdshot or even multiple darts or "flechettes." The poor aerodynamic qualities of these projectiles mean that the projectiles decelerate in air rather rapidly, and the projectiles disperse increasingly widely with distance from the muzzle. These weapons typically have a muzzle velocity of about 400 meters per second, which might be considered low velocity. However, the large mass of projectiles means a 12-gauge shotgun has a muzzle energy of 4 to 5 times that of a 9-millimeter pistol bullet. A 12-gauge shotgun firing a load of 00 buckshot fired from 8 meters or less may shred the tissue for a diameter of up to 10 centimeters.[3] This can cause challenging wounds in locations such as the perineum. Close-range wounds also may contain non-radiopaque wadding, plastic carriers, or sabots used to buffer the projectiles from the propellant or barrel. Multiple pellets can disperse throughout the tissues; when penetrating the kidney, they can cause the peculiar phenomenon of pellet colic.[6,7]

War or terrorist events tend to be dominated by wounds caused by shrapnel and by blast injury instead of gunshot wounds.[8–10] Sixty-eight percent of genitourinary injuries in combat are to the external genitalia.[11,12] Blast injuries due to high-order explosives can cause blunt-type genitourinary injuries by the externally applied acceleration from the supersonic blast wave. These blast injuries frequently are accompanied by penetrating injuries. Most explosive weapons generate shrapnel, which enhances lethality and wounding effect. Shrapnel may have very high initial velocities (over 3000 meters per second), but the irregularly shaped fragments are not aerodynamic and decelerate rapidly in air so that high- or low-velocity wounding effects may be seen.

Antipersonnel mines are a particular threat for genitourinary injury.[13] During the recent war in Bosnia, one field hospital's review of 136 casualties with genitourinary injuries revealed 40% had injuries to the external genitalia, about two-thirds of which were thought to be due to mines.[14] When stepped on, small buried mines typically explode and direct fragments upward to cause severe extremity trauma in addition to missile injuries to the external genitalia and perineum. Bounding mines, those designed to jump into the air before detonating, typically detonate at a height that will cause severe penetrating injury to the abdomen and genitalia.

Penetrating Renal Injuries

Diagnosis

Penetrating renal trauma is diagnosed by clinical, laboratory, and medical imaging. In the hemodynamically unstable patient who must undergo laparotomy to assess abdominal penetration, the evaluation of the genitourinary system may be completed intraoperatively.

Clinical Findings

After ensuring that the patient's airway and ventilatory status is satisfactory, the patient's hemodynamic status is assessed. In one series, 29% of stab wounds and 52% of gunshot wounds to the kidney presented with a systolic blood pressure less than 90 torr.[1] While resuscitating the patient, a history of the wounding is obtained. Determining the size and length of the knife may be helpful in determining the structures at risk in stab wounds. In gunshot wounds, knowing the type of weapon may heighten suspicions of high-velocity–type injury.

Clinical examination of the abdomen should include careful examination of the skin of the back and flanks for multiple penetrations, which may be small and nonbleeding, as well as the skin folds of the perineum and buttocks. Clinical assessment determines those patients who require immediate surgery and those who need further investigation.

Laboratory Findings

Hematuria is defined as microscopic if there is more than 5 red blood cells per high powered field in apparently clear urine, or gross hematuria if blood stained urine is readily visible in the Foley catheter drainage bag. Hematuria of any degree in penetrating injury should raise suspicion of genitourinary injury and mandates investigation. The degree of hematuria does not correlate with the severity of injury. Approximately eighteen percent of stab wounds and 6.8% of gunshot wounds did not have hematuria in the University of California, San Francisco (UCSF) series.[1] Thirty-three percent of patients with penetrating injuries severe enough to require nephrectomy did not have gross hematuria.

Radiological Findings

The intravenous pyelogram (IVP) or excretory urogram is the most thoroughly investigated imaging mode in penetrating renal injury, but it is being replaced at many centers by contrast-enhanced computed tomography (CT) scanning.

The hemodynamic stability of the patient should be considered carefully in choosing imaging modalities. An unstable patient should not be placed in the CT scanner, but may have a one-shot IVP in the resuscitation area or in the operating room prior to laparotomy. The recommended dose is of two milligrams per kilogram of a 50% iodinated contrast material, such as diatrizoate (Hypaque, Amersham Health, Princeton, NJ). This is given at wide open drip, followed by an X-ray in 10 minutes. This can determine bilateral renal function and detect some ureteral injuries.

The utility of the routine use of one-shot IVP before laparotomy in the stable penetrating injury patient has been questioned by Nagy and colleagues, who noted in a study of 240 patients that the prevalence of a unilateral nonfunctioning kidney was less than 1%.[15] In addition, the IVPs were of suboptimal quality in 22% of cases. The IVP was normal in 59% of patients with a proven renal injury, regardless of grade of injury. Nagy and colleagues concluded that the IVP should not be used to exclude renal injuries, but only should be used when the wound trajectory was near the kidney or with gross hematuria.

Patel and colleagues reviewed 40 patients with penetrating abdominal trauma who received one-shot IVP for injuries with proximity to the kidney before laparotomy.[16] Only 2 of 10 patients with proven urologic injuries had positive one-shot IVPs. Seven had renal injuries and 3 had bladder injuries. Two of 9 patients with gross hematuria had a positive IVP, but urologic injuries were found at laparotomy in 6 out of 9 patients. There were 8 false-positive and 6 false-negative one-shot IVPs in this study, yielding a positive predictive value of 20%. The decision of whether or not to perform laparotomy was not influenced in any case. Given the unilateral nonfunctioning kidney rate of less than 1%, Patel and colleagues concluded that one-shot IVP did not influence management of any patient, but did delay definitive management.

It should be noted that concern over the function of a contralateral kidney can be addressed in the operating room after control of bleeding has been obtained by the use of intraoperative IVP or injection of vital dyes such as indigo carmine or methylene blue.

Computed tomography scanning provides superior visualization of renal anatomy and perfusion.[17] Computed tomography scanning also can identify injury to adjacent viscera and the renal vasculature and has eliminated the need for renal angiography. Computed tomography scanning facilitates the nonoperative management of penetrating renal injury.[18] Computed tomography scanning is indicated only in patients who have been hemodynamically stable and without an indication for immediate laparotomy. Delayed images taken 2 to 5 minutes after the initial injection can provide evidence of renal function with contrast seen in the renal pelvis and ureter. Extravasation of contrast aids detection of extravasation of blood and urine.

Nonoperative Management

Nonoperative management of renal injury has been driven by the finding of a higher nephrectomy rate with exploration of blunt kidney injuries versus nonoperative management. Concern exists that opening Gerota's fascia and releasing a perinephric hematoma leads to a higher nephrectomy rate.[19] It has not been possible to determine precisely an American Association for the Surgery of Trauma (AAST) Grade of renal injury that mandates surgical exploration (Table 13-1).[20] Minor injuries such as Grade

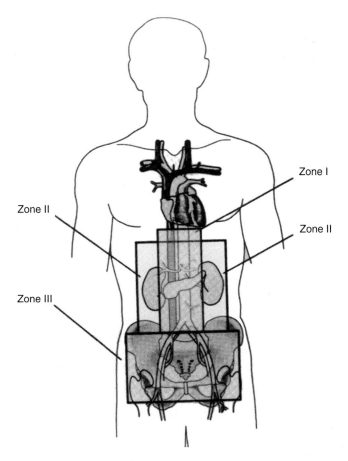

FIGURE 13-1. Anatomic zones of retroperitoneal hematomas. Zone I = periaortic; Zones II = perinephric; Zone III = pelvic. (From: Hoyt DB, Coimbra R, Potenza BM, Rappold JF. Anatomic exposures for vascular injuries. *Surg Clin North Am.* 2001;81(6):1317; with permission).

I and II traditionally have been managed conservatively. Grade IV (renal vascular, pedicle injury) and Grade V (avulsion) injuries usually have been managed operatively. Blunt Grade III injuries (major lacerations) have been managed successfully in a nonoperative manner for three decades.[21]

Gunshot wounds to the abdomen traditionally have been managed by abdominal exploration at laparotomy. Zone I hematomas are explored in blunt or penetrating trauma due to the possibility of abdominal vascular, duodenal, or pancreatic injury. Zone II perinephric nonexpanding retroperitoneal hematomas caused by penetrating injuries found at laparotomy routinely have been explored, whereas in blunt trauma they were not explored (Figure 13-1). However, stable, lateral perinephric Zone II hematomas that have been staged by CT scanning do not require exploration.[22]

Shaftan introduced the concept of "selective conservatism" in the 1960s, which was validated by Nance in later studies.[23,24]

The nonoperative management of penetrating wounds to the kidney is becoming practiced more widely with the use of CT scanning.[25–27] Wounds can be marked with a metallic marker at the wound on the skin or by insertion of a contrast-soaked sponge in the wound. Computed tomography scanning can delineate the tract and can exclude injury to the retroperitoneum in tangential wounds.

In the context of the Level 1 trauma center with an in-house trauma team, selective nonoperative management of civilian abdominal gunshot wounds has been described by several authors. Velmahos and colleagues reported on selective nonoperative management in 1856 patients with abdominal gunshot wounds.[28] Patients who were hemodynamically stable, had no evidence of peritonitis, and who had a reliable clinical examination were observed. Computed tomography scanning was carried out increasingly in all patients undergoing nonoperative management for the first 5 years of the study and in all patients undergoing nonoperative management by the last three years of the study. Seven hundred and ninety-two (42%) patients were selected for nonoperative management. Thirty-four percent of the patients had anterior wounds and 68% had posterior wounds. Eighty (4%) patients failed nonoperative management, no patient died as a result of the delayed laparotomy. Patients with posterior gunshot wounds were more likely to have nonoperative management, but had the same rate of delayed laparotomy and negative delayed laparotomy as anterior abdominal gunshot wounds.

Velhamos and colleagues earlier described the nonoperative management of gunshot wounds to the back.[29] Two hundred and three patients with gunshot wounds were subject to selective nonoperative management. Of the 130 (69%) selected for nonoperative management, four (3%) underwent laparotomy for increasing abdominal tenderness; none of those laparotomies were deemed therapeutic.

Velmahos reported on selective nonoperative management of 52 consecutive renal gunshot wound patients.[25] Patients underwent laparotomy if there was evidence of continued bleeding or a renal hilar injury. Only four patients were managed nonoperatively, three Grade II injuries and one Grade III injury. Of the 48 patients undergoing laparotomy, 32 had Gerota's fascia opened. Two of the two Grade I and two of the five Grade II injuries were deemed to have undergone unnecessary renal exploration. Reconstruction of the kidney was carried out in six of seven Grade III explorations, one Grade III injury underwent nephrectomy, and one Grade III injury did not undergo renal exploration at laparotomy. All grade IV (14 of 52) and V (6 of 52) wounds were explored. Ten of 14 Grade IV injuries were reconstructed. Four Grade IV and all six Grade V injuries underwent nephrectomy. Patients who underwent nephrectomy were more likely to have presented with a systolic blood pressure below 90, a hematocrit less than 30%, an Injury Severity Score greater than 20, or with Grade IV or V injuries.

Santucci and colleagues correlated AAST grade and mechanism of injury (blunt trauma, stab wound, gunshot) in 2467 patients at the UCSF.[30] Grade III stab wounds had an exploration rate of 78% compared to a 93% exploration rate and nephrectomy rate for Grade III gunshot wounds. Grade IV stab wounds had an exploration rate of 94% compared to a 100% exploration rate for Grade IV gunshot wounds. All Grade V penetrating injuries were explored.

Thall reported on 32 penetrating and 13 blunt Grade III renal injuries, 16 stab wounds, and 16 gunshot wounds.[31] Eleven gunshot wounds required immediate exploration, two required renorrhaphy, one had partial nephrectomy, and two had initial nephrectomy. Five gunshot Grade III injuries were managed successfully nonoperatively.

Nonoperative management of Grade IV gunshot wounds has only been described in a few cases. McAninch and colleagues described 2483 renal trauma patients at UCSF. Sixty eight had penetrating Grade IV injuries—of these, 97% required exploration and 10% required nephrectomy.[32] Hammer and colleagues described a policy of restricting renal exploration to patients with exsanguinating hemorrhage with successful nonoperative treatment of two Grade III and three Grade IV gunshot injuries, which in comparison had a 93% and 100% rate of operation in McAninch's series.[33]

These reports of nonoperative management of renal injuries come from major trauma centers. Nonoperative management of penetrating renal trauma appears only to be an option in a defined setting of a hemodynamically stable patient with a CT scan demonstrating a Grade I–III injury with a reliable clinical abdominal exam who can be followed closely in the trauma center. There are limited numbers of patients with Grade IV or Grade V penetrating injuries reported as undergoing nonoperative management. Nonoperative management of such patients only would be appropriate in the setting of a clinical trial.

Before World War I, penetrating torso wounds were managed expectantly. During that conflict, the 53% mortality of abdominal wounds spurred development of abdominal surgery.[34] There are no modern reports on nonoperative management of abdominal gunshot wounds in the austere or conflict environment, where CT scanning, a dedicated trauma team, and skilled nursing units usually are lacking. Occasionally, forward-located military surgeons may have the option of rapid evacuation of a stable penetrating abdominal casualty to a larger rear area hospital, but this not an alternative for humanitarian and developing world surgeons. More often, laparotomy and intraoperative evaluation of the genitourinary tract and associated abdominal injuries will be the prudent action.

Operative Management

Absolute indications for exploration of the kidney are hemodynamic instability due to renal injury, expanding perinephric hematoma, and incomplete radiological assessment of a renal injury. Relative indications include urinary extravasation, nonviable renal parenchyma with a large laceration, and renal vascular injury.

The technique of abdominal exploration requires a midline transabdominal incision. This allows prompt access to the intra-abdominal viscera to allow complete examination and rapid access to the central vasculature of the abdomen, including the renal vessels.

Controversy exists in the need to routinely control the renal pedicle before renal exploration. Carroll and McAnnich obtained vascular control of the renal pedicle before opening Gerota's fascia to reduce the rate of nephrectomy due to uncontrolled hemorrhage.[35,36] They reported that renal pedicle clamping was required in 12% of explorations which resulted in a three-fold increased rate of renal salvage.

If vascular control is desired, the renal pedicle may be accessed anteriorly by reflecting the transverse colon and small intestine superiorly and exposing the retroperitoneum. A vertical incision is made in the peritoneum over the aorta and extended superiorly to the ligament of Treitz. A large retroperitoneal hematoma may obscure these landmarks; however, the inferior mesenteric vein usually is visible, in which case the incision is made medial to that vein. The anterior surface of the aorta is identified and dissection proceeds superiorly to identify the left renal vein, which crosses anterior to the aorta. The vessels ipsilateral to the injured kidney then can be dissected out posteriorly. Vessel loops then can be applied to the renal artery and vein. Gerota's fascia then can be opened lateral to the kidney. Should the release of the tamponade provided by the perinephric hematoma cause uncontrolled bleeding, vascular clamps can be applied to the vessels loops and the injuries identified.

Some surgeons prefer a lateral approach instead of preliminary vascular control in all explorations, believing it saves time without increasing nephrectomy rates.[37,38]

In the unstable patient, a rapid or "scoop" nephrectomy may be required to control exsanguinating hemorrhage. This is accomplished rapidly by incising the peritoneal surface lateral to the injured kidney and then entering Gerota's fascia. The plane behind the kidney is developed with the surgeon's hand and the kidney is reflected anteriorly and medially to allow the renal pedicle to be controlled with digital pressure and vascular clamps.

Renal vascular injuries can be challenging. The kidney cannot tolerate more than an hour of warm total ischemic time, although there may be partial flow from small adrenal and ureteric collaterals. Associated injuries occur in most cases; mortality in a recent series ranged from 2.4%[39] to 54%.[40]

The renal pedicle lies in Zone I along with the renal pelvis and proximal ureter, abdominal aorta, vena cava, duodenum, pancreas, and celiac and superior mesenteric arteries and their branches and tributaries. A small incision in the retroperitoneum directly over the renal vessels may not allow adequate examination of these structures in the setting of a large hematoma or active hemorrhage. Wide access to this area can be obtained by incising the lateral peritoneum widely and performing left or right visceral rotations (Figures 13-2 and 13-3).

Renorrhaphy requires adequate mobilization and exposure of the kidney. Injuries to the parenchyma should have their edges debrided. Bleeding vessels in the renal parenchyma can be ligated with suture ligatures. Injuries in the collecting system should be repaired with continuous fine absorbable suture. Isolated renal lacerations can be repaired by placing an absorbable hemostatic bolster within the laceration. The renal capsule is then loosely approximated over a second bolster (Figure 13-4). Omental or peritoneal flaps can be mobilized to cover extensive defects or to separate the injury from an associated visceral injury. Partial nephrectomy can be used in cases

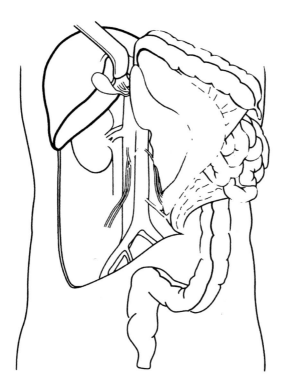

FIGURE 13-2. Left visceral rotation to expose the right kidney, renal vessels, and aorta. (From: Hoyt DB, Coimbra R, Potenza BM, Rappold JF. Anatomic exposures for vascular injuries. *Surg Clin North Am.* 2001;81(6):1318; with permission).

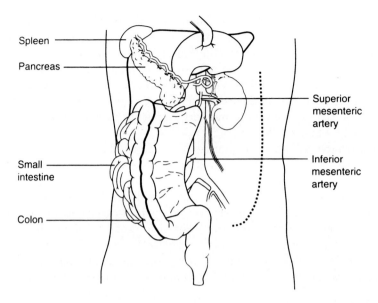

Spleen

Pancreas

Small intestine

Colon

Superior mesenteric artery

Inferior mesenteric artery

FIGURE 13-3. Right visceral rotation to expose the left kidney, renal vessels, and vena cava. (From: Hoyt DB, Coimbra R, Potenza BM, Rappold JF. Anatomic exposures for vascular injuries. *Surg Clin North Am*. 2001;81(6):1322; with permission).

where the pole of the kidney is injured (Figure 13-5). Drains are used when injuries are extensive or involve the collecting system. Gerota's fascia is left open.

Lacerations of the renal vessels may be repaired with fine vascular suture. The left renal vein may be ligated proximal to the vena cava, with the gonadal and adrenal veins acting as collateral venous drainage. Segmental veins also can be ligated safely due to collaterals, but ligation of segmental arteries will result in ischemia to a segment of parenchyma. Associated abdominal injuries, an unreconstructable renal pedicle or kidneys, shock, difficulty in obtaining adequate exposure, and the risk of renovascular hypertension with a stenotic arterial repair are factors that lead to a significant failure rate in repairing renal arterial injuries. Ivatury reported that nephrectomy is the usual outcome in half of renal vascular injuries.[41]

A review of renal vascular injuries by the Western Trauma Association (WTA) described 30 penetrating Grade IV injuries and 14 penetrating Grade V injuries with renal vascular injuries.[39] Penetrating injuries tended to have better outcomes than blunt trauma. Vein repairs had better outcomes than arterial repairs. Hypertension ensued in 4.5% of renovascular repairs, typical of reported rates in recent literature.[42,43] The WTA study suggested that the best outcomes were obtained in penetrating Grade IV injuries with immediate exploration and repair and in Grade V injuries with immediate nephrectomy.

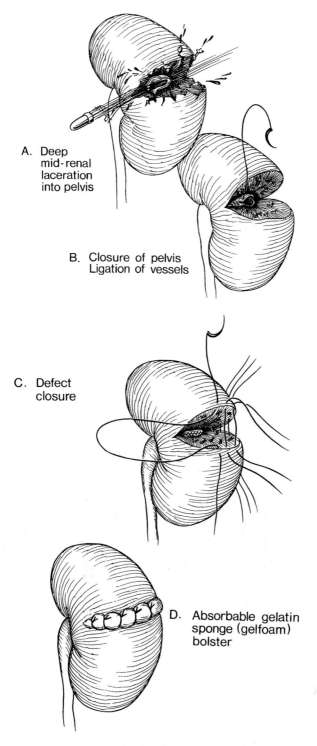

A. Deep mid-renal laceration into pelvis

B. Closure of pelvis Ligation of vessels

C. Defect closure

D. Absorbable gelatin sponge (gelfoam) bolster

FIGURE 13-4. Technique of renorrhaphy. (From: Armenakas NA, McAninch JW. Genitourinary tract. In: Ivatury RR, Cayten CG, eds. *The Textbook of Penetrating Trauma*. Media, PA: Williams and Wilkins; 1996:684; with permission).

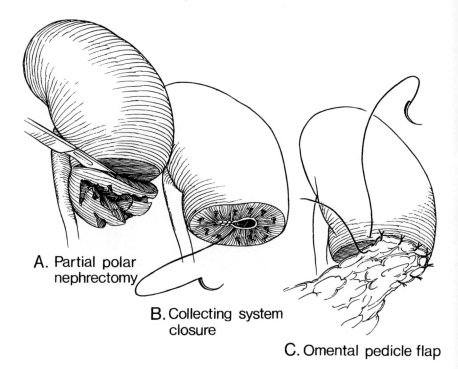

A. Partial polar nephrectomy

B. Collecting system closure

C. Omental pedicle flap

FIGURE 13-5. Technique of partial nephrectomy. (From: Armenakas NA, McAninch JW. Genitourinary tract. In: Ivatury RR, Cayten CG, eds. *The Textbook of Penetrating Trauma*. Media, PA: Williams and Wilkins; 1996:685; with permission).

Patients with a solitary kidney or with bilateral injuries require aggressive management to preserve renal function. In the case of bilateral injuries, the less injured kidney usually is explored, first to reduce the risk of attempting salvage, then performing nephrectomy on a badly injured kidney, and then discovering the contralateral kidney requires considerable time to salvage. Autotransplantation may be required in rare cases.[44,45]

Associated Injuries

Associated injuries to adjacent viscera such as the pancreas or colon may complicate 80% of penetrating renal injury. Patients with combined injuries have a higher rate of complications, including abscess, fistula, urinoma, sepsis, and death. However, the decision whether to perform nephrectomy or renal salvage in these patients should be determined by the nature of the renal injury and the patient's overall condition, rather than by the presence of fecal contamination.

Wessels reported on 62 cases of combined penetrating colon and renal injury with 23% stab wounds and 52% gunshot wounds.[46] Exploration was carried out in 58% of cases and nephrectomy resulted from 16% of those explorations. Twenty-five percent of patients suffered postoperative complications, including abscesses (15%) and one late nephrectomy in a patient with a delayed diagnosis of a colon injury due to blast injury with subsequent abscess after an explored gunshot wound to the kidney. Fecal spillage had no effect on patient outcome or likelihood of urologic complication, nephrectomy, or survival. Despite the higher complication rate in these cases, the rate of renal salvage was felt to justify managing the renal injury based on the degree of renal trauma only.

Outcome and Complications

Complications include delayed bleeding, urinoma and urinary extravasation, perirenal abscess, hypertension, renal failure, and death.

Delayed bleeding occurs in about 18% of nonoperatively managed renal stab wounds.[47] The delayed bleeding rate in nonoperative gunshot wounds is undetermined. The delayed bleeding rate in surgically operated penetrating renal injury is 3.7%.[48]

Computed tomography scanning is sensitive for urinary extravasation. Massive extravasation extending medially (from the renal pelvis) or from a lacerated pole of the kidney suggests a major injury unlikely to stop spontaneously and is managed best with operative repair. Urinomas are large collections of urine in the retroperitoneal space surrounded by a pseudocapsule, best seen on CT scan. They form 14 days to 30 years after injury. Image-guided percutaneous drainage is an effective and safe therapy.[49]

Perirenal abscesses occur when bacteria invade the hematoma, urine, and injured kidney in the perinephric space. The postoperative incidence is low, about 1.5%.[50] These present about 5 to 7 days after injury with spiking fever, ileus, and flank tenderness. Computed tomography scan is diagnostic and percutaneous image-guided drainage is safe and effective.

The most common delayed complication is hypertension, seen in about 5% of renal injuries. Hypertension usually has its onset within 6 months of injury, with some presentation in days and some as late as 20 years.[51] Hypertension may be due to parenchymal ischemia secondary to compression or vascular injury and stenosis. Patients with vascular injuries (Grade IV) appear to be at highest risk. The WTA study noted 15 of 21 renal vascular repairs had poor outcome on follow-up renal scans and recommended obtaining follow-up renal nucleotide scans to screen for poor function that may lead to hypertension and renal failure.[39]

Penetrating Ureteral Injuries

Ureteral injuries from noniatrogenic trauma are rare, comprising about 1% of all genitourinary injuries and about 2 to 4% of all gunshot wounds to the abdomen.[52–54] A recent report from the conflict in Croatia indicated a relatively high incidence of ureteric injury (9.6%) in genitourinary injury, mostly from penetrating fragments.[55] The ureter is small and lies in a relatively protected location. However, it need not be struck directly by a missile to be injured; the cavitation and fragmentation effect by close missile passage may cause significant injury, including disruption or obstruction.

Clinical Findings

There are no classical signs or symptoms in ureteric injury. Frequently, the injury is unrecognized at presentation, and the late signs of flank pain, fever, and fistula formation from urinary leakage prompt investigation. Delay in diagnosis occurs in up to 57% of cases and leads to urinoma, infection, urinary sepsis, and prolonged hospital stays.[52,54,56,57] Ureteric injury must be suspected in all patients with penetrating abdominal injury, and a gunshot wound in proximity to the ureter warrants exploration.

Laboratory Findings

Hematuria is absent in 30 to 47% of cases.[54,56,58]

Radiological Findings

The "complete" IVP (instead of the one-shot IVP) may demonstrate extravasation, delayed function, or ureteral dilation proximal to the injury. There is a significant rate of nondiagnostic studies, which has been reported as about 33 to 37%.[53,56] Computed tomography scanning can be helpful, although the exact sensitivity has not been reported and there is still a significant nondiagnostic study rate. Retrograde pyelogram can be done if time and the patient's condition permits; however, there are cases of non-diagnostic studies reported.[59] The majority of ureteral injuries are diagnosed intraoperatively.[58]

Associated Injuries

Associated injuries are seen in about 97% of ureteric trauma.[60,61] The most common sites are the small intestine, colon, iliac vessels, liver, and stomach. Missed ureteric injuries are seen more commonly in the upper third of the ureter.[62] Missed injuries often are associated with a large retroperitoneal hematoma that may inhibit full exploration of the ureter at laparotomy.

Classification

The ureter is divided into three components according to location:

- Upper, from the pelvic junction to the level of the iliac crest
- Middle, overlying the pelvic bones
- Lower, the segment lying below the pelvic brim to the bladder

The AAST Organ Injury Scale categorizes ureteric injuries as contusions, partial transections, complete transections, and devascularization (Table 13-2).

The most common penetrating injury is a partial transection of the ureter in the middle third.[52,53,63]

Immediate Management

Most patients with ureteral injury require laparotomy for the associated injuries. Preoperative imaging cannot be relied upon to confirm or exclude the diagnosis.[62] Missile injuries can be associated with cavitation with a blunt ureteric injury. The contusion from gunshot injuries may appear minor, but can progress to subsequent ischemic necrosis.[64] Ureteric contusions from shrapnel injury also have a high incidence of subsequent ureteral stenosis if neglected.[55,65] During laparotomy, the ureter must be identified and visualized for evidence of injury, including contusion, discoloration, or lack of bleeding, suggesting devascularization. In cases where exploration of the ureter is unsatisfactory, indigo carmine or methylene blue has been used intraoperatively, although there are cases where injuries were missed despite their use. The appropriate management of an injury depends on the site and severity of injury, delay in diagnosis, the patient's condition, and the surgeon's experience.

Ureteric injuries in an unstable patient in which the time cannot be taken for a careful mucosa-to-mucosa repair over a double-J stent may be managed by cutaneous ureterostomy or exteriorization of a stent passed into the proximal transected ureter and postoperative percutaneous nephrostomy. Poor outcomes and dehiscence of the ureteral repair is more likely in patients presenting with shock, intraoperative bleeding, or associated colon injury. In these patients, temporization is preferable to a lengthy reconstructive procedure. Concomitant renal, ureteric, and associated intra-abdominal injuries may warrant nephrectomy. In a severe life-threatening situation where an expedient damage control approach is indicated, the ureter can be ligated until a subsequent laparotomy is performed in more

TABLE 13-2. Ureteric organ injury scoring system

Grade	Type of injury	Injury description	AIS-90
I	Hematoma	Contusion or hematoma without devascularization	2
II	Laceration	<50% transection	2
III	Laceration	>50% transection	3
IV	Laceration	Complete transection with 2 cm devascularization	3
V	Laceration	Complete transection with >2 cm devascularization	3

Advance one grade for multiple injuries.

Source: Moore et al., 1992.[84] (With permission, Lippincott Williams and Wilkins 2003).

favorable conditions. Operative nephrostomy is not used in management of ureteric trauma.

Ureteral Reconstruction

Urologic consultation should be sought. There are a variety of techniques for reconstruction, all require careful debridement, a watertight, spatulated, and tension-free repair, and adequate ureteral and periureteral retroperitoneal drainage (Figure 13-6).[66]

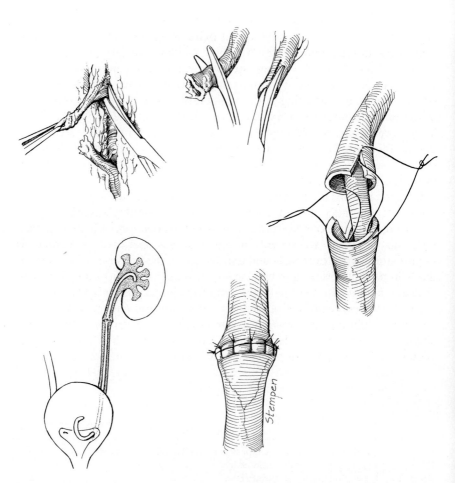

FIGURE 13-6. Ureteroureterostomy showing proximal and distal ureteral segment mobilization, debridement, spatulation, and anastomosis over a double J stent. (From: Presti JC, Carroll PR. Intraoperative management of the injured ureter. In: Schrock TR, ed. *Perspectives in Colon and Rectal Surgery*. St Louis: Quality Medical; 1988:98–106; with permission).

Injuries in the lower third usually are managed by reimplantation into the bladder, either directly or by mobilizing the bladder with a psoas hitch or Boari flap. The ureter is tunneled through the submucosal tunnel with a length three times the ureters diameter and a mucosa-to-mucosa repair is carried out at the neoureterocystostomy. Absorbable sutures (4-0) are used and the anastomosis is stented (Figures 13-7 and 13-8).

Injuries in the middle and upper thirds usually are managed with a primary ureteroureterostomy over a double-J stent. Five to seven centimeters of additional ureteric length can be obtained by mobilization of the kidney. Associated intra-abdominal injury or a tenuous repair may require interposition of omentum to isolate the repair.

Long segmental defects may require transureteroureterostomy, autotransplantation, or interposition with an ileal graft.

All repairs are drained by stents and external drains. Anastomoses can be bolstered by the application of omental flaps. Stents typically are left in for six weeks. Tenuous repairs, and especially those made in the presence of renal, colon, or pancreatic injury, should be protected by percutaneous nephrostomy.[67] A Foley catheter is left in the bladder for five to seven days to avoid backpressure on the anastomosis.

Outcome

Complications after ureteral repair for gunshot wounds occur in 20 to 25% of patients.[62,68,69] Patients with missed ureteric injuries or with ureteric anastomotic dehiscence present with evidence of urinary extravasation with flank pain, fevers, and ileus. Computed tomography scanning is preferred to IVP for diagnosis. Management is with percutaneous nephrostomy, retrograde ureteric stenting, and/or operative repair. Nephrostomy was a definitive treatment in 44% of cases in a report of 63 neglected ureteric injuries in the conflict zone.[70]

Healing is documented by IVP at six and twelve weeks. Delay in diagnosis leads to additional morbidity and cost, and a high index of suspicion is warranted in any patient with penetrating abdominal injury. Dehiscence of the repair is more likely in patients presenting with shock, intraoperative bleeding, or with associated colon injury.

Penetrating Bladder Injuries

Penetrating injury to the bladder accounts for 4 to 25% of bladder injuries and is usually the result of gunshot wounds.[71,72] Extraperitoneal penetration is more common than intraperitoneal penetration.

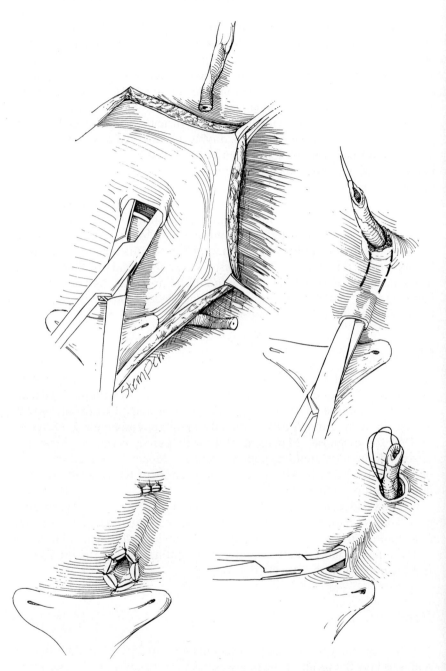

FIGURE 13-7. Ureteral reimplantation by a technique modified from Politano and Leadbetter. (From: Presti JC, Carroll PR. Intraoperative management of the injured ureter. In: Schrock TR, ed. *Perspectives in Colon and Rectal Surgery*. St Louis: Quality Medical; 1988:98–106; with permission).

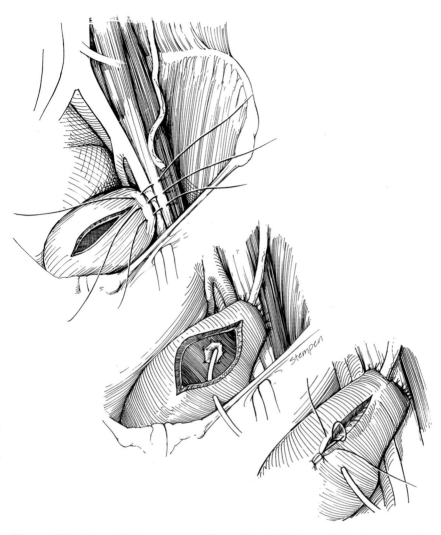

FIGURE 13-8. Psoas hitch maneuver. (From: Presti JC, Carroll PR. Intraoperative management of the injured ureter. In: Schrock TR, ed. *Perspectives in Colon and Rectal Surgery*. St Louis: Quality Medical; 1988:98–106; with permission).

Clinical Diagnosis

The injury is suggested by the location of the wound. Stab or gunshot wounds to the lower abdomen, pelvis, or perineum may injure the bladder. Patients may have lower abdominal pain or tenderness and guarding on palpation.

Laboratory Diagnosis

Gross hematuria is seen in 95% of cases of penetrating bladder injury.

Imaging

Cystography is the most accurate method; it is done by completely distending the bladder via a Foley catheter with 350 milliliters of contrast material and taking an X-ray. The bladder then is emptied and a postdrainage film obtained. The second film is important in that 13% of retroperitoneal extravasations are detected only with this film.[73]

Computed tomography cystography has been reported to have similar predictive value to plain film cystography in blunt trauma, but there are no series evaluating its use in penetrating trauma.

Associated Injuries

Mortality usually is due to associated injuries. The small intestine, colon, rectum, and ureter are commonly involved. Women should have a speculum exam to exclude vaginal injury.

Classification

Bladder injuries can be classified by the AAST Bladder Organ Injury Scale (Table 13-3). In a series of 23 patients by Cass, contusions (Grade I) consisted of about 17% of penetrating injuries. Extraperitonal ruptures were most common at 43%; these are Grade II when less than two centimeters and Grade III when two centimeters or more.[74] Intraperitoneal lacerations comprised 21%; they are Grade III when less than two centimeters and Grade IV when two centimeters or more. Grade V lacerations extend into the bladder neck or ureteral orifice (trigone).

TABLE 13-3. Bladder organ injury scoring system

Grade	Type of injury	Injury description	AIS-90
I	Hematoma	Contusion, intramural hematoma	2
	Laceration	Partial thickness	3
II	Laceration	Extraperitoneal bladder wall laceration <2 cm	4
III	Laceration	Extraperitoneal (>2 cm) or intraperitoneal (<2 cm) bladder wall lacerations	4
IV	Laceration	Intraperitoneal bladder wall laceration >2 cm	4
V	Laceration	Laceration extending into bladder neck or ureteral orifice (trigone)	4

Advance one grade for multiple injuries.

Source: Moore et al., 1992.[84]

Management

Small bladder penetrations can be difficult to find during laparotomy. Hemodynamically stable patients with penetrations in proximity to the bladder should have cystography preoperatively. Care must be taken to look under abdominal retractors during abdominal exploration to examine the bladder adequately.

Contusions can be managed by catheter drainage alone. Intraperitoneal and extraperitoneal penetrating injury should be managed by surgical exploration and primary repair. Nonoperative management of extraperitoneal bladder rupture is well described, but there is limited experience in nonoperative penetrating injury.

Once intra-abdominal injury has been excluded at lower midline laparotomy, the space of Retzius is opened and the anterior bladder dissected away from the pubis. The bladder is opened via an anterior cystostomy to allow examination of the entire interior surface. The ureteric orifices must be examined for injury. Trial insertion of a ureteric stent or use of methylene blue or indigo carmine can ensure ureters are intact.

Extraperitoneal ruptures are closed with absorbable sutures in one or two layers. Intraperitoneal ruptures are closed in two layers, with the peritoneal and muscular bladder wall in one layer and the bladder mucosa in another layer. Injuries extending into the trigone require careful reconstruction of the sphincter or risk incontinence or contracture.

A large suprapubic tube traditionally is used in conjunction with a urethral catheter, especially with a large or tenuous repair, but may not be necessary in many cases.[75] The urethral catheter is removed with the clearing of gross hematuria. The suprapubic catheter is removed at eight to ten days after a cystogram is done to ensure bladder integrity.

Outcome and Complications

Morbidity is related more closely to the associated injuries than to the bladder injury. Infection and continued bleeding are early complications. Long-term complications are uncommon and include incontinence.

Penetrating Genital Injuries

Genital injuries comprised about 68% of genitourinary injuries from combat versus 7% of civilian injuries.[12,67] High-velocity injuries are common in combat; civilian injuries more commonly are low-velocity gunshot wounds than stab wounds. In a civilian series of genital gunshot wounds, the penis was injured most frequently, followed by the testicles and the scrotum only.[76] Thirty percent of civilian patients have multiple gunshot wounds.

Clinical Findings

The external location of the genitalia lends ready inspection. However, associated injuries are seen in over 75% of penetrating genital trauma, including urethra, thigh, buttocks, and hand.[77,78] Injuries to the rectum, iliac vessels, bony pelvis, and hip joint also are possible. Fifty percent of penile gunshot wounds involve the urethra. Most of theses injuries are in the distal, "pendulous" urethra versus the bulbous or proximal urethra. The perineum should be examined for signs of ecchymosis or urinary extravasation.

Radiological Findings

Patients with penetration of the genitalia with blood at the meatus, gross, or microscopic hematuria or inability to void should be suspected of having a urethral injury and require a retrograde urethrogram (RUG). This is done by placing a small Foley catheter just past the meatus and using a Brodny clamp to ensure a seal. Thirty to 50 cubic centimeters of contrast is infused and radiographs taken. If a Foley catheter has already been successfully placed, a small feeding tube can be placed adjacent to the Foley catheter to obtain a useable RUG.

Suspected bladder injuries should be addressed with a static and postdrainage cystogram.

Scrotal injuries should be investigated with ultrasonography to evaluate testicular integrity.[79] Rupture of the testicle reveals an abnormal echo pattern associated with tubular extrusion or contusion with hemorrhage. Color flow Doppler imaging available on most ultrasound machines provides evidence of testicular perfusion.

Management

All penetrating injuries to the genitalia should be explored. Wounds that are seen to be superficial can be debrided and irrigated. Wounds, including high-velocity penetrations, can be closed after exploration.[67]

Penetrating penile injuries require surgical exploration. A circumferential subcoronal incision is made and the skin retracted down the shaft. The rich vascular supply to the area lessens the risk of infection and dehiscence, and therefore does not require extensive debridement, which can impair erectile function. Injuries to the corpora, Bucks fascia, and tunica albuginea are repaired precisely with interrupted absorbable sutures after minimal debridement. Associated urethral injuries are repaired with interrupted fine absorbable sutures and the urethra stented with a silicone Foley catheter. Long segmental defects can be managed by insertion of a suprapubic bladder catheter and delayed urethral reconstruction by a variety of specialized techniques.

Reimplantation of an amputated penis is a specialized microsurgical technique requiring the distal amputated part to be reasonably intact. Results are best if the surgery is performed within six hours of injury.[80]

Penetrating injury to the testes require surgical exploration via a midline scrotal incision. Hematomas are evacuated and the testes, epididymis, and spermatic cord are inspected. Debridement of devitalized tissue or extruded tubules is carried out and hemostasis obtained. The tunica albuginea is re-approximated with absorbable suture. Hematomas in the spermatic cord are associated with arterial injury and require exploration and inspection to obtain hemostasis. A small Penrose drain is left to drain the scrotum, which is closed with absorbable interrupted sutures. Extensive destruction of the testicle or cord requires orchiectomy.

Large skin defects in the perineum may require skin grafting; this can be carried out at the first exploration if the wound is clean and without contamination or devitalized tissue. Otherwise the wound is dressed until delayed grafting is possible onto a granulating wound bed. Loss of the scrotum with viable testicles may require the testes to be placed in skin pockets made through the skin into the subcutaneous tissue of the medial thigh. Thin split-thickness skin grafts are appropriate except on the penis. If the patient is potent, and skin contracture of the graft will complicate erection, then thick split-thickness or full-thickness grafts are appropriate.[81]

Large defects of the perineum may require myocutaneous flaps rotated from the posterior or lateral thigh or from the rectus abdominus.[82]

Outcome and Complications

The external genitalia can be assessed easily and rapidly for injury. Penetrations in this area require exploration after appropriate imaging. Associated injuries are common in genital gunshot wounds and must be considered with a high index of suspicion. The excellent vascular supply of the genitalia ensures rapid healing and the likelihood of acceptable healing and function.[83,85]

Recommended Readings

McAninch JW. *Traumatic and Reconstructive Urology*. Philadephia, PA: WB Saunders; 1996.
Ivatury RR, Cayten CG. *The Textbook of Penetrating Trauma*. Media: Williams and Wilkins; 1996.

References

1. McAninch JW, Carroll PR, Armenakas NA, Lee P. Renal gunshot wounds: Methods of salvage and reconstruction. *J Trauma.* 1993;35(2):279–283.
2. Amato JL, Billy LJ, Lawson NS, Rich NM. High velocity missile injury. An experimental study of the retentive forces of tissue. *Am J Surg.* 1974;127(4): 454–459.
3. Fackler ML. Gunshot wound review. *Ann Emerg Med.* 1996;28(2):194–203.
4. Bowen TE, Bellamy R. Missile cause wounds. In: Bowen TE, Bellamy R. *Emergency War Surgery: Second United States Revision of the Emergency War Surgery NATO Handbook.* Washington, DC: United States Government Printing Office; 1988.
5. Amato JJ, Syracuse D, Seaver PR Jr, Rich N. Bone as a secondary missile: an experimental study in the fragmenting of bone by high-velocity missiles. *J Trauma.* 1989;29(5):609–612.
6. Eickenberg H-U, Amin M, Lich R, Jr. Traveling bullets in genitourinary tract. *Urology.* 1975;6(2):224–226.
7. Harrington TG, Kandel LB. Renal colic following a gunshot wound to the abdomen: the birdshot calculus. *J Urol.* 1997;157(4):1351–1352.
8. Spalding TJ, Stewart MP, Tulloch DN, Stephens KM. Penetrating missile injuries in the gulf war 1991. *Br J Surg.* 1991;78(9):1102–1104.
9. Lovric Z, Kuvezdic H, Prlic D, Wertheimer B, Candrlic K. Ballistic trauma in 1991/92 war in Osijek, Croatia: Shell fragments versus bullets. *J R Army Med Corps.* 1997;143(1):26–30.
10. Ilic N, Petricevic A, Radonic V, Biocic M, Petricevic M. Penetrating thoracoabdominal war injuries. *Int Surg.* 1997;82(3):316–318.
11. Cass AS, ed. *Genitourinary Trauma.* Boston, MA: Blackwell Scientific; 1988.
12. Cass AS. Male genital trauma from external trauma. In: Cass AS, ed. *Genitourinary Trauma.* Boston MA: Blackwell Scientific; 1988:141.
13. Coupland RM, Korver A. Injuries from antipersonnel mines: The experience of the International Committee of the Red Cross. BMJ 1991;303(6816):1509–1512.
14. Hudolin T, Hudolin I. Surgical management of urogenital injuries at a war hospital in Bosnia-Hrzegovina, 1992 to 1995. *J Urol.* 2003;169(4):1357–1359.
15. Nagy KK, Brenneman FD, Krosner SM, Fildes JJ, Roberts RR, Joseph KT, Smith RF, Barrett J. Routine preoperative "one-shot" intravenous pyelography is not indicated in all patients with penetrating abdominal trauma. *J Am Coll Surg.* 1997;185(6):530–533.
16. Patel VG, Walker ML. The role of "one-shot" intravenous pyelogram in evaluation of penetrating abdominal trauma. *Am Surg.* 1997;63(4):350–353.
17. Bretan PN Jr, McAninch JW, Federle MP, Jeffrey RB Jr. Computerized tomographic staging of renal trauma: 85 consecutive cases. *J Urol.* 1986;136(3): 561–565.
18. Meredith JW, Trunkey DD. CT scanning in acute abdominal injuries. *Surg Clin North Am.* 1988;68(2):255–268.
19. Holcroft JW, Trunkey DD, Minagi H, Korobkin MT, Lim RC. Renal trauma and retroperitoneal hematomas—Indications for exploration. *J Trauma.* 1975; 15(12):1045–1052.

20. Moore EE, Shackford SR, Pachter HL, McAninch JW, Browner BD, Champion HR, Flint LM, Gennarelli TA, Malangoni MA, Ramenofsky ML. Organ injury scaling: Spleen, liver, and kidney. *J Trauma*. 1989;29(12):1664–1666.
21. Cass AS, Ireland GW. Trauma to the genitourinary tract: Evaluation and management. *Postgrad Med*. 1973;53(7):63–68.
22. Feliciano DV. Management of traumatic retroperitoneal hematoma. *Ann Surg*. 1990;211(2):109–123.
23. Shaftan GW. Indications for operation in abdominal trauma. *Am J Surg*. 1960;99:657–664.
24. Nance FC, Wennar MH, Johnson LW, Ingram JC Jr, Cohn I Jr. Surgical judgment in the management of penetrating wounds of the abdomen: Experience with 2212 patients. *Ann Surg*. 1974;179(5):639–646.
25. Velmahos GC, Demetriades D, Cornwell EE III, Belzberg H, Murray J, Asensio J, Berne TV. Selective management of renal gunshot wounds. *Br J Surg*. 1998;85(8):1121–1124.
26. Renz BM, Feliciano DV. Gunshot wounds to the right thoracoabdomen: A prospective study of nonoperative management. *J Trauma*. 1994;37(5):737–744.
27. Wessells H, McAninch JW, Meyer A, Bruce J. Criteria for nonoperative treatment of significant penetrating renal lacerations. *J Urol*. 1997;157(1):24–27.
28. Velmahos GC, Demetriades D, Toutouzas KG, Sarkisyan G, Chan LS, Ishak R, Alo K, Vassiliu P, Murray JA, Salim A, Asensio J, Belzberg H, Katkhouda N, Berne TV. Selective nonoperative management in 1,856 patients with abdominal gunshot wounds: Should routine laparotomy still be the standard of care? *Ann Surg*. 2001;234(3):395–402.
29. Velmahos GC, Degiannis, E. The management of urinary tract injuries after gunshot wounds of the anterior and posterior abdomen. *Injury*. 1997; 28(8):535–538.
30. Santucci RA, McAninch JW, Safir M, Mario LA, Service S, Segal MR. Validation of the American Association for the Surgery of Trauma organ injury severity scale for the kidney. *J Trauma*. 2001;50(2):195–200.
31. Thall EH, Stone NN, Cheng DL, Cohen EL, Fine EM, Leventhal I, Aldoroty RA. Conservative management of penetrating and blunt type III renal injuries. *Br J Urol*. 1996;77(4):512–517.
32. McAninch JW, Carroll PR. Renal exploration after trauma. Indications and reconstructive techniques. *Urol Clin North Am*. 1989;16(2):203–212.
33. Hammer CC, Santucci RA. Effect of an institutional policy of nonoperative treatment of grades I to IV renal injuries. *J Urol*. 2003;169(5):1751–1753.
34. Rignault DP. Abdominal trauma in war. *World J Surg*. 1992;16(5):940–946.
35. McAninch JW, Carroll PR. Renal trauma: Kidney preservation through improved vascular control—a refined approach. *J Trauma*. 1982;22(4):285–290.
36. Carroll PR, Klosterman P, McAninch JW. Early vascular control for renal trauma: a critical review. *J Urol*. 1989;141(4):826–829.
37. Atala A, Miller FB, Richardson JD, Bauer B, Harty J, Amin M. Preliminary vascular control for renal trauma. *Surg Gynecol Obstet*. 1991;172(5):386–390.
38. Gonzalez RP, Falimirski M, Holevar MR, Evankovich C. Surgical management of renal trauma: Is vascular control necessary? *J Trauma*. 1999;47(6):1039–1042.
39. Knudson MM, Harrison PB, Hoyt DB, Shatz DV, Zietlow SP, Bergstein JM, Mario LA, McAninch JW. Outcome after major renovascular injuries: A Western Trauma Association multicenter report. *J Trauma*. 2000;49(6):1116–1122.

40. Asensio JA, Chahwan S, Hanpeter D, Demetriades D, Forno W, Gambaro E, Murray J, Velmahos G, Marengo J, Shoemaker WC, Berne TV. Operative management and outcome of 302 abdominal vascular injuries. *Am J Surg.* 2000; 180(6):528–533.
41. Ivatury RR, Zubowski R, Stahl WM. Penetrating renovascular trauma. *J Trauma.* 1989;29(12):1620–1623.
42. Montgomery RC, Richardson JD, Harty JI. Posttraumatic renovascular hypertension after occult renal injury. *J Trauma.* 1998;45(1):106–110.
43. Watts RA, Hoffbrand BI. Hypertension following renal trauma. *J Hum Hypertens.* 1987;1(2):65–71.
44. Wazzan W, Azoury B, Hemady K, Khauli RB. Missile injury of upper ureter treated by delayed renal autotransplantation and ureteropyelostomy. *Urology.* 1993;42(6):725–728.
45. Angelis M, Augenstein JS, Ciancio G, Figueiro J, Sfakianakis GN, Miller J, Burke GW III, Wessells H. Ex vivo repair and renal autotransplantation after penetrating trauma: Is there an upper limit of ischemic/traumatic injury beyond which a kidney is unsalvageable? *J Trauma.* 2003;54(3):606–609.
46. Wessells H, McAninch JW. Effect of colon injury on the management of simultaneous renal trauma. *J Urol.* 1996;155(6):1852–1856.
47. Bernath AS, Schutte H, Fernandez RR, Addonizio JC. Stab wounds of the kidney: Conservative management in flank penetration. *J Urol.* 1983; 129(3):468–470.
48. Carroll PR, McAninch JW. Operative indications in penetrating renal trauma. *J Trauma.* 1985;25(7):587–593.
49. Peterson NE. Complications of renal trauma. *Urol Clin North Am.* 1989; 16(2):221–236.
50. McAninch JW, Carroll PR, Klosterman PW, Dixon CM, Greenblatt MN. Renal reconstruction after injury. *J Urol.* 1991;145(5):932–937.
51. Monstrey SJ, Beerthuizen GI, vander Werken C, Debruyne FM, Goris RJ. Renal trauma and hypertension. *J Trauma.* 1989;29(1):65–70.
52. Rober PE, Smith JB, Pierce JM Jr. Gunshot injuries of the ureter. *J Trauma.* 1990;30(1):83–86.
53. Bright TC III, Peters PC. Ureteral injuries due to external violence: 10 years' experience with 59 cases. *J Trauma.* 1977;17(8):616–620.
54. Brandes SB, Chelsky MJ, Buckman RF, Hanno PM. Ureteral injuries from penetrating trauma. *J Trauma.* 1994;36(6):766–769.
55. Tucak A, Petek Z, Kuvezdic H. War injuries of the ureter. *Mil Med.* 1997; 162(5):344–345.
56. Campbell EW Jr, Filderman PS, Jacobs SC. Ureteral injury due to blunt and penetrating trauma. *Urology.* 1992;40(3):216–220.
57. Peterson NE, Pitts JC III. Penetrating injuries of the ureter. *J Urol.* 1981; 126(5):587–590.
58. Presti JC Jr, Carroll PR, McAninch JW. Ureteral and renal pelvic injuries from external trauma: Diagnosis and management. *J Trauma.* 1989;29(3):370–374.
59. Mendez R, McGinty DM. The management of delayed recognized ureteral injuries. *J Urol.* 1978;119(2):192–193.
60. Carlton CE Jr, Scott R Jr, Guthrie AG. The initial management of ureteral injuries: a report of 78 cases. *Trans Am Assoc Genitourin Surg.* 1970;62:114–122.

61. Holden S, Hicks CC, O'Brien DP, Stone HH, Walker JA, Walton KN. Gunshot wounds of the ureter: A 15-year review of 63 consecutive cases. *J Urol.* 1976; 116(5):562–564.
62. Medina D, Lavery R, Ross SE, Livingston DH. Ureteral trauma: Preoperative studies neither predict injury nor prevent missed injuries. *J Am Coll Surg.* 1998;186(6):641–644.
63. Liroff SA, Pontes JE, Pierce JM Jr. Gunshot wounds of the ureter: 5 years of experience. *J Urol.* 1977;118(4):551–553.
64. Cass AS. Ureteral contusion with gunshot wounds. *J Trauma.* 1984;24(1):59–60.
65. Selikowitz SM. Penetrating high-velocity genitourinary injuries. Part I. Statistics mechanisms, and renal wounds. *Urology.* 1977;9(4):371–376.
66. Presti JC Jr, Carroll PR. Ureteral and renal pelvic trauma: Diagnosis and management. In: McAninch JW, ed. *Traumatic and reconstructive urology.* Philadelphia, PA: WB Saunders; 1996:171–179.
67. Selikowitz SM. Penetrating high-velocity genitourinary injuries. Part II: Ureteral, lower tract, and genital wounds. *Urology.* 1977;9(5):493–499.
68. Perez-Brayfield MR, Keane TE, Krishnan A, Lafontaine P, Feliciano DV, Clarke HS. Gunshot wounds to the ureter: A 40-year experience at Grady Memorial Hospital. *J Urol.* 2001;166(1):119–121.
69. Azimuddin K, Milanesa D, Ivatury R, Porter J, Ehrenpreis M, Allman DB. Penetrating ureteric injuries. *Injury.* 1998;29(5):363–367.
70. al Ali M, Haddad LF. The late treatment of 63 overlooked or complicated ureteral missile injuries: The promise of nephrostomy and role of autotransplantation. *J Urol.* 1996;156(6):1918–1921.
71. Carroll PR, McAninch JW. Major bladder trauma: Mechanisms of injury and a unified method of diagnosis and repair. *J Urol.* 1984;132(2):254–257.
72. Brosman SA, Fay R. Diagnosis and management of bladder trauma. *J Trauma.* 1973;13(8):687–694.
73. Carroll PR, McAninch JW. Major bladder trauma: The accuracy of cystography. *J Urol.* 1983;130(5):887–888.
74. Cass AS, Luxenberg M. Management of extraperitoneal ruptures of bladder caused by external trauma. *Urology.* 1989;33(3):179–183.
75. Parry NG, Rozycki GS, Feliciano DV, Tremblay LN, Cava RA, Voeltz Z, Carney J. Traumatic rupture of the urinary bladder: Is the suprapubic tube necessary? *J Trauma.* 2003;54(3):431–436.
76. Gomez RG, Castanheira AC, McAninch JW. Gunshot wounds to the male external genitalia. *J Urol.* 1993;150(4):1147–1149.
77. Campos JA, Gomez-Orta F. Continent diversion vesicoplasty for the treatment of the irreparable, multi-operated urethral stricture patient. *Arch Esp Urol.* 1993;46(3):255–260.
78. Miles BJ, Poffenberger RJ, Farah RN, Moore S. Management of penile gunshot wounds. *Urology.* 1990;36(4):318–321.
79. Fournier GR Jr, Laing FC, McAninch JW. Scrotal ultrasonography and the management of testicular trauma. *Urol Clin North Am.* 1989;16(2):377–385.
80. Jezior JR, Brady JD, Schlossberg SM. Management of penile amputation injuries. *World J Surg.* 2001;25(12):1602–1609.
81. McAninch JW. Management of genital skin loss. *Urol Clin North Am.* 1989;16(2):387–397.

298 J.J. Doucet and D.B. Hoyt

82. Schlossberg SM, Jordan GH, McCraw JB. Myocutaneous flap reconstruction of major perineal and pelvic defects. In: McAninch JW, ed. *Traumatic and Reconstructive Urology*. Philadephia, PA: WB Saunders; 1996:715–725.
83. McAninch JW. *Traumatic and Reconstructive Urology*. Philadephia, PA: WB Saunders; 1996.
84. Moore EE, Cogbill TH, Jurkovich GJ, McAninch JW, Champion HR, Gennarelli TA, Malangoni MA, Shackford SR, Trafton PG. Organ injury scaling. III: Chest wall, abdominal vascular, ureter, bladder, and urethra. *J Trauma*. 1992; 33(3):337–339.
85. Bandi G, Santucci RA. Controversies in the management of male external genitourinary trauma. *J Trauma*. 2004;56(6):1362–1370.

14
Abdomen and Pelvis

ADAM J. BROOKS, IAN CIVIL, BENJAMIN BRASLOW, and
C. WILLIAM SCHWAB

Introduction

Eighty to ninety-five percent of abdominal gunshot wounds result in an intra-abdominal injury that requires operative repair. Surgeons should treat the wound and not the weapon, yet as the amount of energy transferred to the body from the round increases, so does the incidence, number of wounds (bullets that enter the body), and the severity of the injuries. Organ injury is the rule rather than the exception, even with small muzzle velocity (caliber) handguns. Abdominal viscera, such as the liver, kidneys, and spleen, with their inelastic solid structure and fixed position, are extremely sensitive to the effect of energy transfer and cavitation. Higher-energy rounds will cause massive tissue destruction (see Chapter 9). Consequently, a trauma laparotomy is usually the most appropriate diagnostic and therapeutic procedure.

In war, nearly 90% of penetrating wounds are caused by fragments whereas only 10% are a result of bullets. As a result, 40% of casualties during conventional warfare will have multiple penetrating injuries of the body cavities and limbs. During Gulf War I, fragment-injured patients seen in a British field hospital had on average nine fragments per casualty.[1] The abdomen is the site of injury in approximately 10% of war casualties.[2] Data from the Korean and Vietnam wars presented in the chapter on Ballistic Protection (Chapter 4) reveals that 10 to 27% of casualties killed in action sustained abdominal wounds and 21 to 30% of casualties who died from their wounds had abdominal injuries. Thus, abdominal wounding is common and lethal if not promptly recognized and all injuries repaired.

The increase in civilian gun violence and proliferation of semiautomatic handguns in inner cities during the 1980s and 1990s led to a change in the approach to the management of the casualty with ballistic injury and the advent of the damage control philosophy.[3,4] These changes have led to a fall in mortality even amongst the most severely injured patients in leading civilian trauma centers (see Chapter 10).[5]

This chapter will concentrate on the more physiologically stable patient able to withstand a definitive laparotomy or the Part III damage control patient returning to theater for definitive procedures. The techniques associated with damage control in the critically unstable patient are covered in Chapter 10. The chapter aims to provide the surgeon who is faced with ballistic abdominal trauma only rarely with a framework for the management of the injuries they are likely to encounter.

Initial Management and Assessment

Any penetrating injury between the level of the nipple superiorly and the buttocks inferiorly can lead to an intraperitoneal injury. Therefore, a very high index of suspicion and complete examination is performed in all patients. Fragments and gunshot wounds (GSW) initially may be missed if the "entrance" wound lies in a relatively "inaccessible" location, such as the axilla, beneath the hairline, in the perianal area, or between the buttocks. Wounds in these regions must be sought vigorously.

The basic principles of the Advanced Trauma Life Support (ATLS) course hold in the resuscitation of casualties with abdominal ballistic injuries. Hypotension is the primary concern, as 25% of casualties with abdominal gunshot wounds will have a major intra-abdominal vascular injury. The patient may not progress further than the circulation phase of the primary survey before urgent transfer to the operating theater for definitive hemorrhage control. Because of the multiplicity of wounds, spinal cord injury must be ruled out quickly by a fast and simple motor exam of the upper and lower extremities.

Traditionally, hypotensive patients with penetrating injuries have a high mortality. A number of new strategies and approaches during both resuscitation and surgery have been introduced in an attempt to improve the outcome. Studies undertaken in a large civilian trauma center showed improved survival in patients with penetrating trauma who had low-volume fluid or hypotensive resuscitation.[6] This approach, which has been accepted by the British Army, aims to limit fluid transfusion to maintain the systolic blood pressure at around 90 millimeters Hg so that further bleeding is not precipitated. Vital to this approach is short times from injury to definitive hemorrhage control. Clarke demonstrated that in hypotensive trauma patients with abdominal injuries delays in the emergency department were associated with increased mortality.[7] The surgical philosophy changed radically with the introduction of damage control. The technique initially focused on maximally injured patients with penetrating trauma and clearly demonstrated a survival advantage from the approach.[8] Further refinement of the techniques has continued the improved survival.[9]

Tips and Pitfalls

Do not become distracted by a single injury or body system during the initial assessment. Bullet and fragment wounds are frequently multiple, and it is imperative to prioritize, recognize, and address the patients compelling source of bleeding as the initial surgical step.

Investigations

Laparotomy is the main stay of investigation and management following ballistic injury that penetrates the abdomen, as the rate of significant organ injury following penetration is high. Apparent soft tissue injuries to the abdominal wall, flanks, or back from high-energy rounds may even cause abdominal injury without penetration. Assessment of the gunshot patient might illicit few, if any, signs on examination,[10] as hemoperitoneum may not produce peritonism initially. Directed investigations, when the clinical condition permits, may provide additional diagnostic information so that surgical approaches can be planned or the site of bleeding located in multicavity injury.

Physical Examination

Determining trajectory is the single most important function of a physical examination or radiographs prior to laparotomy. The physical exam should involve a quick thorough survey for all skin wounds, as well as determination of blood at the meatus or in the rectum. Patients should be log-rolled left and right to provide 360 degree inspection of the body. Quick spinal cord function or deficit should be determined by simple motor functions of the arms, hands, legs, and feet. All skin wounds should be marked with metallic flat small objects (e.g., paperclips taped over the wounds, opened widely for posterior wounds, kept closed for anterior wounds) if X-rays are able to be obtained.

Plain Radiographs

X-rays with the addition of "bullet' markers can assist in an approximation of the trajectory of a missile. This information can help build a picture of the likely injuries and therefore may assist in the development of operative strategies. Plain films also demonstrate fractures and secondary missiles from shattered bone, and the location and number of fragments from blast injuries.

Diagnostic Peritoneal Lavage (DPL)

Diagnostic peritoneal lavage (DPL) has limited application in the initial assessment of the trauma patient. In penetrating ballistic trauma, where its role has always been limited, DPLs only use lies in situations where abdominal penetration remains truly equivocal or if there is a low thoracic wound or tangential flank wound and associated abdominal injury that needs to be excluded. Cell counts are reduced compared to blunt trauma (10000 red cells mm^3 and 50 white cells mm^3) to improve the sensitivity of the technique in penetrating injury.

Focused Assessment with Sonography for Trauma (FAST)

FAST has a limited role in the evaluation of penetrating abdominal injury (reported sensitivity is only 46%[11]). However, a positive FAST undertaken during the circulation phase of resuscitation in the ballistic casualty has a positive predictive value of over 90% for the detection of intra-abdominal blood. In multiple fragment or GSW injuries, FAST confirms the site of bleeding and helps direct the surgeon to the appropriate body cavity. Blood on either side of the diaphragm confers diaphragmatic injury.

Computed Tomography (CT)

Computed tomography (CT) has an increasing role in the diagnosis of ballistic abdominal injury in selected stable injured patients. Where there is diagnostic doubt and the patient is hemodynamically stable and CT is immediately available, then its use can exclude intra-abdominal penetration through determination of the trajectory (see Chapter 23). This especially is helpful for wounds of the pelvis, gluteus area, flanks, and occasionally the right upper quadrant of the abdomen.[12] In the right upper quadrant, CT has been used to confirm isolated ballistic abdominal injury to the liver when a conservative approach can be considered.

Laparoscopy

Laparoscopy, similar to CT scan, can have a role in abdominal assessment in the hemodynamically stable patient where there is a significant suspicion that the wound is tangential and doubt that the missile has penetrated the abdomen. In this uncommon situation, laparoscopy may avoid a laparotomy if there is no evidence of peritoneal penetration; however, the detection of peritoneal penetration mandates laparotomy for formal assessment of the viscera.

Wound Exploration

There is little role for wound exploration to detect penetration following ballistic injury to the abdomen. At best, this is an imprecise technique that is unable to rule out injury while, at worst, it may precipitate further hemorrhage as the clot is dislodged. Patients where there is a suspicion of abdominal penetration by bullet or fragment should undergo a laparotomy at the earliest opportunity or be evaluated by one of the above techniques.

Laparotomy

Laporatomy is the definitive investigation and usually is therapeutic following abdominal ballistic injury.

Tetanus and Antibiotics

All patients require tetanus prophylaxis. Patients sustaining abdominal ballistic trauma require preoperative antibiotic prophylaxis. This can be accomplished best by a single dose of a second-generation cephalosporin. Antibiotics can be continued postoperatively based on the injuries found at laparotomy.

Surgical Techniques

Preparation

It is important that the entire operating theater team and anesthetist are adequately prepared, as the initial blood loss on opening the abdomen can be brisk and the patient rapidly can become unstable. A primed rapid fluid infusion and warming device is ideal. Fluid resuscitation should be sufficient to maintain adequate organ perfusion; however, until hemorrhage is controlled, the value of large volume resuscitation is doubtful. Warming devices are vital and should include warm-air convection blankets, fluid warmers, and hats or cotton wool to keep the patient's head warm (see Chapter 8). Two functioning large-volume suction devices and a large number of abdominal packs must be ready and at hand. Adequate retraction and a competent assistant are required. Interaction between the surgical and anesthetic teams and regular communication is vital, especially where maneuvers associated with significant blood loss or reduction in venous return are being contemplated.

Positioning, Draping

The trauma laparotomy usually is undertaken with the patient supine, with arms abducted at 90 degrees. If rectal injuries are suspected (e.g., with a penetrating buttock injury) and the patient is hemodynamically stable, then access to the anus and rectum with the patient's legs in the Lloyd–Davies position can be used. If there are wounds to the left chest or the patient may need a left thoractomy, the patient is placed in the "taxi hailing" position, with the left arm abducted to 110 degrees and forearm and hand placed over the head. All patients are prepped and draped from the chin to the middle of the thigh. This allows access to the chest, abdomen, groins, and upper thighs for saphenous vein harvest if necessary (Figure 14-1).

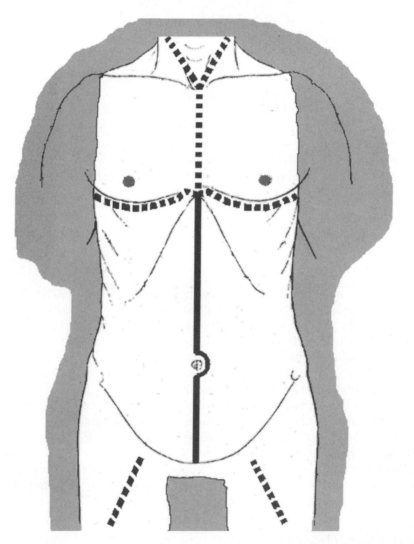

FIGURE 14-1. Prepped and draped for a trauma laparotomy with the initial incision and possible extensions (dotted lines) marked. Groin towel and drapes are shown in grey.

Incision

A full-length midline laparotomy is the incision of choice in ballistic injury to the abdomen. This incision can be extended into the chest as a midline sternotomy or a thoracoabdominal incision by extension of the wound across the costal cartilages if access to the inferior vena cava above the liver or a thoracic procedure is required. Alternatively, the incision can be increased by a right-sided subcostal incison, which may improve access to the liver.

The Trauma Laparotomy

This is a sequential procedure that has three distinct priorities. The initial priority is the control of bleeding; this is followed by systematic exploration of the abdomen for the detection of all injuries.

Priorities of the Trauma Laparotomy
Hemorrhage control
Contamination control
Detection of all injuries

Hemorrhage Control

Free blood and clot is rapidly scooped out of the abdomen and the "quadrants" of the abdomen are packed. Quick examination of the four quadrants and retroperitoneal surface provides key information about location of hematomas or free bleeding. Some information on the source of bleeding may be gained from the location of bullet or fragment wounds and the results of plain films (X-ray). In ballistic injury, the liver, mesentery, and the major retroperitoneal vessels are the most common source of major bleeding. Hemorrhage from the liver and retroperitoneum is controlled by packing while clamps are applied to bleeding mesenteric vessels. If bleeding continues despite initial packing, then this must be urgently addressed.

Systematic Exploration

The abdominal viscera are explored in a systematic fashion. This is a drill that ensures a thorough inspection of the organs for injuries. While ongoing bleeding is addressed during this exploration and contamination temporarily controlled, formal repair is deferred until the abdomen has been thoroughly inspected. A suggested format is shown in Figure 14-2. In ballistic injury, special attention should be made of the track of the missile, taking into account the cavitation effect.

Sequential Approach to the Trauma Laparotomy

Liver
Spleen
Stomach and crura
Right colon
Transverse colon
Descending colon
Rectum
Small bowel including mesentery
Pancreas
Duodenum
Left and right diaphragms
Retroperitoneum
Pelvic structures

OR

Clockwise Examination by Region:

Left Upper Quadrant
Left Lower Quadrant
Right Lower Quadrant
Right Upper Quadrant
Central Abdomen
Retroperitoneum
Small Bowel

FIGURE 14-2. The trauma laparotomy.

Contamination Control

Temporary control of contamination is undertaken as the injuries are discovered; it can be achieved using Babcock clamps, nylon tapes, or staplers applied either side of a bowel injury. If a vascular injury has been discovered, holes in the bowel can be wrapped quickly in towels or pads.

Organ Injury

Although bullet markers on the skin may help in determining the approximate track of a round through the body, bullets and fragments do not necessarily traverse a straight line as they tumble through the abdomen, encounter organs with different densities, or ricochet off bone. This and the cavitation from high-energy transfer seen with military weapons can cause injuries away from the expected track of the round. Therefore, a disciplined and thorough trauma laparotomy must be conducted in every case.

Mobilization

Adequate mobilization of the injured organ is imperative to facilitate evaluation and repair. This may require complete mobilization of the liver in retrohepatic caval injuries or medial visceral mobilization to access the retroperitoneal structures. Details for individual organs are given in the organ injury section later in this chapter.

Special Maneuvers

Temporary Packing

Repopularized by Stone in the 1980s, the placement of laparotomy packs over and around solid organ injuries and on dissected surfaces is an effective method of venous or low-pressure hemorrhage control. It is not effective to control arterial bleeding. Intraparenchymal packing should not be used, as this may precipitate and worsen bleeding. The temporary packs placed as part of the initial trauma laparotomy can be replaced with packs positioned to compress an organ and provide tamponade in natural planes if the packing is felt to be the best definitive treatment at that time. Over-tight packing can occlude venous return and lead to the abdominal compartment syndrome. Liver packing is covered in more detail later.

Damage Control

The surgical techniques associated with damage control include packing, temporary control of contamination, shunting of vascular injuries, and rapid temporary abdominal closure. These are technical aspects of a philosophy that is concerned with the correction of the patients under lying physiology and is part of a coordinated approach that stretches from the emergency department to the intensive care unit. These issues are explored in depth in Chapter 10.

Surgical Adjuncts

A number of adjuncts to trauma surgery have been introduced and others are in development or trials. To date Recombinant Factor VIIa and angiography are the most important.

Recombinant Factor VIIa (RFVIIa) is a procoagulant that is active only in the presence of exposed tissue factor, which is present in the subendothelium of injured vessels. Activated RFVIIa initiates the extrinsic clotting system, and evidence from the management of uncontrollable bleeding in hemophiliacs and an animal model of liver injury[13,14] suggests that RFVIIa reduces blood loss and restores coagulation function without adverse clinical effect. This has been described in several case reports; however, the findings of a randomized double-blind clinical trial investigating RFVIIa in severely injured patients are awaited.

Angiography has become a vital adjunct in the management of the trauma patient. Its use in the control of arterial bleeding following blunt pelvic trauma with fractures and hypotension is widely accepted. It is deployed most widely in the definitive embolization of bleeding vessels that are difficult to access and control with surgery. Besides definitive embolization for hemorrhage control, the interventional radiologist can provide temporary balloon control of major vascular injuries to allow a controlled surgical approach and place vascular stents in select cases. In ballistic injury, angiography and embolization can be used as a valuable adjunct to liver or pelvic packing and may control bleeding in the depths of the liver, large muscle beds of the back, retroperitoneum, or gluteal region that otherwise would be relatively inaccessible.

Crossing Surgical Boundaries

Ballistic injuries do not respect the traditional surgical boundaries that are recognized in surgical specialization. The surgeon managing gunshot wounds, especially in a military field hospital, nongovernmental organization hospital, or other austere location where specialist surgeons are not immediately available, must be prepared to operate in all body cavities and anatomical regions where injury requires control of bleeding.

Abdominal Closure

While complete abdominal wall closure is the ultimate aim, edematous bowel, retroperitoneal hematoma, abdominal packs, the risk of abdominal compartment syndrome, or the requirement for repeat surgery occasionally preclude fascial closure. A number of alternative strategies to fascial closure exist; these are described in more detail in Chapter 10.

Specific Organ Injury and Surgical Management

Management of ballistic injuries to the specific organs is described below in brief. Descriptions of diagnostic findings are included only where directly relevant, as the majority of these injuries will be discovered at laparotomy undertaken as the diagnostic procedure. Injuries to the abdominal organs can be graded using the American Association for the Surgery of Trauma Organ Injury Scales which can be accessed on the web at www.aast.org/injury/injury. The severity of the injury can be used to guide the management.

Intra Abdominal Esophagus

Incidence

Six to ten centimeters of the distal esophagus lie within the abdomen. Although penetrating injury to the intra-abdominal esophagus is rare, any

wound that comes near or crosses near the upper epigastric area needs
to have the diaphragm, cava, proximal aorta, and distal esophagus
visualized.

Management

The patient should be positioned in reverse Trendelenburg and a large nasogastric tube should be placed into the stomach. Visualization and access to
the intra-abdominal esophagus requires excellent lighting, strong upward
retraction of the chest wall, caudal retraction of the stomach, occasionally
mobilization of stomach and spleen from diaphragmatic attachments, and
right lateral rotation of the left lobe of liver.

The esophagus is rotated through 180 degrees from the left to the right
by posterior blunt esophageal mobilization for inspection. If there is a high
index of suspicion of an injury, but a leak is not seen, then normal saline
can be infused into the distal esophagus with the proximal stomach clamped.
Alternatively, methylene blue can be used or air can be infused into
the esophagus with the abdomen filled with normal saline to detect air
leakage.

The options for repair depend on the time since injury, as those less than
six hours can be repaired primarily with two layers of absorbable sutures
and the repair buttressed with pleura. Complex and older injuries can be
repaired, but the addition of a diverting cervical esophagostomy should be
considered. All injuries should be drained with two or more chest tubes. A
feeding gastrostomy or jejunostomy should be inserted.

Outcome

The development of mediastinal sepsis is associated with a poor outcome.
The outcome is worse when injuries are missed or repair delayed.

Tips and Pitfalls

Complete mobilization and exploration of the esophagus is key. Adequate
drainage of the repaired esophagus is required. A feeding gastrostomy
should be inserted at the end of the operative procedure.

Diaphragm

Incidence

The diaphragm may be injured in up to 40% of abdominal GSWs. The
excursion of the diaphragm during respiration places it at risk from injuries
that occur as high as the level of the nipple anteriorly and the tip of lower
scapula posteriorly. Apparent thoracic hemorrhage from wounds at this
level may, in fact, be arising from the abdomen, and evaluation of the
abdomen in this situation is vital. Focused assessment with sonar for trauma
that reveals blood on either side of the diaphragm infers that the diaphragm

has been breached in penetrating trauma. Alternative strategies such as DPL have been shown to be poor in the diagnosis of isolated diaphragmatic injury.

Management

Operative repair is required with a strong nonabsorbable suture through all layers of the diaphragm. Right-sided diaphragmatic injury should be closed unless to do so would incite further bleeding from a liver injury.

Outcome

If recognized and repaired early, morbidity associated with this injury is low. There is a high incidence of morbidity, both early and late, if this injury is missed.

Tips and Pitfalls

Inspection of the diaphragm during the laparotomy is mandatory. Trajectory across or through the thoracoabdominal area predicts a diaphragmatic injury.

Stomach

Incidence

Injury to the stomach occurs in approximately 10% of penetrating abdominal trauma.

Management

Blood in the nasogastric aspirate may provide an early indication of gastric injury. The stomach, including the posterior wall via the lesser sac, must be inspected carefully; repair of wounds can be performed with two layers of absorbable sutures. Formal resection is infrequently required.

Outcome

The stomach usually heals well; however, there is a high risk of abdominal infection following spillage of gastric content.

Tips and Pitfalls

Carefully inspect both the greater and lesser curves, as omentum may obscure these areas. Always look for an exit wound in the posterior wall of the stomach if there is an anterior perforation and consider the possibility of associated pancreatic injury.

Duodenum

Incidence

Duodenal injuries commonly occur in association with injuries to the liver, pancreas, and major abdominal vessels and, because of this, are associated with a high mortality. Gunshot wounds and fragments are more likely to cause duodenal injuries than in blunt abdominal trauma. Surgical awareness and close inspection of the retroperitoneum for bile staining at trauma laparotomy will provide evidence of duodenal perforation.

Management

Kocherization of the duodenum, including mobilization of the hepatic flexure, provides adequate access for assessment and repair of the first, second, and proximal third portion of the duodenum. Mobilization of the fourth portion requires incising the ligament of Treitz and medial rotation. Operative repair is required; however, the technique depends on the severity of the duodenal injury and the presence and severity of associated injuries. The majority of duodenal wounds can be closed transversely with two layers of sutures, ensuring that the lumen is not narrowed, this can be protected by pyloric exclusion where the pylorus is closed with an absorbable suture (or staples) through a gastrostomy. The majority of pyloric exclusions will re-open over a three-week period; meanwhile, a gastrojejunostomy protects the repair by diverting the gastric contents.

In the region of the head of the pancreas, common bile duct (CBD) injury must be excluded. Direct choledocal inspection and a choledochogram can and must be performed. The choledochogram is done best through the gallbladder or with a catheter placed in the CBD. If distal CBD injury is detected, definitive repair or ligation and drainage is selected based on the patient's physiologic condition.

Massive duodenal destruction is associated with significant pancreatic injury and injury to the main duct. In this situation, a Whipple procedure may be required, but damage control principles should be applied.

All injuries to the duodenum require closed suction drainage.

Outcome

The overall mortality of this injury is linked to the number and severity of associated injuries; however, delayed diagnosis of duodenal perforation has a mortality of 40%. The morbidity is also high with more than 50% of patient's developing complications that may include intra-abdominal abscess and fistula formation.

Tips and Pitfalls

Missed injury is associated with high mortality and morbidity. Look for bile staining of the retroperitoneum and mobilize the entire duodenum to allow thorough assessment. Two-layer closure and wide drainage of the injured area is key.

Pancreas

Incidence

Seventy-five percent of pancreatic injuries are caused by penetrating trauma; however, this injury is uncommon, fortunately, and comprises less than 10% of abdominal trauma. The anatomical location and proximity of many vital structures means that pancreatic injuries following ballistic trauma rarely occur in isolation. Injury to the major vascular structures—aorta, portal vein, and inferior vena cava—occurs in up to 75% of penetrating pancreatic injures and account for most of the early deaths. In ballistic trauma, diagnosis relies upon intraoperative inspection during a laparotomy, often performed on an unstable bleeding patient. However, it is important that all pancreatic injuries be detected and any injury to the main duct addressed.

Management

The lesser sac must be opened through the gastrocolic ligament and the duodenum mobilized by a Kocher maneuver to allow bimanual palpation and inspection of the head of the pancreas. To differentiate contusion, partial or complete transaction of the body or tail of the pancreas, the spleen may need to be mobilized by dividing the splenorenal and splenocolic ligaments. Subsequent opening of the retroperitoneum and blunt posterior dissection of the pancreatic tail delivers these structures into the wound. Management strategies can be formed based on the location, severity of the injury, and the presence of a main duct injury (Table 14–1) and evidence of injury to the pancreatic duct. The majority of pancreatic injuries can be managed by drainage alone.

Principles
Hemorrhage control
Mobilization and inspection the entire pancreas, anterior and posterior.
Determine pancreatic duct injury
Debride devitalized pancreas
Preserve maximal amount of viable pancreas
Drain well with closed suction drains
Consider a feeding jejunostomy

TABLE 14-1. Suggested management guidelines for pancreatic trauma by injury severity

Grade	Management
I	Conservative/drainage
II	Conservative/debridement ± drainage
III	Distal pancreatectomy ± splenectomy
IV	Pancreatoduodenectomy (Consider damage control)
V	Pancreatoduodenectomy (Consider damage control)

Contusion/Capsular Laceration, Main Pancreatic Duct Intact

Definitive management is drainage, as attempts at repair may worsen the injury and result in a pseudocyst. Closed suction drains should be placed close to the site of injury.

Injuries to the Tail of the Pancreas

Injuries to the left of the superior mesenteric vessels should be managed by a distal pancreatectomy. A stapler can be used to control the proximal stump and the duct should be sought and over sewn with a nonabsorbable suture. Drains should be placed to the resection line. Preservation of the spleen has been described and this is only an option in the stable patient; most will require concomitant splenectomy.

Injuries to the Head of the Pancreas

These usually are severe, with many associated injuries, and initially require abbreviated surgical techniques. Ductal injury can be managed by drainage to form a controlled fistula or ligation of the ends of the duct and drainage. Severe injury to the head and duodenum needs a Whipple procedure. This may need to be undertaken later according to damage control principles. Packing around the pancreas after closure of the duodenal injury provides control until the patient is stable and can undergo a Whipple procedure.

Outcome

The mortality and morbidity is linked closely to the presence and severity of associated injuries. Specific pancreatic complications are common. The incidence of pancreatic fistula formation is approximately 50%, but most will close spontaneously. Peripancreatic pseudocysts may occur in up to 25% of pancreatic injuries and usually is associated with injury to the bowel.[5] Pancreatic psuedocyst abscesses may develop as a result of retained necrotic pancreatic tissue and require surgical drainage. Postoperative pancreatitis also may occur. The incidence of diabetes and exocrine deficiency is rare unless total pancreatectomy is performed.

There is little evidence that the somatostatin analogue octreotide reduces the incidence or duration of complications.

Tips and Pitfalls

Tailor the management of pancreatic injuries to the physiological status of the patient. Always thoroughly explore the pancreas if ballistic injuries are in close proximity. Adequate drainage is required in all injuries. Determination of pancreatic duct injury is paramount. Staged pancreatic resection is acceptable in unstable patients.

Liver and Hilar Structures

Incidence

The liver is the most frequently injured abdominal organ and may be injured in up to 42%[16] of abdominal GSW. The primary goal of management is the control of bleeding. Terblanche and colleagues reported that the majority of liver injuries (85%) can be managed with simple surgical techniques; however, major injuries require more complex procedures and the overall mortality remains 10 to 17%.[16a]

Management

The main stay of early treatment is hemorrhage control. This usually can be achieved initially with temporary manual compression and perihepatic packing, which compresses the liver parenchyma sufficiently to tamponade bleeding. In deeper wounds or those not entirely accessible, a Pringle maneuver with control of the porta hepatis is the initial maneuver. Bleeding from injuries that are accessible should be managed by direct suture of bleeding vessels using a monofilament nonabsorbable suture and bile ducts with an absorbable suture. The liver wound can be explored gently so that bleeding points are located. Resectional debridement using finger fracture should be used to remove devitalized tissue rather then formal anatomic resection, and closed suction drains should be placed to more severe injuries or those where bile leakage is anticipated.

Juxtahepatic inferior vena cava (IVC) injuries are amongst the most dramatic injuries for a surgeon to manage. The technique of total vascular isolation, control of the cava above and below the liver, is described below. Using this technique, a survival rate of 70% has been reported with direct repair of juxtahepatic IVC injuries.

A policy of selective nonoperative management for isolated Grade I and Grade II gunshot wounds of the liver has been suggested by Demetriades and colleagues.[17] In a study of 52 patients with isolated liver injury diagnosed on CT, the policy was only successful in one-fifth of patients, and 31%

of the patients initially selected for this approach failed and proceeded to laparotomy.

Techniques and Adjuncts

Mobilization

Exposure of the liver injury is vital and, if necessary, the midline wound can be extended by a subcostal incision for better exposure of the posterior aspects of the right lobe. The liver then can be mobilized further, especially for posterior injuries (segments VI and VII), by dividing the ligamentous attachments (falciform ligament, right and left coronary ligaments).

Perihepatic Packing

Perihepatic packing for ongoing bleeding from a liver injury is a valuable technique. Temporary packing as part of the initial trauma laparotomy should be differentiated from formal or therapeutic packing, which is used for definitive control. The falciform ligament should be divided initially to allow placement of packs without tearing the anterior liver capsule. Packs then are inserted around the diaphragmatic surfaces of the liver, providing compression of injuries. Consider using a plastic-covered pack as the initial pack in contact with the liver or laying vicryl mesh on the liver before the packs are applied. These packs are placed tightly around the entire lobe to provide circumferential tamponade and can be left in place for 24–48 hours. Therapeutic packing has been reported to be successful, even in very high-grade injuries.

Inflow Occlusion—The Pringle Maneuver

Occlusion of the portal triad (portal vein, hepatic artery, common bile duct) in the free edge of the hepatoduodenal ligament can provide effective reduction of active bleeding from parenchymal injuries; however, there will be no effect on retrohepatic caval injuries. A tape can be passed around the portal structures and snugged down to occlude flow; alternatively, a vascular clamp can be applied across them. Intermittent occlusion can be tolerated in the previously normal liver for periods of about 60 minutes.

Vena Cava Control

Total vascular isolation of the liver for retrohepatic caval injuries has been described. Clamping of both the infra- and suprahepatic vena cava may lead to cardiovascular collapse and the use of a number of atriocaval shunt devices (e.g., size 8 endotracheal tube or chest drain) have been reported.

The inferior vena cava can be controlled just above the renal veins. Division of the peritoneum lateral to the right side of the IVC is followed by gentle blunt dissection using a finger behind the vessel. The portal vein and bile duct are retracted to the left and the peritoneum incised on the finger passed behind the IVC, taking care not to injure the side wall of the cava or the renal vein. A tape then can be passed around the IVC and snugged tight if required.

Control of the IVC above the liver is more troublesome, as attempts at mobilizing the liver upwards are likely to be met by brisk hemorrhage. Incision of the pericardium and control of the IVC within the pericardium is a valuable technique and usually requires sternotomy.

Tractotomy

Hepatic tractotomy might be required for bleeding from a through-and-through wound of the liver. This is done best with a Pringle maneuver/inflow occlusion in place. Once the tract is opened, individual bleeding points and bile leaks can be sutured directly with figure of eight sutures.

Finger Fracture

Resectional debridement is the rule in liver trauma, rather than formal anatomical resection. Gentle finger dissection of the parenchyma will leave only the vessels and ducts, which then can be ligated.

Fibrin Glue, Topical Hemostatic Agents

Fibrin glue can be sprayed on to the raw liver surface to aid reduction of ooze. Topical hemostatics can be placed on bleeding sites and compressed with packing.

Angiography/Embolization

Interventional radiology can provide a valuable contribution to the management of liver injuries. A policy of angiography for all packed livers may demonstrate ongoing arterial bleeding that can be embolized.[18]

Hepatic Artery Ligation

Hepatic artery ligation has been used as a technique for uncontrollable arterial hepatic bleeding and usually is tolerated.

Track Tamponade

Bleeding from a missile track deep within the liver substance can be managed by an intrahepatic balloon. A Sengstaken esophageal tube or a Penrose drain over a red rubber catheter or tampon made from gel foam and absorbable mesh is inserted through the track and complimented by packing. Angiographic investigation and embolization is required as more than 30% of these injuries have deep intrahepatic arterial bleeding.

Outcome

The mortality from liver injury correlates with the severity of injury. Overall liver injury is associated with a mortality of 10%; however, Grade V and VI injuries have a mortality of 46% and 80%, respectively. The most serious complication is continual bleeding, requiring further laparotomy. Bile leak is a common complication; however, this can be managed nonoperatively in the majority of cases, if drainage is adequate. Prolonged drainage may be reduced by placing a stent across the ampulla.[19] Other rare complications include intrahepatic abscess and late haemobilia.

Tips and Pitfalls

Most liver injuries (85%) require no treatment, 10% require simple therapies with topical pressure, hemostatics, or suturing. Five percent are severe, life-threatening, deep liver injuries requiring innovative, abbreviated techniques to control bleeding. In this select group, packing and angiographic embolization are key.

Extrahepatic Biliary Injuries

These are rare injuries, but amongst the most complex to manage. Wounds of the gall bladder should be managed by simple cholecystectomy. Vascular control and repair of either or both the portal vein and hepatic artery are preferred. Ligation of the artery in extensive injury usually is tolerated, while ligation of the vein can be associated with compromise of both the liver and bowel. Complex injury to the bile duct usually requires a cholecystojejunostomy (preferred initially), choledochojejunostomy, or temporary distal CBD ligation and tube drainage of the biliary tract.

Spleen

Incidence

Infrequently injured by ballistic injury, when injury does occur, it usually results in shattering of the spleen and attempts at repair or salvage of the spleen frequently are futile.

Management

Medial mobilization of the shattered hemorrhaging spleen can be performed using a scoop technique with the hand placed behind the spleen, delivering it up into the wound. Diaphragmatic attachments are divided sharply. A laparotomy pack(s) can be placed behind the spleen to maintain its position. The splenic artery and vein are clamped and ligated individually, ensuring that the tail of the pancreas is not injured or included in the resected specimen. The ties on the short gastric vessels are placed to avoid injury to the stomach wall. Drainage is considered if the tail of the pancreas has also been injured.

Outcome

Mortality and morbidity from isolated splenic injury is low.

Tips and Pitfalls

Prolonged attempts at splenic salvage should be avoided in ballistic injury. Diaphragmatic injury should be identified and repaired.

Small Bowel

Incidence

The location and extent of the small bowel make it the most commonly injured organ following ballistic injury. Wounds can be multiple and widely separated throughout the length of bowel.

Management

Count the number of small bowel perforations. While occasionally wounds may be tangential, this is the exception rather than the rule, and an even number of holes is more reassuring. Plan resections carefully and use a combination of resection and repair to avoid loss of significant lengths of bowel. Mesenteric hematomas close to the small bowel border must be explored to rule out perforation.

Individual enterotomies from low-energy transfer rounds can be repaired after debridement of any dead tissue. Resection is performed following high-energy transfer injuries. Multiple holes require resection and anastomosis. Wounds at or close to the duodenojejunal flexure require distal duodenal mobilization.

Outcome

Small bowel usually heals well, with anastomotic leaks occurring in only a few percent.

Tips and Pitfalls

Small bowel injuries are usually multiple. When in doubt about the extent of injury to the small bowel wall, resection and anastomosis is best performed.

Colon

Incidence

Twenty-five percent of abdominal gunshot wounds involve the colon, with 5% of these involving the rectum. Digital rectal examination is an integral part of the examination of trauma patients and blood on examination in a patient with a penetrating abdominal or buttock wound is evidence of colorectal injury. In suspected rectal injury, further examination by sigmoidoscopy should be performed under general anesthesia, as this may aid planning the operation.

Management

Current management of civilian ballistic injury favors primary repair or resection and anastomosis of most colonic injuries if there is minimal fecal spillage, no hypotension, few other injuries, and no delay to surgery.[17] Conversely, in the face of extensive contamination, significant hypotension, or complex colonic injury (destructive colon injury), colostomy with resection has, to date, been continually advocated. With military or high-energy transfer weapons, the continued use of resection and diverting colostomy is recommended.

Outcome

Complications following colonic injury include abscess and fistula formation.

Rectum

Incidence

Five percent of colon injuries involve the rectum. The location of the injury, intraperitoneal or extraperitoneal, determines the management strategy. Many rectal injuries have concomitant bladder and distal ureter injury. Diagnosis of these occasionally requires cystography.

Management

Intraperitoneal injuries often can be managed following the same approach as with colonic injury. However, extraperitoneal rectal perforations should be managed with a diverting colostomy as either a Hartman's procedure or a loop colostomy with stapled distal end. Unless obvious, the hole in the rectum can be left if it is adequately defunctioned. The role of presacral drainage and rectal irrigation of the rectal stump remain controversial. With higher energy transfer wounds, fecal diversion, presacral drainage, and rectal irrigation are recommended.

Outcome

The complications are similar to colonic injuries Pelvic sepsis, abscess, and death are seen if rectal injury is missed.

Tips and Pitfalls

Injuries to the buttock are intraperitoneal or rectal injuries until proven otherwise.

Kidney/Ureter/Bladder

The management of injuries to these structures is covered in Chapter 13.

Retroperitoneal Hematomas

All Zone I retroperitoneal wounds from ballistic injury require exploration. Chapter 13 gives further details on the management of perinephric haematomas.

Intra Abdominal Vascular Injuries

See Chapter 18.

Postoperative Management

The postlaparotomy trauma patient requires close observation and skilled nursing care. The location, available resources, and further expected casualties may dictate the extent to which this is possible. Multiple casualties may require the patient to be transferred to another facility. Patients with ballistic injury involving the abdomen are at high risk of developing postoperative complications (atelectasis, pneumonia, intra-abdominal infection, etc.). Even when the physiological condition has allowed definitive repair to be performed, at the end of the procedure the patient may be acidotic, cold, and have coagulation abnormalities. These must be urgently addressed. Many civilian facilities will keep these patients intubated and ventilated until these conditions have been reversed; however, this may not be possible in military or austere settings. Issues concerning the critical-care management of ballistic casualties are discussed in the Chapter 22.

The postoperative management centers around the avoidance and early detection of complications, reintroduction of oral diet, removal of drains, and rehabilitation into the community.

Complications and Special Considerations

Abdominal Compartment Syndrome (ACS)

The abdominal compartment syndrome is increasingly being recognized as a cause of postoperative complications on the intensive care unit. Raised intra-abdominal pressure (IAP) has been reported to occur in more than 50% of patients who have direct fascial closure following penetrating abdominal trauma[20] while the incidence was reduced to 22% in those who had mesh or "open" abdomens. Sugrue[16] has recommended that all patients at risk of this syndrome should have eight-hourly measurements of the intra-abdominal pressure using a bladder pressure technique for 24 hours. Absolute criteria for opening the abdomen with raised IAP remain controversial; however, pressures in excess of 25 millimeters Hg with evidence of end organ sequelae are candidates for reopening and conversion to an "open abdomen."

Temporary Abdominal Closure

Techniques for the temporary closure of the abdomen are described in Chapter 10.

Stomas

The move towards primary repair or anastomosis in civilian colonic injuries, as discussed previously, will reduce the number of stomas that are made. When stomas are required, they should be placed laterally away from the wound.

Leaks and Fistulas

Uncontrolled enteric leaks that result in peritonitis require a laparotomy and proximal diversion. Adequately drained anastomotic leaks and localized small bowel fistula can be managed conservatively.

Definitive Treatment vs. Pack and Transfer

Not all surgical facilities will have the necessary equipment, resources, or expertise to definitively manage the whole range of abdominal injuries that may occur from ballistic injury. These patients require a damage control laparotomy with control of hemorrhage and contamination at the initial hospital, then transfer to the nearest suitable tertiary receiving center by an appropriate rapid means of transport. Communication, both written and verbal, between referring and receiving surgeons is vital. The timing of the second laparotomy depends on the injuries and stability of the patient.

Military/Austere Considerations

Sophisticated diagnostic adjuncts are unlikely to be available in austere or operational environments, therefore laparotomy serves as both diagnostic tool and therapeutic intervention. The usual confounders exist, that is, state of battle, numbers of expected casualties, operative resources (theater teams, equipment, resupply, blood, etc.); therefore, triage is imperative. These issues are considered further in the section on resource-limited environments.

Nonoperative Management of Abdominal Ballistic Injury

Selective nonoperative policies for abdominal gunshot wounds and isolated abdominal injuries has been reported. The literature is well reviewed by Saadia and Degiannis, who concluded that although a case for nonoperative management had been made in the group of patients where there was proof that the peritoneum had not been breached, caution should be exercised.[21] This is especially true with wounds from military weapons and fragments (ordnance).

Summary

Ballistic trauma to the abdomen requires decisive intervention. Hemorrhage control is the priority, and the option of damage control always should be considered in the unstable patient. Surgical management depends on the anatomical injury and the available resources.

References

1. Spalding TJ, Stewart MP, Tulloch DN, Stephens KM. Penetrating missile injuries in the Gulf war 1991. *Br J Surg.* 1991;78(9):1102–1104.
2. Roberts P. Patterns of injury in military operations. *Curr Anaesth Crit Care.* 2003;13:243–248.
3. McGonigal MD, Cole J, Schwab CW, Kauder DR, Rotondo MF, Angood PB. Urban firearm deaths: A five-year perspective. *J Trauma.* 1993;35: 532–537.

4. Rotondo MF, Schwab CW, McGonigal MD, Philips GR III, Fruchterman TM, Kauder DR, Latenser BA, Angood PA. Damage control—an approach for improved survival in exsanguinating penetrating abdominal injury. *J Trauma.* 1993;35(3):375–380.

5. Johnson JW, Gracias VH, Schwab CW, et al. Evolution in damage control for exsanguinating penetrating abdominal injury. *J Trauma.* 2001;51:261–271.

6. Bickell WH, Wall MJ, Pepe PE, Martin RR, Ginger VF, Allen MK, Mattox KL. Immediate versus delayed fluid resuscitation for hypotensive patients with penetrating torso injuries. *N Engl J Med.* 1994;331:1105–1109.

7. Clarke JR, Trooskin SZ, Doshi PJ, Greenwald L, Mode CJ. Time to laparotomy for intra-abdominal bleeding from trauma does affect survival for delays up to 90 minutes. *J Trauma.* 2002;52(3):420–425.

8. Rotondo MF, Zonies DH. The damage control sequence and underlying logic. *Surg Clin North Am.* 1997;77(4):761–777.

9. Johnson JW, Gracias VH, Schwab CW, et al. Evolution in damage control for exsanguinating penetrating abdominal injury. *J Trauma.* 2001;51:261–271.

10. Rosuff L, Cohen JL, Telfer N, Halpern M. Injuries of the spleen. *Surg Clin North Am.* 1972;52:667–685.

11. Kahdi F, Rodriguez UK, Chiu WC, Scalea TM. Role of ultrasonography in penetrating abdominal trauma: A prospective clinical study. *J Trauma.* 2001; 50:475–479.

12. Grossman MD, May AK, Reilly PM, McMahon DJ, Rotondo MF, Shapiro MP, Kauder DR, Schwab CW, Frankel H, Anderson H. Determining anatomic injury with computer tomography in selected torso gunshot wounds. *J Trauma.* 1998;45:446–456.

13. Schreiber MA, Holcomb JB, Hedner U, Brundage SI, Macaitis JM, Hoots K. The effect of recombinant factor VIIa on coagulopathic pigs with grade V liver injuries. *J Trauma Injury Infect Crit Care.* 2002;53(2):252–257.

14. Martinowitz U, Holcomb JB, Pusateri AE, Stein M, Onaca N, Freidman M, Macaitis JM, Castel D, Hedner U, Hess JR. Intravenous rFVIIa administered for hemorrhage control in hypothermic coagulopathic swine with grade V liver injuries. *J Trauma Injury Infect Crit Care.* 2001;50(4):721–729.

15. Pitcher G. Fiber-endoscopic thoracoscopy for diaphragmatic injury in children. *Semin Pediatr Surg.* 2001;10(1):17–19.

16. Sugrue M, Danne P, Civil I, eds. *Definitive Surgical Trauma Care Manual.* Liverpool, Australia: 2003.

16a. Marr JD, Krige JG, Terblanche J. Analysis of 153 gunshot wounds of the liver. *Br J Surg.* 2000;87(8):1030–1034.

17. Asensio JA, Roldan G, Petrone P, et al. Operative management and outcomes in 103 AAST-OIS grades IV and V complex hepatic injuries: Trauma surgeons still need to operate, but angioembolization helps. *J Trauma.* 2003;54(4):647–653.

18. Gracias VH, Reilly PM, Philpott J, et al. Computed tomography in the evaluation of penetrating neck trauma: A preliminary study. *Arch Surg.* 2001; 136(11):1231–1235.

19. Hoff WS, Ginsberg GG, Grossman MD, Reilly PM, Kauder DR, Schwab CW. Traumatic choledochogastric fistula: endoscopic evaluation and treatment with a biliary stent. *J Trauma.* 1998;45:1094–1096.

20. Ivatury RR, Porter JM, Simon RJ, Islam S, John R, Stahl WM. Intra-abdominal hypertension after life-threatening penetrating abdominal trauma:

Prophylaxis, incidence, and clinical relevance to gastric mucosal pH and abdominal compartment syndrome. *J Trauma Injury Infect Crit Care.* 1998; 44(6):1016–1021, 1021–1023.

21. Saadia R, Degiannis E. Non-operative treatment of abdominal gunshot injuries *Br J Surg.* 2000;87(4):393–397.

15
Management of Ballistic Trauma to the Head

CHRIS J. NEAL, GEOFFREY S.F. LING, and JAMES M. ECKLUND

Introduction

Historically, the vast majority of penetrating head injuries (PHI) resulted from military combat operations; however, during the latter part of the twentieth century, these injuries have increased in incidence in civilian trauma centers. The difference in military and civilian PHI is often the nature of the penetrating projectile. In a combat situation, a majority of penetrating missile wounds are from either explosive munitions producing low-velocity fragmentation injuries or high-velocity bullets fired from various ranges.[1] Civilian gunshot wounds primarily result from low-velocity bullets fired at close range, typically from handguns.[2] This accounts for a significant proportion of civilian injuries in the form of homicides, suicides, and accidents, with an estimated 2.4 deaths per 100000 each year in the United States.[3,4] With the recent increased threat of terrorist attacks, the penetrating and blast injuries traditionally seen during military conflicts may become more frequently seen in some civilian centers. As a consequence of the large number of patients with PHI treated during wartime, a number of the advances and refinements in the care of these patients have emerged from the military experience.

Prior to 1900, PHIs generally were considered fatal. MacCleod reported a 100% mortality in 86 cases of penetrating or perforating head injury during the Crimean War. During the American Civil War, the death rate from pyremia of wounds to the head was as high as 95% in some series. Few surgical interventions were performed because of the high rate of infectious complications. The introduction of Lister's antiseptic technique in 1867, more sophisticated understanding of cerebral localization during the late 1800s, advances in surgical technique during World War I (WWI), and antibiotics during World War II (WWII) gradually led to new optimism regarding the care of these patients.[5,6]

Major Harvey Cushing encouraged the systematic evaluation and treatment of patients with PHI during WWI. He emphasized the importance of early meticulous debridement of all devitalized tissue and removal of all visualized fragments of bone and/or metal. The application of his techniques reduced the operative mortality from 56% to 28% within 3 months at Base Camp 5.[5-9]

World War II brought with it the broad application of antibiotics and the importance of dural repair. Operative mortality was reduced to 14.5% during this conflict.[10,11]

During the Korean War, an improved medical evacuation system and the eventual placement of neurosurgeons in combat zones resulted in more immediate surgical interventions. This early intervention proved especially efficacious in the treatment of intracranial hematomas and resulted in fewer infectious complications. Surgical mortality was reduced to as low as 10% in some series during this conflict.[12]

As a result of anecdotal reports describing delayed abscess development in PHI from WWII and Korea, the practice of aggressively removing all bone and metallic fragments in an attempt to reduce postoperative infection was mandated in the U.S. Army during Vietnam. This approach sometimes subjected a patient to multiple operations and occasional increased operative morbidity for what was felt to be an "adequate" debridement.[13] Critical review of the results of patients at five and 14 years in the Vietnam Head Injury Study (VHIS) ultimately showed no difference in rates of infection or seizures in those patients with retained bone or metallic fragments as seen on computed tomography (CT).

This data was applied during the Israeli–Lebanese conflict where Branvold and colleagues[14] described a debridement strategy in 113 patients based on preservation of viable tissue with limited debridement. Fragments were removed with gentle irrigation and fragments that were not easily obtainable were left. Of the 43 patients with long-term follow up, there was a 51% incidence of retained fragments and no relationship to the development of intracranial abscess formation. Additionally, there was not an increased incidence of posttraumatic epilepsy with retained bone fragments.[14] These important experiences were instrumental in the evolution of the modern surgical management of PHI.

Ballistics

To understand penetrating trauma, it is important to have a basic understanding of ballistics. Wound ballistics is the study of the projectile's action in human tissue. The ballistic properties of a projectile are dependent primarily on its velocity, size, and shape. The primary injury to the brain is related directly to these properties. Secondary projectiles such as skull fragments may cause further damage.

Penetrating head injury can result from both low- and high-velocity projectiles. Lower-velocity sharp projectiles such as arrows (120 to 250 feet per second) create a tract of primary tissue damage without significant bruising or blunt tearing of surrounding tissue. Higher-velocity projectiles are preceded by a brief (2 ms) sonic shock wave, followed by the penetration of the projectile. In addition to the destruction of tissue in the projectile's path, there is a transmission of kinetic energy resulting in a temporary cavitation effect. In brain tissue, which is relatively inelastic, the cavity is often 10 to 20 times the size of the projectile. After expansion, the cavity collapses under negative pressure that may draw in external debris.

The size of the cavity is dependent on the kinetic energy of the projectile. Kinetic energy (KE) can be expressed in the equation $KE = \frac{1}{2} mv^2$. While mass is directly proportional to the kinetic energy, it is the velocity that is its key determinant.[15,16] The shape of the projectile determines the ballistic coefficient, which is its ability to overcome air resistance and maintain velocity. The shape also influences the yaw, which is the projectile's rotation around its long axis. While small amounts of circular motion (precession and nutation) occur during flight, projectiles often will tumble when striking tissue. Yaw is maximized when the projectile is rotated at 90 degrees to its long axis.[15,16] This imparts more kinetic energy to the tissue, increases the size of the temporary cavity, and increases tissue destruction.

For example, a .45 automatic pistol (muzzle velocity of 869 feet per second and a short round-nosed projectile with little yaw) will create a very small temporary cavity; conversely, a 7.62 millimeter North Atlantic Treaty Organization (NATO) rifle (muzzle velocity 2830 feet per second and a long sharp nose with maximum yaw) will create a very large temporary cavity.

Projectiles also can deform or fragment upon striking tissue. Copper jacketing lead bullets, as mandated for military rounds by The Hague Peace Conference (1899), helps limit the fragmentation potential. Irregularities made by scoring the surface of the bullet (dum dums) lead to increased fragmentation, creating multiple injury tracts as each fragment becomes a new projectile. The Glaser round is filled with small pellets that disperse on impact. Hollow-point rounds, often seen in civilian shootings, expand their diameter in the direction of flight upon impact, thus creating a larger primary wound tract and more destructive temporary cavitation effects. Explosive bullets such as the Devastator round are designed to detonate on impact and thus will produce extensive tissue injury with additional kinetic energy transfer.[17]

Injury Classification

Since WWI, PHIs have been classified in an attempt to correlate the type of injury with prognosis. Cushing's original classification of nine different injury patterns was refined by Matson in WWII to four categories, which are explained in Table 15-1.

Currently, a PHI is described as a tangential wound, a penetrating wound, or a perforating wound.

TABLE 15-1. Cushing and Matson's classification of craniocerebral injuries

Grade	Cushing (WW I) Description	Grade	Matson (WW II) Description
I	Scalp lacerations, skull intact	I	Scalp wound
II	Skull fractures, dura intact	II	Skull fracture, dura intact
III	Depressed skull fracture and dural laceration	III	Skull fracture with dural/brain penetration A: Gutter-type (grazing)—in-driven bone with no missile fragments B: Penetrating—missile fragments in brain C: Perforating—through and through
IV	In-driven bone fragments	IV	Complicating factors: A: Ventricular penetration B: Fractures of orbit or sinus C: Injury of dural sinus D: Intracerebral hematoma
V	Penetrating wound with projectile lodged		
VI	Wounds penetrating ventricles with: A: Bone fragments B: Projectile		
VII	Wounds involving : A: Orbitonasal region B: Auropetrosal region		
VIII	Perforating Wounds		
IX	Bursting Skull Fracture, extensive cerebral contusion		

Tangential Wound

A tangential wound (Figure 15-1) occurs when a projectile strikes the head at an oblique angle and may produce scalp lacerations, skull fractures, and cerebral contusions. The projectile may traverse the subgaleal space and exit or remain lodged in the scalp. The presence of a hematoma, depressed skull fracture, or cerebrospinal fluid (CSF) leak may necessitate surgical intervention. Otherwise, local wound care may be applied. These injuries generally carry a better prognosis with less severe neurological deficits, but they may present with seizures or focal deficit depending on location and extent of injury.

FIGURE 15-1. (A) CT of tangential wound to right occipital region from AK47 while wearing military helmet. Wound was emergently debrided at nearby field hospital. Note the in-driven bone fragments. (B) MRI of same patient revealing underlying contusion after CT confirmation of no residual metal fragments.

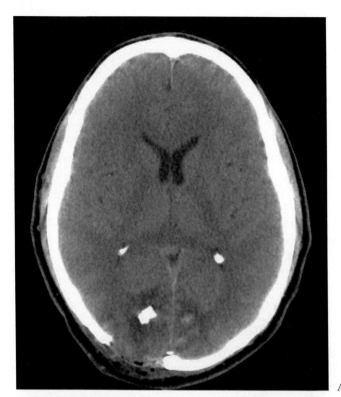

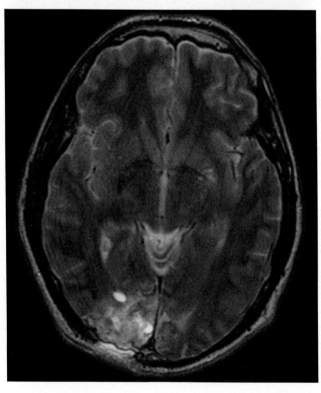

Penetrating Wound

The velocity of the projectile is the main determinant of its energy. If the projectile has enough energy to only penetrate the brain parenchyma, the injury is referred to as penetrating. Energy absorbed by the skull often results in fragments of bone that act as secondary projectiles within the brain. Contusions, lacerations, or hematomas may be caused by these injuries (Figure 15-2).

Depending on the amount of energy, the projectile may produce unusual tracts within the calvaria that may be detected on CT, but missed on plain films. The projectile may ricochet after hitting the inner table opposite of its entry, creating a new tract within the parenchyma. It also may change directions when it hits dura after penetrating the outer and inner tables of the skull. This unusual occurrence is called *careening*. The projectile then travels along the inner table of the skull, with the potential to damage the venous sinuses.

Perforating Wound

The most destructive pattern of injury is the perforating wound (Figure 15-3), which is defined by an entry and exit wound with a tract through brain parenchyma. This injury requires a higher-velocity projectile than with a penetrating injury, and thus imparts a higher amount of kinetic energy to the tissue. Local and distant structures are damaged from the cavitation effect the projectile imparts, resulting in multiple fractures, contusions, and hematomas.

Initial Resuscitation and Management

In civilian trauma, activation of the local emergency medical service (EMS) system allows initial resuscitation efforts to be made in the field to include intravenous (IV) access and intubation when warranted. The use of a helicopter allows for faster transport from the scene or outlying hospital to a neurosurgical center for early intervention.[18,19]

A combat situation provides a different operating environment for PHIs. Initial care is provided by a medic carrying limited supplies and diagnostic equipment. In contrast to civilian systems, combat injuries are triaged in the field and at every level of care. Due to limited capabilities, the goal of combat medicine is to do the greatest good for the most people, thus maintaining the fighting force. If a patient is triaged as expectant, they are not prioritized for rapid evacuation, allowing those resources to be shifted to other, salvageable patients. Military neurosurgeons are viewed as assets, deployed where most beneficial.[20] Depending on the theater of operations, neurosurgical support may be located at a variety of locations or echelons.

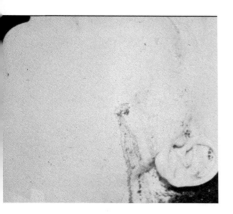
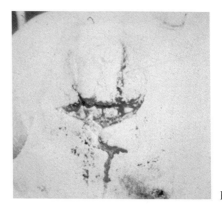

B

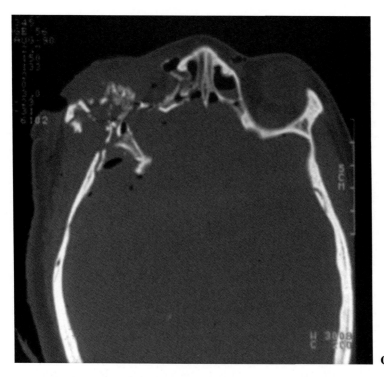

C

FIGURE 15-2. (A) Gun shot entrance wound in left cheek (B) Gun shot exit wounds right periorbital region. Note the increased size of the exit wound compared to the entrance wound. (C) CT demonstrating intracranial involvement.

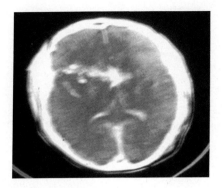 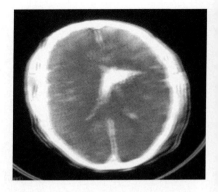

FIGURE 15-3. CT of a perforating GSW with a transventricular tract.

A military neurosurgeon may be located in an austere field hospital. Alternatively, he or she may be in a more sophisticated environment further along the evacuation chain. In urban conflict this may be an urban hospital. Head injuries will need to be triaged and initially managed by medics, general surgeons, or general medical officers at more forward locations. Medical evacuation for these patients, either by ground or air, can be delayed as a result of equipment challenges, the terrain, the weather, or the tactical situation. Proactive training and neurosurgical exposure to far-forward providers and utilization of telemedicine for neurosurgical consultation can greatly facilitate the care of these patients.

In either a civilian or combat environment, patients with a PHI often experience a period of apnea and hypotension. Early intubation and appropriate fluid resuscitation may reduce the secondary complications from these events.[18,19] A challenge to early intubation in the field can be cervical immobilization. Kennedy and colleagues[21] reviewed the incidence of spine injury in patients with isolated gunshot wounds (GSWs) to the head. They found no spine injuries in 105 patients, suggesting that immobilization may not be necessary, facilitating intubation (see also Chapters 7 and 16).

As in any trauma, Advanced Trauma Life Support/Battlefield Advanced Trauma Life Support (ATLS/BATLS) guidelines are followed, with a focus on preventing hypoxia and hypotension. Both of these events significantly worsen the outcome of patients with head injury. Once IV access is obtained, laboratory evaluation to include electrolytes, complete blood count (CBC), prothrombin time/partial thromboplastin time (PT/PTT), type and screen/cross, urinalysis, and toxicology panel should be sent. A brief history from medics, family members, or paramedics is taken to include the mechanism of injury, neurological examination at the scene, periods of hypoxia or hypotension, and known past medical history or allergies. During the primary and secondary survey, the patient is inspected thoroughly for entry and exit wounds, which should also include the oral cavity. A temporary clean, bulky dressing is applied to the wounds.

A brief neurological exam is performed, remembering that the patient should be fully resuscitated before determining a prognosis. The patient's Glascow Coma Scale (GCS) score, the presence of hypotension or hypoxia, and any use of pharmacological agents should be noted.[22] If the patient has a GCS score of less than 8 or cannot otherwise protect their airway, intubation for adequate airway protection, oxygenation, and ventilation should be considered. Brainstem reflexes and pupillary exam, to include size, symmetry, and reactivity, are noted. Evaluation for CSF leak is performed at this point, including inspection of the tympanic membranes and nares. Antiepileptic agents and broad-spectrum antibiotics are administered.

Neuroimaging

Plain radiographic studies of the skull can provide a quick impression of the nature of the injury and evaluate for the presence of intracranial fragments and air, especially in circumstances where a CT scan is unavailable. The true trajectory of the fragment may be misleading in the presence of ricochet or careening fragments (Figures 15-4 and 15-5).[23] If rapid access to a CT scanner is possible, plain films are not required. Noncontrast CT with bone windows allow for precise localization of bone and projectile fragments, identification of the trajectory, and characterization of brain injury (Figure 15-5). The presence of mass effect and classification of hematomas, either epidural, subdural, parechymal, or intraventricular, can be performed.[23]

Angiography is recommended when there is a high suspicion for vascular injury. From Aarabi's experience in the Iran–Iraq war, there was a 4 to 10 time increased risk of traumatic aneurysm development in patients with facio-orbito or pterional entry, intracranial hematoma, or projectile

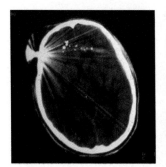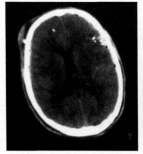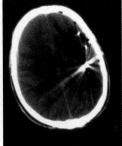

FIGURE 15-4. CT of GSW from close range demonstrating ricochet of fragment posteriorly off contralateral skull. Plain film correlation alone with right fronto-temporal entrance wound would lead to an incorrect assumption of true wound tract.

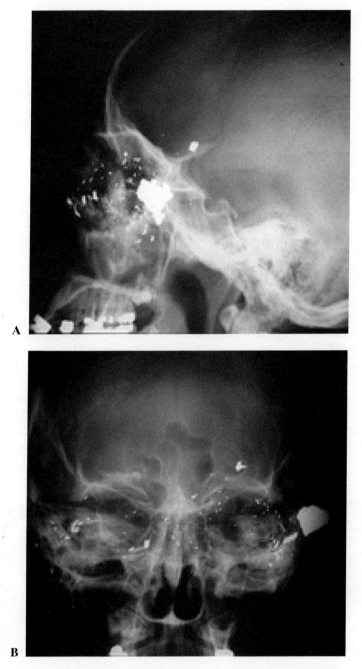

FIGURE 15-5. Lat (A) and AP (B) skull X-rays of GSW provides some information on retained fragments, presumed tract of injury, and involved structures. (C) CT scan gives a much better anatomic delineation of the injury.

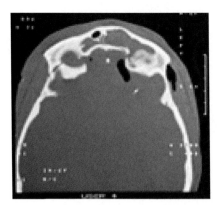 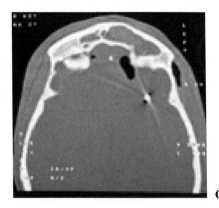

C

FIGURE 15-5. *Continued*

trajectories that cross dural compartments.[24] Haddad and colleagues documented 15 cases of traumatic aneurysms from the Lebanese conflict: 14 from fragmentation injuries and one from a bullet. From their experience, they recommended an angiogram for patients with retained fragments, no associated exit wound, and an intracranial hematoma in the distal portion of the trajectory.[25] Other high-risk injuries include a projectile trajectory through or near the Sylvian fissure, supraclinoid carotid artery, basilar cisterns, or major venous sinuses. After stabilization, any PHI patient who develops a new or unexplained subarachnoid hemorrhage or delayed hematoma should also undergo angiography (Figure 15-6).[23,26]

Magnetic resonance imaging (MRI) currently is not recommended in the acute management of PHI.[23] Retained ferromagnetic fragments produce artifact, distortion, and also can rotate from the magnetic torque.[27–29] Magnetic resonance imaging may be beneficial in certain cases where the projectile is not retained or is known to contain no metallic elements (see chapter 23).

Preoperative Treatment

Increased intracranial pressure (ICP) is common after PHI.[30–33] The exact pathophysiology behind this elevation is not completely understood. The available data suggests that maintenance of an ICP less than 20 mm Hg has a more favorable prognosis than those with uncontrolled intracranial hypertension.[34] Increased intracranial pressure monitoring should be initiated when the clinician is unable to assess a patient's neurological exam, commonly at a GCS score of less than or equal to 8. There are various means to monitor ICP, the most common being intraventricular catheters and intraparenchymal monitors. Intraventricular catheters offer the therapeutic advantage of CSF drainage for treatment of elevated ICP.

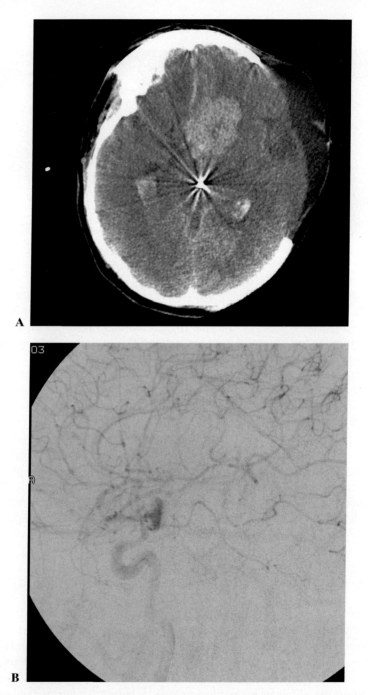

FIGURE 15-6. (A) CT showing delayed hematoma in patient involved in a shrapnel injury to base of skull and orbit. (B) Lateral and (C) AP angiogram revealing pseudoaneurysm of anterior cerebral artery. (D) Pseudoaneurysm was treated by endovascular coiling. The patient's initial angiogram after injury was negative.

Even if ICP monitoring has not been initiated, treatment should be started if the patient demonstrates clinical evidence of herniation or progressive neurological decline. General treatment measures include elevation of the head of the bed to 30 to 45 degrees, keeping the head midline to avoid venous outflow constriction, light sedation, and avoiding hypotension, hypoxemia, or hypercarbia.[35] Cerebral perfusion pressure (CPP) should be kept >60 mm Hg.[36] Elevated ICP affects the CPP through the relationship: CPP = MAP − ICP. More aggressive treatment measures include increased sedation, CSF drainage, and administration of osmotic agents such as mannitol (0.25–1.00 g/kg).[35]

Hyperventilation reduces ICP through cerebral vasoconstriction, and therefore carries the risk of hypoperfusion from decreased cerebral blood flow. Because of this risk, hyperventilation should be employed sparingly, and only for brief periods while other treatment modalities are instituted.

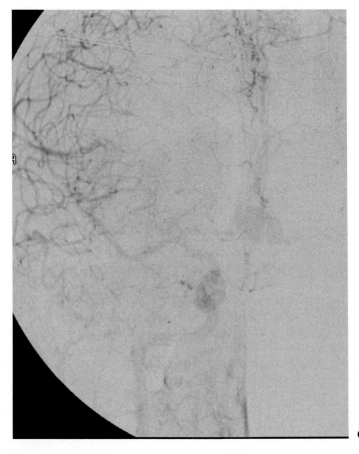

C

FIGURE 15-6. *Continued*

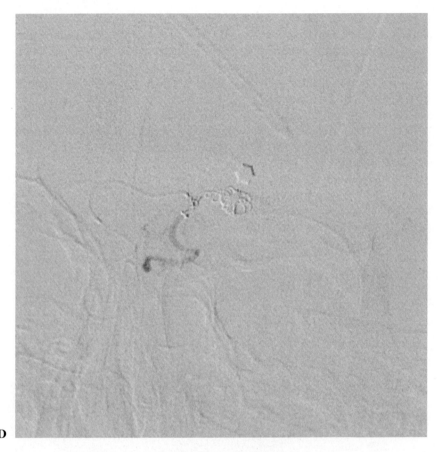

D

FIGURE 15-6. *Continued*

Projectiles can impart various forces on the cerebral vasculature result-ing in arterial wall transection. Depending on the location, the patient may develop a subarachnoid hemorrhage, an intracerebral hematoma, and/or intraventricular hematoma (Figure 15-7). Subarachnoid hemorrhage is seen in 31 to 78% of PHI cases on CT scan.[37] Both Aldrich and colleagues and Levy and colleagues have shown that the presence of subarachnoid hemorrhage correlates significantly with patient mortality.[38,39]

Ten percent of combat-related PHIs are associated with dural sinus involvement.[40] This can lead to massive intraoperative hemorrhage. When the trajectory of the projectile raises the potential of dural sinus injury, preoperative planning should include appropriate hemodynamic support, including blood products and air embolism monitoring, availability of proper equipment, and personnel familiar with surgical techniques for managing venous sinus injury.

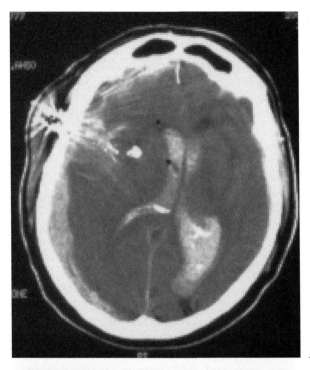

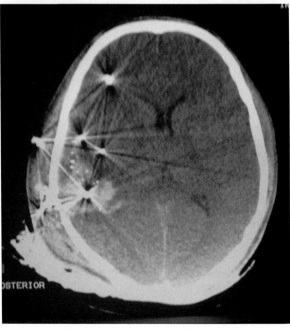

FIGURE 15-7. (A) CT of GSW revealing small intraparenchymal hematoma, intraventricular hemorrhage, and a large subdural hematoma with marked mass effect. (B) CT of shrapnel wound with small intraparenchymal hematoma.

Traumatically induced pseudoaneurysms or traumatic intracranial aneurysms (TICA) may occur, with 0.4 to 0.7% of all intracranial aneurysms caused by trauma, 20% of these from PHI.[24,37] The incidence of TICAs is reported between 3 and 33.3% in PHI patients.[24,26,41,42] Angiography is the standard in detection of vascular injuries, but a single angiogram does not rule out the possibility of a TICA.[24,26,41] Since TICAs are not usually true aneurysms, clipping may not be effective. Endovascular techniques or trapping of the lesion are alternative treatment options.

Seizures are common after PHI. They are typically divided into early and late; early defined loosely in the literature as within the first seven days. Between 30 and 50% of PHI patients develop seizures. Four to 10% of these are early seizures while 80% occur within the first two years.[43,44] Data from the VHIS indicated that after 15 years of follow up, nearly 50% of PHI patients with epilepsy stopped having seizures.[44] If PHI patients do not have seizures within the first three years, 95% will remain seizure free.[45] Few studies exist that examine only PHI patients and the use of prophylactic antiepileptic drugs. The current guidelines extrapolated from those patients with nonpenetrating traumatic brain injury recommend antiepileptic drugs during the first week to prevent early posttraumatic seizures. No data supports the use of these medications prophylatically beyond the first seven days in the PHI population to prevent late posttraumatic seizures.[46]

Penetrating head injury wounds are considered contaminated, both superficially and deep. Negative pressure from the cavity caused by the projectile can draw superficial contaminant and debris deep into the wound. The primary projectile, either bullet or fragment, that remains intracranial is not sterile; insufficient heat is generated from the firing mechanism and high velocity for adequate sterilization.[47,48] Broad-spectrum antibiotics are initiated as soon as possible. In civilian PHI, coverage for Staphylococcus and Streptococcus should be of primary concern. With military combat injuries, coverage should also include Acinetobacter, and may be further broadened depending on the area of operations.[49,50]

Surgical Management

The foundation for surgical management of PHI is found in the work performed by Cushing during WWI: craniectomy, thorough debridement of devitalized scalp, bone, brain, metal and bony fragments, and meticulous closure. This approach remained relatively unchanged through Vietnam. Data from the VHIS and modern military conflicts do not support vigorous removal of all bone and metallic fragments or repeat craniotomies solely for removal of additional fragments. Debridement should be confined to nonviable brain, with removal of readily accessible fragments of bone and metal.[51]

Taha and colleagues reported on a subset of PHI patients that were treated with simple wound closure and a three-day course of IV antibiotics.[52] Patients met the following criteria: initial GCS score greater than 10, presented within six hours of injury, entry wound less than two centimeters, no exit wound, trajectory not through the proximal Sylvain fissure, and no significant intracranial hematoma. These criteria attempted to eliminate patients whose injury would produce a significant amount of devitalized tissue. Out of 32 patients, they reported no deaths and one brain abscess that ultimately was treated without complication. Local wound care and closure is a treatment option recognized by the *Guidelines of Penetrating Brain Injury* for similarly selected patients.

The early identification and evacuation of hematomas is important in effecting the outcome of PBI. Some authors have stated that the only indication for surgery, outside of wound care, is the reduction of mass effect, and thus intracranial pressure, from a hematoma.[33,54] The rapid evacuation of hematomas creating significant mass effect is the standard practice. If a hematoma is not removed in a salvageable patient, ICP monitoring should be considered to confirm the decision and to guide further therapy.

All PHI patients should be evaluated vigorously and monitored continuously for the presence of a CSF leak. In a report based on the VHIS, only 50% of CSF leaks were located at the wound site. The remaining were assumed to be caused by injury from the projectile's concussive effect.[32] Mortality for these patients was 22.8% versus 5.1% for those without a CSF leak. The presence of a CSF leak is the variable most highly correlated with intracranial infection in PHI patients. In the VHIS, 44% of the fistulas closed spontaneously.[55] However, if the leak is persistent or delayed in onset, treatment with either CSF diversion or direct surgical repair should be instituted. During any primary surgical treatment of PHI a meticulous, watertight closure of the dura, including the use of temporalis fascia, fascia lata, or graft material, is essential.

Air sinus injuries present an increased risk for CSF leak, especially with an orbital-facial wound. Analysis of a two-year period during the Korean War revealed a 15% incidence of air sinus injury with combat PHI.[56] Delay in repair of this injury increases the risk of infection.[7,8,10,56] Management may include craniotomy and anterior fossa reconstruction, exoneration of the frontal sinus, and watertight dural closure. For temporal bone injuries, a mastoidectomy or middle ear exploration with Eustachian tube packing may be required.

Postoperative Care

Postoperatively, the patient is monitored in an intensive-care setting. As mentioned, ICP is monitored and treated for a goal ICP of less than 20mmHg and CPP of greater than 60mmHg.[36] Any persistent, unexplained elevation in ICP or deterioration in neurologic status warrants an emergent CT scan of the head to identify a new mass lesion, most typically a delayed hematoma. A new hemorrhage after surgery should raise the suspicion of an underlying vascular injury or coagulopathy. In certain cases, typically young patients with nondominant hemisphere lesions, a decompressive craniectomy, and duroplasty may be considered in refractory increased intracranial pressure.

The development of hydrocephalus is another potential complication. In a patient with a ventriculostomy, the inability to wean over 7 to 14 days with persistent high CSF outflow at normal pressure is a good indication the patient will need CSF diversion. Hydrocephalus also may develop in a delayed fashion with a slowly deteriorating neurological exam. If the CT reveals ventriculomegaly, including an enlarged fourth ventricle with no focal mass effect, a lumbar puncture may be performed to record an opening pressure. The final timing for definitive CSF diversion is determined by the presence of other injuries, nutritional status, and infectious complications.

The presence of fever, elevated white cell count, and meningeal signs are concerns for postoperative meningitis. If a ventriculostomy is in place, CSF may be sent for laboratory inquiry. In addition to evaluating the ICP monitoring system, a thorough examination for a CSF fistula should be performed. Not all CSF leaks are present on admission. In a review of the VHIS, 72% of CSF leaks appear within the first two weeks of injury.[55]

In the initial evaluation and postoperative period, a coagulation panel should be evaluated, as PHI is a known etiology for coagulopathy. The brain parenchyma contains thromboplastin that can activate the extrinsic coagulation cascade. If high levels are released, the patient may develop a disseminated intravascular coagulopathy (DIC). Because the degree of the coagulopathy is related to the amount of thromboplastin released from injured tissue, the presence of DIC represents a large area of parechymal injury and portends a worse prognosis.[19,57]

As discussed above, the patient should remain on antiepileptic medication for seven days post injury for the prevention of early seizures. Antibiotics generally are used for a 7 to 14 day course for isolated PHI. A longer duration may be required based on systemic infection or other complicating factors.

Prognosis

In comparing outcomes with PHI patients and those with nonpenetrating traumatic brain injuries, PHI patients fare worse. They have an overall mortality of 88%, compared to 32.5% in nonpenetrating traumatic brain injury.[38,58] Typically, death occurs soon after the injury, with 70% occurring within the first 24 hours.[58] An accurate assessment of prognosis for each patient is essential to determine the appropriateness of treatment, especially in a military or other resource-constrained environment.

The *Guidelines to Penetrating Brain Injuries* evaluated the literature on five prognostic variables: age, epidemiology, systemic measures, neurological measures, and neuroimaging measures. An understanding of these variables and their outcome can help provide direction in the treatment of the patient and counseling family members on what can be expected.

In general, the older a patient is, the higher mortality they typically have. In the limited studies that evaluated age and prognosis, age greater than 50 years was associated with increased mortality. However, a majority of PHI patients are in their second to third decade.[58]

In the civilian population, gunshot wounds are the most common type of PHI, with a majority of these being suicide attempts. Suicide PHIs are associated with a higher mortality.[58] The question has been raised whether suicide outcomes are based on the injury pattern or the degree of resuscitation based on the belief of a worse outcome.[59] This pattern is different in military PHI, where fragmentation injuries instead of gunshot wounds, are found in those patients who survive transport to higher echelons of care. The high velocity associated with military bullet wounds typically causes a devastating intracranial wound. One series reported a mortality with this wound to be 82% higher than with fragmentation wounds.[14]

Given the velocity, and hence the amount of energy imparted by a projectile to achieve a perforating wound, it is not surprising that these injuries are associated with the highest mortality. While no statistically significant data exists, penetrating wounds tend to have a higher mortality than tangential.[58] Surprisingly, there does not tend to be a correlation between outcome and caliber of weapon. This is likely because the energy imparted to the tissue is also related to the velocity, which can be quite variable.[58]

From the patient's presentation and neurological status, several poor prognostic indicators can be determined. Systemic insults after a PHI can worsen the patient's outcome. Periods of hypotension, respiratory distress, and the presence of a coagulopathy are all associated with increased mortality.[58] From a neurologic perspective, the patient's GCS is one of the strongest predictors of mortality and outcome.[58] In civilian settings, most patients present with a GCS of 3 to 5. These patients have the highest rate of mortality and poor outcome. In military series, more patients present with GCS of 13 to 15, and thus have a better outcome. This reflects more fragment injuries, a more rigid field triage system, and a slower evacuation system. An abnormal pupillary exam is common after PHI and can result from orbital trauma, medications, cerebral herniation, or brainstem injury. Patient who present with unequal or fixed and dilated pupils have an increased mortality.[58] There is little data that exists on the prognostic value of ICP in PHI. What is available suggests that elevated ICP within the first 72 hours predicts higher mortality.[58]

As previously discussed, a CT scan is the diagnostic modality of choice. Three prognostic indicators can be determined from the patient's initial scan: projectile track, evidence of increased ICP, and the presence of hemorrhage or mass lesion. Projectile trajectories associated with increased mortality include bihemispheric lesions, multilobar lesions, and those that involve the ventricular system. One exception may be a bifrontal injury. Basilar cistern effacement on CT, indicative of elevated ICP, is associated with increased mortality. Midline shift alone, however, is not. The presence of large contusions and/or subarachnoid hemorrhage is associated with increased mortality. A stronger correlation, however, exists between increased mortality and the presence of intraventricular hemorrhage.[58]

Given these prognostic indicators, the provider must decide on who would benefit from surgery and aggressive management. Grahm and colleagues reported on 100 consecutive cases of gunshot wounds to the head in an attempt to answer this question.[18] No patient with a postresuscitation GCS of 3 to 5 and only 20% of those with GCS of 6 to 8 had a satisfactory outcome, defined as either good or moderately impaired on the Glasgow Outcome Scale. From their experience, they recommend that all patients with gunshot wounds to the head be resuscitated aggressively and transferred to a trauma center. Patients with a large, extraaxial hematoma, despite their GCS, should undergo surgical therapy. In those patients without a hematoma and a GCS of 3 to 5, no further treatment should be offered. In patients with a GCS score of 6 to 8 and transventricular or dominant hemisphere multilobar injuries in the absence of an extraaxial hematoma, further treatment should not be offered. A patient with a GCS of 6 to 8 without these findings on CT and all those with GCS of 9 to 15 should be offered aggressive therapy, as this is the population with the best chance at a satisfactory outcome.[18]

The management of the patient with ballistic trauma to the head requires aggressive resuscitation and accurate triage based on clinical and CT findings. When surgical intervention is required, strict attention must be paid to the principles of watertight dural closure and wound coverage after an adequate debridement of devitalized tissue and easily accessible fragments is completed. Aggressive intensive care unit management includes avoidance of hypotension, hypoxia, control of ICP and CPP, use of antibiotics and anticonvulsants, and vigilant monitoring for CSF fistulas and pseudoaneurysms. Unfortunately, this current era of terrorist threats mandates that all physicians should have a basic understanding of ballistic trauma to the head.

References

1. Berman JM, Butterworth JF, Prough DS. Neurological injuries. In: Zajtchuk R, Bellamy RF, eds. *Textbook of Military Medicine*. Vol. 1. Washington: Office of the Surgeon General; 1995:375–424.

2. Shaffrey ME, Polin RS, Phillips CD, Germanson T, Shaffrey CI, Jane JA. Classification of civilian craniocerebral gunshot wounds: A multivariate analysis predictive of mortality. *J Neurotrauma*. 1992;9(Suppl 1):S279–S285.
3. Cooper P. Gunshot wounds of the brain. In: Cooper P, ed. *Head Injury*. 2nd ed. Baltimore, MD: Williams and Wilkins; 1987:313–326.
4. Sosin D, Sacks J, Smith S. Head injury associated deaths in the United States from 1979–1986. *JAMA*. 1989;262L:2251–2255.
5. West CGH. A short history of the management of penetrating missile injuries of the head. *Surg Neurol*. 1981;16:145–149.
6. Schmidek, Sweet. Operative neurosurgical techniques. Missile injury to head chapter.
7. Cushing H. Notes on penetrating wounds of the brain. *Brit Med J*. February 1918;221–226.
8. Cushing H. A study of a series of wounds involving the brain and its enveloping structures. *Br J Surg*. 1918;5:558–684.
9. Tilney NL. The marrow of tragedy. *Surg Gynecol Obstet*. 1983:157:380–388.
10. Matson DD. *The Treatment of Acute Craniocerebral Injuries Due to Missiles*. Springfield, IL: Charles C Thomas; 1948.
11. War Surgery Supplement. *Br J Surg*. 1947;34(137).
12. Lewin W, Gibson MR. Missile head wounds in the Korean campaign: A survey of British casualties. *Br J Surg*. 1956;43:628–632.
13. Carey ME, Young HF, Mathis JL. The neurosurgical treatment of craniocerebral missile wounds in Vietnam. *Surg Gynecol Obstet*. 1972;135:386–390.
14. Brandvold B, Levi L, Feinsod M, George E. Penetrating craniocerebral injuries in the Israeli involvement in the Lebanese conflict, 1982–1985. *J Neurosurg*. 1990;72:15–21.
15. Ordog, GJ. Wound ballistics: Theory and practice. *Ann Emerg Med*. 1984; 13(12):1113–1122.
16. Barach E, Tomlanovich M, Nowak R. Ballistics: A pathophysiologic examination of the wounding mechanisms of firearm: part 1. *J Trauma*. 1986; 26(3):225–235.
17. Sykes LN, Champion HR, Fouty WJ. Dum-dums, hollow-points, and devastors: Techniques dsigned to increase wounding potential of bullets. *J Trauma*. 1988;28(5):618–623.
18. Grahm T, Williams F Jr, Harrington T, Spetzler R. Civilian gunshot wounds to the head: A prospective study. *Neurosurgery*. 1990;27:696–700.
19. Kauffman HH, Makela ME, Lee KF, Haid RW Jr, Gildenberg PL. Gunshot wounds to the head: A perspective. *Neurosurgery*. 1986;18:689–695.
20. Knightly JJ, Pullliam MW. Military head injuries. In: Narayan RK, Willberger JE, Povlishock JT, eds. *Neurotrauma*. New York: McGraw-Hill; 1996:891–902.
21. Kennedy FR, Gonzalez P, Beitler A, Sterling-Scott R, Fleming AW. Incidence of cervical spine injury in patients with gunshot wounds to the head. *South Med J*. 1994;87:621–623.
22. Trask T, Narayan RK. Civilian penetrating head injury. In: Narayan RK, Wilberger JE, Povlishock JT, eds. *Neurotrauma*. New York: McGraw-Hill, 1996:869–889.
23. Neuroimaging in the management of penetrating brain injury. *J Trauma*. 2001;51:S7–S11.

24. Aarabi B. Management of traumatic aneurysms caused by high-velocity missile head wounds. *Neurosurg Clin North Am*. 1995;6:775–797.
25. Haddad FS, Haddad GF, Taha J. Traumatic intracranial aneurysms caused by missiles: Their presentation and management. *Neurosurgery*. 1991;28:1–7.
26. Amirjamshidi A, Rahmat H, Abbassioun K. Traumatic aneurysms and arteriovenous fistulas of intracranial vessels associated with penetrating head injuries occuring during war: Principles and pitfalls in diagnosis and management. *J Neurosurg*. 1996;84:769–780.
27. Oliver C, Kabala J. Air gun pellet injury: the safety of MR imaging. *Clin Radiol*. 1997;52:299–300.
28. Smith AS, Hurst GC, Durek JL, Diaz PJ. MR of ballistic materials: Imaging artifacts and potential hazards. *Am J Neruoradiol*. 1991;12:567–572.
29. Teitelbaum GP, Yee CA, Van Horn DD, Kim HS, Colletti PM. Metallic ballistic fragments: MR imaging safety and artifacts. *Radiology*. 1990;175:855–859.
30. Crockard HA. Early intracranial pressure studies in gunshot wounds of the brain. *J Trauma*. 1975;15:339–347.
31. Lillard PL. Five year experience with penetrating craniocerebral gunshot wounds. *Surg Neurol*. 1978;9:79–83.
32. Nagib MG, Rockswold GL, Sherman RS, Lagaard MW. Civilian gunshot wounds to the brain: Prognosis and management. *Neurosurgery*. 1986;18:533–537.
33. Sarnaik AP, Kopec J, Moylan P, Alvarez D, Canady A. Role of aggressive intracranial pressure in management of pediatric craniocerebral gunshot wounds with unfavorable features. *J Trauma*. 1989;29:1424–1437.
34. Intracranial pressure monitoring in the management of penetrating brain injury. *J Trauma*. 2001;51:S12–S15.
35. Bullock R, Chesnut RM, Clifton G, Ghajar J, Marion DW, Narayan RK, Newell DW, Pitts LH, Rosner MJ, Wilberger JW. Guidelines for the management of severe head injury. *Eur J Ernerg Med*. 1996;3:109–127.
36. BTF Website.
37. Vascular complications of penetrating brain injury. *J Trauma*. 2001;51;S26–S28.
38. Aldrich EF, Eisnberg HM, Saydjari C, Foulkes MA, Jane JA, Marshall LF, Young H, Marmarou A. Predictors of mortality in severely head-injured patients with civilian gunshot wound: A report from the NIH Traumatic Coma Data Bank. *Surg Neurol*. 1992;38:418–423.
39. Levy ML, Rezai A, Masri LS, Litofsky SN, Giannotta SL, Apuzzo ML, Weiss MH. The significance of subarachnoid hemorrhage after penetrating craniocerebral injury: Correlations with angiography and outcome in civilian population. *Neurosurgery*. 1993;32:532–540.
40. Kapp JP, Gielchinsky I. Management of combat wounds of the dural venous sinuses. *Surgery*. 1972;71:913–917.
41. Aarabi B. Traumatic aneurysms of brain due to high velocity missile head wounds. *Neurosurgery*. 1988;22:1056–1063.
42. Jinkins JR, Dadsetan MR, Sener RN, Desai S, Williams RG. Value of acute-phase angiography in the detection of vascular injuries caused by gunshot wounds to the head: Analysis of 12 cases. *AJR Am J Roentgenol*. 1992; 159:365–368.
43. Caverness WF, Meirowsky AM, Rish BL, et al. The nature of posttraumatic epilepsy. *J Neurosurg*. 1979;50:545–553.

44. Salazar AM, Jabbari B, Vance SC, Grafman J, Amin D, Dillon JD. Epilepsy after penetrating head injury, I: Clinical correlates—a report of the Vietnam Head Injury Study. *Neurology*. 1985;35:1406–1414.
45. Weiss GH, Salazar AM, Vance SC, Grafman JH, Jabbian B. Predicting post-traumatic epilepsy in penetrating head injury patients. *Arch Neurol*. 1986;43: 771–773.
46. Antiseizure prophylaxis for penetrating brain injury. *J Trauma*. 2001;51:241–243.
47. Thoreby FP, Darlow HM. The mechanism of primary infection of bullet wounds. *Br J Surg*. 1967;54:359.
48. Wolf AW. Autosterilization in low-velocity bullets. *J Trauma*. 1978;18:63.
49. Taha JM, Saba MI, Brown JA. Missile injuries to the brain treated by simple wound closure: Results of a protocol during the Lebanese conflict. *Neurosurgery*. 1991;29:380–383.
50. Taha JM, Haddad FS, Brown JA. Intracranial infection after missile injuries to the brain: Report of 30 cases from the Lebanon conflict. *Neurosurgery*. 1991;29:864–868.
51. Surgical management of penetrating brain injury. *J Trauma*. 2001;51:S16–S25.
52. Suddaby L, Weir B, Forsyth C. The management of .22 caliber gunshot wounds of the brain: A review of 49 cases. *Can J Neurol Sci*. 1987;14:268–272.
53. Shoung HM, Sichez JP, Pertuiset B. The early prognosis of craniocerebral gunshot wounds in civilian practice as an aid to the choice of treatment. *Acta Neurochir (Wien)*. 1985;74:27–30.
54. Arendall REH, Meirowsky AM. Air sinus wounds: an analysis of 163 consecutive cases incurred in the Korean War, 1950–1952. *Neurosurgery*. 1983;13:377–380.
55. Kearney TJ, Bentt L, Grode M, Lee S, Hiatt JR, Shabot MM. Coagulopathy and catecholamines in severe head injury. *J Trauma*. 1992;32:608–612.
56. Part 2: Prognosis in penetrating brain injury [review]. *J Trauma*. August 2001;51(suppl 2):S44–S86.
57. Marshall LF, Maas AI, Marshall SB, Bricolo A, Fearnside M, Iannotti F, Klauber MR, Lagarrigue J, Lobato R, Persson L, Pickard JD, Piek J, Servadei F, Wellis GN, Morris GF, Means ED, Musch B. A muticenter trial on the efficacy of using tirilazad mesylatein cases of head injury. *J Neurosurg*. 1998;89:519–525.
58. Kaufman HH, Schwab K, Salazar AM. A national survery of neurosurgical care for penetrating head injury. *Surg Neurol*. 1991;36370–377.

16
Spinal Injury

Neil Buxton

Introduction

A spinal cord injury can be devastating to the victim. The management of spinal cord injury secondary to gunshot wounds or other ballistic injuries is still controversial. In the United States of America, a gunshot wound is the second most common cause of spinal cord injury. In one civilian series, up to 25% of all spinal cord injuries were secondary to gunshot wounds. This is a condition affecting mainly young people under 30 years of age, more than 90% of whom are males. Over a third will be under the influence of alcohol or drugs, and nearly half will be shot from behind. Over half of such injuries will present with complete paraplegia. By the nature of the inflicting injury, more than one quarter will have associated injuries. The majority of the gunshot wounds affect the thoracic spine, with the lumbar spine being second most common.

History

In World War I, only patients with incomplete injuries survived. Overall mortality rate was 71.8%, with urinary sepsis being the main cause of death. At this time there was also a 62.2% operative mortality rate. Complete injuries were only treated with wound debridement. Laminectomy was reserved for incomplete injuries that were experiencing further neurological deterioration.

In World War II, surgery was offered to all, but the mortality rate had been reduced to 11.4%. In the Korean War, operative mortality was only one percent. Improved casualty evacuation times seen in the Vietnam War did nothing to further improve neurological recovery.

Civilian series have been even less encouraging. Stabbings have been found no less devastating than gunshot wounds to the spine.

Pathophysiology

A complete spinal cord injury is one whereby there is no function below the level of the injury. Some spinal cord reflexes may return. A physiologically complete injury does not require complete transection of the spinal cord.

With modern high-velocity weapons, it is not necessary to hit the spinal cord directly to cause a spinal cord injury; hitting the bony components of the spine can cause microscopically detectable spinal cord injury up to 15 centimeters from the level of the primary injury. There is usually intramedullary hemorrhage and more rarely extradural or subdural haemorrhage, even with a direct cord injury.

Initial Management and Assessment

Each victim of such an injury should undergo a full normal resuscitation protocol with appropriate management of life-threatening injuries along Advanced Trauma Life Support/Battlefield Advanced Trauma Life Support (ATLS/BATLS) guidelines. In such an injury, it is important to remember that, until proven otherwise, hypotension is due to blood loss and not spinal cord shock.

Having resuscitated the patient, stabilized them, and treated the other life-threatening injuries, the patient is then ready to be assessed by the neurosurgeon, and, in times of conflict, this may take many hours to days to achieve. However, it generally is agreed that early assessment of the neurological status is deemed vital and ideally should be carried out within 24 hours of the injury, always after the resuscitation. This is important because the presenting neurological and autonomic status have considerable implications for the prognosis. Therefore, the first medical attendant who sees the casualty after resuscitation needs to fully examine them from a neurological point of view, and, of course, this should be recorded with care. This is of paramount importance for prognostication, as 90% of presenting neurological deficits are permanent.

The neurological examination needs to record the sensory status, strength of muscle groups, tone in the limbs, reflexes, and sphincter status.

Simple measures such as nasogastric tube, bladder catheterization, and nursing management to prevent decubitus ulcers and deep venous thrombosis are vital for the overall care of such an injured patient. For the medical attendant, the neurological examination should be repeated periodically in order to document recovery and/or deterioration.

Spinal Shock

This results in flaccid paralysis distal to the injury. The reflexes and tone return to become hyperactive by six to twelve weeks. The more rapid the return of the reflexes, the poorer the prognosis for neurological recovery in patients with complete injuries.

Neurogenic shock with bradycardia, hypotension, and hypothermia is due to autonomic paralysis and is managed with fluid replacement and active warming. Atropine may even be required, especially if the pulse rate drops below 40 beats per minute.

Investigations

Plain X-ray

This will demonstrate the bony anatomy and the presence and position of any retained foreign bodies.

Computed Tomography (CT)

Computed tomography provides good bony detail, but in the presence of metal fragments will have significant artifact. Computed tomography is excellent for three-dimensional reconstruction of the bony anatomy, but in the face of a fragment injury, the radiological artifact may be too great to make the pictures meaningful.

Magnetic Resonance Imaging (MRI)

Magnetic resonance imaging is extremely useful for the soft tissues, in particular spinal cord anatomy. This is a particularly important modality, as early realization that complete transection of the cord has occurred is extremely useful for prognostication. The problem with MRI scanning is that there is a theoretical risk of the magnetic field causing foreign body movement, as well as artifact, even though there are records of the MRI being used safely in patients with fragmentation injuries. Magnetic resonance imaging is essential to investigate delayed deterioration (see chapter 23).

Myelography

This may be necessary where metal fragments and metal artifact prevent the use of CT or MRI.

Angiography

With respect to penetrating neck injuries, it is recommended that cervical angiography be undertaken before any surgical exploration. Late deterioration in some penetrating spinal cord injuries may need spinal angiography as the deterioration may be due to the development of an arteriovenous fistula.

Instability

Battlefield gunshot wounds to the neck causing neurological deficit have a high fatality rate. In those surviving, it generally is accepted that the neck injury is not unstable.

It is important that the mechanism of injury be elicited during the history as, especially during the transition to war phase, there are many motor-vehicle accidents and those injured in them would be expected to have potentially unstable spinal injuries. It is essential to treat any person so injured who has reduced or impaired levels of consciousness due to intoxication or the injury as having a spinal injury until positively proven otherwise. In such an instance, where practical, full ATLS-type management should be initiated. In a mass casualty situation, or where the tactical situation is unsafe, the expediency of life-saving treatment may necessitate reduced diligence with respect to spinal immobilization.

It is important to remember that some penetrating injuries, if treated as unstable, may actually be to the detriment of the casualty as, for example, putting on a cervical collar for a penetrating neck injury has in some instances been found to mask significant deteriorations. Indeed, in these casualties, subsequent investigation have found that the spinal injury was, in fact, not unstable after all. Quite clearly, if an unstable injury is missed, the consequences for the casualty are potentially devastating; this is why the mechanism of injury is important in the history. In fact, in a purely penetrating injury of the neck, it is recommended that a supportive collar not be used at all (see Chapter 7 and Chapter 11).

Operation?

There is considerable controversy regarding whether or not to decompress the spinal cord or theca. The initial neurological status remains the most important factor for overall expected outcomes. Initial military experience from the major wars of the twentieth century suggested that highly aggressive surgical therapy should be the approach; however, in recent years, with increasing civilian experience, a more conservative approach has been adopted. With regard to incomplete spinal cord injuries alone, it has been found that removal of the penetrating fragment, if impinging upon the spinal cord, does improve overall motor function in some reported series. In some published studies where surgery was undertaken in nearly all cases, there have been some instances where the neurological status has actually been made worse by surgery.

For foreign bodies present in or around the cauda equina, many studies have supported the removal of the foreign body, but this can be a technical challenge at operation because the foreign bodies can move. Having the patient positioned slightly head up and using fluoroscopy to aid identification of the foreign body position is recommended.

There is considerable agreement that where there is cerebrospinal fluid leakage, progressive neurological deficit, or spinal instability, surgery should be undertaken, although surgery for instability may be controversial to some authorities. In war, if casualty evacuation is needed, the spinal injury casualty will need to be made stable by surgical fixation so transfer can be made more easily and safely. The removal of the foreign body to prevent later sepsis remains controversial, as many studies have indicated that foreign body retention does not actually increase the risks. In cases were the penetrating fragment traverses the abdominal cavity, and therefore possibly the bowels, prior to entering the spinal canal, the life-threatening injuries are recommended to be dealt with first, followed by thorough wash out from anteriorly with a prolonged high-dose usage of antibiotics. It is hardly surprising that penetration of the colon is associated with the highest risks of infection, although some studies have suggested that transoral is higher still. Retained foreign bodies can cause problems in other areas, in particularly plumbism (lead poisoning), but this is an infrequent complication of lead fragments. It has been recognized that lead fragments in joint spaces or disc spaces should be removed, as toxicity is likely. Of more concern are copper-jacketed projectiles, as these are particularly toxic and it is recommended that, whatever the situation, any copper-jacketed projectile be removed at surgery as soon as possible.

Role of Antibiotics and Other Drugs

It is recommended that high-dose broad-spectrum antibiotics be administered intravenously for seven to ten days, especially if there is a retained foreign body or if the projectile has traversed a hollow viscous.

Antacids are recommended to minimize the risk of stress ulceration.

Methylprednisolone has been advocated in the management of blunt spinal cord injury, but a number of studies have not found methylprednisolone to be of any clinical benefit in gunshot-wound–induced spinal cord injury. Indeed, in one series, increased rate of complications was found and attributed to the use of steroids. There is currently ongoing controversy regarding the use of steroids, even in the previously advocated blunt spinal cord injury; therefore, at this moment in time, the use of steroids in penetrating spinal cord injury cannot be recommended.

General Nursing Care/Postoperative Care

The management of a spinally injured patient, whether it be due to penetrating injury or blunt, are virtually identical from the nursing and postoperative management aspects. The casualty needs a nasogastric tube, bladder management, aseptic management of catheters, careful pressure area care, and early physiotherapy and rehabilitation. Careful fluid management and catheter management needs to be maintained with avoidance of urinary tract infections and catheter blockage in the long-term care. With increasing sophistication in the management, these patients are living significant lengths of time and represent a considerable nursing challenge.

Care of such a casualty needs to be addressed at identifying missed injuries, such as peripheral fractures, but with emphasis on ruling out a second spinal injury. Other severe injuries, such as abdominal trauma and head injury, should have been recognized in the primary or secondary survey and dealt with accordingly. A low threshold for investigating for other injuries should be maintained throughout the care of such a patient.

Other important considerations include hypovolemia; ruling out active bleeding may be difficult, but is vital. Once a sinister cause is excluded, then fluid resuscitation to maintain a blood pressure between 80 and 100 millimeter Hg systolic is appropriate. Adequate urine output is the best marker.

Hypothermia due to sympathetic failure causing peripheral vasodilatation should be actively managed.

Bradycardia due to decreased sympathetic drive can be so severe as to lead to asystolic arrest. Atropine may be necessary. Hypoxia and tracheal toilet can be enough to exacerbate the bradycardia to produce arrest.

Autonomic dysreflexia (mass reflex) can occur in over 50% of those with injuries higher than T6. There is an uncontrolled sympathetic reflex to usually only mildly noxious stimuli such as a full bladder or bowel. There is flushing, headache, sweating, anxiety, and hypertension with bradycardia. Removal of the stimulus and elevation of the head of the bed are needed. Failure to resolve the hypertension may require drug therapy such as hydralazine. Untreated, this hypertension can be fatal. Therefore, prevention by nursing diligence is necessary.

Prophylaxis for DVT and PE is essential.

Care to prevent chest problems due to reduced chest excursions, poor cough reflex, etc., is important. Chest infections are common. Breathing control is impaired.

There may be ileus, constipation, gastric reflux, and gastric stress ulcers. All need appropriate management and, in the case of bowel motility and ulcers, prophylaxis. Nutritional advice and support is required early to minimize the effects of posttraumatic catabolism.

Improved urological care has reduced the long-term death rate. Improved catheter technology and the introduction of intermittent self-catheterization have brought about significant improvements. There should be a low threshold for treating urinary tract infections and periodic renal tract ultrasound to assess bladder capacity and any ureteric reflux.

Pressure area care and prevention of ulcers can make the difference between a relatively normal life and a prolonged hospital stay. The worst cases end up with osteomyelitis and major plastic and reconstructive surgery.

Pain can be a long-term problem. It may be due to spasm, or it can be neurogenic or analogous to phantom limb pain. Multidisciplinary pain team management is recommended.

Delayed deterioration should always prompt urgent investigation for posttraumatic syringomyelia, arachnoid adhesions, etc. Appropriate therapy is indicated to preserve function above the original level of injury. Therefore, any complaint of neurological change no matter how bizarre or minor must be taken seriously, and ideally, periodic complete physical examination of the patient is needed.

Early physiotherapy and transfer to a dedicated spinal injury facility is essential for their optimal rehabilitation. This will include psychosocial, sexual, vocational, educational, and recreational rehabilitation in a multi-disciplinary setting.

Evacuation/Transfer

The patients having such an injury in an austere military environment will need careful and well-managed nursing care in order to facilitate their safe evacuation and transfer. As previously mentioned, they should be transferred to a dedicated spinal unit at the earliest opportunity for appropriate rehabilitation and management. It is reasonable to suggest that in the presence of a spinal fracture that an operative fixation will facilitate the early and easier transfer of such an injured patient, as less emphasis would need to be placed on prevention of further injury in the presence of an unstable spine.

Summary

The management of penetrating spinal cord injuries due to gunshot wounds or fragment injuries is, in the initial phase, as for any ATLS/BATLS protocol. In the battlefield, the chances of the injury being unstable in survivors due to a penetrating injury is very small. It is important to recognize the mechanism of injury and manage the patient accordingly. For example, a casualty involved in a motor-vehicle accident will be at higher risk of an unstable spinal injury than one who has just been shot by a 5.56-millimeter round. Surviving casualties who have such penetrating neck injuries are extremely unlikely to have an unstable neck, and therefore the application of a stabilizing collar may in fact be detrimental to their care. As with the majority of spinal cord injuries and spinal injuries in general, other life-threatening injuries always take priority. North Atlantic Treaty Organization (NATO) guidelines are specific regarding the management of spinal injuries; they state that complete injuries do not require surgery, surgery being indicated for progressive neurological deficit and spinal instability. To this recommendation should be added that surgery should be applied in the presence of CSF leaks, delayed infections or foreign body reactions, and/or the presence of copper-jacketed rounds or lead foreign bodies in a joint or disc space. In addition, if there is radicular pain where the foreign body can clearly be demonstrated to be compromising a root on appropriate imaging, then this also should be removed. Decompressive laminectomy and foreign body removal for the sake of it is no longer justified. The use of steroids is not recommended at this time. High-dose antibiotics for at least seven to ten days are indicated.

Overall, the most important factor for a prognosis is the presenting neurological status. In 90% of casualties, the presenting neurological deficit is permanent. However, the mortality from a spinal cord injury alone is low, and with the best long-term care available, life expectancy can be virtually normal and that life can be fruitful and useful to society.

Further Reading

Tator CH, Benzel EC, eds. *Contemporary Management of Spinal Cord Injury: From Impact to Rehabilitation*. Park Ridge, IL: AANS; 2000.

17
Limb Injuries

Jonathan C. Clasper

Introduction

Limb wounds are the most common injuries seen during military conflict, accounting for up to 70% of all wounds, with the lower limb most commonly involved. In general, the majority of penetrating injuries are due to fragments, although in some conflicts, such as in recent years in Northern Ireland, bullet wounds predominate. The wounds can range in severity from superficial low-energy wounds caused by shrapnel, some of which can be managed conservatively, to high-energy bullet wounds when as many as half of the injuries are associated with a fracture, and complex surgical reconstruction may be required.

Although some limb injuries, particularly femoral fractures or vascular trauma, can be life threatening, the majority are not and treatment can be delayed. However, all limb injuries can be associated with considerable morbidity, and therefore adequate early assessment and appropriate treatment is necessary. This applies not only to military injuries, but also to civilian ballistic trauma that is being seen increasingly worldwide.

It is important to realize that the true assessment of most wounds can only be made at the time of surgery and cannot be made on external appearances, particularly if there are no exit wounds. Figure 17-1 shows a high-energy wound to the upper arm from several bullets; the skin wounds are small, but despite the external appearance, an extensive soft tissue and bony wound is present (Figure 17-2) and the outcome was relatively poor. Figure 17-3 illustrates an apparently more severe wound, and yet there is a simple fracture (Figure 17-4), relatively minimal soft tissue damage, and early internal fixation and flap coverage was possible (Figure 17-5) with a good functional outcome.

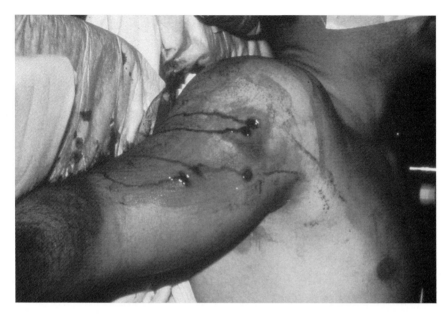

FIGURE 17-1. Multiple gunshot wounds to the upper arm; despite the small wounds, extensive soft tissue and bony damage is present.

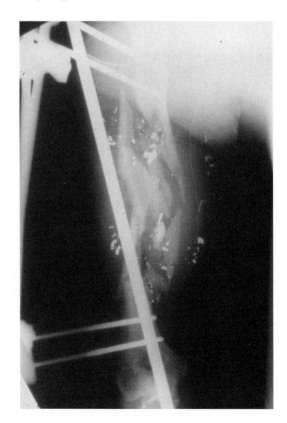

FIGURE 17-2. Radiograph of the humerus of Figure 17-1; extensive fracture has been stabilized by external fixation.

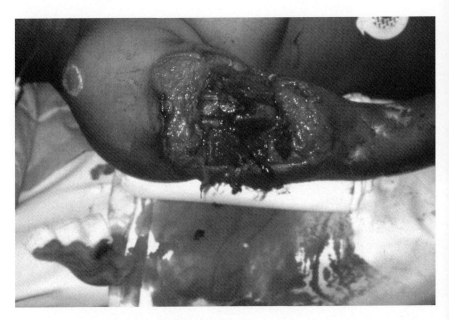

FIGURE 17-3. Shotgun wound to the upper arm; despite the appearances, relatively little soft tissue or bony damage is present.

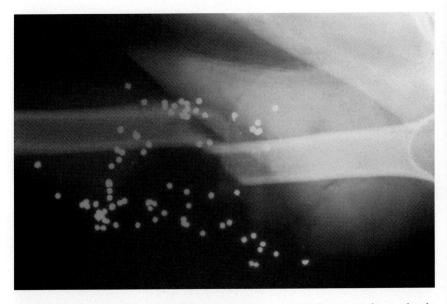

FIGURE 17-4. Radiograph of the humerus of Figure 17-3 demonstrating a simple complete fracture.

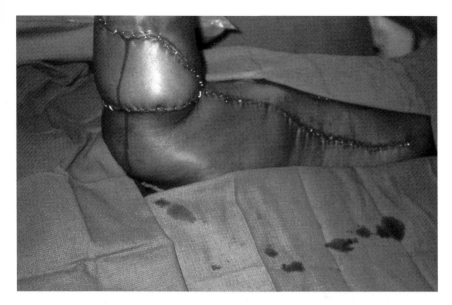

FIGURE 17-5. Patient shown in Figure 17-3 (upper arm at top abducted away from the side) showing early closure using a local (latisimus dorsi) flap.

Differences Between Military and Civilian Injuries

As well as the extensive soft tissue damage and the multifragmentary nature of high-energy ballistic fractures, the morbidity is also due to the highly contaminated nature of some (particularly military) wounds. Although ballistic injuries are being seen increasingly in the civilian environment, these injuries usually differ considerably from military injuries. These differences include:

– Military wounds are more heavily contaminated. Reports from the Second World War, Korea, and Vietnam have documented that military wounds are more heavily contaminated than civilian wounds, with three to four different species of bacteria isolated from most military wounds, and up to six different species in some reports. This compares to only one species from most civilian wounds, even when the wounds have been caused by gunshots. The species of aerobic bacteria appear to be very similar, but anaerobic bacteria contaminate most military wounds and are rarely isolated from acute civilian wounds.[1]

The only civilian equivalents of military wounds are those injuries occurring in agricultural or sewage settings.

- Delays in evacuation, which averaged 10 hours between wounding and starting appropriate care during the 1991 Gulf War. Wounds can be considered *contaminated* for up to six hours; after this the bacteria are actively dividing and have spread via the lymphatic system. Wounds older than six hours should be considered *infected* rather than contaminated.
- Military wounds are more likely to be associated with penetrating trauma to the abdomen and torso, which may be associated with the *spillage of abdominal contents*. This is due to the multiple penetrating wounds seen during conflict. Civilian wounds, in contrast, are associated with far fewer wounds. Abdominal injuries may result in further contamination with Gram negative pathogenic bacteria.
- Military wounds will frequently be treated in less-than-ideal circumstances, with *limited resources* and *possible mass casualties*. This may impose further delays on the initiation of treatment.

This means that although the principles in the management of military and civilian ballistic injuries are the same, in general, military wounds require more radical local surgery in an attempt to reduce the infection rate.

Management

Overview

The principles of treatment for ballistic injuries remain the same as any trauma, with the initial aim being to identify and treat any life-threatening injuries. Unless there is an obvious source of major hemorrhage, limb wounds will not be dealt with until the secondary survey, after the patient has been stabilized.

The principles of wound care are also similar to the civilian environment:

- surgical debridement and adequate lavage,
- stabilization of the limb, and
- use of appropriate antibiotics.

Of these, adequate surgery is by far the most important factor. Antibiotics, although an important factor, are secondary to early surgery and should not be considered as an alternative form of treatment.

Resuscitation

The priorities in the management of any casualty remain the ABCs (see Chapter 7 and Chapter 8).

- The airway must be secured (with cervical spine control if required, see Chapters 7, 11 and 16).
- Adequate breathing confirmed, with the application of dressings and chest drains as appropriate.
- External bleeding should be stopped, usually by compressive dressings, and intravenous fluids started as necessary.

The majority of patients with limb injuries, however, will not have major life-threatening injuries, will usually be conscious, and some may even be able to walk. All wounds should be covered with a sterile dressing, appropriate antibiotics should be commenced, and tetanus prophylaxis considered. Although heavily contaminated wounds can be lavaged, the majority of wounds should be left until the patient has been anesthetized.

If clinically there is suspicion of a fracture, the limb should be reduced and immobilized as appropriate. The diagnosis of a fracture will often be straightforward, as the limb will be flail at the site of the wound. Incomplete fractures can occur (see below).

Surgical Treatment

The aim of local surgery is to reduce the risk of infection, one of the most important factors in the morbidity after ballistic injuries. All military bullet wounds must be formally explored to reduce the infection risk, although civilian trauma centers have reported the successful nonoperative management of bullet wounds. These, however, were low-energy wounds, evacuated rapidly to a hospital, and not associated with the factors discussed above.

When small shrapnel wounds, particularly multiple wounds, are present, not all need debridement. If wounds are small, there is no evidence of fracture or joint penetration, and they appear to be superficial and low energy, then a conservative approach can be adopted provided regular review is possible (see also Chapter 9).

Surgical Technique

The principle of debridement is to remove all foreign and nonviable tissue.[2]

Debridement starts with the skin, and often excision of the skin margins is all that is required; degloving injuries may require more extensive debridement of skin. Although minimal excision is required, the wound should be extended to allow its full extent to be visualized. For high-energy wounds, considerable extension may be required. This should be in the long axis of the limb, with the exception of the flexor surface of a joint, when oblique incisions should be used.

Subcutaneous fat should be excised, but additional areas of degloving must not be created by over-generous debridement.

The deep fascia should be incised along the complete length of the wound, including any extensions. Fasciotomies with complete longitudinal division of the deep fascia along the full length of the compartment should be carried out in most high-energy wounds.

Adequate debridement of muscle is essential, and often a large amount of necrotic muscle may have to be excised. The aim is to remove all non-viable tissue, with the aim of leaving only pink, healthy-looking contractile muscle.

Lack of capillary bleeding or contractility, color, and consistency (the 4 Cs) are guides, but experience is the best way of judging viability of muscle. Debridement of muscle may result in considerable bleeding from the wound, and both the surgeon and anesthetist should be prepared for this.

Nerves and patent blood vessels should be left, as can tendons in continuity with muscles. Often, the tendons may become desiccated and may have to be excised at a later date. Divided nerve ends should be marked with a nonabsorbable monofilament suture.

Difficulties often can occur in the debridement of bone, particularly the fate of the many small fragments. Bone fragments without any soft tissue attachments are avascular and should be removed. Often, periosteal and other soft tissue attachments are present and the viability of the fragment can be difficult to determine. Experience is probably the most important factor in deciding the viability of a bone fragment or muscle. Experimental work has suggested that there is the limited spread of contamination beyond the fracture site and, therefore, exposure of intact bone beyond the fracture site is not necessary. The fracture site itself must be well visualized and washed out (Figure 17-6).

All wounds should be washed with copious amounts of fluid. It has been recommended that nine liters be used for open fractures. In a military environment, it may impossible to use this quantity of sterile fluids, but potable water can be used with a final washout of one liter of sterile saline. With high-energy transfer wounds, contamination can be spread along tissue planes, and these should be thoroughly irrigated.

Amputation

Primary amputation may be required as part of the initial debridement. Although the decision may be easy with a limb that is hanging off and obviously nonviable, the viability of less-severe injuries can be difficult to determine. The following criteria can be used in deciding to amputate:

– The presence of a large bony defect.
– Extensive skin wounds that will require flap coverage.

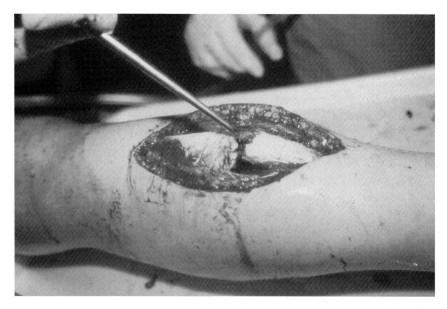

FIGURE 17-6. Open fracture after debridement, with all dead and foreign material excised and the fracture site fully exposed.

- Soft tissue injury (including vein injury) that will impair function.
- Vascular injury that requires repair.
- Neurological injury, particularly involving the hand or sole of the foot.

Although scoring systems have been developed for civilian limb injuries, there is still no reliable predictor of the need for amputation. Even in the military environment, a second opinion should be obtained, if possible, before amputation. If the viability of the limb cannot be determined initially, it may be reassessed after 48 hours. However, with military casualties, a return to the operating theater cannot be guaranteed, as problems with evacuation or mass-casualty situations may occur. The decision to perform bilateral or upper limb amputations will often be delayed, but infection may threaten the life of the casualty and this must be considered.

Closure of the Wound

Delayed primary closure of ballistic wounds is the rule. Wounds are left open to allow for swelling and to prevent raised tissue pressures, which will impair microcirculation and lead to further tissue death, predisposing to infection. Although certain injuries, such as wounds to the face or genitals may need to be closed primarily, this should be the exception. High-energy transfer wounds, with comminution of the bone, should never be closed primarily and will often require plastic surgical techniques several days after the initial debridement (Figure 17-5). Delayed primary closure can be carried out between two and fourteen days after initial surgery depending on the nature of the wound, evacuation of the casualty, and available resources and casualty numbers. Heavily contaminated wounds and limbs that may require amputation can be reassessed at 48 hours, but for most wounds, four to five days is the optimum period until the wound is closed.

Low-energy injuries are associated with small wounds and require minimal debridement. Often they can be left to close by secondary intention, but should not be closed primarily.

Exposed joint surfaces should be covered at the initial operation to reduce the risk of infection. Ideally this should be achieved by closure of the joint capsule, but in cases of tissue loss, part of the skin wound can be closed. Although the wound has been sutured, the patient should still be returned to the operating theater after several days for a further inspection and washout. Exposed bone or tendon does not have to be covered at the initial operation, but consideration should be given to early closure of these wounds to prevent desiccation. Bone or tendon that is left exposed for long periods usually will require further debridement despite appearing viable at initial surgery.

Wounds can be dressed with plain gauze, which can be fluffed up, but the wound should not be packed. The purpose of the dressing is to allow absorption of fluid and not to hold the wound open. Packing will increase wound pressure, leading to further tissue death.

Following debridement, antiseptic-soaked dressings should not be used. If debridement has been adequate, antiseptics are unnecessary and potentially toxic, particularly to bone cells. Bandages and tape can be used to secure the dressing but must not be allowed to encircle and constrict the limb.

Use of Tourniquets

For wounds of the forearm, hands, and feet, a pneumatic tourniquet should be used if possible (Figure 17-7). Home-made or nonpneumatic devices should not be used due to the inability to control the pressure and possible local tissue damage. A pressure of approximately 250 to 300 millimeters Hg should be used and the tourniquet should not be inflated for longer than 90 minutes.

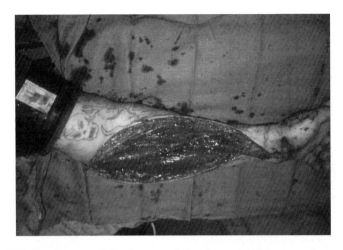

FIGURE 17-7. Fasciotomy of the forearm following a gunshot wound; a tourniquet has been used and the wound continued into the palm to include the carpal ligament.

Extent of Bony Injury[3]

Bone is less elastic than skin and muscle. This rigidity produces a greater resistance and results in greater energy transfer, and commonly bone fracture is a sequel to ballistic injury. In addition to the soft tissue injury, instability of the limb may occur, requiring stabilization of the fracture site.

Fractures can be divided into complete or incomplete, depending on whether some continuity of the bone is maintained.

Complete fractures can be further divided into:

– Simple: when only two main fragments are present (Figure 17-8).
– Comminuted: when multiple fragments are present (Figure 17-9).

Incomplete fractures can also be subdivided into:[4]

– Drill-hole type: when a channel is created through the bone (Figure 17-10).
– Divot or chip type: when part of the cortex is removed, but no channel exists (Figure 17-11).

High-energy weapons such as military or hunting rifles usually result in complete fractures, which are often comminuted (multifragmentary). Low-energy weapons, such as handguns, often result in incomplete fractures and even when complete, are not usually multifragmentary. High-energy wounds are also more likely to have greater contamination, and it is these unstable, highly contaminated injuries that have to be managed appropriately.

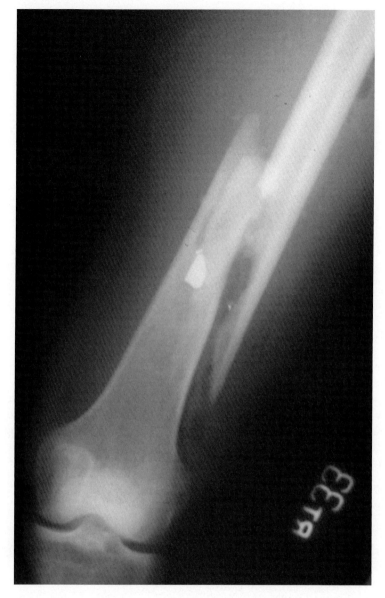

FIGURE 17-8. Complete simple fracture.

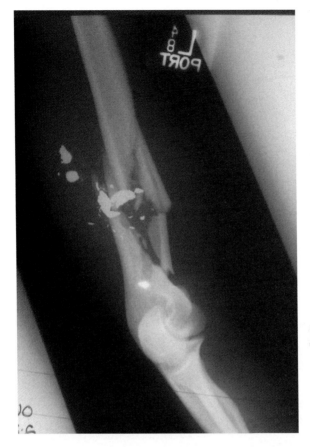

FIGURE 17-9. Complete multifragmentary fracture.

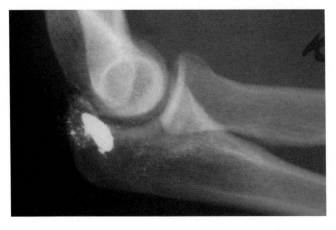

FIGURE 17-10. Incomplete drill-hole fracture of the elbow; the channel and bullet communicated with the joint and had to be removed.

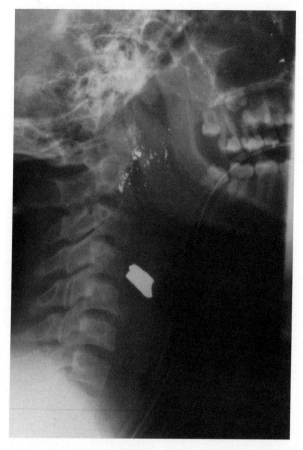

FIGURE 17-11. Incomplete divot fracture; the bullet "bounced off" the upper cervical vertebrae and passed further down the neck. No major structure was damaged and the patient survived.

Stabilization of the Fracture

The majority of fractures and all extensive soft tissue wounds should be splinted. Stabilization of fractures provides pain relief and helps to prevent further bone and soft tissue injury. Stabilization, with the fracture reduced, allows functional use of the limb, and this is of particular concern during war, as it may allow casualties to help to care for themselves. Despite debates on the pros and cons of the various methods of splinting, adequate local surgery is more important than the method of stabilization.

Plaster

Plaster was originally developed for use on the battlefield and remains the best method of splinting limb injuries. Little additional equipment is required, and personnel can be readily trained in its use. Although plaster is often considered inadequate for extensive wounds, the technique of encasing the wound in plaster and allowing the wound to heal on its own was used extensively during the Spanish Civil War, with a good outcome reported. In addition, plaster can be combined with other external splints and has been used to facilitate evacuation of casualties with fractures of the femur (see below).

Plaster backslabs should be used, and these can be supplemented with lateral slabs when used in the lower limb, particularly with the knee and ankle joints. In the acute situation, or after initial debridement, plaster must not be allowed to encircle the limb. If cylinders are used, they must be split down to skin along their complete length. Tight dressings are one of the most common causes of severe postoperative pain, and this must be avoided, particularly as patients may undergo prolonged evacuation with limited medical care available.

The disadvantages of plaster are its inability to control movement at the fracture site, and shortening and malunion are common with multifragmentary fractures. This would be a particular problem with high-energy wounds, but plaster is certainly suitable for low-energy wounds. Difficulty of access to the wounds can also be a problem with the use of plaster.

Other External Splints

The Thomas splint was specifically designed for the evacuation of patients with ballistic fractures of the femur during the First World War. With the increased use of intramedullary nailing of civilian femoral fractures, its use has diminished. It is a useful method of stabilizing fractures in the military environment, either alone or in combination with plaster, and can be used in the definitive management of military fractures. The disadvantages of the Thomas splint are related to the prolonged immobilization necessary and the difficulty with access to wounds.

Other splints are available, including malleable wire and inflatable devices, but their main role is the short-term stabilization of fractures treated in civilian hospitals.

Traction

Before the advances in both internal and external fixation, traction was used widely to control fractures that were difficult to manage in plaster, particularly unstable or open fractures. It still has a place in the management of fractures when limited resources are available and has been used extensively by the Red Cross. It is less than ideal when rapid, prolonged, or repeated evacuation is necessary. To obtain good results, experience in the use of traction and regular adjustments may be required, and this may be difficult to achieve in the military environment. It does have potential in both the initial and the definitive treatment of ballistic fractures.

Internal Fixation

Plates

The advantages of internal fixation with plates and/or screws are the accurate reduction and rigid fixation that can be achieved. However, internal fixation of ballistic fractures can be technically demanding and has been associated with a high infection rate. Delayed internal fixation has been shown to have a lower complication rate than acute plating. Despite this, the complication rate of both infection and delayed healing is still high, and with the other advances that have been made, internal fixation probably has little place in the management of most ballistic fractures, especially of the lower limb. Plate fixation of upper-limb fractures has been used for civilian injuries and is particularly suitable when the fracture is near a joint (Figure 17-12).

Intramedullary Fixation

Intramedullary (IM) fixation with a nail is currently considered the method of choice for the stabilization of open tibial and femoral fractures in the civilian environment. The advantages of IM nailing are the high rates of healing for both wound and fracture. No additional splints are necessary, and this allows full access to the wound for inspection, dressings, or plastic surgical procedures.

Its main disadvantage is that the operation is technically very demanding. It requires even more equipment than plating, including image intensification, making it relatively unsuitable for use in most military facilities.

In a report from the Vietnam War, the results of open fractures that required a vascular repair were discussed[5] and the method of stabilization of the fracture analyzed. It was reported that when IM nailing was used, 50% of the nails required removal for complications directly related to the implant. The most common complication was infection, and the authors concluded that, in the military environment, external splints with the use of transfixion pins was a safer option for the stabilization of fractures associated with vascular injuries. The possible reasons for the high infection rate are discussed above. In the civilian environment, particularly in the United States, IM nailing is used extensively in the treatment of ballistic long bone fractures (Figure 17-13), but these are low-energy, minimally contaminated fractures that are usually treated within six hours of wounding.

FIGURE 17-12. Ballistic fracture of the humerus (as shown in Figure 17-9) stabilized by internal fixation with a plate; the fragments of the bullet did not need to be removed.

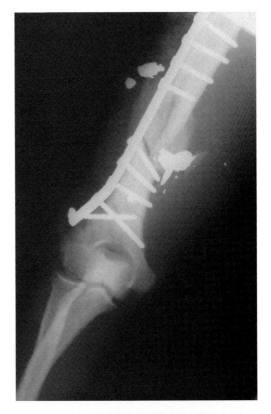

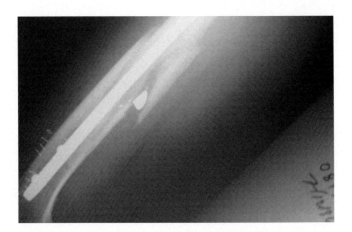

FIGURE 17-13. Ballistic fracture of the femur (as shown in Figure 17-8) stabilized by internal fixation with an IM nail; the fragments of the bullet did not need to be removed.

External Fixation

External fixation (Figure 17-14), together with plaster, is one of the main methods of stabilizing military ballistic fractures. Indications for external fixation rather than plaster include:

– extensive bone loss,
– large soft tissue wounds,
– vascular injuries that require repair,
– fractures in association with burns,
– multiple injuries,
– facilitating casualty evacuation.

External fixators often are considered easy to apply, but for ballistic injuries, they may be technically difficult to apply well due to the multifragmentary nature of many of the fractures; consequently, they will be associated with a high complication rate.

Technique of External Fixation

If possible, pins should be inserted into the subcutaneous surface of a bone. Although the pins can be inserted through "stab" incisions, these should be at least one centimeter in length. One of the complications of external fixation is damage to adjacent structures, and larger incisions should be used,

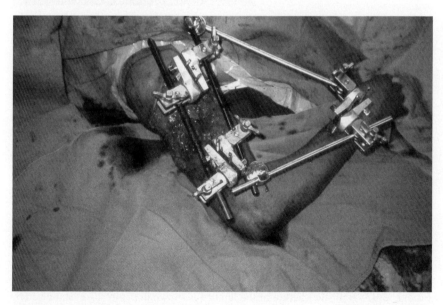

Figure 17-14. Ballistic fracture of the elbow stabilized by a bridging external fixation.

if necessary, to ensure safe insertion of pins. Open insertion should be used for distal humeral and distal radial pins.

Bicortical pin placement, where the pin passes through the medullary canal before penetrating the far cortex, must be ensured. With many fixators, predrilling is essential; with the British military pattern fixators, the pins have been designed to be self-drilling and self-tapping.

Ideally, all pins should be connected to the same bar. This can be achieved by inserting the most proximal and distal pins first. These are connected to a single bar and the fracture reduced as accurately as possible. Further pins can then be inserted by connecting pin-to-bar connectors to the bar and using these as guides for further pin insertion. In most circumstances, a second bar should also be used to increase the stability of the frame. Following fracture reduction, the skin wounds should again be checked, and any tenting of the skin released.

Specific Injuries

Upper Limb

Upper Arm

This has two compartments, the flexor, which contains the biceps and related muscles, and the extensor, which contains the triceps. Both can be decompressed by longitudinal incisions, which may be possible through the wound.

Extensive soft tissue wounds and all fractures of the humerus must be splinted, usually with the elbow at 90 degrees. Plaster is ideal, but simple splints, particularly when worn under the clothes, are also very effective. Following debridement, plaster should be used for the majority of fractures, avoiding external fixation unless there are specific indications.

If external fixation is considered necessary:

– Pins should not be inserted into the proximal humerus; there is a poor hold and significant risk of neurovascular damage.
– In the shaft they should be inserted through the lateral aspect of the bone, with particular care to avoid the anteromedial neurovascular bundle.
– Distal pins should also be inserted laterally, but under direct vision, through an open incision to avoid the radial nerve.

For distal fractures or severe soft tissue injuries around the elbow joint, a bridging fixator, with pins inserted into the distal humerus and ulna shaft, should be considered (Figure 17-14). With low-energy wounds, particularly in the civilian environment, internal fixation with plates (Figure 17-12) or even an IM nail may be considered.

If the initial treatment is with external fixation, later conversion to internal fixation may be considered, although continuing with plaster or external fixation may be appropriate. Early bone grafting should be considered for fractures with bone loss.

Forearm

Surgical debridement of the forearm should be carried out with care due to the close proximity of neurovascular structures, but excision of all non-viable tissue must be carried out.

Although the forearm also has a flexor and extensor compartment, release of individual muscles may be required at the time of fasciotomy.

If fasciotomy is required, consideration should also be given to releasing the carpal tunnel.

Both soft tissue and bony injuries can be splinted with plaster, which should include the wrist and, for proximal injuries, the elbow.

Definitive stabilization with plates may be considered for civilian injuries or as a secondary procedure at a base hospital for military injuries. External fixation will rarely be required in the civilian environment due to the availability and safety of internal fixation techniques. Even in the military environment, it will seldom be used, as vascular injuries in the forearm are unlikely to be repaired at a forward surgical facility, and for severe soft tissue and bony injuries, primary amputation may be required.

If required, pins should be inserted through the subcutaneous border of the ulna, and only the distal radius should be considered for pin placement, and then only using an open technique.

Hand

Ballistic injuries to the hands can be complex and the cause of significant morbidity. Adequate conditions are essential—appropriate anesthesia, good light, tourniquet, and experience. All injuries must be fully assessed, and many may require exploration under an anesthetic. Although this is not life-saving surgery, it should be carried out early to optimize functional recovery. Skin excision should be kept to the minimum and extensive debridement is usually not necessary. In particular, skin flaps should be preserved even if they appear degloved; they may be required for wound closure.

Compartment syndrome of the hand is rare except for crush injuries. The techniques of release are outwith the scope of this chapter, and with the possible exception of carpal tunnel, release should only be carried out by surgeons with experience in hand trauma.

All injuries should be splinted by plaster, with the wrist slightly extended, the MCP joints at 90 degrees, and the interphalangeal joints extended. The hand *must* be elevated in a sling to reduce swelling and the tips of the fingers should be visible.

Early expert input must be obtained.

Lower Limb

Thigh

Casualties with extensive thigh wounds will have lost a considerable amount of blood, particularly if associated with a fracture. Although these patients may initially appear to be stable, they may deteriorate, particularly if there were delays in evacuation. All patients must be adequately assessed and resuscitated as appropriate (Figure 17-15).

The thigh contains three compartments, the flexor, the extensor, and a medial adductor compartment. In civilian practice, release of anterior and posterior compartments through a single lateral incision may be sufficient, but penetrating injuries to the thigh may require release of the medial compartment. This will require a separate incision.

Extensive soft tissue wounds and fractures of the femur should be managed by splinting. Plaster on its own is unsuitable, but can be used in combination with a Thomas splint, known as a Tobruk splint.

External fixation should be avoided unless there are specific indications. Although it is a satisfactory method of stabilizing femoral fractures (providing sufficient bone is present both proximally and distally), there is a high complication rate.

Three good pins must be inserted into each segment, and at least two, and preferably three or four bars should be used to connect the pins. The

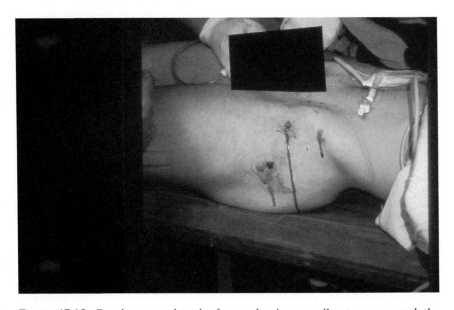

FIGURE 17-15. Gunshot wound to the femur; despite a small entrance wound, the patient was profoundly shocked, and there was extensive soft tissue, bone, and vascular injury.

pins can be inserted through the anterior, lateral, or posterolateral surface of the bone, but pins above the lesser trochanter or below the flare of the distal femur should be avoided.

Injuries around the knee can also be immobilized in a Thomas splint, but plaster is also effective. For extensive injuries, bridging external fixation, with pins in the distal femur and proximal tibia, can be very effective.

For civilian low-energy injuries, IM nailing has been used widely with low complication rates.

Lower Leg

This is the most common site of injury during war and is frequently seen in civilian practice. The prognosis for open fractures of the tibia is worse than that of other long bones; therefore, adequate local treatment of these injuries must be carried out as soon as practicable.

There are four compartments: anterior, lateral, superficial, and deep posterior compartments. Failure to release the deep posterior compartment is the most common error in lower limb fasciotomy, and occurs when releasing the soleus muscle from the posterior aspect of the tibia is mistaken for releasing the compartment. The posterior tibial artery is located between the two posterior compartments, and this can be used as a landmark during surgery. A two-incision technique should be used in the lower limb, decompressing the posterior compartments through an incision just posterior to the medial border of the tibia. The anterior and lateral compartments can be decompressed through an incision between the lateral border of the tibia and the fibula.

Plaster provides sufficient stabilization for many fractures, although external fixation is commonly required. Pins should be inserted into the subcutaneous surface of the bone. Care should be taken to ensure bicortical placement due to the triangular shape of the tibia.

Foot Injuries

Although these are not life threatening, they should never be dismissed as minor injuries. Significant injuries can occur (Figure 17-16), and inadequate management will cause later morbidity and functional limitations.

The principles of management remain the same, but stabilization of severe foot injuries can be difficult. Plaster is inadequate for severe injuries, except in the short term, and external fixation or wire fixation should be considered (Figure 17-16).

External fixator pins can be inserted into the tibial shaft, a transfixion pin can be inserted through the calcaneus, and pins inserted into the great toe metacarpal. This triangulation frame, in addition to stabilizing fractures, also maintains the foot at 90 degrees to the leg, preventing an equinus deformity, which can be a cause of significant later morbidity.

As with hand injuries, the foot must be elevated to reduce swelling.

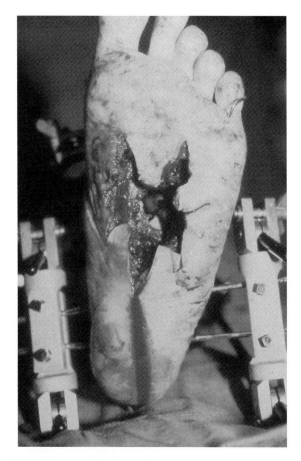

FIGURE 17-16. High-energy gunshot wound to the foot with significant soft tissue and bony damage; extensive local surgery with external fixation was necessary to avoid amputation.

The later management of severe foot injuries is outwith the scope of this chapter. Flap coverage may be required, as may bone grafting, local fusions, and partial amputations.

Miscellaneous Issues

Radiographs

Plain radiographs should be obtained for all ballistic limb injuries in the civilian environment, and although not essential in the management of military limb injury, they are very useful. With direct high-energy fractures, endosteal spread is universal and the spread of infection is more extensive than with indirect fractures. As the fracture pattern is different, the extent of contamination can be estimated on radiographs before debridement. In addition, the extent of the fracture can be assessed, and this may determine the technique of stabilization. External fixator pins should not be inserted within two to three centimeters of a fracture. Not only is there a risk of propagating cracks from the fracture site, but also this region will be contaminated, predisposing to a pin tract infection.

If used, radiography must not be allowed to delay the management of patients, particularly in a mass casualty situation.

Retained Fragments

As many bullet wounds will be associated with an entrance and exit wound, the issue of retained fragments will not arise. Most of the remaining fragments will be removed at the time of initial debridement, but some will be left behind and often are diagnosed on later radiographs.

Retained fragments can usually be left with only a small risk of subsequent infection. If the wound does develop an infection, secondary surgery will often be required, and the fragments can be removed at this stage. Consideration must be given to the removal of retained bullets.

Civilian data suggests that intra-articular and intra-bursal bullets should be removed due to the risk of lead arthropathy. This can be delayed and arthroscopic techniques can be used.

Bullets retained in soft tissues, including muscle, can be observed, and the current evidence would suggest that bullets retained in bone can also be treated conservatively (Figures 17-12 and 17-13).

Nonoperative Management of Ballistic Fractures

While it is true that in certain circumstances low-energy missile wounds involving bone can be treated nonoperatively, much of the data derives from American trauma centers. As discussed above, there are significant differences between civilian wounds and those seen during military conflicts, and the infection rate with military wounds is higher than with civilian wounds.

Secondary Management of the Fracture

Initial Treatment in Plaster

For fractures treated by plaster, if a satisfactory position is confirmed on subsequent radiographs, plaster can be used as the definitive treatment. If any delay in healing occurs, early bone grafting with or without appropriate internal fixation should probably be carried out.

Initial Treatment by External Fixation

For the more complex injuries, an external fixator may have been applied. However, the long-term outcome of external fixation in the treatment of military fractures is not known, and complications do occur with the civilian use of external fixators. Many of the problems associated with external fixation are due to its prolonged use, and it is possible that initial external fixation should be used followed by conversion to a different method of stabilization at a later date, when better facilities are available.

Fractures with Joint Involvement

If the fracture involves a joint surface and the fragments are displaced, plaster, external fixation, and IM nailing are not suitable methods of definitive treatment. If reconstruction is possible and suitable facilities are available, early fixation with screws and/or plates should be carried out. If reconstruction of the joint is not possible, the position should be accepted and early mobilization carried out. Fusion of the joint is an alternative for some joints, particularly the ankle and wrist, but should be avoided at the hip and knee, and particularly the elbow, if possible.

Red Cross Wound Classification

The International Committee of the Red Cross (ICRC) has developed a scoring system to allow the classification of military wounds. This classification was designed not only to permit wound assessment, but also to allow surgical audit, and to attempt to determine the relationship of war wounds to experimental ballistic injuries. The grading is based on the size of both entry and exit wounds, as well as the presence of a fracture, cavity, metallic fragments, or damage to a vital structure. This allows a grading and subtyping of wounds and can be used to help in the treatment, as well as an outcome measure. Further information can be found in specific ICRC publications.

References

1. Lindberg RB, Wetzler TF, Marshall JD, Newton A, Strawitz JG, Howard JM. The bacterial flora of battle wounds at the time of primary debridement. *Ann Surg.* 1955;141:369–374.
2. Coupland RM. Technical aspects of war wound excision. *Br J Surg.* 1989;76: 663–667.
3. Clasper JC. The interaction of projectiles with bone and the management of ballistic fractures. *J R Army Med Corps.* 2001;147:52–61.
4. Rose SC, Fujisaki CK, Moore EE. Incomplete fractures associated with penetrating trauma: Etiology, appearance and natural history. *J Trauma.* 1988;28:106–109.

5. Rich NM, Metz CW, Hutton JE, Baugh JH, Hughes CW. Internal versus external fixation of fractures with concomitant vascular injuries in Vietnam. *J Trauma.* 1971;11:463–473.

Further Reading

Cooper GJ, Dudley HAF, Gann DS, Little RA, Maynard RL. *Scientific Foundations of Trauma.* Oxford: Butterman-Heinemann; 1997.

Coupland RM. The Red Cross wound classification. In: *War Wounds of Limbs: Surgical Management.* Oxford: Butterworth Heinemann; 1993.

Dufour D, KromannJensen S, Owen-Smith M, Stening GF, Zetterström B. *Surgery for Victims of War.* 3rd ed. International Committee of the Red Cross; 1998.

18
Vascular Injury

ELIAS DEGIANNIS and MARTIN D. SMITH

The local and regional effect of ballistic trauma to the arterial system is directly related to the velocity of the missile. In high-energy–transfer gunshot wounds, the bullet creates a cavitational effect on impact, which can produce massive soft tissue injury for several centimeters around the missile tract. In this case, debridement of the injured artery is required. On the other hand, low-velocity gunshot wounds behave similarly to stab wounds, with minimal soft tissue injury, and debridement of the injured vessels is not usually necessary.

Close-range shotgun wounds can also cause extensive soft tissue injury. In addition, parts of the cartridge may penetrate the wound, increasing the possibility of severe infection if the parts are not recovered with the initial debridement. Exsanguination can follow complete or partial transection of the artery, particularly if it is related to a large soft tissue wound. In complete transection, it is possible for the two ends of the severed artery to retract and for thrombosis to occur, preventing extensive blood loss. On the contrary, in partial transection, retraction is not possible; therefore there is a greater possibility of exsanguination. If the blood loss is contained in the perivascular tissues, a pseudoaneurysm can be formed. In contiguous wounds of both the artery and the adjacent vein, an arteriovenous fistula may develop.

Acute interruption of arterial blood flow can produce regional ischemia to the limb or organ. The vulnerability of a tissue to ischemia depends on its basal energy requirement and substrate stores. Peripheral nerves, having a high basal energy requirement and no glycogen stores, can undergo damage after a relatively short period of ischemia. Therefore, altered neurology is often the first manifestation in a patient with arterial injury.[1]

Skeletal muscle is much more tolerant of ischemia. Extremity muscle can often survive without nutrient blood flow for up to four hours without developing any permanent changes. If the ischemia extends for six hours or longer, there is a risk of sustaining irreversible tissue changes in spite of reperfusion. Incomplete interruption of arterial flow combined with good collateral circulation will substantially extend the tolerance of the ischemia, and therefore the ischemia time. In these cases, basic aerobic metabolism is maintained for a longer period of time and oxygen-free radical formation is contained. As a result, the risk of reperfusion injury is diminished.

Reperfusion injury is directly related to biochemical events occurring with ischemia. During ischemia, oxygen-free radicals are produced in a cascade of biochemical processes, resulting in injury of the microvascular endothelial membrane. The loss of its integrity results in interstitial edema with muscle swelling inside the compartment encased by the deep fascia of the limb, followed by occlusion of capillaries resulting *in a no-reflow phenomenon* and irreversible nerve and muscle damage.[2] Therefore, reperfusion after complete ischemia can aggravate the initial ischemic insult.

The consequence of skeletal muscle necrosis includes the release of potassium and myoglobin into the circulation, resulting in acute tubular necrosis and renal failure. Therefore, apart from the possibility of limb loss, complications of acute traumatic ischemia can result in death if not timely recognized and treated.

Diagnosis

A high degree of suspicion is of paramount importance to avoid missing vascular injuries, as delay in diagnosis and treatment increases the risk of irreversible ischemic damage. The aim is to diagnose and treat the injury within the "golden period" of six hours. Although, as mentioned above, in the presence of collateral circulation, the limb is more tolerant of arterial disruption and the "golden period" can be extended; the earlier the vascular repair takes place the better the results.

Physical examination remains the cornerstone of the diagnosis, and arteriography is reserved for the selected patient. The physical examination will reveal "hard" or "soft" signs of arterial injury. "Hard" signs are indicative of ischemia or ongoing hemorrhage and include absent distal pulses, extensive external bleeding, expanding or pulsatile hematoma, palpable thrill, continuous murmur, and signs of distal ischemia such as pain, pallor, paresthesia, paralysis, and coolness. The presence of "hard" signs mandates immediate surgical exploration, as virtually all will have injuries requiring operative repair.[3]

Significant vascular injuries can be associated with *poly-trauma* and varying degrees of shock from other sources, resulting in diminished or absent peripheral pulses. In hypotensive patients, it may not be possible to determine whether or not arterial or venous injury is present until the shock has been reversed and the peripheral pulses in the uninjured limbs have returned. Absent peripheral pulses in the nonhypotensive patient and the presence of neurological findings indicate severe ischemia. On the other hand, if neurological function is intact, there is virtually no risk of gangrene. However, with the loss of neurological function, gangrene is probable unless circulation is rapidly restored. With concomitant ballistic injury to peripheral nerves, neurologic function as an index of the severity of anoxia is less useful. It should be remembered that ischemia produces a more global neurologic deficit in the involved extremity while injuries to peripheral nerves produce a deficit limited to specific dermatomes or muscle groups.[1]

"Hard" signs of arterial injury mandate immediate intervention. Sending these patients to the Radiology Department for formal angiograms is dangerous and unnecessary. Angiography is only done on stable patients if there is uncertainty as to the site of injury (e.g., multiple gunshot wounds, shotgun wounds, or to select the exposure for distal subclavian or proximal axillary arteries). For lower limb injury, emergency room or intraoperative arteriography is practiced if it is considered helpful in planning the operative approach by providing the location and extent of the arterial injury.

A significant percentage of arterial injuries presents with "soft" signs—history of active bleeding at the trauma scene, diminished but palpable pulses, and peripheral nerve deficit. Radiology Department arteriography is practiced in all these patients.

As recommended by Frykberg and colleagues[3,4] "proximity" of the injury alone (without any other signs) is not considered an indication for arteriography except in cases of suspected axillary artery trauma, where extensive collateral circulation can mask severe arterial injury.

In the last few years, Doppler studies have been used in our department as an adjunct for stratifying risk in patients with ballistic trauma. In the absence of "hard" signs, a Doppler pressure deficit of greater than ten percent (compared with the opposite side) is considered a "soft" sign of arterial injury and we proceed to arteriography.

Preoperative Control of Bleeding

Control of external torrential hemorrhage is usually the first priority in the presence of peripheral vascular injuries. Direct focal pressure is the most effective way to control bleeding. This is done initially by direct digital pressure, which must be maintained until definitive operative exposure is obtained. Extraluminal balloon tamponade is a very useful adjunctive measure for preoperative control of hemorrhage with peripheral vascular trauma. A Foley catheter is inserted into the tract of the missile and the balloon is inflated until hemorrhage is controlled. A large skin wound is rapidly sutured around the catheter to prevent dislodgement during balloon inflation and to assist in creating a tamponade. Balloon catheters are especially useful in controlling hemorrhage from surgically inaccessible sites, such as Zone III in the neck, and in sites where direct digital pressure is ineffective. Such sites include the supraclavicular area, the axilla, and the groin. The technique of balloon tamponade for controlling supraclavicular bleeding was first described from Chris Hani Baragwanath Hospital.[5] The Foley catheter is inserted into the wound towards the estimated source of bleeding. The balloon is then inflated until the bleeding stops or moderate resistance is felt. For supraclavicular wounds with associated hemothorax, a combination of two Foley catheters may be necessary. The first catheter is inserted as deeply as possible into the chest, the balloon is inflated, and the catheter is pulled back firmly and held in place with an artery clip. This compresses the injured subclavian vessels against the first rib or the clavicle and prevents further bleeding. If external bleeding continues, a second Foley catheter is *inserted more superficially into the wound tract and inflated.* Blood through the lumen of the Foley catheter suggests distal bleeding and repositioning or further inflation of the balloon or clamping of the catheter should be considered.[6]

Operative Management

At operation, when surgically approaching a peripheral arterial injury, the entire extremity should be prepared, draped, and included in the operative field. The contralateral uninjured lower or upper extremity should also be included in the operative field if it is anticipated that an autologous graft will be required. The incision in most patients with extremity wounds should follow the course of the neurovascular bundle and remain between natural anatomical planes to reduce the chance of causing inadvertent injury to adjacent structures. It is of paramount importance to obtain proximal and distal control early in the course of the operation. Failure to achieve this before exposing the site of injury of a large vessel may convert a careful anatomical dissection into a frantic attempt to stop massive bleeding. After obtaining proximal and distal vascular control, one can gradually dissect along the vessel toward the site of the injury, and at the same time replace the vascular tapes closer to the injury until the distance between the proximal and distal tapes is reduced to the area of injury plus two centimeters on each end.[7] Once control has been established, the injured vessels are inspected and debrided up to macroscopically normal intima (Figure 18-1). Before definitive repair, one must ensure that any clots that may have formed proximally or distally have been removed. Fogarty catheters are carefully passed both proximally and distally to the arterial injury in order

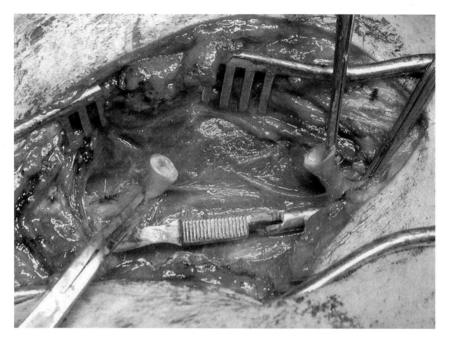

FIGURE 18-1. The injured part of the femoral artery has been resected in preparation for graft repair.

to remove intraluminal thrombus. Good back bleeding from the distal artery does not exclude intravascular thrombus beyond the first patent collateral vessels, thus routine distal insertion of the Fogarty catheter is essential. Care should be exercised not to over-inflate the balloon, thus damaging the endothelial lining and producing spasm of the vessel or thrombosis.[8] The passage of the Fogarty's balloon catheter should be repeated as many times as necessary to obtain pulsatile flow proximally and steady back flow distally. This is particularly important with distal lower-extremity arterial lesions where there has been some delay in operative treatment. After clot extraction, local anticoagulation can be obtained by instilling 10 to 15 milliliters of a heparin solution containing 50 units per milliliter. This is done proximally and distally using a Fogarty irrigating catheter. If systemic heparinization seems preferable and is safe, it can be obtained with 50 to 100 units of heparin per kilogram body weight. This has the advantage of producing a more complete and effective anticoagulation; however, if there is little or no distal blood flow, additional heparin will have to be injected into the injured vessels to prevent distal thrombosis.[7]

The repair of an arterial injury in ballistic trauma should always be accomplished with the use of a graft.[3] There is no role for lateral repair and patch angioplasty. It is believed that an end-to-end anastomosis after proper debridement will be unlikely to result in a tension-free anastomosis, and the use of a graft is the safest choice. Reversed autogenous saphenous vein graft from an uninjured lower extremity is the conduit of choice for extensive peripheral arterial injuries. Long-term patency in smaller arteries of the extremities has simply never been shown with synthetic prosthesis. Polyte-trafluoroethylene (PTFE) prosthesis should be available for the patients in which the saphenous vein cannot be used. Examples include saphenous vein of inadequate size to maintain patency; when it is absent, fibrotic, or thick-ened; when there is a significant size discrepancy between the injured artery and vein graft; or when such severe truncal or extremity injuries exist that a synthetic prosthesis will save operating time. Whereas the long-term patency rates with prosthetic material is less than with autologous vein, par-ticularly distal to the knee or elbow, previous concerns about the increased potential for infection with prosthetic grafts were probably exaggerated. All completed vascular repairs should be free of tension and covered with avail-able viable soft tissues. Monofilament 5-0 or 6-0 sutures are suitable for most peripheral vascular repairs. The spatulated technique in which the artery on each end is cut in an elongated oblique spatulated manner is always followed with the length of the spatulated extension approximately equal to the diameter of the distal vessel (Figure 18-2). It is advisable to vent the anastomosis of air or clots or both before the last one or two sutures are tied. The vessel is occluded just distally to the distal suture line and then the proximal clamp is removed to allow proximal air or clots to be vented. After this has been accomplished, the suture is tied.

Small bleeding anastamotic points at a completed vascular anastomosis can be dealt with by properly placed digital pressure and a little patience, which will usually obviate the need for repair sutures. After the vascular anastomosis has been completed, the heparin is allowed to metabolize. Giving protamine to counteract the remaining heparin is generally unnecessary and probably unwise because it may cause a rebound hypercoagulability.

After proper and timely vascular reconstruction, excellent distal flow should be apparent by the restoration of normal peripheral pulses. If there is any question about the successful restoration of flow, as may occur in patients with peripheral vasoconstriction from prolonged ischemia, intra-operative completion arteriography is indicated. Intraoperative completion angiography should be performed in theater with the repair exposed. It is extremely helpful in documenting the adequacy of the vascular recon-struction and in detection of persistent distal thrombi. It is performed via vessel cannulation with a small catheter proximal to the repair, proximal occlusion during the injection of full-strength contrast, and exposing the film during active injection (two-thirds complete). If a technical defect is

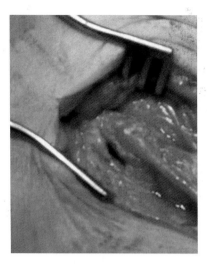

FIGURE 18-2. The proximal anastomosis to the femoral artery with a saphenous vein graft, after spatulation of the two ends being anastamosed.

identified, the anastomosis should be revised. In the occasional patient with severe spasm distal to the arterial repair and with significant disruption of collaterals, adjuncts exist that may help salvage "borderline" distal viability. These include arterial infusion with a mixture of heparin (1000 units)–saline (1000 milliliters)–tolazoline (500 milligrams) at 30 millilters per hour; venous infusion with low molecular weight dextran (500 milliliters per 12 hours); if there is clinical or radiological evidence of multiple distal thrombi, infusions of urokinase may be helpful if the patient has no other injuries that may bleed.

The current consensus favors repair of the veins unless life-threatening problems exist that preclude further surgery or more complex repairs other than simple lateral suture and end-to-end anastomosis are required.

Copious irrigation of the wound with saline and appropriate debridement of all devitalized tissue and foreign material are essential to reduce the risk of postoperative infection. When the arterial injury is associated with massive soft tissue loss, the muscle and subcutaneous tissue normally overlying the neurovascular bundle may be absent. If a vein graft is exposed or covered only by ischemic or contaminated tissue, it will necrose and rupture.[9] If a prosthetic graft becomes infected, a false aneurysm can develop at the site of anastamosis, or sometimes in the artery proximal or distal to the anastomosis where clamps had been applied.[10] Therefore, it is of paramount importance to cover the area of the repair. These wounds should be closed with vascularized tissue,[11] preferably a transposed muscle flap or a free tissue transfer (muscular or myocutaneous).[12,13] Local fasciocutaneous flaps have also been used.[14] Rarely, the soft tissue defect will be so enormous that a local flap or free tissue transfer will be inadequate to completely cover the vascular repair. In such circumstances, the application of biological dressing such as split-thickness porcine skin graft may be the only solution. This is likely to be successful as long as one wall of the vein is lying on healthy muscle, with oxygenated interstitial fluid that flows by capillary action between the exposed vein wall and the covering split-thickness porcine graft (oxygenation of vein grafts is provided not from the red cells that flow through the lumen, but from oxygen dissolved in the interstitial fluid bathing the outside of the vein).[15,16] The porcine graft can be changed every 48 hours at the bedside without the need to administer general anesthetic. Over a period of four to six weeks, the "exposed" vein graft will gradually become covered with pink granulation tissue, after which the vein wall will no longer be seen. At this time, the vein graft and the covering granulation tissue will accept an autologus split-thickness skin graft. Extra anatomic bypass of large defects is also a consideration, especially when there is extensive contamination or a graft infection has occurred.[7]

At the time of closure, meticulous hemostasis is extremely important and obviates the need for drains. Drains should never be placed adjacent to vascular repairs because they may erode or infect the suture line.

In patients with a high risk of developing a compartment syndrome, the addition of a fasciotomy is of paramount importance. These are the patients with a prolonged period of shock or arterial occlusion, combined arterial and venous injuries, or a need for arterial or venous ligation. Fasciotomy should be performed before arterial exploration, when an obvious compartment syndrome exists or when intracompartmental pressures are significantly elevated (greater than 30 millimeters Hg) before reperfusion. In such instances, fasciotomies in the distal extremity can be performed rapidly and may be invaluable in preventing subsequent neurological disability.

Lateral and medial straight incisions are used to decompress the anterior and posterior compartments of the arm, respectively. Dorsal and volar skin incisions are used for the forearm. The dorsal incision is straight, but the volar incision should preferably form a "lazy S" to avoid contractures caused by scar formation. The incision should start from the medial side of the upper part of the forearm, curve towards the radius at mid arm, and return towards the ulnar side close to the wrist. The incision may extend over the mid proximal wrist to decompress the carpal tunnel.

The standard incisions to complete a four-compartment leg fasciotomy are lateral and medial. The lateral incision is placed slightly anterior to the fibula and the medial approximately five centimeters posterior to the tibia. They should both run from the upper part of the tibia or fibula to the medial or lateral malleolus. The anterior and lateral compartments are decompressed through the lateral incision and the superficial and deep posterior compartments through the medial incision. Every effort should be made to elevate the extremity after performing the fasciotomy to decrease the edema of the exposed muscles. At five to seven days, closure of the most exposed lateral fasciotomy site with vertical mattress skin sutures is possible in over 50% of patients.

The surgical treatment of combined vascular and orthopedic injuries is one of the most challenging problems in the management of patients with vascular trauma. In general, the arterial repair should be performed first, with circulation to the limb restored prior to orthopedic stabilization. However, massive musculoskeletal trauma from a high-velocity gunshot wound may render the limb so unstable that external fixation is required prior to the vascular procedure. Selective use of intraluminal shunts and rapid placement of external fixation devices minimizes limb ischemia. If the vascular repair is performed prior to orthopedic fixation, it is incumbent on the surgeon to inspect the vascular reconstruction prior to final wound closure.

Apart from its use in combined orthopedic and vascular injury, intraluminal shunts can be used in the context of damage control in the physiologically unstable patient. A shunt is best inserted after proximal and distal control of the injured artery is achieved. The choice of shunt material and configuration are matters of personal preference. Many surgeons are comfortable using carotid shunts (i.e., those used for carotid endarterectomy), although polyvinyl chloride endotracheal suction tubing is easily available and can be rapidly cut to a convenient length to provide an inexpensive and effective shunt. T-shaped carotid shunts allow repeated checking of shunt patency, as well as serving as an irrigation port. The key technical maneuver in the insertion of a temporary shunt is securing the shunt. This can be done either with silk or with a vessel loop that is passed twice around the vessel and then held in place with a silver clip or a Rummel tourniquet. The vessel can be easily injured at the point where it is secured; thus, it is always safer not to rely on this potentially traumatized segment of wall during subsequent reconstruction. The shunt provides distal perfusion while other life-threatening injuries are addressed or during subsequent resuscitation in the trauma intensive care unit. The two major post-insertion complications are dislodgement and occlusion. Shunts are not indicated for venous injuries.[17]

Ligation of a gunshot artery is a valid technical option in the critically injured patient who is rapidly approaching his/her physiological limits. This is especially true if the injured vessel is relatively inaccessible—a complex repair is required or a temporary shunt cannot be inserted. The external carotid artery can be ligated with impunity. The internal carotid can be ligated as a life-saving maneuver with a reasonable chance of neurological recovery. In most patients, ligation of the subclavian artery does not result in critical ischemia if no major soft tissue destruction has occurred around the shoulder. A significant risk of critical limb ischemia is present following ligation of the common and superficial femoral arteries. When a major limb artery is ligated in the context of damage control surgery, an adjunctive open fasciotomy is often in the patient's best interest.[17]

Nerve injury in association with vascular trauma is a formidable obstacle to the restoration of a functional limb. Primary repair of nerves is superior to delayed repair, but ballistic injury may cause laceration and a variable zone of neural contusion for which primary repair is contraindicated.[6]

There is a small group of close-range high-velocity injuries that present with vascular disruption in combination with severe, open, comminuted fractures and moderate loss of soft tissue. These "mangled limbs" are associated with a high morbidity and a poor functional prognosis and often require late amputation despite initial limb salvage. The decision to proceed to primary amputation is usually easier in the significantly unstable patient with multiple gunshot wounds because very often the patient's physiological reserves preclude the option of a prolonged multidisciplinary reconstructive effort. The decision to proceed to immediate amputation should ideally be made by a team that includes vascular, orthopedic, and plastic surgeons.

Specific Arterial Injuries

Subclavian/Axillary Artery

The patient is placed in the supine position with the arm abducted at 30 degrees and the head turned to the opposite side. Excessive abduction should be avoided because it distorts the local anatomy and makes the exposure more difficult. The chest should always be included in the preparation of the surgical field. The recommended incision for injuries of the first part of the *right* subclavian is a median sternotomy with right supraclavicular extension. For the first part of the *left* subclavian, a left lateral thoracotomy combined with a left supraclavicular incision is recommended. These approaches to access the origin of the subclavian artery are practiced in all our physiologically unstable patients regardless of the injured anatomical part of the subclavian artery. The recommended incision (in stable patients) for injury to the second and third parts of the subclavian artery on both sides is a supraclavicular incision with lateral infraclavicular extension (S-shaped incision). If difficulty in gaining proximal control is encountered at any stage of the operation, there should be no hesitation to extend the incision as recommended with injuries of the first part of the subclavian. To expose the subclavian artery at the clavicular level, it is usually necessary to resect the middle third of the clavicle or divide the clavicle in half. Care should be taken to divide the clavicle in the subperiosteal plane so as to avoid injury to the subclavian vein located at the inferior border of the clavicle. The artery is located fairly deep, and in the absence of pulsations due to thrombosis or retraction of the transected ends, it might be difficult to locate and identify. In these cases, it is easier to expose the axillary artery and proceed proximally. Similarly, in the presence of a large hematoma or severe active bleeding, the vascular exposure may start distally and proceed proximally toward the site of the vascular injury. If the scalenus anterior muscle needs to be retracted or divided, special precautions must be taken to avoid injury to the phrenic nerve, which lies on the anterior surface of the muscle.[18,19]

In hemodynamically stable patients, arteriography and stent graft treatment should be considered. Encouraging results are emerging from South-African centers; however, this modality is less readily available because of resource constraints. Du Toit and colleagues have recently published results of 10 stable patients with penetrating vascular injury at the root of the neck.[20] Seven had arteriovenous fistulas and three had pseudoaneurysms. Stent graft treatment was successful in all 10 patients with no procedure-related complications, and no complications were encountered with clinical and sonographic follow up at a mean of seven months. Naidoo and colleagues, from Durban, South Africa, reported on 41 patients with injuries to "noncritical" peripheral arteries treated by endovascular techniques, with successful outcome in 97% of cases.[21] Long-term outcomes with this method of treatment are still unclear.

The axillary artery is approached through a horizontal infraclavicular incision, with division of the pectoralis major muscle about two centimeters from its attachment to the humerus. Proximal supraclavicular control of the subclavian artery may be necessary for injuries of the subclavian/axillary junction. Resection of the middle third of the clavicle is rarely necessary, but may be required for injuries of the axillary/subclavian junction.[22]

Brachial/Radial/Ulnar Artery

Brachial artery injuries are always repaired because if left untreated claudication results in a significant number of patients. Fashioning of the anastomosis with interrupted sutures is also advised due to the small caliber of the artery.[23] Single-vessel injury in the forearm need not be repaired and may be ligated. Repair is mandatory if one of the vessels has been previously ligated, if the palmar arch is incomplete, or if Allen's test is positive. In injuries of both radial and ulnar arteries, the ulnar, which is the dominant and larger vessel, should preferably be repaired.

Femoral Artery

The common femoral, profunda femoris, and superficial femoral arteries are exposed by a longitudinal incision over the femoral triangle. The common femoral artery lies within the femoral sheath, with the common femoral vein located medially and the femoral nerve laterally. If proximal control of the external iliac artery is needed, the retroperitoneal approach is ideal. A separate incision parallel to and three centimeters above the inguinal ligament is made, the muscles lateral to the rectus abdominis are divided with diathermy, and the transversalis fascia is incised. The peritoneum and its contents are reflected medially and proximally, and the external iliac artery and vein are well visualized posteriorly.[24,25]

Popliteal Artery

The entire lower limb should be included in the operative field to be able to visualize the foot and palpate distal pulses. The patient should be supine, with a support under the knee in slight flexion and the hip abducted and externally rotated. The incision is made parallel to the sartorius muscle. Division of the gracilis, semimembranous, semitendinosus, and medial head of the gastrocnemius is possible and will expose the entire popliteal artery.[26]

Tibial Arteries

Isolated injury to one of the interpopliteal arteries (anterior tibial, posterior tibial, or peroneal arteries) rarely causes limb-threatening ischemia because of the collateral supply through the plantar arch. Therefore, an occlusive injury of a single infrapopliteal artery does not require therapeutic intervention if signs and symptoms of ischemia are absent.

Carotid Artery

Most carotid artery injuries are best managed by primary arterial repair, regardless of neurological status.[27] Zone II injuries are relatively easy to expose by a neck incision overlying and parallel to the anterior border of the sternocleidomastoid muscle. Zone I injuries frequently require median sternotomy to expose the more proximal portions of the common carotid artery or to address concomitant arch injuries. Zone III injuries are a surgical challenge (Figure 18-3). Division of the digastric muscle provides

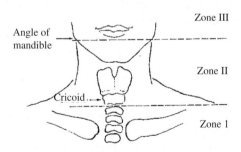

FIGURE 18-3. The zones of the neck.

exposure of the distal internal carotid artery. Access to the artery above the digastric muscle also may be facilitated by anterior subluxation of the mandible.[27-29] Osteotomy of the angle of the mandible also can be helpful in achieving additional distal exposure. Vascular control should be achieved proximally and distally before approaching the arterial injury. Unexpected or ongoing hemorrhage can be arrested by digital compression. Control of bleeding from distal internal carotid artery injuries may be difficult, particularly if encountered prior to complete surgical exposure. In such cases, a vascular balloon catheter can be inserted into the vessel, either through the injury or through a proximal arteriotomy. The balloon is inflated to occlude the arterial lumen. Once hemorrhage is controlled, exposure can be completed and the injury definitively addressed. Small carotid injuries that can be repaired rapidly do not need shunts. However, in more complex injuries requiring graft repair, the role of shunting is controversial. The existing studies are small and nonrandomized, and the recommendations made are anecdotal. Based on the available data and the safety of modern shunts, it is reasonable to employ shunting for complex injuries requiring graft reconstruction, especially in the presence of preoperative neurologic deficits or severe hypotension.

Vertebral Artery

Vertebral arterial injuries can be challenging to tackle operatively, and interventional radiology for control of lesions in these vessels is highly desirable. In 1988, Hatzitheofilou and colleagues, from Chris Hani Baragwanath Hospital, described the application of clips proximally and distally within the intervertebral foramina to control the injury.[30] Although this was described from our institution, our more recent experience has found this very difficult and rarely successful. Tight packing and closure of the neck without drains and the endotracheal tube left *in situ* for ventilation successfully controls most cases of severe hemorrhage found in this situation. At re-exploration, rebleeding is almost never encountered. The surgical management of very high vertebral artery injuries at the level of exit from the cervical vertebra immediately before or after entering the skull can be taxing to the most experienced trauma surgeon. The presence of a neurosurgeon for the management of this injury is mandatory because a suboccipital craniectomy may be required for distal ligation.[31]

References

1. Shackford SR, Rich NH. Peripheral vascular injury. In: Mattox KL, Feliciano DV, Moore EE, eds. *Trauma*. 4th ed. New York: McGraw-Hill; 2000:1011–1044.
2. Menger MD, Pelikan S, Steiner D, Messmr K. Microvascular ischemia-reperfusion injury in striated muscle: Significance of "reflow paradox". *Am J Physiol*. 1992;263:1892–1900.

3. Degiannis E, Levy RD, Sofianos C, Florizoone MGC, Saadia R. Arterial gunshot injuries of the extremities: A South African experience. *J Trauma*. 1995; 39:370–376.
4. Frykberg ER, Crump JM, Dennis JW, Wines FS, Alexander RH. Nonoperative observation of clinically occult arterial injuries: A prospective evaluation. *Surgery*. 1991;109:85–90.
5. Gilroy D, Lakhoo M, Charalambides D, Demetriades D. Control of life-threatening hemorrhage from the neck: A new indication for balloon tamponade. *J Trauma*. 1992;23:557–559.
6. Bowley D, Degiannis E, Goosen J, Boffard KD. Penetrating vascular injuries in Johannesburg. *Surg Clin N Am*. 2002;82:221–236.
7. Wilson RF. Vascular injuries. In: Wilson RF, ed. *Handbook of Trauma*. Philadelphia: Lippincott Williams and Wilkins; 1999:515–527.
8. Weaver FA, Papanicolaou G, Yellin AE. Difficult peripheral vascular injuries. *Surg Clin N Am*. 1996;76:843–859.
9. Rich NM, Baugh JH, Hughes CE. Acute arterial injuries in Vietnam: 1,000 cases. *J Trauma*. 1970;10:359–369.
10. Feliciano DV, Mattox KL, Graham JM, Bitondo CG. Five-year experience with PTFE grafts in vascular wounds. *J Trauma*. 1985;25:71–82.
11. Strinden WD, Dibbell DG, Tirnipspeed WD, Archer CW, Rao VK, Mixter RC. Coverage of acute vascular injuries of the axilla and groin with transposition muscle flaps: Case reports. *J Trauma*. 1989;29:512–516.
12. Melissinos EG, Parks DH. Post-trauma reconstruction with free tissue-transfer—Analysis of 442 consecutive cases. *J Trauma*. 1989;29:1095–1102.
13. Khouri RK, Shaw WW. Reconstruction of the lower extremity with microvascular free flaps: A 10 year experience with 304 consecutive cases. *J Trauma*. 1989;29:1086–1094.
14. Hallock GG. Local fasciocutaneous flaps for cutaneous coverage of lower extremity wounds. *J Trauma*. 1989;29:1240–1244.
15. Artz DP, Rittenbury MS, Yarbrough DR III. An appraisal of allografts and xenografts as biological dressings for wounds and burns. *Ann Surg*. 1972; 175:934–938.
16. Ledgerwood AM, Lucas CE. Biological dressings for exposed vascular grafts: a reasonable alternative. *J Trauma*. 1975;15:567–574.
17. Ancar JA, Hirschberg A. Damage control for vascular injuries. *Surg Clin N Am*. 1997;77:853–862.
18. Demetriades D, Asensio JA. Subclavian and axillary vascular injuries. *Surg Clin N Am*. 2001;81:1357–1373.
19. Degiannis E, Velmahos GC, Krawczykowski D, Levy RD, Souter I, Saadia R. Penetrating injuries of the subclavian vessels. *Br J Surg*. 1994;81:524–526.
20. Du Toit DF, Strasuss DC, Blaszczyk M, De Villiers R, Warren BL. Endovascular treatment of penetrating thoracic outlet arterial injuries. *Eur J Vasc Endovasc Surg*. 2000;19:489–495.
21. Naidoo NM, Corr PD, Robbs JV. Angiographic embolisation in arterial trauma. *Eur J Vasc Endovasc Surg*. 2000;41:760–762.
22. Degiannis E, Levy RD, Potokar T, Saadia R. Penetrating injuries of the axillary artery. *Aust N Z J Surg*. 1995;65:327–330.
23. Degiannis E, Levy RD, Sliwa K, Potokar T, Saadia R. Penetrating injuries of the brachial artery. *Injury*. 1995;26:249–252.

24. Degiannis E, Levy RD, Velmahos GC, Potokar T, Saadia R. Penetrating injuries of the femoral artery. *Br J Surg*. 1995;82:492–495.
25. Degiannis E, Levy RD, Hatzitheofilou C, Florizoone MGC, Saadia R. Arterial gunshot injuries to the groin. Comparison of iliac and femoral trauma. *Injury*. 1996;27:315–318.
26. Degiannis E, Velmahos GC, Florizoone MGC, Levy RD, Ross J, Saadia R. Penetrating injuries of the popliteal artery: the Baragwanath experience. *Ann R Coll Surg Engl*. 1994;76:307–310.
27. Ram Kumar S, Weaver F-A, Yellin AE. Cervical vascular injuries. *Surg Clin N Am*. 2001;81:1331–1344.
28. Sofianos C, Degiannis E, van den Aardweg MS, Levy RD, Naidu M, Saadia R. Selective surgical management of zone II gunshot injuries of the neck: a prospective study. *Surgery*. 1996;119:785–788.
29. Velmahos GC, Souter I, Degiannis E, Mokoena T, Saadia R. Selective surgical management in penetrating neck injuries. *Can J Surg*. 1994;37:487–491.
30. Hatzitheofilou C, Demetriades D, Melissas J. Surgical approaches to vertebral artery injuries. *Br J Surg*. 1988;75:234–237.
31. Demetriades D, Asensio JA, Velmahos G, Thal E. Complex problems in penetrating neck trauma. *Surg Clin of N Am*. 1996;76:661–683.

19
Ballistic Trauma in Children

GRAEME J. PITCHER

Epidemiological Background

The natural inquisitiveness and vulnerability of early life predispose children to penetrating injury; varying in severity from a minor laceration or foreign body penetration to life-threatening impalement, stab wound, or missile injury. Ballistic injuries, defined as injuries caused by thrown or projected missiles, comprise an important proportion of pediatric penetrating injury. Penetrating injuries are responsible for approximately 15% of pediatric trauma deaths in developed countries.[1] Injury patterns differ widely between different communities, socioeconomic groups, cities, countries, and cultures. Such injuries are also more common during times of revolution or sociopolitical change.

Missile injuries may be intentional (homicidal or suicidal intent) or unintentional. In younger children, most are unintentional or homicidal. Suicidal attempts are confined mainly to adolescence. In developed countries, most children are injured unintentionally, occurring as a result of the child playing with the firearm or during firearm sports. These injuries appear to be declining in incidence, but they are still a prominent cause of death in the pediatric population.[2] In 1988, gunshot wounds were the eighth leading cause of unintentional injury deaths among persons in all age groups in the United States, and the third leading cause of such deaths among children and teenagers aged 10 to 19 years.[3] This underscores the importance of educating gun owners in the safe use and storage of their weapons, as this has been shown to be a contributory factor in the decline of this type of injury.[4]

The incidence of serious penetrating injuries, and of gunshot wounds in particular, seems to be on the increase worldwide.[5-7] The incidence of pediatric gunshot injuries varies according to the number and availability of firearms in the community, with the United States having the greatest incidence amongst developed countries.[8,9] Homicide and suicide in pediatric age groups appears to be increasing in incidence in most countries worldwide. From 1950 through 1993, the overall annual death rate for U.S. children aged less than 15 years declined substantially, primarily reflecting decreases in deaths associated with unintentional injuries, pneumonia, influenza, cancer, and congenital anomalies. However, during the same period, childhood homicide rates tripled and suicide rates quadrupled. In 1994, among children aged one to four years, homicide was the fourth leading cause of death; among children aged five to 14 years, homicide was the third leading cause of death, and suicide was the sixth.[6] In America, the factors that have been identified with increased risk of intentional injury include: urban resident, age group 10 to16 years, male gender, lower socio-economic group, poor family support systems, and African-American race.[10,11] In male adolescents, gang activities with alcohol and drug abuse account for the bulk of injuries in many cities.[2, 12] The emergence in the last few decades of the phenomenon known as "family murders"—where an adult member of the family, usually the father executes the entire family and then commits suicide—has perhaps also contributed to this disturbing trend. In general, the perpetrator of firearm injuries in young children tends to be an adult, whereas in adolescents, peers are usually responsible. Overall, the child's status as a protected and cherished member of the community appears to be increasingly threatened.

In developing countries, particularly in times of social instability and change such as is being experienced currently in South Africa, children too young to be able to participate in crime and violence are frequently shot as innocent bystanders or in retaliation for the perpetrator's grudge against a parent. These patients often suffer severe injuries, and almost inevitably, there is a delay in reaching the hospital, with resultant high mortality rate and significant long-term major morbidity.[13]

In Cape Town, South Africa, homicide is the single leading cause of non-natural death in the under-19 age group.[12] An exponentially increasing incidence of childhood gunshot wounds over the last twenty years has been reported from another South African province—KwaZulu-Natal. The mean age of pediatric gunshot victims in that province is 6.4 years. Experience here also shows that for every child admitted to hospital with a gunshot wound, four were delivered to police mortuaries in the province during the same period. This statistic underscores the wounding and killing potential of modern weapons when used against children.

It is abundantly clear that urgent preventative measures are required in all communities to protect children from this senseless litany of violence.

Weapons and Patterns of Penetrating Injury

Ballistic weapons are designed to inflict bodily damage to adult victims. The severity of injury sustained by the pediatric victim is therefore not un-expectedly much higher. This is particularly true for the soft and vulnerable tissues of the neonate and infant. In addition, the bony skeleton is incompletely mineralized, providing less resistance to the passage of missiles. A positive effect of this is that injury due to secondary bony missiles is rarely seen. Anecdotal experience on the effect of high-velocity military weapons such as rifles, grenades, and shrapnel, on children is that these weapons have extraordinary wounding and killing potential in the young child. During times of war, these injuries are particularly devastating and have a high mortality, particularly in young children. The tragedy of large populations of amputees, many of whom are children, in countries such as Angola and Mozambique is well known. They are the victims of antipersonnel mines laid in times of civil conflict. Some areas still have a multitude of unexploded mines lying in wait for innocent civilian victims. These weapons usually are designed to maim an adult soldier, but not necessarily to kill. Their effect on a young child is devastating and often fatal—for every amputee consigned to a life of disability in these under-resourced countries, there are many unpublicized fatalities.

In peacetime, children are often injured by air-powered missiles such as air rifle pellets. The wounding potential of these has become apparent. They frequently are responsible for injuries to the globe of the eye and have been documented to cause body cavity penetration, head injury, major vascular injury, and death. A significant number of patients experience long-term morbidity.[14-16] The ability of these weapons to inflict serious injury should not be overlooked. In the urban environment, especially in high-risk areas, children are usually injured by handguns. Shotgun wounds are not infrequently seen in both urban and rural areas. They are associated with high mortality rates.[17] High-velocity rifle injuries are uncommon, usually occurring in rural areas and usually as a result of hunting accidents. Children are frequently injured by arrows, crossbow bolts, darts, marine spearguns, and a miscellany of other penetrating missiles due to their intrinsic inquisitiveness and desire to experiment. Home-made bombs are well known to cause bizarre missile injuries, as well as thermal and chemical burns.

Prehospital Care and Resuscitation

Much debate still continues regarding the optimum approach to the prehospital care of trauma victims. Proponents of the "scoop and run" approach maintain that prolonged efforts at on-scene treatment only delays the arrival of the patient at the definitive care establishment and are deleterious, particularly in the patient with penetrating thoracic injury.[18] Most formal studies evaluating the efficiency of pediatric prehospital care have contained an overwhelming majority of blunt trauma victims.[19] Major penetrating injury in early life is frequently associated with hypovolemia and severe instability. It is precisely this group of patients who require rapid definitive surgical hemostasis for a successful outcome. On-scene fluid resuscitation has never been shown to be of value in this group of patients, and may indeed be detrimental. Venous access by any technique other than intraosseous puncture is difficult and likely to delay hospital transfer. In most areas, experience shows that effective prehospital care of children is only provided by personnel with advanced training who have the opportunity to regularly practice and update their skills. In many developed countries, prehospital personnel attend to severely injured children infrequently so that the individual practitioner has difficulty developing the necessary experience.[20]

In the case of the child with life-threatening penetrating injury, the prehospital staff should be able to provide airway interventions, effectively control external hemorrhage, establish venous access (with the use of intraosseous infusion if necessary), initiate *appropriate* fluid resuscitation, and rapidly transfer the patient safely to an appropriate "child capable" institution. The on-scene time should not exceed 10 minutes. If the above cannot be achieved for whatever reason, a "scoop and run" approach will probably ensure a better outcome, particularly if the transport time to a surgical facility is short.

The concept of delayed or hypotensive resuscitation for adult patients with penetrating truncal trauma is currently being investigated. In patients with ongoing blood loss requiring surgical hemostasis (e.g., major vascular injuries), the endpoints of resuscitation are not clear. It has been suggested recently that minimal volume resuscitation prior to surgical hemostasis in adults with penetrating abdominal trauma or ruptured abdominal aortic aneurysms may be beneficial.[21-24] It appears as if prolonged fluid resuscitation to attempt to produce hamodynamic normality—particularly if this resuscitation delays definitive surgical repair—is deleterious to the patient and is associated with a greater incidence of coagulopathy, hypothermia, and a poorer outcome. This approach may be unsuitable to blunt trauma patients with head injury, as it may decrease critical cerebral perfusion during the period of delay; conventional endpoint resuscitation is currently recommended in this group.[25] Prospective trials researching minimal volume resuscitation in the paediatric trauma population need to be done before any firm conclusion can be reached. In the patient with ongoing massive bleeding (without head injury) where it is clear that surgery will be required for hemostasis, resuscitation should probably be of *minimal duration*, with a goal of ensuring adequate venous access and the administration of sufficient fluid or blood to ensure adequate end organ perfusion. This patient should be transferred to the operating room without delay, where definitive hemostasis and further resuscitation can occur concurrently.

Head Injury

This is fortunately a rare injury in childhood. The prehospital mortality of cranial gunshot wounds in children is high. Pellet penetrations occur more commonly, and even these have been associated with fatal outcomes. Resuscitation of the severe cases should proceed along normal lines and often will include endotracheal intubation and ventilation. In the young baby with a compliant skull, life-threatening hypovolemia can ensue from intracranial bleeding. Vigorous arterial bleeding from injuries at the base of the skull often portends a poor prognosis.

After stabilization, all cases should be investigated by an emergency cranial computed tomography (CT) scan (Figure 19-1). This will provide important prognostic information and guide surgical intervention. Cranial arteriography is used less frequently today and is usually reserved for specific circumstances when deemed necessary by the attending neurosurgeon. Examples include deep-seated hematomas, traumatic arteriovenous fistulae or false aneurysms, and prior to the removal of retained blades or large missiles.

Children are uniquely susceptible to raised intracranial pressure caused by progressive cerebral edema with blunt injury. The role of intracranial pressure monitoring is well established in this situation, although its impact on survival remains unproven. Trans-hemispheric wounds commonly cause massive brain destruction, especially in young children, often causing death (Figure 19-2). In survivors, cerebral edema can occur and appears to be more frequently seen with higher-velocity missile injuries. It is currently recommended that intracranial pressure transducers be used whenever cerebral edema requires active treatment.[26] The development of posttraumatic hydrocephalus, although rare, should always be sought in the recovery

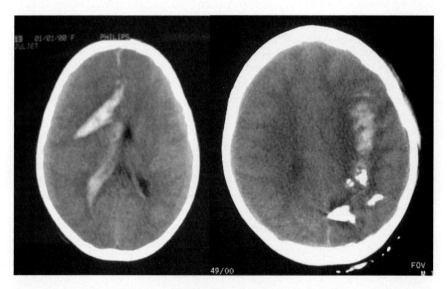

FIGURE 19-1. Left: A CT scan showing a linear intracerebral hemorrhage with intraventricular hemorrhage after an assault with a broad bladed knife (panga). Right: the bullet tract created by a 9-millimeter bullet traversing the left cerebral hemisphere of a three-year-old boy who was the victim of a family murder.

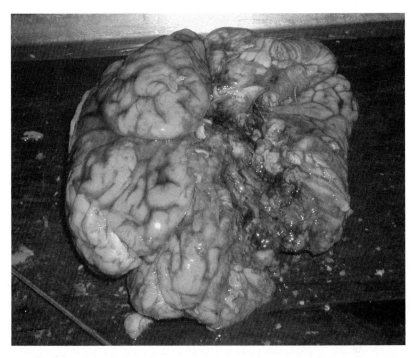

FIGURE 19-2. Autopsy findings in five-year-old sibling of patient B in Figure 19.1 showing massive damage to the frontal and temporal lobes after passage of a 9-millimeter missile.

period. Prophylactic antibiotics are used universally and should be of a broad spectrum. Anticonvulsant medication should be used to treat convulsions, but there is little evidence for their use prophylactically beyond the second week post injury. Specifically, they have not been shown to reduce the risk of post-injury epilepsy in the long term.

The surgical management of penetrating brain injury is controversial. In many instances the first decision to be taken is whether the patient's prospects for meaningful neurological recovery warrant aggressive surgery. Some patients with a poor neurological prognosis after thorough assessment are best treated by minimal local wound care. Generally accepted factors associated with a poor prognosis are presented in Table 19-1.

For civilian injuries, there is a tendency towards less-aggressive debridement without an apparent increase in infective complications. The decision to operate is best left to the attending neurosurgeon. Most will operate for significant intracranial hematomata, severely depressed skull fractures, and large open wounds with brain and dura exposed. The principles of wound debridement and cleaning, dural closure, and primary or flap closure are usually adhered to. For children with small penetrating wounds without

TABLE 19-1. Poor prognostic factors in patients with cranial gunshot wounds

Type of variable	Variable
Demographics	Younger age
Epidemiology	Suicide attempt
	Military injury
	High-caliber and -velocity weapon
	Perforating (through and through) injury
Systemic secondary insults	Hypotension
	Hypoxia
	Coagulation abnormalities
Neurological assessment	Level of consciousness (GCS 3-5)
	Fixed dilated or unequal pupils
	Raised intracranial pressure
Imaging features	Missile track through both hemispheres
	Passage through ventricle
	Evidence of raised intracranial pressure
	Hemorrhage or lesion with mass effect

Source: Modified from Florin RE, J Trauma. 2001;51:S44–S86.

severe tissue destruction, simple closure appears adequate. Prophylactic broad-spectrum antibiotics should be used. In most instances, no attempt is made to remove bullets during the acute phase, as this can result in worse cerebral edema and can be harmful. Bullets causing symptoms or seizures can be removed later as the clinical situation demands it.

Neck Injury

Selective conservatism of cervical stab injury is becoming increasingly more common in adult patients. The safety of this approach has been documented for Zone II stab injuries in children.[27] Its safety for gunshot and other missile injuries has not been satisfactorily ascertained and the clinician should use their discretion tempered with common sense. The proximity of vital structures in the small child's neck rarely permits its safe application in this group. If a conservative approach is adopted, angiography, endoscopy, and contrast esophagography should be used liberally (Figure 19-3). Angiography is recommended for Zone I and Zone III injuries, including in stable patients where surgery is planned. The need for angiography to assess the vasculature in patients with Zone II injuries being treated conservatively who do not have clinical signs of vascular injury is controversial. The approach should be individualized in each case, bearing in mind the risk of iatrogenic vascular injury that is present in young children. Air rifle pellet injuries, even those involving the retropharyngeal space, have successfully been treated conservatively.[28]

Penetrating vascular injuries in the cervical area generally require surgical exploration and repair. Venous injuries are treated by direct repair or ligation, and injuries to the carotid artery complex are treated by repair whenever feasible. Patency rates for arterial repairs and grafts of the internal carotid artery in children under five years of age are not good. In stable patients, repair using the operating microscope is an option if the injury lends itself to this. Most young healthy children have adequate vertebrobasilar collateral flow, allowing ligation as a safe, more practical alternative.

Spinal cord injury is not uncommon after gunshot wounds in the neck and torso. In the absence of other indications for cervical exploration, these patients are investigated by magnetic resonance scanning. Usually, direct cord injury is confirmed to be the cause of neurological deficit, but rarely an intraspinal hematoma is shown to be present, which should be decompressed. Unstable cervical bony injuries are rare and usually can be treated in a traction device at this age.

The use of methylprednisone therapy in these injuries is not supported by any evidence and is not recommended.

The recommended incisions for exploration of the child's neck are as follows:

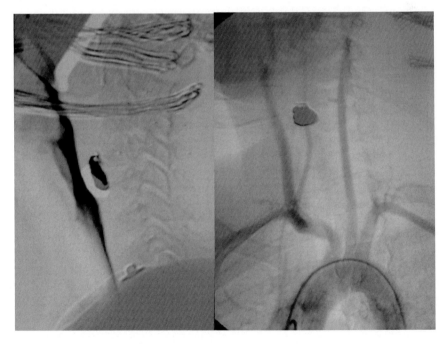

FIGURE 19-3. Ten-year-old boy with a bullet in the prevertebral space after Zone II injury. Barium swallow and angiogram performed as part of nonoperative management.

1. Anterior sternomastoid incision as the standard incision, especially where the need for exploration of the vascular structures of Zone I and III is anticipated. This incision affords optimal exposure of the internal carotid artery at the base of the skull and can easily be extended to a median sternotomy for control of mediastinal vascular structures.

2. Transverse collar incision is useful for transverse injuries in Zone II, especially where through-and-through injury exists to the upper trachea, larynx, and pharynx. Most concurrent vascular injuries are easily dealt with through such an incision, but it should be used with caution and is not advised in patients suspected of having vascular injuries of the skull base or root of the neck.

Thoracic Injury

Penetrating thoracic injuries carry a mortality of approximately 15% in early life and the thoracic injury is directly responsible for the death.[29] The small size of the child and the proximity of organs in the abdomen and chest make thoracoabdominal injuries more common in the younger age groups. High-velocity missile wounds to the chest can be devastating in early life, but these patients rarely reach the hospital alive. With the increasing incidence of pediatric gunshot wounds, the spectrum of injuries seen in childhood mirrors that seen in the adult population.

Technique of Insertion of a Chest Drain

The standard position recommended for intercostal drain placement is the fifth intercostal space in the anterior axillary line. It can be expected that the young child will be uncooperative with regard to the drain during the recovery period. For this reason, the drain should be well secured by both suture and skin strapping to ensure that the patient does not remove it prematurely. The skin incision should be placed one intercostal space below the intended space of chest entry to ensure a tunneled subcutaneous tract. This facilitates removal of the drain later to allow for direct pressure on the subcutaneous tract, thereby preventing air entering the pleural space and causing iatrogenic pneumothorax in a crying child. The drain should be placed primarily by blunt dissection; trocars are not used to avoid iatrogenic injury. The recommended size of intercostal drains at various ages is shown in Table 19-2.

Special Investigations Required

Every patient should have a chest X-ray in the erect position, if possible. The use of radiopaque markers (Figure 19-4) on any entrance or exit wounds facilitates interpretation of the films. In the unstable patient with clear signs of thoracic injury, chest decompression should be performed for

TABLE 19-2. Recommended chest drain sizes by age

Age	Size (Fr)
0–3 months	10–12
3–18 months	12–16
18–24 months	18
2–4 years	20–22
4–6 years	22–24
6–8 years	24–28
8–12 years	28–30
12–16 years	30–34

a suspected tension pneumothorax and a chest drain can be placed without radiological confirmation of the presence of an injury. For stable patients, treatment should be delayed until a chest X-ray can be obtained.

If the chest X-ray or the patient's clinical signs are suggestive of specific organ injury, further investigations may be needed. Sometimes thoracic ultrasonography is helpful to detect small collections of blood in the pleural

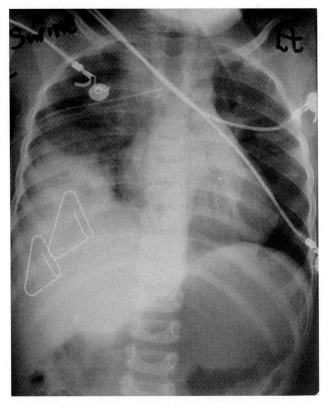

FIGURE 19-4. Four-year-old male with gunshot wound right lower chest showing use of radiopaque markers.

space. Echocardiography is requested whenever there is a possibility of cardiac injury in a stable patient. Liquid-soluble contrast swallows and esophagoscopy are used to diagnose suspected esophageal injury and bronchosopy is used to diagnose major airway injury.

All patients who have evidence of trans-mediastinal wounds without clear clinical indications for thoracotomy are subjected to arch aortography, esophagoscopy, and bronchosopy, if indicated, in order to exclude serious injury.

Computed tomography (CT) scanning has little place in the acute investigation of the child with a penetrating chest injury.

Thoracoscopy

Thoracoscopy is increasingly being used to assess the diaphragm or intrathoracic structures after penetrating injury in children. It should be reserved for those patients without clinical indications for emergency thoracotomy (see below), and only in stable patients. Studies in adult patients have indicated that the use of thoracoscopy may exclude injuries and reduce the need for formal thoracotomy in equivocal cases.[30] It is probably the most efficient modality to assess the diaphragm for injury, which can be easily repaired using a stapling device[31] or intracorporeal suturing. In this situation, there is always the risk of a missed abdominal injury. Either the abdomen can be assessed concurrently by laparoscopy or the thoracoscopy can be used as a screening test, mandating an exploratory laparotomy when a diaphragmatic injury is found. Laparoscopy has its advocates, and in skilled hands is an option for stable patients without a large hemoperitoneum. In most, a laparotomy seems the safest and simplest option.

In our environment, a sterilized fiberoptic gastroscope has been used to assess the integrity of the diaphragm in cases of blunt and penetrating trauma. The intercostal drain is removed and the scope is passed through the drain tract into the chest. This allows any residual hemothorax to be evacuated by suction and the lung can be collapsed by air insufflation and the diaphragm inspected. The procedure is well tolerated and can be performed without general anesthesia in the emergency room.[32]

Indications for Thoracotomy

Resuscitative Thoracotomy

The place of emergency department thoracotomy is one of the ongoing controversies in the management of the injured patient. It is probably better termed Resuscitative Thoracotomy (RT), indicating its role as an adjunct to resuscitation when the patient does not respond to conventional resuscitation. A number of studies have addressed the role of RT in pediatric trauma.[33-36] Previously, children were assumed to have greater physiological reserve and hence RT was applied liberally in an attempt to salvage desperate situations. Cumulative experience to date indicates that RT should be reserved for the following categories of pediatric patients after penetrating trauma:

1. Penetrating thoracic injury with deterioration or poor response despite vigorous resuscitation;
2. Patients with penetrating thoracic injury who present with no signs of life to the emergency room but with a recently witnessed cardiac arrest.

Under these circumstances, salvage rates of between four and 26% can be expected depending on the mechanism of injury and local circumstances.[33,35] Children with penetrating abdominal trauma who do not respond to resuscitation should be transferred immediately to the operating room where the operation and prompt surgical hemostasis can be carried out concurrently with further fluid resuscitation. Results of RT for patients with penetrating abdominal injuries who present without vital signs are so dismal that it cannot be advocated.

Definitive Thoracotomy

Most (approximately 80%) penetrating thoracic injuries in children can be satisfactorily managed by placement of an intercostal drain alone.[37] Patients with gunshot injuries may require surgery more frequently, especially in the younger age groups.[38,39] Accepted indications for emergency thoracotomy include:

1. Brisk thoracic hemorrhage and ongoing hemodynamic instability or deterioration.
2. Evidence of cardiac tamponade or posttraumatic pericardial effusion.
3. Evidence of major airway injury.
4. Evidence of esophageal injury.

Ongoing bleeding requiring blood transfusion of greater than 50% of blood volume or at a rate of greater than one to two milliliters per kilogram per hour may be an indication for thoracotomy depending on the circumstances.

Incisions for Access

Children tolerate all types of incisions for thoracic access better than their adult counterparts. Their inherent good health and cardiopulmonary reserves mean that postoperative ventilation is usually not necessary and intensive care stays are much shorter. Complications related to the wound, pleural fluid collections, and atelectasis occur infrequently, and children can usually be mobilized out of bed as early as the first postoperative day without any difficulty. Pain is easily controlled by a combination of intercostal nerve blocks and opiate analgesia.

The incision used for access to the chest varies depending upon the side of injury and the anticipated surgery required.

Resuscitative Thoracotomy

Performed by a left anterolateral thoracotomy through the fifth intercostal space. If there is a penetrating injury to the right hemithorax with obvious bleeding from that cavity, then a right anterolateral thoracotomy is preferred. The anterolateral approach gives adequate emergency room access to the heart, aorta, and pulmonary hilum, and can always be extended posteriorly for better definitive access in the operating room.

Definitive Thoracotomy

Is usually performed through a sixth or seventh intercostal space approach in the posterolateral position.

Median Sternotomy

In the young child with flexible ribs, the degree of exposure that can de achieved gives excellent access to the heart, major vessels, trachea, both lungs, and pleural cavities. The sternum can quickly and easily be divided by using a pair of Mayo-type scissors in the younger child or osteotomy shears in the older child. Sternotomy is therefore an excellent incision for general access to the child's chest in the trauma situation and should always be used if there is a suspicion of cardiac or major vessel injury, or if the side of the injury is not clinically obvious.

"Clam Shell" Incision

Extending an anterolateral thoracotomy transversely across the sternum and through the opposite intercostal space (sometimes referred to as a sternothoracotomy) gives excellent exposure to the chest contents, with the possible exception of the mediastinal great vessels. This option can be used in instances where a resuscitative anterolateral thoracotomy suggests an injury such as a cardiac or contralateral pulmonary hilar injury that cannot comfortably be dealt with through the initial incision. This situation is not encountered commonly, but the incision is becoming increasingly popular for elective surgical procedures such as bilateral pulmonary metastasectomy and lung and heart transplantation,[40,41] and it has been used in children and infants for cardiac surgery with good results.[42] Care must be taken when closing the incision to achieve careful approximation of the sternum by using K-wires or stainless steel wires, otherwise unsightly overlapping of the sternum may result.

Abdominal Injury

No specific distinction is made between high-velocity gunshot wounds and low-velocity injuries sustained typically from handgun injuries except to recognize the devastating wounding potential of the former weapons in small children. High-velocity injuries from weapons such as military assault rifles and hunting rifles are fortunately rare in children, but carry a high mortality, with most patients dying at the scene of injury. Clinical experience is therefore mainly derived from the management of civilian handgun injuries.

In adults, the policy of selective conservative management for penetrating abdominal stab wounds and other low-velocity penetrating injuries is well established.[43] Data documenting the safety of selective conservative treatment strategies for penetrating injuries in children are sparse. This is probably a result of the relative rarity of these injuries and the inability of single centers to compile a sufficient number of cases in order to construct prospective controlled trials. It has been our policy and those of other units to adopt a policy of selective conservatism in pediatric abdominal stab wounds. The usually thin anterior abdominal wall of the child favors accurate clinical assessment of peritonism. With bullet wounds, shrapnel injuries, and other high-velocity missiles that penetrate the peritoneal cavity, the chance of visceral injury requiring operative intervention is much greater and exploratory laparotomy is mandatory.

Diagnostic Peritoneal Lavage (DPL)

Diagnostic peritoneal lavage has little role in the assessment of the child with suspected penetrating abdominal injury. It requires a general anesthetic in the conscious child and compromises the clinical assessment of the abdomen by virtue of the associated pain thereafter. Stab and other low-velocity missile wounds are usually treated by selective conservatism and abdominal gunshot wounds are submitted to laparotomy. Two potential indications for DPL in penetrating injury in children are the assessment of the diaphragm and the assessment of peritoneal penetration. Thoracoscopy and laparoscopy, respectively, are superior in this situation and provide more specific information.

Incisions

The infant and young child (up to three years of age) has a round abdomen. The transverse supra-umbilical laparotomy incision serves very well as the standard incision for access to the abdomen for non-trauma surgery in this age group. It suffers from two main disadvantages in the trauma situation when the nature of the required surgery is notoriously unpredictable:

1. It does not allow for extensions of the incision in a cranial or caudal direction to gain access to the pelvic area and epigastrium, if required. Exposure of the bladder and rectum can be awkward in a child outside the neonatal period.

2. It cannot be extended directly into a median sternotomy to allow for direct cardiac massage, deal with any unexpected cardiac injury, or allow access to the great vessels. If a transverse laparotomy is extended upwards into a sternotomy, this results in a cosmetically unsatisfactory wound and the problem of having to close the abdominal wall at the junction of the two incisions.

For these reasons, one should consider the use of a midline incision as the standard access to deal with penetrating and ballistic injuries in children (Figure 19-5).

Special Situations for Consideration

Is the Injury Penetrating?

In the case of stab wounds and other low-velocity injuries, it is not critically important to determine whether penetration has occurred or not, as these wounds will usually be managed by selective conservatism in the absence of bleeding or peritonitis (although they may penetrate the abdominal cavity). In the case of patients with gunshot or missile wounds, our approach has been to operate if there is any suspicion of abdominal cavity penetration.

The Patient Presenting in Shock

Children presenting with penetrating abdominal injury and shock should be prepared for immediate exploratory laparotomy. Blood should be urgently crossmatched, initial venous access obtained, and the patient transferred as rapidly as possible to the operating room. where surgical hemostasis and further resuscitation should occur together. There should be no undue delays for X-rays or ultrasound investigations. These patients should always be sent to the nearest capable institution and never spend prolonged time in transportation and transfer between hospitals, if at all possible.

Workup of Penetrating Injuries with Hematuria

Stable patients with hematuria and penetrating abdominal injuries are investigated by contrast studies of the lower tract or emergency room excretory urography, or both if deemed clinically relevant. The information obtained is useful to plan operative strategy and to localize the site of injury; it also confirms the function and position of the contralateral kidney in case nephrectomy is required.

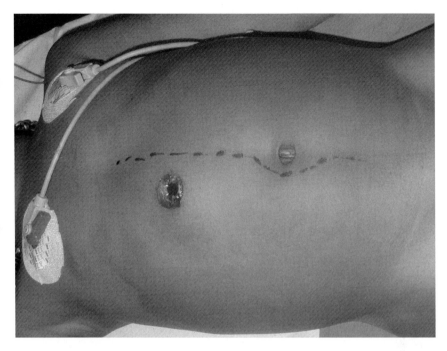

FIGURE 19-5. Two-year-old girl with epigastric gunshot wound illustrating the use of the midline incision.

Peripheral Vascular

Gunshot wounds causing major peripheral vascular injury are an unusual clinical problem in children. The challenges of vascular repair procedures in the under-five age group are significant, with poor patency rates being the historical norm. The ongoing evolution of microvascular techniques has resulted in recent improvements in results in small children.

The Role of Angiography

The diagnosis of a vascular injury usually is clinically evident, presenting with vigorous bleeding, an expanding hematoma or false aneurysm, or signs of vascular insufficiency. In general, clinical examination is sufficient to make the diagnosis and to decide on the need for operative intervention.[44] The use of Doppler Artery Pressure Index (the systolic arterial pressure measured by Doppler in the injured limb divided by the systolic pressure in the uninjured limb) has been shown to reliably exclude extremity major vascular injury in adults.[45] A threshold of 0.9 is used to indicate a probable arterial injury. This technique is simple, quick, and inexpensive, and it should be a routine part of the vascular assessment of any limb in which an arterial injury is not clinically evident but needs to be ruled out.

In specialized centers, arteriography can be safely performed with low complication rates, even in young children. It is associated with higher complication rates when performed by the inexperienced or occasional operator and should only be performed when the presentation is atypical or the physical signs are equivocal. The role of angiography to detect arterial injury when a penetrating injury is anatomically in proximity to the vascular structures, but in the absence of signs of vascular injury, has largely been discredited in adult trauma practice,[46,47] and studies have confirmed this for the pediatric population as well.[48] The reason for this is that injuries are rarely found and are usually not of sufficient severity to require repair. There is some controversy as to whether it is important to detect such minor arterial injuries in children[49] (where their presence may result in growth retardation), but these are usually treated conservatively in any event. There are no long-term follow-up studies to give guidelines for the management of these occult arteriographically detected lesions in children. The current practice in most units is to keep the patient under surveillance and to intervene if patients experience claudication or growth retardation in the affected limb.

Conservative Management

It is generally accepted that all major vascular injuries in childhood are treated by prompt exploration and repair with revascularization. This is true for all cases of penetrating trauma where there are signs of ischemia or where the surgeon needs to control bleeding or repair traumatic arteriovenous fistulae.

The generally excellent cardiovascular status of the young child provides for the establishment of an efficient collateral circulation after acute injury. Even when complete vascular occlusion has occurred, there may be no signs of acute ischemia. This is particularly true in the axillary and brachial arteries. Many children present with clear signs of an arterial injury, but with no evidence of ischemia or limb threat. If these patients are operated on in an attempt to restore flow, the surgeon may do harm by interfering with the collateral circulation and converting a stable situation where neither the limb nor patient is threatened to one of limb threat. This is particularly likely in the young child, where the vascular anastamosis is most technically challenging. It is recommended that under these circumstances, if there is no other urgent need for operation, that the patient be observed.[50] The Doppler Arterial Pressure Index (API) is helpful under these circumstances. An index of greater than 0.6 indicates sufficient arterial perfusion by collaterals. These patients must be carefully followed. If the patient develops claudication or growth retardation of the affected limb, elective vascular repair can be performed at a later date. In the small number of patients that we have treated in this way, chronic ischemia has not occurred.

Arterial Spasm

Arterial spasm is said to occur with greater frequency in pediatric arterial injury than in the adult. The frequency with which it is reported varies from series to series. It is usually reported to be present in patients with blunt trauma where arteriography demonstrates an abnormality, but where, at exploration, there is narrowing of the vessel but no macroscopically visible injury.[44] Vasospasm is thought to occur when there is a shear injury or contusion to a blood vessel. This results in anatomical or functional separation of the endothelium and the media. The constant vasodilatory effect maintained by endothelial production of nitric oxide is therefore lost and the vessel goes into prolonged spasm.[51] The small caliber of pediatric vessels makes them particularly vulnerable to the spasm thus produced.[52] The role of spasm in penetrating arterial trauma is less clear. Generally, exploration for penetrating injury reveals a clearly injured vessel. Spasm certainly occurs in the artery being anastamosed, but this usually resolves after successful anastamosis or can be diminished by the topical application of papaverine.

It is important that all patients with clinical or arteriographic signs of a vascular injury after penetrating injury are assumed to have a vascular injury and treated appropriately. If signs of ischemia are present, the area of injury must be promptly explored. It is dangerous and usually erroneous to assume that the condition is due to spasm and therefore self-limiting. This may delay exploration and repair of the vessel and decrease the chances of successful revascularization (Figure 19-6).

Techniques of Repair and Revascularization

Many injuries can be managed by mobilization of the vessel ends, excision, and primary end-to-end anastamosis. If this is not possible without tension, then bypass grafting should be performed. Reversed vein grafts are preferred because they have better patency rates in small vessels and have the potential to grow with the patient. Anastamoses in children should be performed by using an interrupted suture technique to allow for an increase in the vessel diameter with growth. Most peripheral vessels are best sutured with 6-0 or 7-0 polypropylene and the use of magnification is mandatory. Systemic heparinization generally is not used.

Venous injuries when encountered are treated by simple repair if this is feasible without significant narrowing of the vein. In most peripheral venous injuries, there is an excellent system of venous collaterals, which makes complex repairs of venous injuries unnecessary. The superior vena cava and the suprarenal inferior vena cava are the only veins that should

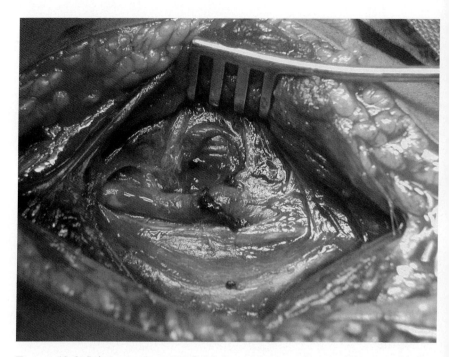

FIGURE 19-6. Injury to the superficial femoral artery in an eight-year-old boy. Appearance at the time of exploration for "spasm."

always be repaired. The injured vein should be ligated if repair with a reasonable chance of success cannot be achieved without compromising the patient (by excessive blood loss and prolonged operating time). Any postoperative venous engorgement that ensues will be manageable by supportive treatment. One notable exception is the popliteal artery and vein injury where, like in adults, every attempt should be made to restore both arterial and venous flow because of the well-known risks of venous hypertension in this situation.

Fetal Injury

Occasionally, the surgeon is called upon to treat a preterm baby injured during penetrating maternal trauma. This situation is typically seen in the third trimester, is usually a stabbing injury, and the mother often knows the perpetrator. Although pregnant mothers do suffer abdominal gunshot wounds, the survival prospects for these fetuses are slim.

References

1. Vane D, Shedd FG, Grosfeld JL, Franiak RJ, Ulrich JC, West KW, Rescorla FJ. An analysis of pediatric trauma deaths in Indiana. *J Pediatr Surg.* 1990;9:955–960.
2. From the Centers for Disease Control. Unintentional firearm-related fatalities among children, teenagers—United States, 1982–1988. *JAMA.* 1992;268:451–452.
3. Unintentional firearm-related fatalities among children and teenagers—United States, 1982–1988. MMWR Morb Mortal Wkly Rep, 1992 Jun, 41:25, 442–5, 451.
4. Cummings P, Grossman DC, Rivara FP, Koepsell. State gun safe storage laws and child mortality due to firearms. *JAMA.* 1997; 278:1084–1086.
5. Powell EC, Tanz RR. Child and adolescent injury and death from urban firearm assaults: Association with age, race, and poverty. *Inj Prev.* 1999;5:41–47.
6. Nance ML, Stafford PW, Schwab CW. Firearm injury among urban youth during the last decade: An escalation in violence. *J Pediatr Surg.* 1997;32:949–952.
7. Copeland AR. Childhood firearms fatalities: The Metropolitan Dade County experience. *South Med J.* 1991;84:175–178.
8. Rates of homicide, suicide, and firearm-related death among children—26 industrialized countries. *MMWR Morb Mortal Wkly Rep.* 1997;46:101–115.
9. Krug EG, Dahlberg LL, Powell KE. Childhood homicide, suicide, and firearm deaths: An international comparison. *World Health Stat Q.* 1996;49:230–235.
10. Patterson PJ, Holguin AH. Firearm-related deaths among children in Texas: 1984–1988. *Tex Med.* 1990;86:92–97.
11. Dowd MD, Knapp JF, Fitzmaurice LS. Pediatric firearm injuries, Kansas City, 1992: a population-based study. *Pediatrics.* 1994;94:867–873.
12. Wigton A. Firearm-related injuries and deaths among children and adolescents in Cape Town—1992–1996. *S Afr Med J.* 1999;89:407–410.
13. Hadley GP, Mars M.S. Gunshot injuries in infants and children in KwaZulu-Natal—an emerging epidemic? *Afr Med J.* 1998;88:444–447.
14. Scribano PV, Nance M, Reilly P, Sing RF, Selbst SM. Pediatric nonpowder firearm injuries: Outcomes in an urban pediatric setting. *Pediatrics.* 1997;100:E5.
15. Bratton SL, Dowd MD, Brogan TV, Hegenbarth MA. Serious and fatal air gun injuries: more than meets the eye. *Pediatrics.* 1997;100:609–612.
16. Bhattacharyya N, Bethel CA, Caniano DA, Pillai SB, Deppe S, Cooney DR. The childhood air gun: Serious injuries and surgical interventions. *Pediatr Emerg Care.* 1998;14:188–190.
17. Nance ML, Sing RF, Branas CC, Schwab CW. Shotgun wounds in children. Not just accidents. *Arch Surg.* 1997;132:58–62.
18. Ivatury RR, Nallathambi MN, Roberge RJ. Penetrating thoracic injuries: In field stabilisation vs prompt transport. *J Trauma.* 1987;27:1066–1072.
19. Paul TR, Marias M, Pons PT, Pons KA, Moore EE. Adult vs paediatric prehospital trauma care. Is there a difference? *J Trauma.* 1999;47:455–459.
20. Gaffney P, Johnson G. Paediatric prehospital trauma care. *Trauma.* 1999;1:279–284.
21. Bickell WH, Wall MJ Jr, Pepe PE, Martin RR, Ginger VF, Allen MK, Mattox KL. Immediate versus delayed fluid resuscitation for hypotensive patients with penetrating torso injuries. *N Engl J Med.* 1994; 331:1105–1109.

22. Bickell WH, Barrett SM, Romine Jenkins M, Hull SS Jr, Kinasewitz GT. Resuscitation of canine hemorrhagic hypotension with large-volume isotonic crystalloid: Impact on lung water, venous admixture, and systemic arterial oxygen saturation. *Am J Emerg Med*. 1994;12:36–42.

23. Bickell WH, Bruttig SP, Millnamow GA, O'Benar J, Wade CE. Use of hypertonic saline/dextran versus lactated Ringer's solution as a resuscitation fluid after uncontrolled aortic hemorrhage in anesthetized swine. *Ann Emerg Med*. 1992;21:1077–1085.

24. Bickell WH. Are victims of injury sometimes victimized by attempts at fluid resuscitation? *Ann Emerg Med*. 1993;22:225–226.

25. Wright JL. Patterson MD. Resuscitating the pediatric patient. *Emerg Med Clin North Am*. 1996;14:219–231.

26. Sarnaik AP, Kopec J, Moylan P, Alvarez D, Canady A. Role of aggressive intracranial pressure control in management of pediatric craniocerebral gunshot wounds with unfavorable features. *J Trauma*. 1989;29(10):1434–1437.

27. Hall JR, Reyes HM, Meller JL. Penetrating zone-II neck injuries in children. *J Trauma*. 1991;31(12):1614–1617.

28. Mitchell RB, Pereira KD, Younis RT, Lazar RH. The management of asymptomatic firearm injuries in children. *J R Coll Surg Edinb*. 1997;42(6):418–419.

29. Cooper A, Barlow B, Di Scala C, String D. Mortality and truncal injury: the pediatric perspective. *J Pediatr Surg*. 1994;29:33–38.

30. Mineo TC, Ambrogi V, Cristino B, Pompeo E, Pistolese C. Changing indications for thoracotomy in blunt chest trauma after the advent of videothoracoscopy. *J Trauma*. 1999;47:1088–1091.

31. Chen MK, Schropp KP, Lobe TE. The use of minimal access surgery in pediatric trauma: A preliminary report. *J Laparoendosc Surg*. 1995;5:295–301.

32. Pitcher GJ. Fiber-endoscopic thoracoscopy for diaphragmatic injury in children. *Semin Pediatr Surg*. 2001;10:17–19.

33. Powell RW, Gill EA, Jurkovich GJ, Ramenovsky ML. Resuscitative thoracotomy in children and adolescents. *Am J Surg*. 1988;54:188–191.

34. Rothenberg SS, Moore EE, Moore FA, Baxter BT, Moore JB, Cleveland HC. Emergency department thoracotomy in children—a critical analysis. *J Trauma*. 1989;29:1322–1325.

35. Beaver BL, Moore VL, Peclet M, Haller JA, Smialek J, Hill JL. Efficacy of emergency room thoracotomy in paediatric trauma. *J Pediatr Surg*. 1987;22:19–23.

36. Sheikh AA, Culbertson CB. Emergency department thoracotomy in children: Rationale for selective application. *J Trauma*. 1993;34:323–328.

37. Inci I, Ozcelic C, Nizam O, Eren N, Ozgen G. Penetrating chest injuries in children: A review of 94 cases. *J Pediatr Surg*. 1996;31:673–676.

38. Nance ML, Sing RF, Reilly PM, Templeton JM, Schwab CW. Thoracic gunshot wounds in children under 17 years of age. *J Pediatr Surg*. 1996;31:931–935.

39. Peterson R, Tepas JJ 3rd, Edwards FH, Kissoon N, Pieper P, Ceithaml EL. Pediatric and adult thoracic trauma: Age-related impact on presentation and outcome. *Ann Thorac Surg*. 1994;58:14–18.

40. Bains MS, Gisnberg RJ, Jones WG 2nd, Mc Cormack PM, Rusch VW, Burt ME, Martini N. The clamshell incision: An improved approach to bilateral pulmonary and mediastinal tumor. *Ann Thorac Surg*. 1994;58(1):30–33.

41. Shimizu J, Oda M, Morita K, Watanabe S, Ohta Y, Hayashi Y, Murakami S, Watanabe Y. Evaluation of the clamshell incision for bilateral pulmonary metastases. *Int Surg.* 1997;82(3):262–265.
42. Luciani GB, Starnes VA. The clamshell approach for the surgical treatment of complex cardiopulmonary pathology in infants and children. *Eur J Cardiothorac Surg.* 1997;11(2):298–306.
43. Shorr RM, Gottlieb MM, Webb K, Ishiguro L, Berne TV. Selective management of abdominal stab wounds: Importance of the physical examination. *Arch Surg.* 1988;123:1141–1145.
44. Mills RP, Robbs JV. Paediatric arterial injury: Management options at the time of injury. *J R Coll Surg Edinb.* 1991;36:13–17.
45. Johansen K, Lynch K, Paun M, Copass M. Non-invasive vascular tests reliably exclude occult arterial trauma in injured extremities. *J Trauma.* 1991;31:515–522.
46. Gahtan V. The role of emergent arteriography in penetrating limb trauma. *Am Surg.* 1994;60:123–127.
47. Weaver FA, Yellin AE, Bauer M, Oberg J, Ghalambor N, Emmanuel RP, Applebaum RM, Pentecost MJ, Shorr RM. Is arterial proximity a valid indication for arteriography in penetrating extremity trauma? A prospective analysis. *Arch Surg.* 1990;125:1256–1260.
48. Reichard KW, Hall JR, Meller JL, Spigos D, Reyes HM. Arteriography in the evaluation of penetrating pediatric extremity injuries. *J Pediatr Surg.* 1994;29:19–22.
49. Itani KM, Rothenberg SS, Brandt ML, Burch JM, Mattox KL, Harberg FJ, Pokorny WJ. Emergency center arteriography in the evaluation of suspected peripheral vascular injuries in children. *J Pediatr Surg.* 1993;28:677–680.
50. Frykberg ER, Crump JM, Dennis JW, Vines FS, Alexander RH. Nonoperative observation of clinically occult arterial injuries: a prospective evaluation. *Surgery.* 1991;109:85–96.
51. Kuo PC, Schroeder RA. The emerging multifaceted roles of nitric oxide. *Ann Surg.* 1995;221:220–235.
52. Reichard KW, Reyes HM. Vascular trauma and reconstructive approaches. *Semin Pediatr Surg.* 1994;3:124–132.

20
Injuries in Pregnancy

PAUL D. WALLMAN and ADAM J. BROOKS

Introduction

Trauma is an increasing cause of morbidity and mortality in pregnancy, accounting for approximately seven percent of maternal fatalities, and is the most common case of non-obstetric maternal death. Even minor trauma can result in serious fetomaternal complications, including premature labor, placental abruption, and fetal injury. In most communities, blunt trauma accounts for the majority of injuries in pregnant women; however, in some series, penetrating trauma is responsible for 20% of the injuries seen in pregnant patients.

As pregnancy progresses, a series of specific anatomical and physiological adaptations occur that bring with them altered injury patterns, unique complications, and a change in the response to injury. It is essential that those involved in the management of ballistic injury in a pregnant patient understand these changes so that appropriate care can be provided for both the mother and her unborn child.

All female trauma victims of child-bearing age must be considered to be pregnant until proven otherwise.

Relevant Anatomy and Physiology of Pregnancy

The most striking anatomical alteration during pregnancy is the development of the uterus from a pelvic organ in the non-pregnant female to an intra-abdominal organ as the pregnancy develops. By the twentieth week, when the uterus has reached the umbilicus, the abdominal viscera are displaced up toward the diaphragm and the uterus becomes exposed to the same hazards as the intraperitoneal structures. As the pregnancy progresses, the uterus shields the mother from penetrating trauma, with the incidence of maternal organ damage following gunshot wounds being quite low. At this stage, the uterus is thin walled, the amniotic fluid volume is decreased, and *the full-term pregnant uterus is highly vulnerable to ballistic trauma.*

A series of physiological adaptations occur during pregnancy that may complicate the resuscitation and can alter the physiological response to injury.

Cardiovascular System

- 50% increase in plasma volume
- slight increase in hemoglobin, but not as marked as the plasma volume, therefore the hematocrit is decreased (*physiological anemia of pregnancy*)
- increase in cardiac output by 1.0 to 1.5 liters per minute
- increase in heart rate by 5 to 15 beats per minute
- 5 to 15 millimeters Hg decrease in blood pressure during the second trimester, returning to normal by term
- during the later stages of pregnancy, in the supine position, the gravid uterus can compress the inferior vena cava, reducing the venous return and hence cardiac output (supine maternal hypotension)

The maternal volume expansion allows for a greater absolute volume loss, up to 1.5 liters, prior to signs of maternal shock, although the fetus may already be in distress.

Respiratory System

- hyperventilation due to increased oxygen requirements
- 50% increase in tidal volume and minute ventilation
- functional residual capacity is reduced
- partially compensated respiratory alkalosis

The other organ systems are also affected during pregnancy. Displacement of the abdominal viscera leads to delayed gastric emptying and failure of the lower esophageal sphincter. This combination increases the risk of aspiration of stomach contents.

Initial Assessment and Management

The initial assessment and management of the pregnant patient with ballistic injury should follow the doctrine provided throughout this book. In order to optimize the outcome of both mother and fetus, it is essential to assess, identify, and resuscitate the mother first, and then subsequently address the needs of the fetus. Early consultation with an obstetrician is vital to the outcome of both patients.

The adaptations of pregnancy described previously can alter the patterns and manifestation of injury. The alterations that have a potential impact on the resuscitation of the pregnant patient are highlighted below.

Airway

- There is an increased risk of aspiration due to gastric reflux and delayed gastric emptying; therefore, the stomach should be decompressed early with a nasogastric tube.
- Endotracheal intubation can be complicated by edema of the neck or epiglottis.

Cervical Spine Control

- Cervical spine management remains as detailed in the chapters on pre-hospital care and spinal injury.

Breathing

- The pregnant patient is resuscitated in the standard way and high-flow oxygen should be administered to ensure a high FiO_2.

Circulation

- Due to an increased circulatory volume, the mother may compensate for a long period before signs of hypovolemia become apparent.
- The utero-placental circulation will be sacrificed to maintain the mother's cardiovascular status. The fetal circulation will therefore be reduced and may result in a poor fetal outcome.
- Early intravenous access and volume replacement are essential prior to definitive control for minimal morbidity and mortality to the patient and fetus.
- These procedures should not delay early surgical intervention or early cesarean section when required (see *Surgical and Obstetric Intervention*).

The maternal physiological preference may result in the fetus being in shock while the mother's cardiovascular vital signs and condition remains stable.

- Supine maternal hypotension exacerbates cardiovascular compromise. In the absence of spinal injury requiring immobilization, the patient can be managed in the left lateral position; alternatively, the right pelvis can be tilted upwards on a spinal board or with a rolled towel. Otherwise an individual can be allocated to manually displace the uterus to the patient's left-hand side, thus holding the uterus "off" the inferior vena cava (IVC).

In addition to the usual blood tests, serum beta human chorio-gonadotrophin and analysis for the Rhesus antibody should be performed. Full monitoring of the mother's physiological parameters is required and electronic fetal monitoring is an essential adjunct if available.

Assessment of the Pregnant Abdomen

The change in position of the intra-abdominal organs that occurs as pregnancy progresses must be considered when abdominal ballistic wounds and likely injury patterns are being evaluated. As part of the abdominal examination, a thorough examination of the perineum, vagina, and rectum must be performed, in addition to an assessment of the uterus and upper abdomen. Free drainage of clear amniotic fluid, cervical dilatation, fetal presentation, and concealed or occult bleeding must be excluded. Rectal examination may add information regarding bowel, uterine/fetal, and pelvic injury.

Investigations

In ballistic trauma to the abdomen, little investigation is usually required, as laparotomy is usually indicated; however, ultrasound is a useful diagnostic tool in the evaluation of the pregnant abdomen, as it can be used to assess for fetal well being and intrauterine pathology, as well as intra-abdominal bleeding. CT can also be considered where trajectory is in doubt in the stable patient in the late stages of pregnancy.

If peritoneal penetration is truly in doubt, diagnostic peritoneal lavage may rarely be used to guide the decision for laparotomy, but it is invasive and should be performed well above the umbilicus by an experienced surgeon.

Plain radiography is indicated as for the non-pregnant patient; however, the minimum number of X-rays should be performed to obtain maximum information. Bullet markers can be used to help determine uterine penetration and therefore the chance of fetal injury.

A Pinnard's stethoscope or Doppler fetoscopy should be immediately available to identify the presence of a fetal heartbeat. Continuous electronic fetal heart-rate monitoring is the modality of choice in most institutions and provides information on the fetal heart rhythm, including abnormal rate, decelerations, accelerations, and beat-to-beat variability. A normal fetal heart-rate pattern has at least a 95% correlation with good fetal perfusion.

Surgical and Obstetric Intervention

Early involvement of an experienced surgeon and obstetrician is central to the reduction of morbidity and mortality in these patients. Risk assessment involves balancing the well being of the mother versus the well being of the fetus. In addition, fetal well being must be assessed in terms of the risk in utero versus the risk of premature delivery.

As pregnancy progresses, the bowel is displaced and compressed upwards by the uterus, making it vulnerable to gunshot wounds to the upper abdomen and liable to multiple perforations. The enlarged uterus acts as a shield for the mother; lower abdominal wounds nearly exclusively involve the uterus and its contents, which act to absorb the energy of the missile. This clearly places the fetus in jeopardy; gunshot wounds to the uterus are associated with a fetal mortality of 70%, with a maternal mortality of less than ten percent. Fetal survival following ballistic injury is also dependent on gestation, with gestations less than 37 weeks having much worse survival.

Extra-uterine abdominal ballistic injuries are managed as previously discussed in this book, although in the later stages of pregnancy the uterus can impede access and mobilization of the viscera. Abdominal injuries and the need for a laparotomy do not alone justify cesarean section (c-section). Urgent c-section has only been recommended in cases of severe maternal shock in near-term pregnancies, fetal distress in excess of the risk of premature delivery, exsanguinating injury, and unstable thoracolumbar spine injury.

Ballistic Injuries in the Pregnant Patient: Special Considerations

All torso ballistic injuries in the pregnant patient may give rise to spillage of fetal blood into the maternal circulation. If the fetus is Rhesus antibody positive and is being carried by a Rhesus antibody negative mother, then there is the potential for maternal sensitization to occur even with minimal volume. Isoimmunization, the production of antibodies against the Rhesus positive fetus, can result, and appropriate treatment should be considered all cases.

Post-mortem cesarean section is only justified where there is a viable (greater than 26 week gestation) fetus and the mother is dead or moribund. Under optimal conditions, there is a 40 to 70% chance of fetal survival without major disability. However, as the elapsed time increases, the chance of survival falls and 70% of surviving infants will be delivered within five minutes of maternal death.

Summary

All members of the trauma team must appreciate the unique differences in caring for the pregnant victim of ballistic trauma.

- All female trauma victims of child-bearing age must be considered to be pregnant until proven otherwise.
- Early involvement of both a surgeon and obstetrician is required to minimize morbidity and mortality in both patients.
- Members of the trauma team should have a basic knowledge of the anatomical and physiological alterations that occur in pregnancy.

- The initial trauma approach remains the same as all other patients—the mother is treated first and the fetus second.
- Rapid and meticulous assessment must exclude general life-threatening pathologies, and those injuries unique to pregnancy must be considered.
- The fetus may be in jeopardy despite apparent minor injury to the mother.

Further Reading

Buschbaum HJ. Penetrating injury of the abdomen. In: Buschbaum HJ, ed. *Trauma in Pregnancy*. Philadelphia: WB Saunders Co; 1979:43–87.

Franger AL, Buchsbaum HJ, Peaceman AM. Abdominal gunshot wounds in pregnancy. *Am J Obstet Gynecol.* 1989;160:1124–1128.

Advanced Trauma Life Support for Doctors. American College of Surgeons Committee on Trauma. Student Course Manual. 6th ed. 1997:313–323.

Higgins SD. Trauma in pregnancy. *J Perinatol.* 1988;8(3):288–292.

Rozycki GS, Knudson MM. Reproductive system trauma. In: Felicinao DV, Moore EE, Mattox KL, eds. *Trauma.* 3rd ed. Stamford, CT: Appleton & Lange; 1996.

Nash P. Trauma in pregnancy. In: Skinner DV, Swain A, Robertson C, Peyton JWR, eds. *Cambridge Textbook of Accident and Emergency Medicine.* Cambridge, MA: Cambridge University Press; 1997:702–707.

21
Burns

ALAN R. KAY

Introduction

Burn injury is seen with ballistic trauma both in isolation and as part of multiple injuries. It is important that those dealing with victims of ballistic trauma understand the nature of burn injury and be able to manage it effectively.

Although modern definitive burn care is based on large multidisciplinary expert teams working in centers of excellence, much of the success in treating burn injury is dependent on the adequacy of initial management performed before arrival at a definitive care facility. Burn-injured casualties are trauma victims, and early care does not deviate from Advanced Trauma Life Support (ATLS) principles. Lack of familiarity with burns and the unpleasant nature of the injury, however, often distract the caregiver from following these basic management techniques.

This chapter aims to provide a framework for assessment and initial management, guidelines for who requires transfer to a specialist facility, and an overview of the principles of definitive care.

In all environments, treating a severe burn draws heavily on resources and a small number of casualties can stretch the capability of any facility. Unlike many other types of trauma injury, burn victims can become progressively more unstable for several days, even with appropriate management. This on-going burden needs to be appreciated in circumstances where resources are constrained. Triage decisions can be difficult.

Epidemiology

The pattern of burn injury related to ballistic weaponry is very variable. Traditional munitions use an explosive charge to create the energy to injure, which, by its nature, produces heat. The energy is often transferred to the victim via a projectile. If a casualty is close enough to the detonation to sustain serious burns, they are normally killed. Where infantry alone are used, the incidence of burns is low. This changes with the use of vehicles, aircraft, and ships. Weapon systems designed to defeat armor normally will not primarily cause significant burns in survivors. The predominant cause of burn injury is the secondary ignitions of fuel and munitions in the vehicle. The incidence of burns is therefore high in armored, air, and sea warfare.

There has been little published data about the incidence of burns in terrorist bomb attacks. Recent atrocities in Omagh, Northern Ireland, in 1998, and in Bali in 2002 seemed to have a larger proportion of significant burns. Victims from the latter overwhelmed the burn services of Australasia.

There are, of course, weapons such as Napalm, phosphorus, and flame-throwers that by their nature are designed to inflict burns.

The majority of burns encountered in conflicts will be accidental. Fifty-eight percent of all burn injuries in the Vietnam War were not related to fighting. The background incidence of noncombat-related burns in the civilian population may rise as normal social habits are changed, for example, the use of kerosene to cook when electricity supplies are disrupted. Combatants are particularly at risk of accidental burns in transition to war due to lack of familiarity and incorrect use of equipment and ignoring safety procedures. The type of injuries will be similar to those seen in normal civilian practice, where there is a low incidence of concomitant non-burn injury.

In war fighting, burn injury rates vary significantly with the type of conflict. In the 1982 Falklands conflict, 34% of those injured on ships sustained burns compared to 14% of total U.K. casualties. Burns were seen in 10% of injured troops in the 1973 Yom Kippur war, but in up to 70% of Israeli tank casualties. Up to 50% of battlefield burn casualties may have concomitant non-burn injury.

Thermonuclear detonations will cause large numbers of burns. Radiation doses sufficient to cause cutaneous burns will generally be fatal. Combined thermal burns and radiation exposure reduces chances of survival, but the poor outcome from burns in Hiroshima and Nagasaki would have had as much to do with the massive degradation of the health services.

Newer enhanced blast weapons, such as thermobaric explosives, produce significantly higher amounts of heat, but their impact on survivable burn incidence has yet to be seen.

Pathophysiology

Thermal injury causes burns to the skin and upper airway. This is associated with inflammation that can be systemic. Inhalation of the products of combustion can injure the lungs and cause systemic toxicity.

Systemic Injury

Direct thermal injury causes cell death progressively with temperatures over 45°C and almost instantaneously above 60°C. Heat is also conducted into surrounding tissues, causing injury. Tissues non-fatally injured by heat exhibit very marked inflammation, with increased capillary permeability and loss of fluid from the intravascular space. The clinical impact of the inflammation evolves for several hours and is related to the total volume of tissue injured. This is best expressed as the percentage of total body surface area burned (%TBSAB).

The most superficial of burns cause only erythema, with no effect on capillary leakage, and as such should not be considered when calculating the %TBSAB.

Injuries over 15%TBSAB in adults and 10% in children cause sufficient loss of intravascular fluid for compensatory mechanisms to be overwhelmed. Additional fluids need to be administered to prevent shock from developing.

Injuries above about 25 to 30%TBSAB cause massive activation of inflammatory mediators and a potentially fatal Systemic Inflammatory Response Syndrome (SIRS) develops. This is a progressive process and the clinical signs of SIRS can be delayed for several hours after the burn. Toxins released from the burn wound further stimulate the SIRS.

Inhalation Injury

This consists of a variable combination of the following:

The True Airway Burn

This is caused by inhalation of hot gases, be they flame, smoke, or steam. The resulting injury is thermal in nature and normally only affects the supraglottic airway. The initial manifestation is upper airway edema, which develops over a period of hours and is maximal between 12 and 36 hours. The edema can be severe enough to obstruct the airway.

Lung Injury

The upper airways are efficient at dissipating heat and, along with reflex laryngeal closure, protect the lower airways from direct heat injury. If, however, the products of combustion are inhaled into the lower airways, they dissolve into the fluid lining the bronchial tree and alveoli. This leads to a chemical injury to the lungs that produces varying degrees of pulmonary failure, often delayed by hours or even days. The pulmonary complications of SIRS add a further insult to the inhalation injury.

Systemic Toxicity

Absorption of the products of combustion into the circulation through the alveoli leads to systemic toxicity. The most important agents are carbon monoxide and cyanides. This is the most common cause of death due to fires in enclosed spaces. Carbon monoxide competes with oxygen for binding to hemoglobin, having 240 times the affinity. It therefore displaces oxygen, effectively causing hypoxemia. It also binds to the intracellular cytochrome system, causing abnormal cellular function. A low level of carboxyhemoglobin (<10%) causes no symptoms and can be found in heavy smokers. Above 20%, feelings of fatigue and nausea can start and higher mental functions are impaired. Levels above 40% lead to progressive loss of neurological function, and death occurs with levels over 60%. Note that in the presence of carboxyhemoglobin, pulse oximeter readings are unreliable indicators of oxygen saturation ($\%SaO_2$).

There is no measure to quantify the severity of an inhalation injury, but its presence significantly worsens the prognosis following a burn.

Blast Lung is an injury secondary to the passage of a shock wave through the lungs and, although in some ways clinically similar, is not part of inhalation injury.

Cutaneous Injury

The severity of a cutaneous burn is difficult to qualify. The %TBSAB will be reflected by the degree of systemic inflammation and will dictate resuscitative needs. The depth of burn has less of an effect on the systemic response, but dictates wound management needs. The extent and distribution of any residual burn scarring can have devastating social and psychological effects. The personal impact of burn scarring on an individual is very variable and has been shown to be unrelated to the size or location of scars. The interactions of the burn survivor in society are complex.

Classification of the burn wound is purely descriptive and indicates the %TBSAB and depth involved. Methods of calculating %TBSAB are described later.

With respect to depth, burns either involve the full thickness of the skin and are called full-thickness burns or involve only part of the thickness of the skin and are called partial-thickness burns. Partial-thickness burns are sub-classified depending on which parts of the skin are involved.

Epidermal Burns

These cause local inflammation of the epidermis, leading to erythema alone, like sunburn. No blistering is seen. They can be extremely painful. Spontaneous resolution in about 48 hours is expected. They are not included when calculating %TBSAB.

Partial Thickness Burns

These are subdivided into the following two categories.

Superficial Dermal

The skin blisters and oozes clear fluid. When the blisters are removed, the underlying surface has marked erythema, which blanches on pressure and has an intact capillary refill. The deeper skin adnexal structures survive, providing a source of epithelial cells for healing. If managed correctly, these burns should heal in less than two weeks.

Deep Dermal

When the blisters are removed, the underlying surface has a darker red color, which does not blanch. This "fixed staining" is caused by damage to deeper blood vessels. There is no visible capillary refill. Due to loss of deeper epithelial elements, these burns rarely heal in two weeks and often require skin grafting.

Full Thickness Burns

The thermal damage causes total destruction of dermis, leaving a firm, leathery necrotic layer known as eschar. This can be waxy white or have lobster red fixed staining. Soot or charred tissue may mask the true appearance and will need to be cleaned off. Surgery is required except for very small areas.

The level of pain from a wound and the pinprick test of sensation are poor discriminators of depth and should not be relied on.

Burn wounds are not homogenous and a mixed pattern may be seen.

The inflammation surrounding the burn wound alters the local circulation and can lead to further necrosis. This burn wound progression can account for the deepening seen in some wounds originally thought to be superficial. Early cooling of a burn wound can reduce the magnitude of the local inflammatory injury and lower the chance of progression.

Deep dermal and full-thickness burns can constrict deeper structures, particularly if circumferential. Around the torso this can restrict respiration. In the limbs, a similar picture to compartment syndrome will be seen. In these situations, surgical release of the constriction (escharotomy) is indicated.

Managing the Burn Victim

Burn victims are trauma victims and the initial assessment is the same as for any other seriously injured patient. There may be injuries other than the burn, and these must be treated or excluded. Some common sense should prevail because not every patient needs to be treated as a major trauma case. As a general principle, though, any burn involving more than 10% of the total body surface area should be regarded as significant.

Whatever the cause of the burn, the severity of the injury is proportional to the volume of tissue damage. In terms of survival, the %TBSAB is the most important factor. Functional outcome is more often dependent on depth and site of the burn.

At all levels of care, the broad principles of management are: anticipate and preempt any potential of airway problem, estimate likely fluid requirements and administer them to prevent burn shock, monitor the adequacy of fluid replacement, perform initial burn wound care, prevent hypothermia, and transfer appropriate cases for definitive care.

Burns are painful and the victims are often terrified. With large burns, there are tangible levels of anxiety in caregivers, even those familiar with such cases. Relatives and friends of the victim are usually distraught. The whole atmosphere surrounding the initial care of a burn-injured patient is frequently highly charged. It is vital that the patient receives early adequate analgesia, anxiolytics, and sedation. Intravenous opiates are the obvious choice. This should be supported by the professional staff acting in a manner that will instill confidence.

First Aid

With safety of the rescuer in mind, the immediate priority is to stop the burning process. This is best achieved by dousing the effected area in cold water and removing smoldering clothes and those soaked in scalding fluids. All constricting items such as jewelry, watches, and tight clothing should be removed.

Carry out any necessary standard Basic Life Support first aid.

There is evidence that immediate cooling of the burn wound modifies local inflammation and reduces progressive cell necrosis. This is best achieved by the topical application of cool water, preferably flowing. Proprietary wet gels may have a role in this respect. Cooling the wound also has a beneficial analgesic effect. Very cold water and ice cause local vasoconstriction and are to be avoided.

Ideally, the cooling should be started immediately and continue for about twenty minutes. It is uncertain if there is any benefit beyond this time. Protracted cooling and cooling large areas may lead to systemic hypothermia, particularly in small children, and a degree of common sense should prevail. The maxim "cool the burn but warm the patient" is true, but is difficult to achieve with large burns.

A clean nonstick dressing can then be placed on the burn. Clingfilm is ideal, and there are several proprietary "first burn dressings" available. The dressing does not need to be sterile and clean moistened linen is a satisfactory alternative. Air movement over a fresh burn causes pain and this initial dressing removes that stimulus. Do not wrap the burn, as this can lead to constrictions; merely lay the dressing on.

Give adequate analgesia as soon as possible.

Further management at the scene or in transit depends on the local capabilities and proximity of the medical facility. For burns over about 20% in adults and 10% in children, administer oxygen if possible and obtain intravenous access if feasible.

Initial Medical Care

On arrival at a medical facility, the burn victim should be assessed by standard Advanced Trauma Life Support/Battlefield Advanced Trauma Life Support (ATLS/BATLS) principles.

Perform a primary survey using the ABCDE approach.

A–Airway

Airway swelling occurs progressively for many hours following inhalation injury and may not be evident when the casualty is first seen. It is important to anticipate those at risk of developing airway obstruction.

The presence of any of the following indicate the possibility of an inhalation injury:

- a history of exposure to fire and smoke in an enclosed space,
- exposure to blast,
- collapse, confusion, or restlessness at any time,
- hoarseness or any change in voice,
- harsh cough,
- stridor,
- flame or steam burns to the face,
- singed nasal hairs,
- soot in saliva or sputum,
- an inflamed oropharynx.

Oxygen should be administered in the highest concentration feasible, preferably humidified.

It can be very difficult to decide on how severe an upper airway burn is. Experienced senior help should be sought as soon as possible.

If any degree of upper airway obstruction is present, endotracheal intubation is mandatory. Remember that the swelling is likely to be increasing. The majority of cases will be conscious and intubation will be impossible without first anesthetizing the patient.

In areas where anesthetic expertise may not be available, judgement is required in cases where there is a high suspicion of inhalation injury but without evidence of upper airway obstruction. If it is considered safe to observe a casualty with a possible inhalation injury unintubated, they should be nursed sitting up. In high-risk cases, it may be necessary to perform a surgical airway on an awake patient. If there is any doubt, endotracheal intubation (by whichever route) should be performed.

B–Breathing

The pulmonary manifestations of burn injuries rarely occur early. If the airway is clear, the only likely effect of a burn that will cause compromise of respiration in the first few hours is a restriction of chest excursion by a deep circumferential torso burn. This is an indication for emergency escharotomy (see below).

A terrified patient gasping for air may have a blast lung injury.

C–Circulation

Hypovolemic shock secondary to a burn takes some time to produce measurable physical signs. If the burn victim is shocked soon after injury, other causes should be excluded. A history of a blast, vehicle collision, or a fall while escaping the fire should raise suspicion of other injuries.

If the patient has hypovolemic shock, they should be treated according to current shock protocols independent of the severity of burn.

Establish intravenous access with two large-bore cannulae. It is possible to cannulate through burnt skin, but this should be avoided if possible. If necessary, use cut-downs, intraosseous or, as a last resort, central routes. Commence an intravenous infusion of crystalloid.

D–Disability

A reduced level of consciousness, confusion, or restlessness normally indicates hypoxia; in the burn victim, this can be secondary to an inhalation injury. Do not, however, overlook the possibility of other injuries. Drug and/or alcohol ingestion should be considered.

E–Exposure/Environment

The entire body surface area should be inspected for burns and other injuries, but care should be taken to avoid hypothermia. Unwrap one limb at a time to avoid excessive cooling. It may be possible to assess the burn without removing previously applied Clingfilm. Ensure that no constricting items of clothing remain. If possible, keep the ambient temperature high.

Other Initial Interventions

Ensure the casualty has received adequate analgesia.

If the facilities are available, measure the full blood count, urea and electrolytes, and blood gases. If there is a suspicion of inhalation injury, obtain a chest X-ray and measure carboxyhemoglobin levels. Even in severe inhalation injury, the chest X-ray and blood gases may initially be normal.

In burns over 20% TBSA in an adult and 10% in a child, insertion of a nasogastric tube and urinary catheter will be required.

Reassess the patient's ABCD and perform a full secondary survey.

Initial Specific Burn Management

Inhalation Injury

Regularly reassess those with suspected inhalation injury. Beyond keeping a patent airway and delivering the maximally achievable oxygen concentration, little can be done without critical care intervention. Any patient with a suspected inhalation injury should be closely observed in an area equipped for intubation. If there is a definite inhalation injury, then the patient should be managed by an experienced anesthetist before and during transfer.

Remember to interpret pulse oximetry readings with caution.

There is no evidence that administration of steroids is beneficial (although pre-injury users should continue their steroids).

There should be an extremely low threshold for elective intubation if the patient is going to be transferred to another hospital.

Establish the Size of the Burn

Accurate assessment of the size of burn can be difficult. When seen early, it may not be possible to tell whether or not areas of erythema will progress to blistering. Soot may mask an underlying burn. Initially, an estimate should be made upon which to base the fluid requirements.

Aids to estimating the %TBSAB are serial halving (see box) and "Rule of Nines" (Figure 21-1). In very large burns, it is often easier to work out how much is not burnt. The palmar surface of the patient's hand, including the fingers, equates to 1% TBSA and can be used to estimate small areas of burn.

FIGURE 21-1. The rule of nines—for estimating the %TBSAB.

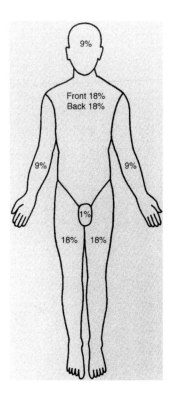

Serial Halving

This is designed to be a quick method of triaging the burn victim into one of four groups to describe the size of the burn.

Look at the front of the patient. This represents half of their TBSA. Estimate if more or less than half of the front is burned. If it is less than half, is it more or less than half of a half? Repeat the same for the rear of the patient.

You can then describe the burn as being:

– More than half of the body (>50% TBSAB)
– Between a quarter and a half (25–50% TBSAB)
– Between an eighth and a quarter (12.5–25% TBSAB)
– Less than an eighth (<12.5% TBSAB)

At this stage, it is not necessary to evaluate burn depth apart from identifying circumferential deep burns. Consideration should be given for the need of emergency escharotomies (see below).

As soon as is possible, an accurate assessment of the burn should be made. For this, a Lund & Browder chart should be used (Figure 21-2). If there is to be no undue delay in transfer, this can safely be left until arrival at a definitive care facility.

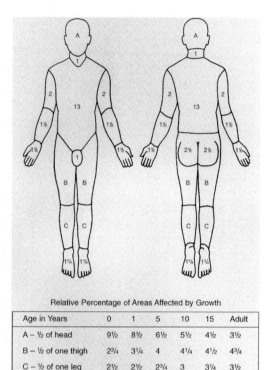

Relative Percentage of Areas Affected by Growth

Age in Years	0	1	5	10	15	Adult
A – ½ of head	9½	8½	6½	5½	4½	3½
B – ½ of one thigh	2¾	3¼	4	4¼	4½	4¾
C – ½ of one leg	2½	2½	2¾	3	3¼	3½

FIGURE 21-2. Lund and Browder chart—for accurate assessment of the %TBSAB. (Lund CC, Browder NC. The estimate of area of burns. Surg Gynecol Obstet 1944; 79:352–8.)

Calculate the Fluid Requirements

Prophylactic intravenous fluids above normal requirements should be administered to prevent burn shock in injuries greater than 15 %TBSAB (10% in children). The fluid calculations are based on an assumption that the need for additional fluids starts at the time of injury, not the time of assessment. Several formulae have been developed over the years, all based on retrospective analysis of fluids administered. It should be remembered that all formulae provide only an estimate of needs. The ultimate guide to adequacy is the patient's physiological response. The most widely used formula at present estimates the likely volume of crystalloid needed in the first 24 hours.

> Volume of crystalloid needed in first 24 hours (milliliters)
> = 2 × Weight (Kg) × %TBSAB
> In children this should be; 3 × Weight (Kg) × %TBSAB

Half this volume is given in the first eight hours from injury, then the second half in the following 16 hours.

Hartmann's/Ringer's Lactate solution is recommended. Normal saline can be used if necessary, but it produces a hyperchloremic acidosis.

The rate of administration must take in to account that the requirement of fluids starts at the time of injury.

Other fluid requirements are not accounted for in this regime. Administer additional fluids where indicated for losses due to other injuries and normal daily maintenance.

Monitor

The calculated volume for fluid administration is an initial guide only. The individual's physiological response should be monitored to assess its adequacy. Large full-thickness burns and those with an inhalation injury often require very large volumes of fluid over what is expected. An accurate fluid-balance record should be maintained and updated at least hourly.

The simplest guide to adequacy of fluid administration is urine output. Aim to keep the urine output between 0.5 and 1.0 milliliters per kilogram body weight per hour in adults and double this for children. Do not be afraid to adjust the fluid input to keep the urine output within these limits. It is equally as important to reduce fluid administration when indicated. Full blood count and urea and electrolytes should be measured at least twice in the first 24 hours.

In children, a reduced capillary refill time and tachypnea are also good indicators of inadequate perfusion.

Use pulse oximetry to monitor $\%SaO_2$ and pulse rate. Carbon monoxide poisoning can give anomalously high $\%SaO_2$ readings.

The Burn Wound

Apart from small superficial burns, wound management needs to be supervised by experienced surgeons. Beyond stopping the burning process and cooling the burn as described above, there is rarely any indication for the initial team to interfere with the burn wound.

If the patient is going to be transferred to another facility, Clingfilm is a more than adequate dressing. Do not apply ointments or creams, as this can make later accurate wound assessment more difficult. If there is to be a delay in planned arrival at definitive care beyond about twelve hours, then the burn wound should be thoroughly cleaned as described below.

Burns are usually sterile initially and infection is uncommon for the first few days. In uncomplicated civilian-type burns, there is no requirement for antibiotic prophylaxis. In the battlefield situation, wound contamination is assumed and antibiotics should be administered. Make sure the casualty is tetanus immune.

A circumferential full-thickness burn can act like a tourniquet and compromise circulation. Division of the constriction is known as escharotomy. This is not a straightforward undertaking and should be performed in an operating theater by skilled persons. There is rarely a need to perform an escharotomy within the first few hours. The exception is full-thickness burns of the entire trunk that are compromising respiration by restricting chest excursion. This constitutes a surgical emergency, and in this situation, it is appropriate to perform torso escharotomies in any setting.

Transfer to Definitive Care

Burns are complex injuries and the occasional burn practitioner will not be in a position to achieve optimal recovery.

Referral Criteria

The following injuries should be referred to a facility able to provide definitive burn care:

- burns greater than 10% TBSA in an adult,
- burns greater than 5% TBSA in a child,
- full-thickness burns greater than 1% TBSA,
- burns of special areas; face, hands, feet, genitalia, and major joints,
- electrical burns,
- chemical burns,
- presence of an inhalational injury,
- circumferential burns (except where superficial),
- burns in the very young and very old,
- burns associated with any condition that may affect outcome such as pre-existing disease, other injuries, social circumstances, and non-accidental injury.

Early contact with a burn center should be made. Further advice on initial management and transfer will be given. There may be specific local guidelines that need to be followed.

Preparation for Transfer

All patients at this stage will have had a primary survey with appropriate resuscitative interventions, an assessment of the burn, and initial burn management, as outlined above, commenced. Before transfer, it is important to ensure the following:

- a thorough secondary survey has been performed and any other injuries identified be appropriately managed,
- oxygen is being administered,
- if there is any suspicion of an inhalational injury, the patient has been assessed by an experienced anesthetist and intubated if necessary,
- adequate intravenous access is secured and appropriate fluid resuscitation has started,

- the burn wound is covered appropriately and the patient is being kept warm,
- there is adequate analgesia,
- there is a urinary catheter in place,
- there is a free draining nasogastric tube in place,
- all findings and interventions, including fluid balance, are clearly and accurately documented.

With the interventions described above, a burn casualty should remain stable and fit for transfer for about 12 hours. In many areas of the world, arrival at a definitive care facility within this time is unlikely. If it is likely that transfer will exceed this time, then the situation needs to be discussed further with the receiving burn center. In this circumstance, it may be deemed necessary for:

- escharotomies to be performed,
- the burn wound to be cleaned and a specific dressing applied,
- the commencement of maintenance intravenous fluids and/or nasogastric feeding.

All patients should be transferred with appropriately trained escort staff.

Experience has shown that burn-injured casualties tolerate long-distance aeromedical transfer satisfactorily if carried out early. As the SIRS evolves, such transfers become more complicated. This becomes very significant progressively beyond 48 hours.

Principles of Definitive Care

Definitive burn care should be delivered by a multidisciplinary team in a facility capable of providing all aspects of care simultaneously. The process of full rehabilitation of the burn survivor back into society can be long and complicated.

The initial goal, though, is to achieve burn wound healing while managing any systemic response. Deep dermal and full-thickness burns need surgery and the management of SIRS requires critical care facilities. Inhalation injury will normally be managed in intensive care. Ideally, all these capabilities should be found within a Burn Center.

A full description of the definitive management of burn care is beyond the scope of this chapter. Below is a summary of important aspects that those providing care outside of specialized facilities may need to consider.

Ongoing Care

Using the system of care described above with good monitoring and fine adjustment of the advocated fluid regime where appropriate, the majority of cases up to about 40% TBSAB will pass through the phase of systemic inflammation fairly smoothly. Burn injury does produce changes in normal physiology that do not resolve even with adequate management. These include a tachycardia, pyrexia of up to 38.5°C and a leucocytosis, and can persist for several days, even in uncomplicated burns.

Deep burns cause loss of red blood cells and transfusion may be required. Breakdown products of the lost red cells are excreted in the urine and increase the risk of acute tubular necrosis. If dark red pigmentation of the urine is seen, increase fluid input to achieve a urine output of 1.5 to 2.0 milliliters per kilogram per hour.

Nasogastric feeding should be started as early as possible, ideally, immediately on admission. This helps maintain gut function, lowers the risk of peptic ulceration, and may have a benefit in reducing bacterial translocation. If it is not possible to start nasogastric feeding, give either a H_2 antagonist or proton pump inhibitor to prevent peptic ulceration.

The patient should be nursed partially sitting up, with arms elevated on pillows to help reduce edema. Physiotherapy should start early with the aim of maintaining the range of motion of all joints. This may need to be compromised to avoid damage to recent skin grafting.

Once a casualty's burns are dressed, analgesia requirements decrease. High levels of anxiety remain, so good psychological support is important. Anxiolytics can help, along with a balanced analgesia regime. Nonsteroidal anti-inflammatory drugs (NSAIDs) should be avoided in the first 24 hours.

Additional fluid requirements extend beyond the first 24 hours. With nasogastric feeding, a standard regime will provide for the majority of cases. Five-hundred milliliter boluses of colloid (10 milliliters per kilogram for children) should be used if hypovolemia becomes apparent. Again, the patient's physiological response is the main indicator of fluid requirement. In general, a low urine output is an indicator of hypovolemia, and diuretics should not be used.

In large burns and those with inhalation injury, the SIRS can be severe and management becomes complicated. The general strategies of intensive care become necessary.

Inhalation Injury

The management of inhalation injury requires experience in respiratory intensive care.

Actual upper airway edema is an indication for endotracheal intubation. High-risk cases not yet showing signs should be nursed sitting up in a high-dependency area equipped for intubation. Supplementary oxygen should be administered as necessary to keep the PaO_2 above 10 kilopascal.

Even in severe injuries, initial blood gas and chest X-ray results may be normal. The normal clinical picture is that of deterioration up to several days following injury.

Fiberoptic bronchoscopy is the investigation of choice. The use of pulmonary toilet and various ventilation strategies will depend on the experience of clinicians and equipment available. Chest physiotherapy should be commenced early in all cases.

Systemic intoxication is treated with general supportive measures and administration of 100% inspired oxygen until signs resolve or carboxyhemoglobin levels fall below 15%.

Current practice suggests that there is no role for prophylactic antibiotics, steroids, or hyperbaric oxygen in inhalation injury.

Accurate Assessment of the Burn

To do this properly causes pain and adequate analgesia will normally need to be supplemented with sedation. In large burns, a general anaesthetic is appropriate and the best environment is in a warm (30°C) operating theater.

Thoroughly clean all involved areas with copious volumes of warm aqueous-based antiseptic solution. All blister roofs, loose skin, debris, and soot should be removed. This has to be a vigorous process using large gauze swabs. Gentle wiping of the burn is ineffectual.

Once cleaned, the full extent of the burn will be clear. Draw the burn areas on a Lund & Browder chart (Figure 21-2) and calculate the %TBSAB. Do not include simple erythema. Recalculate expected fluid requirements if this accurate assessment is widely different from a previous estimate, but at this stage, it is the patient's physiological response that is the primary guide to fluid-administration rates.

Identify deep areas that may cause circumferential constriction. This is the time to perform escharotomies (see below). The need for accurate assessment of burn depth depends on the surgical strategies to be used.

Escharotomies

The necrotic layer of firm and unyielding deeply burnt skin is known as eschar. As edema forms in the deeper tissues, the eschar resists swelling, and tissue pressure rises. When circumferential, this can compromise perfusion and, in the torso, restrict ventilation. Surgical division of the eschar, escharotomy, is then indicated.

The restriction of chest excursion constitutes a surgical emergency. It is unusual, however, for there to be a need for escharotomies of the limbs within the first couple of hours. It is best to perform the procedure under controlled conditions in an operating theater. To adequately relieve the constriction, it is necessary to extend the incisions just into unburned tissue; the procedure, therefore, does cause pain and bleeding. A general anesthetic is indicated.

The lines of election for escharotomies are shown in Figure 21-3. As much normal ventilation is performed diaphragmatically, it is important to ensure the horizontal torso release is over the upper abdomen. There is a risk of damaging the ulnar nerve at the elbow and peroneal nerve around the fibular head. Dorsal hand and mid-lateral finger releases may be needed.

Cutting diathermy should be used to carefully incise down until the constriction is released along the full length of the deep burn. Slashing down into unburned fat is not required. As with letting down a tourniquet, a period of local hyper-perfusion follows, and significant bleeding can occur. It is important to ensure good hemostasis.

When there has been prolonged delay in performing escharotomies, compartment syndrome may be encountered, necessitating fasciotomies.

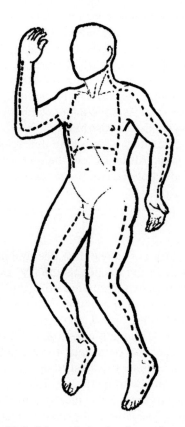

FIGURE 21-3. Lines of election for escharotomies.

Achieving Burn Wound Healing

Following a basic surgical premise that dead tissue needs to be debrided, necrotic burnt skin should be removed. In deep dermal and full-thickness burns, this requires surgical excision and takes the form of tangential shaving. It is now recognized that leaving necrotic burn provides a stimulus for SIRS and early excision (certainly within the first couple of days) is advocated. Indeed, in the case of life-threatening SIRS, it should be the view that debridement is essential rather than that the patient is too sick for surgery. The resultant post-excision wound is closed by various strategies depending on its extent. Autogenous split skin grafting is the mainstay with supplementary use of allograft, cultured, and artificial skin.

In superficial dermal burns where it is anticipated that uncomplicated wound healing will be achieved within two weeks, the vigorous cleaning described above should suffice as debridement. Various dressings can be applied to maintain an optimum healing environment.

Between the obvious superficial and deep burns lies the common situation of the "indeterminate depth" burn. In this situation, newer biologically active dressings are used to try to achieve as much healing as possible without surgery.

Where it is not possible to excise deep burns, the use of topical agents can help reduce the risk of wound infection and possibly diminish the effect on SIRS. Examples are cerium in silver sulphadiazine cream (Flammacerium®), normal silver sulphadiazine cream (Flammazine®), and mafenide acetate. Burn wounds produce a large volume of exudate. The dressings need to be changed when soaked through or, if possible, at least daily.

Infections in Burns

Burn wounds are initially sterile but become progressively contaminated, increasing the risk of invasive infection. In large burns, there is marked immunosupression. Several of the traditional signs of infection are also seen as part of the normal systemic response to burn injury (tachycardia, pyrexia, and leucocytosis). Positive surface wound cultures do not necessarily indicate invasive infection. It can therefore be difficult to diagnose infection in burn injury.

With a lack of any clear evidence of benefit and the risk of resistance emergence, it is not normal practice to use prophylactic antibiotics in uncomplicated civilian-type burn injuries. Where wounding is secondary to ballistic trauma, contamination is potentially significant and prophylaxis is indicated. Early burn wound excision and the antimicrobial activity of the topical agents is the main strategy for reducing infection.

Streptococcal and Staphylococcal infections predominate in the first five days, with gram negative organisms becoming evident beyond this time.

If infection is apparent, antibiotics should be given according to micro-biological culture results. In cases of extremis, blind therapy should be:

- First five days: Benzylpenicillin and flucloxacillin
- Beyond five days: Third generation cephalosporin and gentamicin

Special Burns

Phosphorus Burns

These are almost exclusively a military phenomenon. The metal sponta-neously ignites in air and is prevented from doing so by immersion in water. The majority of phosphorus burns are caused by secondary ignition of clothing and are treated as for normal burns.

To prevent further ignition of phosphorus imbedded in wounds, visible lumps should be removed and the area irrigated with water. Soaking dress-ings are then applied and kept wet until arrival at a surgical facility.

To help identify further particles during wound debridement, an ultra-violet lamp will highlight phosphorescence. Irrigation of the wound with one-percent copper sulphate solution will coat the fragments with a layer of black cupric phosphide. This reduces the chance of ignition and makes them easier to see. Copper sulphate is toxic and should be thoroughly washed from the wound. It must never be used as part of a dressing. Debrided particles must be immersed in water to prevent ignition in the operating theater.

Vesicant Burns

Various chemical-warfare agents cause cutaneous burns. The main aim of these agents is to produce large numbers of surviving casualties who require significant medical input. Typically, irritation and erythema appear several hours after exposure, followed by blistering. Wound healing is significantly slower than with a comparable thermal injury. There may be associated pulmonary, systemic, and ocular injury.

Full decontamination procedures must be carried out before admission to any medical facility.

Thorough cleaning with removal of all blisters is performed. There is usually no active agent in blister fluid. The exception is Lewisite, but this is easily neutralized by using a weak hypochlorite solution.

Dressings and fluid resuscitation are then the same as for thermal burns. The loss of fluid can be delayed in vesicant burns and the need for replace-ment starts when blisters appear as opposed to the moment of injury.

Pulmonary involvement is treated as for an inhalation injury. Sulphur mustard causes bone marrow suppression, increasing the risk of infection.

British anti-Lewisite (BAL) is a specific antidote for systemic Lewisite toxicity.

Despite the long healing time, vesicant burns will often do well without skin grafting. Debridement of the wound using either dermabrasion or laser has been shown experimentally to accelerate healing.

Burns in Mass Casualty Scenarios

With optimal care, survival with good quality of life can be achieved even in massive burn injury. It is no longer appropriate to arbitrarily choose a certain % TBSAB above which it is assumed care is futile. The high demand of burn care, however, necessitates careful use of triage when resources are stretched.

The factors that significantly reduce survival rates are:

- inhalation injury (except isolated oropharyngeal swelling),
- deep burns over 80% TBSA,
- age over 60,
- significant concomitant illness or injury.

Burns that need skin grafting of over about 40% TBSA require a very high level of surgical input and will draw heavily on time and manpower.

In mass casualty scenarios, the prime importance of a Burn Assessment Team consisting of an experienced surgeon, anesthetist, and nurse is in making the appropriate triage decisions, not just delivering care.

Oral fluid therapy can be used for burns at least up to 20% TBSA, and may be even higher if the nasogastric route is used. Moyer's solution or proprietary oral rehydration formulae can be used. A normal diet with extra water to drink is probably as efficacious.

Further Reading

Herndon DN, ed. *Total burn care.* 2nd ed. London: WB Saunders; 2002.

Specific Articles

Arturson G. The pathophysiology of severe thermal injury. *J Burn Care Rehabil.* 1985;6:129–146.

Bellamy RF. The medical effects of conventional weapons. *World J Surg.* 1992; 16:888–192.

Baxter CR. Fluid volume and electrolyte changes in the early post-burn period. *Clin Plast Surg.* 1974;1:693–703.

Chapman P. Operation Corporate—the Sir Galahad bombing. Woolwich Burns Unit experience. *J R Army Med Corps.* 1984;130(2):84–88.

Jackson DM. The diagnosis of the depth of burning. *Br J Surg.* 1953;40:588–596.

Jandera V, Hudson DA, deWet PM, Innes PM, Rode H. Cooling the burn wound: Evaluation of different modalities. *Burns.* 2000;26:265–270.

Leonard LG, Scheulen JJ, Munster AM. Chemical burns: Effect of prompt first aid. *J Trauma.* 1982;22:420–423.

Levine BA, Petroff PA, Slade CL. Prospective trials of dexamethasone and aerosolized gentamicin in the treatment of inhalational injury in the burned patient. *J Trauma* 1978;18:188–193.

Moritz AR, Henriquez FC. Studies of thermal injury II. The relative importance of time and surface temperature in the causation of cutaneous burns. *Am J Pathol.* 1947;23:695–720.

Pruitt BA Jr. Fluid resuscitation of extensively burned patients. *J Trauma.* 1981; 21(Suppl):690–692.

Richards T. Medical lessons from the Falklands. *Br Med J.* 1983;286:790–792.

Scheinkestel CD, Bailey M, Myles PS, Jones K, Cooper DJ, Millar IL, Tuxen DV. Hyperbaric or normobaric oxygen for acute carbon monoxide poisoning: A randomised controlled clinical trial. *Med J Aust.* 1999;170:203–210.

Smith JJ, Scerri GV, Malyon AD, Burge TS. Comparison of serial halving and rule of nines as a pre-hospital assessment tool. *Emerg Med J.* 2002;19(suppl):A66.

22
Intensive Care of the Trauma Patient with Ballistic Injuries

Spiros G. Frangos, Marilee Freitas, and Heidi Frankel

Introduction

This chapter is composed of three sections.

First, routine care in the intensive care unit (ICU) will deal with how to manage, reexamine, and continue to resuscitate the injured patient after surgery. The chapter will reemphasize the need for a tertiary examination, continuous monitoring, and surveillance for missed injury or physiologic deterioration.

The second section provides a brief review of the damage control patient and their special needs in the critical care unit.

This will be followed in the third section by a review of several contemporary critical care issues and their relevance to managing the ICU phase of patients with severe penetrating injuries.

Routine ICU Care

Upon Arrival—The First Six Hours

Admission of the ballistic injured patient to the ICU should be accompanied by a careful reassessment of all details of the history surrounding the event and operative intervention. A thorough repeat physical examination should be conducted, searching carefully for wounds that may have been of less priority during rapid transit to the operating theater. Attention needs to be called to the type of weaponry, ordnances, the care provided in the prehospital arena, as well as during the emergency resuscitation and evaluation. However, completion of a tertiary survey may be made difficult by altered sensorium due to medication, mechanical ventilation, or return to the operating theater.

Repetitive, comprehensive physical examination and radiographic imaging may be necessary, especially with multiple wounds or multiple body regions wounded.

The ICU team should strive to understand all ballistic trajectories to ensure that all injuries have been identified. Once identified, planned repair or conservative management is selected and documented. Performance of a tertiary survey by the ICU team serves as a checks-and-balances system to avoid missed injuries; additionally, at this time, all prior laboratory and radiographic studies should be reviewed, as should the anesthetic and surgical operative records quantifying blood loss and fluid replacement.

Attention also should be directed to routine medication administration that may have been neglected with the patient in extremis, such as tetanus toxoid, pain medication, and antibiotics. Family members who may not have seen the patient preoperatively should be counseled and allowed to visit once the patient is stable, or as soon as is practical. The family may also be a valuable resource to obtain accurate medical, surgical, and social histories. Documentation of any and all new findings is imperative. Review of prehospital, trauma resuscitation area, and operating suite documentation, as well as the resuscitative and operative surgeon's note, is key to minimizing unrecognized injuries. Attention should be directed to drawings and descriptions of wounds with concern to laterality and correlated with actual wounds and oral reports from the surgical team. Standardized admitting orders, especially if computerized, reduce the rate of missed orders and medication error.[1]

Physical examination in the tertiary survey should proceed in Advanced Trauma Life Support (ATLS) fashion, starting with the ABCs and progressing to a head-to-toe evaluation. This should be supplemented by addressing issues unique to the ICU environment:

- An endotracheal tube, when present, may require more definitive anchoring, and its intratracheal position should be verified by a portable chest radiograph.
- Bilateral breath sounds should be auscultated and chest tubes inspected for the rate, quantity, and quality of fluid output, function, and the presence or absence of an air leak.
- Intravenous (IV) and intra-arterial catheter patency and location should be assessed.
- Urinary drainage catheters should be secured without tension and appropriate hygienic care given.
- If possible, a complete neurological examination should be performed that includes documentation of spinal cord deficits on an American Spinal Injury Association form, if applicable, to assay for progression of disease.
- Cervical collars and splints should be opened to afford full inspection, and, if required for longer than a few hours, treatment plans used to relieve skin pressure under all devices. Finally, patients should be

log-rolled and hidden areas examined for gunshot wounds and/or palpable retained bullets.

Damage control patients display many clinical variables that may confound the tertiary survey and result in delayed or missed diagnoses (Table 22-1). In these patients, repeated physical examination and liberal use of general radiographs and computed tomography (CT) scans may be warranted. This radiographic tertiary survey, especially if it cannot be accomplished in the ICU, should be prioritized based on the hemodynamic and respiratory stability of the patient. Although portable CT scanning is now possible, most ICUs do not have this technology available, and the ability to perform ultra-fast scans with three-dimensional reconstruction may not be achievable with portable scanners. Alternate modes of radiographic diagnosis should be entertained, including sonography with or without duplex scanning, fluoroscopy, and/or echocardiography. Generally, only anteroposterior and lateral projection radiographs are possible with a patient in an ICU specialty bed, and completion of high-quality lateral and oblique films require a trip to the radiology suite.

Endpoints of Resuscitation

Trauma resuscitation implies minute-to-minute bedside management of evolving pathophysiology. Furthermore, it is important that the communication between the trauma team and surgical ICU team be efficient and precise.

Any IV catheters that were placed at the time of the initial emergency room resuscitation should be changed to clean new sites as soon as possible, and ideally within the first 24-hour period. Large-bore upper extremity IV catheters should be the preferred access sites throughout the course of the resuscitation, and any central catheters should be discontinued as soon as the information gained ceases to affect decision making. Subclavian and internal jugular venous catheters are preferred to femoral venous catheters, as they have a smaller risk of infection and thrombosis.

TABLE 22-1. Factors that may confound the tertiary survey

– Field intubation
– Hemodynamic instability
– Closed head injury
– Intoxication
– Use of analgesics, anxiolytics, and/or paralytics
– Incomplete information, i.e., transfer from outside facility
– High injury severity score
– Multiple wounds, trajectories

The ICU resuscitation may be guided by monitoring vital signs—heart rate, blood pressure, and temperature. Hourly urine output must be assessed with an indwelling Foley catheter. Bedside physical examinations must be performed to further assess adequacy of resuscitation (e.g., warming of extremities) and to rule out the emergence of any central or peripheral compartment syndrome. Laboratory tests, including hemoglobin/hematocrit, bicarbonate, pH, base deficit, lactate, and coagulation parameters, need to be evaluated, especially in the first 24 to 48 hours to ensure adequacy of the resuscitation and rule out continued blood loss.

Pulse oximetry is an integral part of the care of the trauma patient within the ICU. It allows for a rapid continuous assessment of systemic oxygenation and allows for early interventions if compromised. Gastric tonometry, a method used in some ICUs, allows for organ-specific oxygenation assessment using the splanchnic circulation as a marker for oxygenation deficits.

Resuscitating trauma patients to specific fixed-target endpoints of cardiac index, oxygen delivery, and oxygen consumption are not universally advocated. As serum lactate values represent the balance between peripheral accumulation of lactate in underperfused tissues and its hepatic elimination, lactate clearance represents reestablishment of tissue oxygen demands. The time needed to clear lactate, rather than the initial lactate value, predicts a successful resuscitation and appears to correlate exceedingly well with survival. In the same manner, the base deficit acts as a sensitive measure of the degree of inadequate perfusion. Both lactate and base deficit levels should be used as supportive rather than conclusive parameters of resolving shock alongside each individual patient's overall clinical picture.

A pulmonary artery catheter is often useful to assist in guiding the anticipated large-volume resuscitation and to determine the need for inotropes. There is no clear evidence as to whether or not there are morbidity and mortality benefits derived by the use of these catheters, with a number of small studies producing mixed results. There is good evidence, however, that elderly high-risk surgical patients in the ICU may obtain no benefit when care is directed by pulmonary artery catheters over standard care,[2] although this study was not limited to trauma patients. Attaining a pulmonary artery capillary wedge pressure of 18 millimeters Hg and a cardiac index of 3.5 (or greater) liters per minute per square meter may assist in optimizing oxygen delivery.

Failure to clear elevated lactate levels should prompt the ICU team to employ invasive monitoring techniques. Pulmonary artery pressures, pulmonary capillary occlusive pressures, cardiac indices, and mixed venous oximetry provide helpful parameters for *guiding* a large-volume resuscitation and confirming that all efforts are moving in the right direction. There is evidence that even young patients in hemorrhagic shock secondary to penetrating trauma may benefit from such invasive hemodynamic monitoring.

The controversy over isotonic crystalloid or colloid as the ideal resuscitation fluid persists. In a recent systematic review comparing crystalloid versus colloid resuscitation, it was determined that crystalloid is associated with a lower mortality rate in trauma patients. However, due to limitations in the methodology of the reviewed randomized clinical trials, no definitive recommendations could be made.

Understanding which resuscitation strategy best prevents cellular injury is imperative. Neutrophil activation and adhesion varies depending on the type of resuscitation fluid used.

Lactated Ringer's (LR) solution has been shown to produce neutrophil activation and an increased immediate cell death by apoptosis in animal models following hemorrhagic shock and resuscitation. It has also been shown that LR leads to an increased production of reactive oxygen species by neutrophils and influences the expression of leukocyte genes in humans. These studies began to question the use of LR as the current Advanced Trauma Life Support (ATLS) standard for resuscitation.

Hextend is a plasma volume expander that contains six percent hydroxyethyl starch in a physiologically balanced medium of electrolytes, lactate, and glucose. Compared with 0.9% saline, volume resuscitation with Hextend has been shown to be associated with longer short-term survival in an animal model of septic shock. The use of hydroxyethyl starch, as well as other colloid solutions, continues to be studied in hemorrhagic shock in the hope of finding evidence for an improved survival in humans.

Packed red blood cells should be readily available as transfusion requirements may be exceedingly high. The hospital's blood bank should be aware of the imminent demand and urgency for multiple blood products. Many hospitals have approved massive transfusion protocols to efficiently and effectively allow blood products to reach those in the direst need. In the face of uncontrolled nonsurgical bleeding, the hemoglobin may need to be pushed to a level of 10 grams per deciliter to maximize peripheral perfusion. Hypovolemia is the norm in these patients and transfusion requirements at this stage of care should be liberal in the face of ongoing nonsurgical blood loss. This, of course, need not be the case in those patients whose bleeding has been controlled and whose resuscitation requirements are beginning to level off, as euvolemia will likely not benefit from a liberal, overzealous transfusion policy. As for the subset of patients with evidence for ongoing surgical bleeding, re-operation is mandated.

Daily Maintenance Care in the ICU

Adequate pain control using intermittent or continuous narcotics (e.g., morphine, 1–5 milligrams IV hourly; fentanyl, 25–150 micrograms IV hourly) is essential. Sedation is best accomplished with benzodiazepines (e.g., midazolam, 1–3 milligrams IV hourly), in dosages intended to provide optimal levels of comfort and safety. Propofol (0–3 milligrams per kilogram per hour titrated to goal) should be reserved for trauma patients who are hemodynamically stable with primarily neurosurgical injuries or in those patients in whom early extubation is intended.

Muscle relaxation may be necessary to achieve satisfactory mechanical ventilation in some patients. The requirement for muscle relaxation must be reviewed regularly. There is evidence that when pain and sedation protocols are used to guide ICU care, the duration of mechanical ventilation is shortened and costs are kept down.[3]

Attention must also be directed to management of drug and alcohol dependence, which is common in the civilian penetrating injury patient population. Identifying patients at risk for abuse dependency withdrawal occurs by assaying drug and alcohol levels upon admission and interviewing family members or, if possible, the patient. Simple screening tests and interventions need not be lengthy. Alcohol withdrawal symptoms are managed by judicious use of benzodiazepines, alpha agonists and beta antagonists, the latter two to blunt sympathetic responses. Narcotic and benzodiazepine addiction is best managed by use of these agents until the patient is medically stable for detoxification.

Prophylaxis for deep venous thrombosis should be provided only when the risks of bleeding are small. This can be in the form of intermittent subcutaneous (SQ) heparin or low molecular weight heparin, as well as sequential compression devices. Very careful decision making about the risks versus benefits of any form of anticoagulant use is needed, especially in patients with CNS, spinal cord, or solid organ injury. Stress gastritis prophylaxis using histamine-2 blockers is also important. Prophylactic antibiotics may be necessary, but should be narrow spectrum, of short duration, and selected on a case-by-case basis.

Continuous cardiac monitoring and intermittent electrocardiography is mandatory for the early detection of arrhythmia or cardiac ischemic injury. Frequent chest radiographs are often beneficial for detecting evolving pulmonary processes, such as pneumonia, pneumothorax, effusion, and the acute respiratory distress syndrome (ARDS).

If ventilator support is necessary, this should be provided by using the lowest necessary fractional inspired oxygen and positive end-expiratory pressures (PEEP) that will maintain oxygen saturations in the mid to upper 90s. Difficulty with oxygenation and elevations in peak airway pressures may be indicative of a developing abdominal compartment syndrome; therefore, a high index of suspicion is warranted.

In high-risk patients, bladder pressure should be checked every four hours or so, especially in the first 24 hours of the resuscitation, when the incidence of abdominal compartment syndrome appears to be highest. This is important in all patients who have received a large volume resuscitation (more than 8 liters over 24 hours) or with major abdominal injuries or in the presence of a poor nutritional state. The prevention of intra-abdominal hypertension contributes to an improved survival.[4]

Specific Missed Injuries When Performing the Tertiary Survey

The missed injury rate has been estimated at around ten percent. A recent study indicated that the tertiary survey with reevaluation of radiographs can identify 90% of clinically significant missed injuries. Nonetheless, in trauma populations with a high incidence of penetrating trauma, both vascular and visceral missed injuries have been reported.

Abdomen

Abdominal injury may be missed even in patients who have undergone laparotomy. Particular areas of vulnerability include the diaphragm, where small posterior wounds may have gone undetected (and are likely more significant on the left side); the retroperitoneum (including kidneys, ureters, duodenum, and colon) and deep pelvis, where rectal lacerations may be missed (less important if drained and diverted, see Rectal exam revisited, Hard lesson 1). Furthermore, "disease progression" may occur from the time of laparotomy. Blast injuries to hollow viscera may become full thickness and result in stricture or, more often, perforation. Additional surgical bleeding may be revealed as the patient is warmed and resuscitated. The ICU team should be attentive to development of these complications by monitoring drain output, hemodynamic parameters, serial hemoglobin, and creatinine. Continued bleeding, particularly in relation to pelvic, liver, or retroperitoneal injury, may be best treated by angiographic embolization. Finally, mechanical and infectious complications of laparotomy and repair may occur and include pancreatitis, obstruction, fistulae, and abscesses.

Thorax

The chest cavity may be a source of new or renewed bleeding and missed injury. In addition, delay in recognition of injuries such as pulmonary contusion is common. Attention should be directed to both continued chest tube output (in excess of 200 to 300 cubic centimeters per hour) and undrained collections noted on serial chest radiographs. More slowly accumulating hemothoraces may be amenable to thoracoscopic drainage. This diagnosis is best made on a CT scan at 48 hours, as chest radiographs may miss clinically significant collections.

Thoracoscopy or laparoscopy are excellent methods for diagnosing diaphragmatic injuries. Diaphragm injuries are common ($\approx 40\%$) in patients with penetrating thoracoabdominal injury and need repair to avoid long-term complications. Pulmonary contusion can be protean in presentation.

This can occur with direct lung injury from bullets or blast effect. Other non-thoracic injuries take priority early after wounding. Close monitoring of gas exchange, pulmonary dynamics and chest x-ray appearances are recommended.

Vascular

Extremity vascular injuries may be delayed in diagnosis in patients requiring emergent treatment of torso or head trauma. Injuries most frequently missed result from the sequelae of blast trauma such as intimal flaps, pseudoaneurysms, or arteriovenous fistulae. Rarely, vascular insufficiency may result from bullet embolization from more proximal entry.

Spine

The work-up of spinal trauma is often left to the ICU team for penetrating injured patients who present in extremis to the emergency department (ED). Literature is rapidly accumulating that CT scanning, which is expeditious and highly accurate, is the modality of choice to image the cervical and thoracolumbar spine. Three-dimensional computer reconstruction of images further improves diagnostic accuracy and provides better guidance for spine injury.

Extremity/Orthopedic

The most common site of injuries delayed in diagnosis or management is the distal extremity. Most important is the surveillance for the development of extremity compartment syndrome, which may occur in patients with even minor blunt extremity injury, but who require large volume resuscitation for other injuries.

Combined Penetrating and Blunt Injury

Consideration should be given to the possibility that the penetrating injured patient may also be a victim of blunt trauma. Gunshot victims may suffer an antecedent fall or have been assaulted, which may bring other injury constellations into play. These include closed head trauma, facial fractures, renal contusions, and other solid viscus injuries. Special attention should be given to blast injury in victims of high-velocity wounds or explosions, particularly in a confined space. Air-containing structures are at risk. Eardrums may rupture at two pounds per square inch (psi) and lungs at 70 psi, with death likely above 80 psi. Hollow viscera are also at risk with significant blast, as are extremities, which may be injured when the patient becomes a projectile and sustains injury after falling.[5]

Damage Control in the ICU

The progression of hemorrhage and hypovolemic shock following severe trauma leads to the initiation of a deadly triad of metabolic acidosis, hypothermia, and coagulopathy. In both civilian and military trauma, damage control has become a valuable tool in the armamentarium of the surgeon. Damage control (Figure 22-1), which will be discussed in detail further in the chapter, refers to a management approach that involves three distinct stages and is designed to interrupt and reverse the progression of the deadly triad.

A patient with penetrating injury and hemodynamic instability should be taken immediately to surgery for control of hemorrhage and contamination.

This is the first stage of damage control. The recognition of the deadly triad during surgery should lead to the early termination of the procedure as soon as surgical bleeding is controlled.

The aspects of care that follow can be just as formidable. This second stage of damage control occurs in the ICU and poses a different set of challenges—attempts at restoration of normal physiology and reversal and correction of acidosis, hypothermia, and coagulopathy.

Once these goals have been met, proceeding to the third stage of damage control—reoperation, packing removal, and definitive repair—may be considered.

Reversing the Deadly Triad

Acidosis

The state of hemorrhagic shock involves a shift from aerobic to anaerobic metabolism, secondary to poor perfusion and end-organ oxygen deficits.

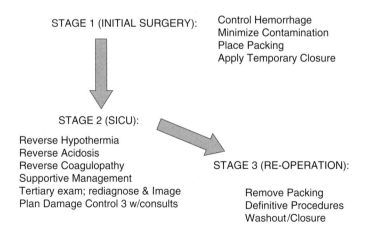

STAGE 1 (INITIAL SURGERY):   Control Hemorrhage
Minimize Contamination
Place Packing
Apply Temporary Closure

STAGE 2 (SICU):
Reverse Hypothermia
Reverse Acidosis
Reverse Coagulopathy
Supportive Management
Tertiary exam; rediagnose & Image
Plan Damage Control 3 w/consults

STAGE 3 (RE-OPERATION):
Remove Packing
Definitive Procedures
Washout/Closure

FIGURE 22-1. Damage control.

Anaerobic metabolism leads to a buildup of lactate and an anion gap acidosis. The reversal of this metabolic acidosis relies on optimizing the delivery of oxygen to ischemic tissues and providing intensive supportive care to get the patient beyond this life-threatening physiologic insult.

Normal cellular function relies on the maintenance of serum pH within a narrow range. As pH decreases below this physiologic range (7.36–7.44), visceral homeostasis and intracellular enzymatic reactions are compromised. All organ systems are affected, although the detrimental effects to the cardiovascular system, with loss of vasomotor tone and impaired myocardial contractility, often lead to an irreversible and unsalvageable state.

The ICU team's goal is to reestablish adequate oxygen delivery, whose primary components are cardiac output, oxygen saturation, and hemoglobin. A drop in hemoglobin concentration can have a significant influence on the arterial oxygen content and hence on oxygen delivery; therefore, anemia must be avoided in these critically ill patients. Hypovolemic shock warrants a sustained and continuous volume resuscitation to optimize cardiac indices. Inotropic drugs, especially dobutamine, may be indicated in order to optimize cardiac performance once adequate preload has been established.

Coagulopathy

The coagulopathy of hemorrhagic shock has a multifactorial etiology, including severe hemorrhage, massive resuscitation with hemodilution of clotting factors, hypothermia, dysfunctional platelets, increased fibrinolysis, and acidosis. Platelets and fresh frozen plasma (FFP) usually are necessary to reverse the coagulopathy. Platelets are transfused to keep counts above $50\,000/mm^3$, and FFP is administered to maintain prothrombin time and partial thromboplastin time as normal as possible. This supportive management is beneficial as long as the resuscitation and rewarming proceed successfully. Failure to correct the hypothermia and acidosis prevents correction of the coagulopathy with blood products alone. If the coagulopathy persists despite an appropriate resuscitative response, the possibility of ongoing hemorrhage must be entertained.

When bleeding results from hypofibrinogenemia or disseminated intravascular coagulation (in which both fibrinogen and factor VIII are low), cryoprecipitate may be indicated. DDAVP, or desmopressin, a synthetic analog of vasopressin, may be helpful in those patients who have dysfunctional platelets, secondary to renal failure, or aspirin ingestion. There may also be a role for recombinant activated factor VII as an adjunctive hemostatic measure in trauma patients suffering from uncontrolled hemorrhage.[6] Its potential advantage stems from the fact that it acts predominantly at the site of injury without systemically activating the coagulation cascade. A true benefit must, however, be validated by larger studies.

Hypothermia

The most important immediate management rests in the correction of hypothermia. The cessation of nonsurgical bleeding relies on a rapid progressive reversal of the hypothermic state, since a low temperature strongly inhibits the enzymatic reactions of the coagulation cascade. An aggressive approach to correcting hypothermia reduces coagulopathy and contributes to an improved survival in patients with exsanguinating penetrating abdominal injuries.[4] Furthermore, there is evidence of an association between postoperative hypothermia and myocardial ischemia.

The patient's temperature may be monitored in a variety of ways, but invasive core temperature monitoring is the most accurate. This may be accomplished by using a pulmonary artery catheter thermistor or urinary catheter thermal probe. The ICU room should be warmed to 28°C and a convective warming blanket should be placed around the patient's torso and extremities to provide active external warming. Using passive external warming techniques (e.g., blankets) mandates that the patient's intrinsic heat generation is sufficient to reverse the hypothermia and in most cases is not efficient.

Internal warming techniques are an important means of restoring normothermia. All IV fluids and blood products should be administered through a rapid infusion device capable of warming fluids to body temperature. The ventilator circuitry should also provide warmed humidified air. These methods are usually sufficient to provide for the appropriate rewarming in the majority of patients who are mildly hypothermic. Body cavity lavage may also be employed if more rapid rewarming is deemed necessary. This entails administering warm, sterile crystalloid solutions into the pleural or peritoneal cavities and allowing them to equilibrate with body temperature prior to drainage. This, of course, is limited by the fact that injured and/or packed cavities are off-limits for employment of this technique. Continuous arteriovenous or veno-venous hemofiltration may also be employed in the more severe cases or in those unresponsive to less invasive means.

Management of the Open Abdomen

Over the last fifteen years, a number of temporary abdominal closure techniques have been used. The vacuum pack technique allows for rapid closure, reduces tissue injury, minimizes contamination, and is inexpensive. For the purposes of ICU care, it allows for effective, yet simple maintenance of the open abdomen by the ICU staff. The vacuum pack technique is one of the few closures that successfully keeps the area around the open abdomen dry. The vacuum pack method, or a modification thereof, is an ideal closure with minimal postoperative complications, and therefore it is recommended. Recent reports of the development of abdominal compartment syndrome with a vacuum pack in place stress the need for continuous use of bladder pressure monitoring.

In a well-supplied surgical ICU with experienced nursing staff, it is possible (and often necessary) to perform bedside washout and dressing changes for patients with an open abdomen using conditions and lighting that mimic the operating room itself. Such capability allows for care that may have otherwise been delayed, as in those patients who manifest continued respiratory instability, but who require packing removal and exchange.

Planned and Unplanned Returns to the Operating Room

The average time prior to planned formal reexploration is usually 24 to 36 hours; this amount of time allows for substantial correction of acidosis, hypothermia, and coagulopathy in those patients whose surgical bleeding has been controlled. Delaying the operative takeback greater than three days is not advocated since it contributes to higher rates of infection within the retained sponges and temporary closures; packing for greater than 72 hours contributes not only to significantly higher intra-abdominal abscess rates, but also to higher mortality rates, as compared with lesser duration.

There are times when the patient must be returned to the operating room or go to the interventional suite prior to a completed resuscitation. This is especially true if the temperature and coagulopathy are not corrected despite adequate efforts and there is evidence for ongoing surgical bleeding. This is suggested by a higher-than-expected rate and volume of transfusion and the need to continuously provide volume to maintain near normal pulse, blood pressure, and urine output. It becomes a futile endeavor to attempt to fully correct a coagulopathy when there is ongoing bleeding. A missed injury and ongoing blood loss should be presumed if a patient's lactate fails to clear or return to normal within the first 24 hours. These are patients who have the most to gain from early intervention directed at stopping bleeding.

Close attention must be paid to the potential development of abdominal compartment syndrome in the ICU. Intra-abdominal packing and significant visceral edema from large volume fluid requirements contribute to its occurrence. An open abdomen in itself does not protect against the development of compartment syndrome, although it occurs much more frequently if the fascia or skin are closed during the initial damage control surgery.

Bladder pressures greater than 25 millimeters of Hg suggest intra-abdominal hypertension significant enough to cause the syndrome. When elevated intravesicular pressures is less than ~20 millimeters Hg, but is associated with high peak airway pressures and oliguria, prompt decompression is appropriate and often therapeutic.

Contemporary ICU Issues

Significant advances continue to be made in the care of the surgical ICU patient (Table 22-2). In the remainder of this chapter, we will briefly discuss several of these developments that may be useful in the care of the penetrating injured patient. These include:

- strategies to treat renal failure and Adult Respiratory Distress Syndrome (ARDS),
- methods to prevent and treat common ICU infections such as pneumonia, catheter-related infections, and sepsis,
- optimal nutrition management,
- aggressive glycemic control.

Pulmonary/ARDS

Severe penetrating trauma with exsanguinating hemorrhage and large-volume resuscitation are risk factors for ARDS. Clinical ARDS occurs primarily as a result of acute inflammation, leading to diffuse alveolar damage. The lungs are particularly vulnerable to damage secondary to inflammatory mediators released in response to tissue destruction, bleeding, and shock. Normal barriers to alveolar edema are lost, leading to alveolar collapse with impaired gas exchange and compliance.

ARDS is defined as:

- a PaO_2/FiO_2 <200
- absence of left atrial hypertension (pulmonary capillary wedge pressure <18)
- chest radiographic findings of bilateral fluffy infiltrates.

TABLE 22-2. Recent advances in SICU care

Field	Advance
Nutrition	Early enteral feedings
	Immune-modulating formulations
Acute renal failure	Continuous veno-venous hemo-filtration/dialysis
	Acetylcysteine for contrast nephropathy prophylaxis
Pulmonary/ARDS	Low-volume ventilation
Infection	
Ventilator associated pneumonia	Early diagnosis via bronchoalveolar lavage
	Early, directed antibiotic therapy
Catheter-related blood stream infection	Antibiotic-coated catheters
	Maximum barrier precautions
Sepsis/MODS	Activated protein C (if no bleeding predisposition)
Glycemic control	Intensive insulin therapy

Patients experience severe initial hypoxemia and tachypnea. Pulmonary dysfunction typically develops within 24 to 48 hours of the inciting event,[7] with most patients ultimately requiring prolonged ventilatory support.

Complications include nosocomial pneumonia, multiple-organ dysfunction syndrome (MODS), and barotrauma.

Evidence from animal studies suggests that ventilation with excessive tidal volumes may exacerbate the damage by over-stretching the lung parenchyma. The ARDSNet trial, a retrospective analysis of data from 718 patients with ARDS, questioned the traditional approach of providing 10 to 15 milliliters per kilogram tidal volumes and suggested that lower tidal volume ventilation (6 milliliters per kilogram) improved clinical outcome. Mortality was reduced by 22%. Furthermore, the number of ventilator-free days was increased, and the lung inflammation with subsequent systemic inflammation was less in the lower tidal volume group. Priority should be given to preventing excessive stretch during mechanical ventilation. There has been an improved survival in ARDS patients in recent years, although mortality remains high, approximating 35 to 40%. Diverse modalities of therapy to improve shunt and recruit alveoli (such as proning and use of inhaled nitric oxide, perfluorocarbons, and surfactant) have all not affected mortality. The presence of infection and multiple organ failure predict survival better than respiratory parameters alone.

Pneumonia

Nosocomial pneumonia, a complication of prolonged mechanical ventilation, is an important cause of morbidity and mortality in the critically ill patient.

It is defined as an infection of the lower respiratory tree occurring 48 hours after admission, excluding any process incubating at the time of admission.

Early ventilator-associated pneumonia (VAP) is more often caused by *Streptococcus pneumoniae* and *Haemophilus influenza*, while *Staphylococcus aureus* and gram-negative rods are organisms frequently found in patients with VAP with greater than 72 hours of hospitalization. Multitrauma patients are at particularly higher risk for VAP.

Bronchoscopy to obtain bronchoalveolar lavage specimens from the affected lung area has been advocated by some, allowing for a therapeutic strategy better than one based on clinical evaluation alone and a reduction in excessive antibiotic use.[8]

Effective prevention strategies for VAP include semirecumbent patient positioning, adequate hand washing between patient contacts by health care workers, and avoidance of unnecessary antibiotics. Available data suggests that withholding antibiotic therapy in some patients without infection may have a distinct long-term advantage because it minimizes the emergence of resistant organisms in the ICU and redirects the search for the true infection site. However, for patients with clinical evidence of sepsis, initiation of antibiotic therapy should not be delayed, and effective antimicrobial therapy supplemented by adequate supportive measures remains the mainstay of treatment.[8]

Blood Stream Infections

Many patients with penetrating trauma require central venous access and invasive monitoring. The central venous circulation provides convenient, beneficial access and is commonly used for parenteral nutrition and fluid and drug administration. The use of central venous catheters does increase the risk of nosocomial blood stream infections. These infections are a serious complication leading to increased mortality, length of hospital stay, and hospital costs. In the ICUs in the United States, infection occurs in three to seven percent of catheters, with anywhere from 500 to 4000 patients dying annually of catheter-related blood stream infections. Microbial organisms that colonize catheter hubs and the skin surrounding the catheter insertion site are the source of infection. Priority should be given to cutaneous antisepsis with povidone-iodine and to maximum barrier precautions, namely sterile gloves, gowns, caps, masks, and drapes. Additionally, the site of catheter insertion can reduce the risk of infection with the subclavian vein being preferred. Subcutaneous tunneling of short-term catheters further minimizes potential colonization because catheter hubs are not frequently manipulated. Antibiotic-coated or impregnated catheters are important additions to preventative strategies and are recommended when catheterization is expected to last more than two weeks.[9]

Sepsis and Multiple Organ Dysfunction Syndrome (MODS)

Systemic inflammatory response syndrome (SIRS) is characterized by systemic inflammation, with increases in pro-inflammatory cytokines and complement factor activation leading to widespread tissue injury. The presence of two or more of the following clinical signs characterize the syndrome:

- a temperature greater than 38°C or less than 36°C,
- a heart rate greater than 90 beats per minute,
- a respiratory rate greater than 20 breaths per minute,
- a $PaCO_2$ less than 32 millimeters Hg,
- a white cell count greater than 12000 cells/mm^3, less than 4000 cells/mm^3, or greater than 10% immature forms.

Sepsis affects up to 25% of all ICU patients, and current estimates indicate that there are more than 600000 cases per year, with greater than 100000 deaths per year within the United States.[10]

It is clinically important to distinguish between underlying disease (infection, renal failure) and the host inflammatory response (SIRS). It is this host response and not the specific organ injury that accounts for MODS seen in critically ill patients. Multiple-organ dysfunction syndrome and septic shock are the most severe consequences of sepsis and SIRS.

Despite modern interventions and advances in supportive care, the prognosis of sepsis remains poor. There are a number of factors including site of infection, causative organism, and the presence of organ dysfunction that influence outcome. Abnormalities in coagulation have been noted in MODS and several reports suggest protein C supplementation may be beneficial in sepsis. A multi-center trial in February 2001 supported the efficacy of recombinant human activated protein C (Xigris®) for patients with septic shock.[11] Incidence of multi-organ failure was lower for patients treated with activated protein C with a more rapid recovery of cardiopulmonary function. The drug appears to be most beneficial in the acutely septic patient, resulting in a significantly lower mortality rate.

However, the use of this antithrombotic medication in the penetrating trauma patient 48 hours or less from surgery is not FDA approved or advocated at this time, as this population maybe predisposed to bleeding with CNS or solid viscus injury.

Nutrition

Malnutrition in hospitalized patients is well documented. Nutritional therapy is frequently instituted, but it often remains unclear when and how to intervene. The stress of trauma and surgery creates a hypermetabolic state with high protein and energy requirements. The resulting protein–calorie malnutrition increases susceptibility to infection, immune system dysfunction, poor wound healing, and bacterial overgrowth in the gastrointestinal tract. Sepsis and poor wound healing are of particular concern in the postoperative trauma patient.

Before formulating a nutritional approach to a critically ill patient, it is important to assess the patient's underlying nutritional status. This is best accomplished by history and physical exam, although certain laboratory tests provide important additional information. In general, most favor early nutritional support, even in young, theoretically well-nourished patients. As number and severity of injury increases, so does need for nutritional support. With its long half-life of 18 to 20 days, serum albumin reflects nutritional status over a two to three month period. Pre-albumin, with a half-life of two to three days, is less helpful in assessing overall nutritional status, but acts as a practical marker of nutritional repletion in the critically ill patient. Bedside metabolic carts are useful for performing nutritional assessments by measuring the carbon dioxide in expired gas and estimating metabolic demands.

Many animal and clinical studies have advocated the use of the gastrointestinal tract whenever possible. Using the gut leads to improved mucosal structure and function, as well as enhanced immunity.[12] This is also the case in penetrating injury. Parenteral nutrition is recommended if the gastrointestinal tract is not functional or seven to ten days of bowel rest is anticipated.

Several nutrients have been shown to influence immunologic and inflammatory responses in humans. These nutrients, which are normally considered nonessential, become essential under conditions of stress. Glutamine, an important precursor for nucleotide synthesis and fuel for rapidly dividing cells, can prevent gastrointestinal mucosal atrophy and facilitate its prompt healing. Glutamine has been suggested as an important factor in decreasing the rate of sepsis, bacteremia, and pneumonia in trauma patients. Arginine, an amino acid important in nitrogen metabolism, has been shown in animal studies to improve rates of wound healing and to facilitate the synthesis of acute phase reactant proteins in sepsis. Proprietary "immunonutritional" formulas are associated with significant decreases in nosocomial infection, ventilator days, and length of stay.

Acute Renal Failure

The development of acute renal failure in the intensive care unit is a common problem, but one that carries a mortality of over 30%. Pre-renal azotemia and acute tubular necrosis are the most frequent causes, and optimization of renal perfusion is the most current renal preservation strategy. Patients with sepsis have a worse prognosis. Injured and critically ill patients frequently undergo a variety of diagnostic studies. Radiographic contrast dye-induced renal insufficiency is one of the leading causes of acute renal failure in this population. Correction of volume deficits should be initiated prior to the study unless the patient needs the study immediately for life-saving interventions. The antioxidant acetylcysteine, along with hydration, has been shown to prevent the renal dysfunction induced by contrast agent in patients with chronic renal insufficiency.[13]

To date, no intervention has been shown to definitively prevent acute renal failure in the critically ill patient. Supportive treatments include traditional hemodialysis[14] and continuous veno-venous hemodialysis (CVVH). The latter produces less hypotension and is effective for patients with multiorgan system failure. Furthermore, continuous renal replacement therapy has advantages, including its ease of initiation and maintenance within an ICU setting.

Hyperglycemia

Hyperglycemia and insulin resistance are common in critically ill patients. The stress and hypermetabolism following severe trauma also raises blood glucose levels. It is reported that pronounced hyperglycemia predisposes to complications such as increased susceptibility to infection, multiple-organ failure, and death.[15] Immune function is impaired during marked hyperglycemia. Enteral and parenteral feedings often elevate serum glucose concentrations, compounding these problems.

A prospective, controlled trial of more than 1500 ventilated patients in the surgical ICU found that tighter blood glucose control reduced mortality.[15] Patients were randomly assigned to either intensive insulin therapy via insulin infusion (target blood glucose 80 to 100 milligrams per deciliter) or to standard care with target glucose levels between 180 and 200 milligrams per deciliter. The use of intensive insulin therapy to keep serum glucose levels less than 110 milligrams per deciliter substantially reduced mortality and morbidity. It also reduced the overall hospital mortality by 34%. Tight glycemic control reduced the risk of acute renal failure by 41% and is the only strategy, other than optimization of hemodynamic status, that has proven to be effective. There was also a reduction in septicemia and the consequent need for long-term antibiotics. Furthermore, there was a reduced need for mechanical ventilation, which is attributed to the decreased rate of ICU polyneuropathy.

Travel from the ICU

Travel from the ICU with the trauma patient has risks. The need to know the information sought from studies must be balanced with the patient's physiologic status. Patients can suffer oxygen desaturation, hypotension, changes in intracranial pressure, and device dislodgment as a result of any movement, but especially during transport. Safe transport involves consideration of the risks versus benefits and preparation. Transport ventilators, drug administration kits, and transport personnel should accompany the patient. This is also true for transport back to the operating suite. Patients on high PEEP settings should not just be "bagged" without an in-line PEEP valve, but should be transported on a ventilator capable of accomplishing present settings. Coordination of studies to consolidate and limit travel is key. At times, it may be necessary to defer additional imaging (e.g., head CT scan) in patients who are critically ill and unstable after injury. Protocols should be in place to expedite transport of the patient from the ED to the operating room to radiology and the ICU.

Summary

Careful attention to "details" in the ICU is the necessary complement to expeditious management in the operating room of the critically ill penetrating injured patient. A thorough examination should be accompanied by review of pre-ICU care with appropriate resuscitation, analgesia, thromboembolism prophylaxis, and monitoring.

Successful correction of acidosis, coagulopathy, and hypothermia suggests that resuscitation with blood products and other fluids is successful and surgical bleeding is controlled. Vacuum pack closure is effective in minimizing leakage and the risk of abdominal compartment syndrome. Nonetheless, elevated bladder pressures and persistent anemia suggest that earlier operative intervention is warranted.

Various evidence-based strategies that have improved outcome in ICU patients are applicable to penetrating injured patients. These include ventilator strategies to improve ARDS outcome, infection control methods to lower the risk of ventilator-associated pneumonias and blood stream infections, use of activated protein C in severe sepsis (but not until 48 hours after surgery), early use of enteral immunonutrition, strict glucose control, and techniques to prevent and treat renal failure.

References

1. Pronovost P, Wu AW, Dorman T, Morlock L. Building safety into ICU care. *J Crit Care.* 2002;17:78–85.
2. Sandham JD, Hull RD, Brant RF, et al. A randomized, controlled trial of the use of pulmonary-artery catheters in high-risk surgical patients. *N Engl J Med.* 2003;348:5–14.
3. Jacobi J, Fraser GL, Coursin DB, et al. Clinical practice guidelines for the sustained use of sedatives and analgesics in the critically ill adult. *Crit Care Med.* 2002;30:119–141.
4. Johnson JW, Gracias VH, Schwab CW, et al. Evolution in damage control for exsanguinating penetrating abdominal injury. *J Trauma.* 2001;51:261–271.
5. Leibovici D, Gofrit ON, Stein M, et al. Blast injuries: bus versus open-air bombings- a comparative study of injuries in survivors of open-air versus confined-space explosions. *J Trauma.* 1996;41:1030–1035.
6. Martinowitz U, Kenet G, Segal E, et al. Recombinant activated factor VII for adjunctive hemorrhage control in trauma. *J Trauma.* 2001;51:431–439.
7. Hudson LD, Milberg JA, Anardi D, et al. Clinical risks for development of the acute respiratory distress syndrome. *Am J Respir Crit Care Med.* 1995;151:293.
8. Chastre J, Fagon JY. Ventilator-associated pneumonia. *Am J Respir Crit Care Med.* 2002;165:867–903.
9. Mermel LA. Prevention of intravascular catheter-related infections. *Ann Intern Med.* 2000;132:391–402.
10. Martin GS, Mannino DM, Eaton S, Moss M. The epidemiology of sepsis in the United States from 1979 through 2000. *N Engl J Med.* 2003;348:1546.
11. Bernard GR, Vincent JL, Laterre PF, et al. Efficacy and safety of recombinant activated protein C for severe sepsis. *N Engl J Med.* 2000;344:699–709.
12. Braga M, Gianotti L, Vignali A, et al. Artificial nutrition after major abdominal surgery: Impact of route of administration and composition of the diet. *Crit Care Med.* 1998;26:24.
13. Tepel M, van der Giet M, Schwarzfeld C, Liermann D, Zidek W. Prevention of radiographic-contrast-agent-induced reductions in renal function by acetylcysteine. *N Engl J Med.* 2000;343:180–184.
14. Schiffl H, Lang SM, Fischer R. Daily hemodialysis and the outcome of acute renal failure. *N Engl J Med.* 2002;346:305–310.
15. Van den Berghe G, Wouters P, Weekers F, et al. Intensive insulin therapy in the critically ill patients. *N Engl J Med.* 2001;345:1359.

Further Readings

Surgical critical care in the new millennium. In: Schwab CW, Reilly PM, eds. *Surgical Clinics of North America*. 2000;80(3).

Rabinovici R, Frankel H, Kaplan L. Trauma evaluation and resuscitation. *Curr Probl Surg*. 2003;40(10):599–681.

Stott S. Recent advances in intensive care. *BMJ*. 2000:320:358–361.

23
Imaging Triage for Ballistic Trauma

STEPHEN C. GALE and VICENTE H. GRACIAS

Introduction

The initial evaluation of victims of ballistic trauma is largely dependent on the physical examination and physiologic status of the patient. Patients are fully exposed and wounds are carefully examined in an attempt to determine trajectory. Based on the suspected path of the missile, determinations can be made as to what structures are likely injured and what interventions may be needed.

All who care for the injured patient agree that there is a limited role for radiologic assessment in hemodynamically unstable patients. However, in those patients without physiologic compromise, radiologic evaluation can serve as a very useful adjunct in the triage of patients toward more invasive studies, surgical intervention, or nonoperative management. Routine plain film radiographs remain an essential tool in the initial evaluation of all victims of penetrating trauma. Nevertheless, an increasing role has developed for additional diagnostic modalities including surgeon-performed ultrasound, computed tomography (CT), and angiography in those who are stable and have a questionable need for operation or uncertain trajectory. With the expansion of these accurate and versatile imaging modalities, many traditional principles in the management of ballistic trauma patients are being redefined.

Chest Films

All gunshot victims, irrespective of the area injured, should routinely undergo portable anteroposterior (AP) radiography of the chest. This important and inexpensive screening tool quickly excludes many life-threatening conditions. When possible, every effort should be made to perform this study with the patient's torso in the upright, seated, or reverse Trendelenberg position. This may allow earlier diagnosis of perforated viscus with the visualization of free intraperitoneal air, or may help demonstrate a hemothorax by the dependent layering of fluid in the chest.

Wound Markers

In order to maximize information gained from plain radiographs or CT scans, radiopaque markers should be placed on all external wounds to aid in locating skin perforations and their relevance to retained foreign bodies, projectiles, and fragments. Simple items such as self-adherent electrocardiogram electrodes or taped-on paper clips serve as useful reference points when viewing multiple anatomic projections of plain films and multiplanar CT images.

Computed Tomography

In particular, there has been an increasing interest in defining the role of helical CT in the evaluation of selected patients. In hemodynamically stable patients, the use of helical CT as a triage tool has become a standard diagnostic modality. Many centers have studied the role of CT in determining missile trajectory in various anatomic regions, including the neck, chest, and abdomen and pelvis.[1-5] The constantly improving resolution of modern CT imaging allows accurate characterization of soft tissue planes and contrast-enhanced vasculature. The growing consensus is that by accurately defining missile trajectory and demonstrating it to be distant from vital structures, some patients can avoid further invasive testing or unnecessary operative exploration.

The phrase "Accurate trajectory determination equals injury identification," is a summary of this concept and is a growing axiom in the evaluation of ballistic trauma.[2]

Magnetic Resonance Imaging

The role of magnetic resonance imaging (MRI) in the evaluation of ballistic trauma victims remains poorly defined. There are reports of its use in the evaluation of cranial and extremity trauma. The issue of greatest concern is whether the projectile fragments have ferromagnetic properties and thus will move under the influence of the MRI magnet. Hess and others[6] recently performed an extensive evaluation of the ferromagnetic properties of 56 different projectiles fired from various air guns, handguns, rifles, and shotguns. They concluded that while not all bullets were ferromagnetic, the only current method of determining if a gunshot victim qualifies for MRI is by pretesting identical missiles before scanning. At present, these limitations certainly prevent the widespread use of MRI in the acute evaluation of ballistic trauma victims.

Imaging Away from the Emergency Room

There are a number of important considerations for the trauma team leader in choosing to obtain imaging studies outside the resuscitation area. In some settings, most or all of these advanced diagnostic modalities are available in close proximity to the Emergency Department and Trauma Bay. However, this level of technology is not universal. Diagnostic studies should not delay or prevent ongoing resuscitation and rewarming of the injured patient. Intensive care of the patient is a philosophy that drives optimal care and should not be constrained by location. Patients must be continuously and adequately monitored while imaging studies are being performed. Patients with potentially life-threatening injuries should be accompanied by a physician-member of the trauma team who is capable of identifying and immediately acting upon changes in the patient's condition. In all situations, the decision to obtain advanced diagnostic studies should weigh the potential utility of the information gained versus the risk of transporting the patient out of the "safety" of the resuscitation area or directly moving the patient to the operating room.

Imaging of Specific Anatomical Regions

Craniofacial Injury

The initial diagnostic study of choice to assess victims of penetrating injury to the head or face is non-enhanced CT.[1,7,8] The accuracy of this modality to assess the extent of brain injury and to diagnose or exclude a transcranial trajectory allows rapid triage of patients to surgical intervention, medical management, or expectant observation (Figure 23-1). Multiplanar reconstruction of facial CT scans allows assessment of ocular, maxillofacial, or mandibular injuries and planning for reconstructive surgical intervention. It should be noted that, in cases of severe bullet fragmentation, the scatter effect created by metallic foreign bodies might limit image resolution. Patients with ongoing arterial hemorrhage from gunshot wounds to the face may benefit from early angiographically guided embolization of bleeding vessels.[9,10]

In patients with penetrating injuries to both the head and torso, hemodynamic stability should guide decision making with regard to diagnostic imaging. In unstable patients, operative interventions aimed at controlling the compelling source of bleeding should take priority as hypotension significantly increases the mortality associated with traumatic brain injury.[11] In hemodynamically stable patients with combined injuries, there may be some benefit to obtaining a head CT prior to operative intervention provided that the study can be rapidly obtained, patients are adequately

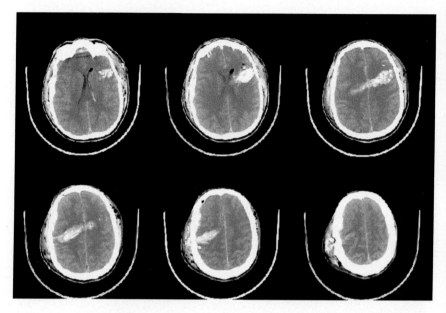

FIGURE 23-1. Self-inflicted gunshot wound to the head with demonstration of transcranial trajectory.

monitored, and the team is prepared to urgently transport the patient to the operating room if their condition deteriorates.

Specific knowledge of intracranial pathology allows necessary neurosurgical intervention to occur concurrently with laparotomy or thoracotomy, or prior to leaving the operating room. Of note, patients who have sustained isolated craniofacial gunshot wounds do not routinely require immobilization or radiographic evaluation of the cervical spine; however, caution is advised if the complete mechanism of injury is not known or the patient cannot be fully examined.[12]

Neck Injury

The evaluation of hemodynamically stable patients with penetrating neck injuries continues to evolve. By tradition, the management of this complex anatomic region has relied upon classification of the penetration into one of the classic cervical "zones" as described in 1979 by Roon and Christensen (Figure 23-2).[13]

Evaluation and management of patients with gunshot wounds to Zones I or III traditionally includes urgent aortic arch and great vessel angiography, bronchoscopy, and esophagoscopy to exclude significant injury to the great vessels or aerodigestive tract.[14,15] In the past, those victims with Zone

II injuries have undergone mandatory complete diagnostic neck exploration or more recently, "selective management," which requires angiography and panendoscopy.[16–19]

These nonspecific algorithms, while highly accurate at identifying and
excluding injuries, are quite labor/resource intensive and demand multiple
procedures performed by different specialists. In addition, in stable patients,
the positive yield is often low, with approximately 15% of patients requiring operative intervention.[20]

Finally, these invasive diagnostic procedures carry a small but real
rate of complications and take considerable time.[21] In the evaluation of
less-invasive diagnostic techniques, Montalvo found cervical color duplex
sonography to be an accurate alternative to angiography in stable patients
with Zone II or Zone III injuries who were not actively bleeding.[22] Accurate cervical duplex ultrasound is often not readily available, is operator
dependent, and requires specialist expertise in interpretation. In addition,
this technology is limited by patient habitus, does not image skull-base
injuries, and does not impact the need for evaluation of the aerodigestive
tract. These issues have led a number of surgeons to question whether rigid
algorithmic protocols for invasive evaluation of victims of gunshot wounds

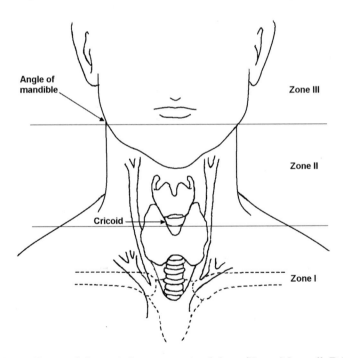

FIGURE 23-2. Zones of the neck for penetrating injury. (From Maxwell, RA. Penetrating Neck Injury. In: Peitzman AB, Rhodes M, Schwab CW, Yealy DM, Fabian
TC, eds. *The Trauma Manual*. Philadelphia: Lippincott Williams & Wilkins; 2002:192,
with permission) (See also Figure 11-3.)

to the neck should apply to all patients, most importantly to those with normal physical examination[23] and normal chest radiograph.[21]

These controversies, and the ever-increasing incidence of multi-zone penetration, the profession-wide trend toward less-invasive diagnostic approaches, and the improved resolution and speed of current-generation CT scanners, have changed the algorithm for penetrating neck injuries.

The initial diagnostic study of choice in hemodynamically stable patients with cervical gunshot injuries appears to be helical CT with timed contrast injection.[2] This imaging modality can serve as a definitive diagnostic tool in cases where injury requiring surgery is identified or where the visualized trajectory clearly places sensitive structures out of "harm's way." In those patients in whom trajectory suggests proximity to vital structure or where trajectory is unclear, helical CT serves as a triage tool to select further individualized invasive diagnostic evaluation.

There is a growing body of literature to support the use of CT angiography in penetrating cervical trauma. Ofer[24] reported a series of patients in whom CT angiography was highly accurate in determining vascular injury with successful nonoperative management of patients with negative CT scans.

In 2001, a prospective study of Zone II penetrations by Mazolewski[25] demonstrated a 100% sensitivity of trauma-surgeon–evaluated neck CT in identifying injuries requiring operative intervention. That same year, Gracias[2] reported the first series that included patients with gunshots to any of the three neck zones and found that CT was a safe and effective modality "to direct or eliminate further invasive studies in selected stable patients with penetrating neck injury."

In 2002, a prospective study by Munera[26] evaluated 175 patients with penetrating neck injury by CT angiography. They were able to accurately characterize vascular injuries in 27 (15.6%) patients and direct them to appropriate therapy. The other 146 patients were successfully observed without further intervention and without missed injury.

In 2003, Gonzalez[27] prospectively evaluated helical CT scan in stable victims of penetrating neck trauma. The study reported equivalent accuracy of helical CT to esophagography in the evaluation of penetrating injury to the cervical esophagus, but noted that the sensitivity of helical CT was similar to physical examination. Of note, in this study, 86% of the patients sustained stab injuries. Due to the difficulty in determining stab wound trajectory with CT scan, these data and conclusions likely do not apply to ballistic trauma.

Recommendations

Based on the current evidence, irrespective of zone of penetration, stable patients without hard signs of vascular (pulsatile bleeding, expanding hematoma, bruit) or of aerodigestive injury (subcutaneous emphysema, wound bubbling, airway compromise) after gunshot wound to the neck are candidates for trajectory determination and injury identification by contrast-enhanced CT (Figure 23-3). Injuries to the trachea, oropharynx, cervical esophagus, and important vascular structures can be readily identified. Using helical CT as a triage tool, trauma surgeons can choose to pursue operative intervention as necessary or obtain further individual diagnostic studies where appropriate, including interventional angiography for definitive endovascular repair in selected cases.[10] If helical CT is not available, or if the findings on CT scan are inconclusive or do not match clinical findings, traditional methods of evaluating penetrating neck trauma with diagnostic angiography, endoscopy, esophagography, or operative exploration should be pursued.

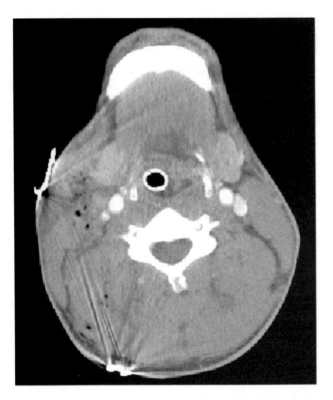

FIGURE 23-3. Computed tomography after gunshot wound to the neck with clear demonstration of trajectory. Injury to the patient's carotid artery, oropharynx, and tracheobronchial tree are excluded. (See also Figure 11-5.)

Chest Injury

The evaluation of penetrating chest injuries has also continued to evolve. As with all victims of penetrating trauma, hemodynamic stability remains the most important triage criteria. Patients in extremis often have injuries to the heart or great vessels requiring immediate intervention and making diagnostic imaging impossible. If permitted by the patient's condition, a single anteroposterior (AP) plain radiograph can provide valuable information about trajectory and insight into what vital structures may be injured. This information may also be useful when planning the operative approach.

In most cases, hemodynamically stable victims of thoracic gunshot wounds have sustained simple unilateral "through-and-through" injuries resulting only in damage to the pulmonary parenchyma. These patients are usually evaluated with plain chest radiographs and are managed with a tube thoracostomy alone. Plain abdominal X-rays to exclude subdiaphragmatic pathology are also sometimes helpful in these patients.

Ultrasound

Surgeon-performed ultrasound in the resuscitation area plays an increasingly valuable role in the noninvasive evaluation of patients with penetrating chest trauma. In hemodynamically unstable patients, ultrasound can serve as a rapid, repeatable triage tool to identify significant hemothorax[28] and to exclude an abdominal source of blood loss. In addition, pericardial ultrasound reliably excludes cardiac tamponade and, in the absence of hemothorax, significant injury to the heart.[29–31] Thoracic ultrasound has also been shown to accurately identify pneumothorax in penetrating chest trauma.[32]

At the discretion of the trauma surgeon, patients with continued significant bleeding are taken to the operating room for definitive treatment.[31] Rarely is more advanced imaging needed in the initial evaluation of these patients.

Angiography

Angiography is indicated for stable patients sustaining periclavicular injuries who have physical or radiographic findings, such as pulse or neurologic deficit, suggestive of subclavian or axillary vascular injury. Patients with no signs of vascular compromise do not require angiography based on proximity alone.[33,34]

Transmediastinal Injury

Hemodynamically stable patients with transmediastinal gunshot wounds, multiple penetrations, or with gunshot woundings of unknown trajectory represent a controversial injury subset in which the appropriate diagnostic pathway continues to evolve. The crucial information that must be obtained from advanced imaging modalities is the status of the mediastinal structures. Patients sustaining transmediastinal trajectories may have injuries to the heart, great vessels, esophagus, or tracheobronchial tree. Each of these injuries is life threatening and delays in diagnosis significantly increase morbidity and mortality.[35]

After undergoing primary and secondary surveys, including chest radiograph and thoracostomy tube placement as needed, *stable* patients with suspected transmediastinal gunshot wounds must quickly proceed to advanced imaging to exclude injury to vital structures and aid in timely triage of secondary interventions (Figure 23-4). Traditionally, this diagnostic algorithm includes formal angiography, bronchoscopy, esophagography, esophagoscopy, and pericardial window.[36,37] Transesophageal echocardiography has also been described to assist in the evaluation of the heart and great vessels.[38,39] While accurate, this multi-specialty evaluation is highly invasive, time consuming, and expensive, it may be best reserved for unstable patients requiring immediate operation.

Recently, contrast-enhanced helical CT scan has emerged as an accurate triage tool to guide further organ-specific evaluation as needed.[31] Missile trajectory can be determined with the exclusion or identification of injuries to specific structures (Figure 23-5).[3] While helical CT may also help identify cardiac injuries,[40] the addition of thoracoabdominal ultrasound to this approach reliably excludes hemopericardium and cardiac injury.[30] Two recent studies reflect the utility of this approach. In 2000, Hanpeter and

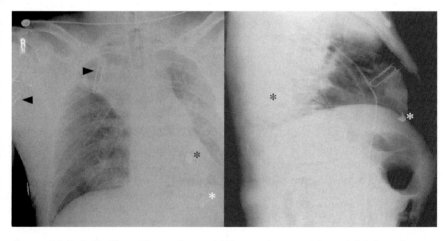

FIGURE 23-4. Left: Chest X-ray after multiple gunshot wounds to right chest. Arrows demonstrate entrance wounds. Anterior (white asterisk) and posterior (black asterisk) foreign bodies are seen in the left chest having traversed the mediastinum.

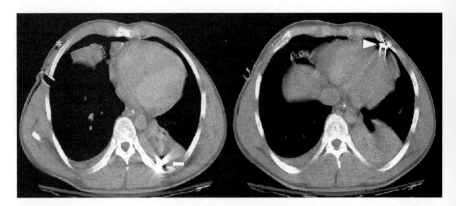

FIGURE 23-5. Chest CT of patient in Figure 23-4. Asterisk demonstrates one entrance wound. Anterior and posterior foreign bodies are seen (arrow). The mediastinal structures are clearly at risk for injury and further studies are needed.

others[4] evaluated 24 stable patients with transmediastinal gunshot wounds with contrast-enhanced CT scan. Further work-up was indicated in 12 patients based on missile trajectory; one patient required operative intervention. The remaining 11 patients were successfully observed with no further work-up and had no missed injuries. Stassen,[41] in 2002, reviewed 22 patients with transmediastinal gunshot wounds who underwent contrast-enhanced CT scan as the initial diagnostic study. Seven patients required further diagnostic work-up based on CT scan findings and two patients required operation. No further evaluation was required in 15 patients and no injuries were missed. These studies reflect the ability of contrast-enhanced CT scan to accurately and efficiently screen patients with trans-mediastinal gunshot wounds for life-threatening injuries, direct further diagnostic studies, and avoid unnecessary invasive procedures.

It is important to emphasize that while contrast-enhanced CT scan has emerged as a useful triage tool in the evaluation of patients with trans-mediastinal gunshot wounds, positive findings must be followed with traditional studies to guide therapeutic decision making. Patients with suspected vascular injury based on identified missile trajectory, contrast extravasation, or the presence of mediastinal blood should undergo formal angiography, either as a diagnostic modality to direct operative intervention or as a therapeutic modality for embolization or stent placement at the discretion of the interventional radiologist.

In patients suspected of sustaining esophageal perforation, contrast esophagography, first with water-soluble contrast (Gastrograffin), then with thin barium if needed, is performed to accurately identify injuries. Flexible or rigid endoscopy can also be used as an initial diagnostic modality to exclude or identify thoracic esophageal injuries or to confirm negative esophagography where high clinical suspicion still exists.

Computed tomography findings or missile trajectory that suggests tracheobronchial injury mandates bronchoscopy to identify the level of injury and guide operative intervention. Formal echocardiography should be used to exclude pericardial violation in patients with questionable findings on surgeon-performed ultrasound or to follow studies limited by emergency department ultrasound equipment, operator inexperience, or patient body habitus.[42]

Finally, after penetrating chest trauma, a subset of hemodynamically normal victims has a normal chest radiograph and no suspected mediastinal involvement. While more common in stab victims, this presentation does occur in gunshot wounds as well. After initial evaluation, a three- to six-hour period of observation in a monitored setting followed by repeat chest radiograph is a safe approach.[43,44] Patients with normal follow-up chest radiograph can be reliably discharged without further diagnostic studies. While CT can more reliably exclude small pneumothoraces and identify trajectory in these patients, it may not be as cost effective as the above approach.[43]

Abdominal Injury

Few would argue that abdominal gunshot victims who arrive to care with hemodynamic instability or with evidence of peritonitis (rigidity, pain distant from missile tract, distention) should be urgently taken to the operating room for thorough abdominal exploration and definitive repair of injuries. For these patients, little more than a plain radiograph of the chest is needed to exclude multicavity trauma. In some centers, if hemodynamic parameters allow, plain films of the abdomen are also obtained to help identify trajectory and give surgeons some insight prior to exploration. If readily available, an ultrasound exam may be performed to document the presence of fluid in the abdomen consistent with the clinical picture and to exclude pericardial violation as previously discussed. Patients with penetrating abdominal injuries and obvious indication for laparotomy *rarely* benefit from preoperative or on-table "one-shot" intravenous pyelogram (IVP). This practice delays definitive treatment and does not usually alter the course of therapy.[45]

While many patients with abdominal gunshot wounds are easily triaged toward exploratory laparotomy, this is not true in all cases. Victims of ballistic abdominal trauma represent perhaps the most controversial group of patients to which the concept of advanced imaging-based triage is being applied. Since the late nineteenth century, the traditional and uniform approach to the evaluation of victims of abdominal gunshot wounds has been with mandatory exploratory laparotomy. Using this approach, the acceptance of a nearly 20% negative laparotomy rate has been considered necessary to avoid potentially life-threatening missed injuries. Fundamental to this concept had been the long-held belief that nearly all patients with torso gunshot wounds, irrespective of trajectory, are likely to have significant intra-abdominal injuries. Surgical dogma maintained that any delay in the diagnosis and treatment of intra-abdominal injuries led to an unacceptable increase in morbidity and mortality. The perception existed that abdominal exploration as a diagnostic procedure was rarely associated with complications.[46] An ever-increasing body of literature continues to examine these enduring principles with the goal of decreasing the incidence of unnecessary laparotomy and taking a more individualized approach to patients with ballistic abdominal trauma.

In 1995, Renz and Feliciano[47] prospectively reported 254 "unnecessary laparotomies" for trauma. They noted a negative laparotomy rate of 23.4% (128 of 548) for patients with abdominal gunshot/shotgun wounds. Complications occurred in 43% of these patients. Demetriades and others[48] published prospective data in 1997 on their selective-management protocol for gunshot wounds to the anterior abdomen. Using a combination of physical exam and imaging, they successfully managed 29.8% of their patients nonoperatively.

Based on the work of these groups and others, there has been great interest in the use of abdominal imaging to select the subset of stable patients with ballistic abdominal trauma who can be managed nonoperatively. Of particular interest are those patients who appear to have sustained either tangential abdominal wounds or wounds isolated to the soft tissue of the flank, back, or pelvis. Both ultrasound[49–53] and CT[3,54–58] have been studied for use in the evaluation of these patients.

Ultrasound

Although most commonly used to evaluate victims of blunt abdominal trauma, focused abdominal sonography for trauma (FAST) is a useful and readily available modality for the evaluation of all patients with abdominal trauma.[52] Furthermore, the use of ultrasound is being increasingly incorporated into surgical training worldwide.[49–51,59]

In the evaluation of the trauma victim, dependent areas of the abdomen are interrogated for the presence of free intraperitoneal fluid. Any fluid identified is assumed to be either blood or enteric contents. Ultrasound has the advantage of being easy to perform and free of radiation risk to the patient or the hospital staff. In many institutions, this modality is present in the trauma resuscitation area and has become part of the routine physical examination of all patients.

In 2001, Udobi and colleagues[60] prospectively examined 75 stable patients with penetrating trauma to the abdomen, flank, or back with FAST. Their data revealed a sensitivity of 46%, a positive predictive value of 90%, and negative predictive value of 60% for the need for laparotomy based on ultrasound findings. That same year, Boulanger and others[61] reported their experience with FAST in 72 patients. A sensitivity of 67%, a positive predictive value of 92%, and a negative predictive value of 89% were reported for detecting significant intra-abdominal injury with FAST.

Recommendations

Based on these two prospective studies it would appear that *a positive FAST exam is clinically useful in the triage of patients toward laparotomy while a negative study does not reliably exclude injury and warrants further diagnostic imaging.*

Contrast Enhanced CT Scan

For this reason and others, contrast-enhanced CT scan has emerged as a highly useful diagnostic study to assist trauma surgeons in the evaluation and triage of stable victims of ballistic abdominal trauma (Figure 23-6).

In 1998, Grossman and others[3] retrospectively reviewed their experience in evaluating patients with torso gunshot wounds and found that contrast-enhanced abdominal CT is an effective method of determining missile

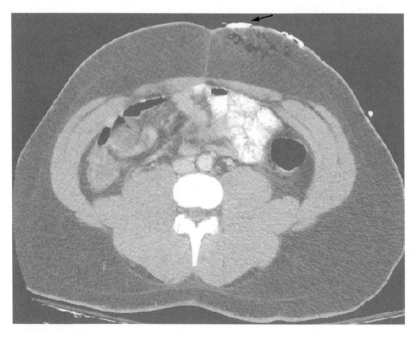

FIGURE 23-6. Computed tomography of patient with gunshot to the abdomen. Trajectory through adipose tissue without peritoneal violation is demonstrated. Paperclip (arrow) marks one skin wound.

trajectory, and therefore anatomic injury, in selected patients. In 2001, Shanmuganathan and colleagues[56] reported their prospective data on the evaluation of 104 stable patients with penetrating torso trauma with triple-contrast abdominal CT. Computed tomography scans were positive in 35 patients (34%), of which 22 underwent laparotomy and 19 (86%) were therapeutic. Of those patients with negative CT scans, 97% (67/69) were successfully managed nonoperatively. They reported a negative predictive value of 100% and 97% accuracy of triple-contrast CT scan in selected patients.

Patients who sustained isolated gunshot wounds to the back or flank are particularly well-suited for evaluation by helical CT scan to identify or exclude significant injury and to avoid unnecessary laparotomy[55,58] with a reported negative predictive value of 100% (Figure 23-7).[57] In 1987, Hauser reviewed 40 stable patients with posterior penetrating injuries who had been initially evaluated with CT to determine trajectory and identify injuries.[58] Six patients were found to have scans diagnostic of injuries that were confirmed at laparotomy. The other 34 patients were successfully managed nonoperatively based on CT exclusion of significant injury.

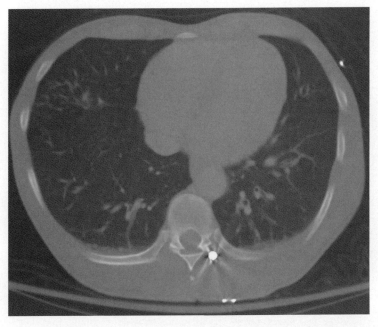

FIGURE 23-7. Computed tomography of patient with gunshot to the back. The missile is seen in the para-spinous region without violation of the chest or spinal canal.

Ginzburg and colleagues[55] reviewed 83 stable patients with abdominal and flank gunshot wounds who were initially evaluated by CT scan. They demonstrated that in 53 patients with no evidence of peritoneal penetration on abdominal CT, nonoperative management could safely be pursued.

The use of contrast-enhanced CT scan to triage patients with abdominal gunshot wounds has been further expanded to include selected stable patients with isolated right upper quadrant wounds (Figure 23-8).[62] Based on lessons learned from the management of blunt abdominal trauma, nonoperative management of these patients can be attempted if there is confidence that the bullet trajectory is isolated to the liver and lung parenchyma.

Demetriades and colleagues,[63] in 1999, published a series of 52 patients with gunshot wounds to the liver as diagnosed by CT scan. Of these patients, 16 remained hemodynamically stable, had no other indication for laparotomy, and were successfully managed nonoperatively. Although a

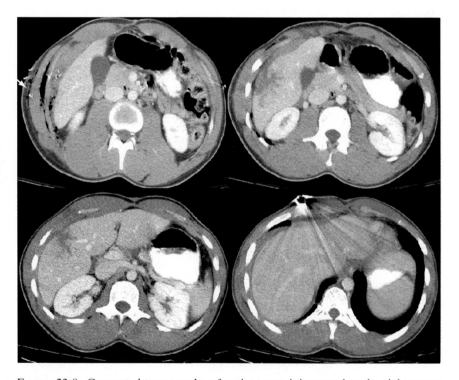

FIGURE 23-8. Computed tomography of patient sustaining gunshot the right upper quadrant/flank demonstrating isolated hepatic injury. Arrow marks entrance wound and foreign body (bullet) is seen in the last image of the sequence. This patient was successfully managed nonoperatively.

diaphragmatic injury may be present in these patients, the presence of the liver abutting the right hemi-diaphragm prevents clinically significant complications. In selected patients with isolated liver injuries, angiographic embolization is another option to avoid unnecessary laparotomy and worsening of bleeding in patients with isolated hepatic gunshot wounds.[62,64,65]

Diaphragm Injuries

While CT has clearly added to the diagnostic accuracy of trauma evaluation, injuries to the diaphragm are often missed by this modality.[66-68] Nau found CT to be no better at identifying diaphragmatic injury than plain chest X-ray.[66] Definitive diagnosis by direct visualization at laparoscopy or laparotomy is often the only method of accurately excluding diaphragm injury in penetrating trauma victims. While right-sided injuries to the diaphragm can be treated conservatively, left-sided injuries are still at high risk for herniation and must be repaired operatively. Some questions remain as to the appropriate management of anterior right-sided injuries involving the diaphragm that are not isolated by hepatic parenchyma.

Extremity Injury

Many patients arrive to the trauma center with extremity gunshot wounds. These patients must be quickly assessed for signs or symptoms of bony and vascular injury. In hemodynamically stable patients, plain radiographs can quickly determine if bony injury is present. Additional views assist in determining injury severity and the need for orthopedic intervention.

More important is the need to identify or exclude significant vascular injury. Hard signs of vascular injury, such as absent/diminished pulse, pulsatile bleeding, expanding hematoma, or signs of distal ischemia, are indications for immediate operative intervention and repair. There is no indication for preoperative angiography in these patients if needed; angiography can be performed "on-table" as part of the operative procedure.[69]

Patients without hard signs of vascular injury should have ankle-brachial indices (ABIs) performed using hand-held Doppler and compared to the non-injured extremity. Formal angiography is indicated for the further evaluation of patients with no signs of vascular injury, but who have an ABI of less than 0.9. Soft signs of penetrating vascular trauma, such as proximity to an artery, nonexpanding hematoma, or extremity neurologic deficit, are not indications for angiography.

Patients with shotgun injuries with multiple penetrations are an exception and may benefit from injury exclusion by angiography if clinically warranted. The role of CT angiography in relation to extremity ballistic injury triage is currently being explored.

Imaging in Battlefield Conditions

While many of the options for the imaging of ballistic trauma victims discussed above are easily accessed in the medical center setting, it is obvious that such technology is often not available in the austere conditions of the battlefield and in military forward surgical units. Computed tomography and interventional radiology are likely to be options only at the higher echelons of care. Moreover, the radiologic expertise to assist in interpreting radiographic studies is usually not available in the field. Despite this "handicap" to the modern trained surgeon, those clinicians evaluating ballistic trauma patients under these conditions are often able to gain significant information regarding missile trajectory with the use of plain radiographs alone. Furthermore, the evolving use of teleradiology by the military in forward settings may allow the addition of both radiologist and trauma surgeon's clinical experience to aid in the interpretation of these images.[70,71]

The development of small, portable, battery-powered ultrasound machines such as the SonoSite (SonoSite Inc., Bothell WA) has recently made ultrasound technology available to the battlefield surgeon.[72] The use of this technology for the FAST exam evaluation of the abdomen and pericardium as described previously, as well as its use for additional soft tissue imaging depending on the experience of the operator, is ideal for the isolated and often in-hospitable conditions experienced by the battlefield surgeon.[73] Prehospital transmission of images by properly trained medics in the field may also have useful triage applications.[74]

While diagnostic imaging is often helpful in the evaluation of ballistic trauma victims, certainly the trauma surgeon must always maintain the perspective that direct visualization and operative inspection to diagnose or exclude injury to vital structures is the gold standard. In the absence of advanced technologies and in the multiple patient scenarios of battlefield surgery, deviation from this axiom can be fraught with peril.

Summary

The role of ancillary imaging tools in the evaluation of victims of ballistic trauma continues to evolve. While physical exam and plain radiographs are the mainstays of evaluation, there is an increasing role for advanced imaging techniques to identify injuries in hemodynamically normal patients. In properly selected patients, CT and ultrasound are excellent triage tools and can be alternatives to more invasive testing and can help prevent unnecessary procedures or operations. A growing body of evidence supports the use of these modalities to evaluate stable gunshot wound victims with injuries to the neck, chest, or abdomen. Continued clinical research is needed to further define the role of advanced imaging in ballistic trauma and to possibly expand its use as technology evolves.

References

1. Besenski N. Traumatic injuries: Imaging of head injuries. *Eur Radiol.* 2002; 12(6):1237–1252.
2. Gracias VH, Reilly PM, Philpott J, Klein WP, Singer M, Schwab CW. Computed tomography in the evaluation of penetrating neck trauma: A preliminary study. *Arch Surg.* 2001;136:1231–1235.
3. Grossman MD, May AK, Schwab CW, et al. Determining anatomic injury with computed tomography in selected torso gunshot wounds. *J Trauma.* 1998;45: 446–456.
4. Hanpeter DE, Demetriades D, Asensio JA, Berne TV, Velmahos G, Murray J. Helical computed tomographic scan in the evaluation of mediastinal gunshot wounds. *J Trauma.* 2000;49(4):689–695.
5. Demetriades D, Velmahos G. Technology-driven triage of abdominal trauma: The emerging era of nonoperative management. *Annu Rev Med.* 2003;54:1–15.
6. Hess U, Harms J, Schneider A, Schleef M, Ganter C, Hanning C, et al. Assessment of gunshot bullet injuries with the use of magnetic resonance imaging. *J Trauma.* 2000;49(4):704–709.
7. Anonymous. Neuroimaging in the management of penetrating brain injury. *J Trauma.* 2001;51(2 Suppl):S7–S11.
8. Kim PE, Go JL, Zee CS. Radiographic assessment of cranial gunshot wounds. *Neuroimaging Clin N Am.* 2002;12(2):229–248.
9. Demetriades D, Chahwan S, Gomez H, Falabella A, Velmahos G, Yamashita D. Initial evaluation and management of gunshot wounds to the face. *J Trauma.* 1998;45(1):39–41.
10. Diaz-Daza O, Arraiza FJ, Barkley JM, Whigham CJ. Endovascular therapy of traumatic vascular lesions of the head and neck. *Cardiovasc Intervent Radiol.* 2003;26(3):213–221.
11. Chesnut RM. Avoidance of hypotension: Conditio sine qua non of successful severe head-injury management. *J Trauma.* 1997;42(5 Suppl):S4–S9.
12. Kaups KL, Davis JW. Patients with gunshot wounds to the head do not require cervical spine immobilization and evaluation. *J Trauma.* 1998;44(5):865–867.
13. Roon AJ, Christensen N. Evaluation and treatment of penetrating cervical injuries. *J Trauma.* 1979;19(6):391–397.
14. Jurkovich GJ, Zingarelli W, Wallace J, Curreri PW. Penetrating neck trauma: Diagnostic studies in the asymptomatic patient. *J Trauma.* 1985;25(9):819–822.
15. Back MR, Baumgartner FJ, Klein SR. Detection and evaluation of aerodigestive tract injuries caused by cervical and transmediastinal gunshot wounds. *J Trauma.* 1997;42(4):680–686.
16. Asensio JA, Valenziano CP, Falcone RE, Grosh JD. Management of penetrating neck injuries. The controversy surrounding zone II injuries. *Surg Clin North Am.* 1991;71(2):267–296.
17. Biffl WL, Moore EE, Rehse DH, Offner PJ, Francoise RJ, Burch JM. Selective management of penetrating neck trauma based on cervical level of injury. *Am J Surg.* 1997;174(6):678–682.
18. Klyachkin ML, Rohmiller M, Charash WE, Sloan DA, Kearney PA. Penetrating injuries of the neck: Selective management evolving. *Am Surg.* 1997;63(2): 189–194.

19. van As AB, van Deurzen DF, Verleisdonk EJ. Gunshots to the neck: Selective angiography as part of conservative management. *Injury.* 2002;33(5):453–456.
20. LeBlang SD, Dolich MO. Imaging of penetrating thoracic trauma. *J Thorac Imaging.* 2000;15(2):128–135.
21. Eddy VA. Is routine arteriography mandatory for penetrating injury to zone 1 of the neck? Zone 1 Penetrating Neck Injury Study Group. *J Trauma.* 2000; 48(2):208–214.
22. Montalvo BM, LeBlang SD, Nunez DB, Jr., et al. Color Doppler sonography in penetrating injuries of the neck. *AJNR Am J Neuroradiol.* 1996;17(5):943–951.
23. Azuaje RE, Jacobson LE, Glover J, et al. Reliability of physical examination as a predictor of vascular injury after penetrating neck trauma. *Am Surg.* 2003;69(9):804–807.
24. Ofer A, Nitecki SS, Braun J, et al. CT angiography of the carotid arteries in trauma to the neck. *Eur J Vasc Endovasc Surg.* 2001;21(5):401–407.
25. Mazolewski PJ, Curry JD, Browder T, Fildes J. Computed tomographic scan can be used for surgical decision making in zone II penetrating neck injuries. *J Trauma.* 2001;51:315–319.
26. Munera F, Soto JA, Palacio D, et al. Penetrating Neck Injuries: Helical CT angiography for initial evaluation. *Radiology.* 2002;370:366–372.
27. Gonzalez RP, Falimirski M, Holevar MR, Turk B. Penetrating zone II neck injury: Does dynamic computed tomographic scan contribute to the diagnostic sensitivity of physical examination for surgically significant injury? A prospective blinded study. *J Trauma.* 2003;54:61–65.
28. Ma OJ, Mateer JR. Trauma ultrasound examination versus chest radiography in the detection of hemothorax. *Ann Emerg Med.* 1997;29(3):312–316.
29. Blaivas M. Triage in the trauma bay with the focused abdominal sonography for trauma (FAST) examination. *J Emerg Med.* 2001;21(1):41–44.
30. Rozycki GS, Feliciano DV, Ochsner MG, et al. The role of ultrasound in patients with possible penetrating cardiac wounds: a prospective multicenter study. *J Trauma.* 1999;46(4):543–552.
31. Demetriades D, Velmahos GC. Penetrating injuries of the chest: Indications for operation. *Scand J Surg.* 2002;91(1):41–45.
32. Dulchavsky SA, Schwarz KL, Kirkpatrick AW, et al. Prospective evaluation of thoracic ultrasound in the detection of pneumothorax. *J Trauma.* 2001;50(2): 201–205.
33. Gasparri MG, Lorelli DR, Kralovich KA, Patton JH, Jr. Physical examination plus chest radiography in penetrating periclavicular trauma: The appropriate trigger for angiography. *J Trauma.* 2000;49(6):1029–1033.
34. Gonzalez RP, Falimirski ME. The role of angiography in periclavicular penetrating trauma. *Am Surg.* 1999;65(8):711–714.
35. Asensio JA, Berne J, Demetriades D, et al. Penetrating esophageal injuries: Time interval of safety for preoperative evaluation—how long is safe? *J Trauma.* 1997;43(2):319–324.
36. Richardson JD, Flint LM, Snow NJ, Gray LA Jr, Trinkle JK. Management of transmediastinal gunshot wounds. *Surgery.* 1981;90(4):671–676.
37. Demetriades D. Penetrating injuries to the thoracic great vessels. *J Card Surg.* 1997;12(2 Suppl):173–180.
38. McIntyre RC, Jr., Moore EE, Read RR, Wiebe RL, Grover FL. Transesophageal echocardiography in the evaluation of a transmediastinal gunshot wound: Case report. *J Trauma.* 1994;36(1):125–127.

39. LiMandri G, Gorenstein LA, Starr JP, Homma S, Avteri J, Gopal AS. Use of transesophageal echocardiography in the detection and consequences of an intracardiac bullet. *Am J Emerg Med.* 1994;12(1):105–106.
40. Nagy KK, Gilkey SH, Roberts RR, Fildes JJ, Barrett J. Computed tomography screens stable patients at risk for penetrating cardiac injury. *Acad Emerg Med.* 1996;3(11):1024–1027.
41. Stassen NA, Lukan JK, Spain DA, et al. Reevaluation of diagnostic procedures for transmediastinal gunshot wounds. *J Trauma.* 2002;53:635–638.
42. Aaland MO, Bryan FC, 3rd, Sherman R. Two-dimensional echocardiogram in hemodynamically stable victims of penetrating precordial trauma. *Am Surg.* 1994;60(6):412–415.
43. Kiev J, Kerstein MD. Role of three hour roentgenogram of the chest in penetrating and nonpenetrating injuries of the chest. *Surg Gynecol Obstet.* 1992; 175(3):249–253.
44. Shatz DV, de la Pedraja J, Erbella J, Hameed M, Vail SJ. Efficacy of follow-up evaluation in penetrating thoracic injuries: 3- vs. 6-hour radiographs of the chest. *J Emerg Med.* 2001;20(3):281–284.
45. Patel VG, Walker ML. The role of "one-shot" intravenous pyelogram in evaluation of penetrating abdominal trauma. *Am Surg.* 1997;63(4):350–353.
46. Nance ML, Nance FC. It is time we told the Emperor about his clothes. *J Trauma.* 1996;40(2):185–186.
47. Renz BM, Feliciano DV. Unnecessary laparotomies for trauma: A prospective study of morbidity. *J Trauma.* 1995;38(3):350–356.
48. Demetriades D, Velmahos G, Cornwell E, et al. Selective nonoperative management of gunshot wounds of the anterior abdomen. *Arch Surg.* 1997;132(2): 178–183.
49. Pak-art R, Sriussadaporn S, Vajrabukka T. The results of focused assessment with sonography for trauma performed by third year surgical residents: A prospective study. *J Med Assoc Thai.* 2003;86(Suppl 2):S344–S349.
50. Gracias VH, Frankel H, Gupta R, et al. The role of positive examinations in training for the focused assessment sonogram in trauma (FAST) examination. *Am Surg.* 2002;68(11):1008–1011.
51. Gracias VH, Frankel HL, Gupta R, et al. Defining the learning curve for the focused abdominal sonogram for trauma (FAST) examination: Implications for credentialing. *Am Surg.* 2001;67(4):364–368.
52. Rozycki GS, Ballard RB, Feliciano DV, Schmidt JA, Pennington SD. Surgeon-performed ultrasound for the assessment of truncal injuries: Lessons learned from 1540 patients. *Ann Surg* 1998;228(4):557–567.
53. Davis JR, Morrison AL, Perkins SE, Davis FE, Ochsner MG. Ultrasound: Impact on diagnostic peritoneal lavage, abdominal computed tomography, and resident training. *Am Surg.* 1999;65(6):555–559.
54. Federle MP, Goldberg HI, Kaiser JA, Moss AA, Jeffrey RB Jr., Mall JC. Evaluation of abdominal trauma by computed tomography. *Radiology.* 1981;138(3): 637–644.
55. Ginzburg E, Carillo EH, Kopelman T, et al. The role of computed tomography in selective management of gunshot wounds to the abdomen and flank. *J Trauma.* 1998;45:1005–1009.
56. Shanmuganathan K, Mirvis SE, Chiu WC, Killeen KL, Scalea TM. Triple-contrast helical CT in penetrating torso trauma: A prospective study to deter-

mine peritoneal violation and the need for lapartotomy. *AJR Am J Roentgenol.* 2001;177:1247–1256.
57. Himmelman RG, Martin M, Gilkey S, Barrett JA. Triple-contrast CT scans in penetrating back and flank trauma. *J Trauma.* 1991;31(6):852–855.
58. Hauser CJ, Huprich JE, Bosco P, Gibbons L, Mansour AY, Weiss AR. Triple-contrast computed tomography in the evaluation of penetrating posterior abdominal injuries. *Arch Surg.* 1987;122(10):1112–1115.
59. Kern SJ, Smith RS, Fry WR, Helmer SD, Reed JA, Chang FC. Sonographic examination of abdominal trauma by senior surgical residents. *Am Surg.* 1997;63(8):669–674.
60. Udobi KF, Rodriguez A, Chiu WC, Scalea TM. Role of ultrasonography in penetrating abdominal trauma: A prospective clinical study. *J Trauma.* 2001;50(3): 475–479.
61. Boulanger BR, Kearney PA, Tsuei B, Ochoa JB. The routine use of sonography in penetrating torso injury is beneficial. *J Trauma.* 2001;51(2):320–325.
62. Carrillo EH, Richardson JD. The current management of hepatic trauma. *Adv Surg.* 2001;35:39–59.
63. Demetriades D, Gomez H, Chahwan S, et al. Gunshot injuries to the liver: The role of selective nonoperative management. *J Am Coll Surg.* 1999;188(4): 343–348.
64. Velmahos GC, Demetriades D, Chahwan S, et al. Angiographic embolization for arrest of bleeding after penetrating trauma to the abdomen. *Am J Surg.* 1999;178(5):367–373.
65. Dondelinger RF, Trotteur G, Ghaye B, Szapiro D. Traumatic injuries: Radiological hemostatic intervention at admission. *Eur Radiol.* 2002;12(5): 979–993.
66. Nau T, Seitz H, Mousavi M, Vecsei V. The diagnostic dilemma of traumatic rupture of the diaphragm. *Surg Endosc.* 2001;15(9):992–996.
67. Patselas TN, Gallagher EG. The diagnostic dilemma of diaphragm injury. *Am Surg.* 2002;68(7):633–639.
68. Shackleton KL, Stewart ET, Taylor AJ. Traumatic diaphragmatic injuries: spectrum of radiographic findings. *Radiographics.* 1998;18(1):49–59.
69. Arrillaga A, Bynoe R, Nagy K, Frykberg ER. Practice management guidelines for penetrating trauma to the lower extremities. 2002. The EAST Practice Management Guidelines Work Group. Available at http://www.east.org/tpg/lepene. pdf. Accessed January 5, 2004.
70. Cawthon MA, Goeringer F, Telepak RJ, et al. Preliminary assessment of computed tomography and satellite teleradiology from Operation Desert Storm. *Invest Radiol.* 1991;26(10):854–857.
71. Levine BA, Cleary K, Mun SK. Deployable teleradiology: Bosnia and beyond. *IEEE Trans Inf Technol Biomed.* 1998;2(1):30–34.
72. Sonosite Inc. Web site. Available at http://www.sonosite.com/home.html. Accessed January 5, 2004.
73. Wherry DC. Potential of a hand-held ultrasound in assessment of the injured patient. *Cardiovasc Surg.* 1998;6(6):569–572.
74. Strode CA, Rubal BJ, Gerhardt RT, Bulgrin JR, Boyd SY. Wireless and satellite transmission of prehospital focused abdominal sonography for trauma. *Prehosp Emerg Care.* 2003;7(3):375–379.

24
Training to Manage Ballistic Trauma

Kenneth D. Boffard and Nigel R.M. Tai

Nothing worth knowing is ever taught
Stella Rimington, Ex Director of MI5

Train hard, fight easy
British Army Maxim

Introduction

Historically, the provision of trauma care has attracted little political interest,[1] with the result that many present-day trauma care systems are the product of chance evolution rather than thoughtful design.[2] Many countries lack a unified and integrated system for trauma training and trauma care, an issue only partially addressed by widespread uptake of the Advanced Trauma Life Support (ATLS) course. Even countries such as the United States, with mature, organized systems of trauma care and well-established programs of postgraduate surgical education, have reported a reduction in the opportunities for trauma education as levels of violent crime diminish, motor-vehicle accident rates fall, and new, conservative modalities of treatment emerge.[3] The resultant paradox is that in many industrialized states there are reduced prospects for trainees to develop and sustain the skills necessary to manage ballistic trauma, despite the harsh truth that such injuries are particularly unforgiving of suboptimal or belated treatment. Furthermore, the capacity to train surgeons and others in this demanding field has been limited by the reduction of military medical infrastructure following the end of the cold war.[4]

Clearly, there is a pressing requirement to train, but the means and mode of training are contentious. The experiential approach, embodied by the first quotation given in the start of this chapter, maintains that the best-remembered lessons are those learnt through hard experience rather than didactic instruction. The second motto asserts the advisability of intensive, focused, and relevant tutelage if a good outcome is to result, especially under adverse circumstances. Each argument has its merits and shortcom-

486

ings: the short-term cost of the experiential approach is usually paid for by the patient; however, a shortened more-focused training leaves surgeons with little competence to solve multi-system injury inflicted by ballistic trauma. This latter problem has become an increasingly important training issue, as the recent drive towards sub-specialization and shorter training timelines has effectively killed the traditional apprenticeship that surgical training once resembled. Hence, it has been argued that the precise but restricted expertise that modern trainees accumulate will be of little benefit to the victim of missile injury seeking timely, competent intervention.[4,5] However, brute experience by itself does not necessarily endow competence. Therefore, the best compromise is to carefully train surgeons and other providers in the principles of trauma care and surgical decision making and to endow them with as much appropriate experience as possible.[5] The purpose of this chapter is to define the goals of training and to examine the strategies available to produce proficient trauma practitioners, civilian and military, working in either the prehospital or hospital environment.

Attributes of the Ideal Trauma Practitioner

Defining the desired skills of personnel managing ballistic injury is a necessary first step if one aspires to design a scheme of training. One must also identify which personnel or specialties require education, quantify the degree to which trauma must form a part of the emergency syllabus, and then tailor the training so that it is consistent with role, setting, and the local trauma epidemiology. Such a template is given in Table 24-1, using the "trauma surgeon" as an example. Notably, trauma in the United Kingdom and Europe is managed by multidisciplinary teams frequently led by non-surgical specialists dealing with a predominantly blunt pattern of injury, and the concept of the utility "trauma surgeon" or "trauma unit" as understood in North America and South Africa does not exist.[6] As such, it generally is accepted that the specialty of the coordinating trauma team leader is not important provided that the leader has been trained to consultant level in an acute specialty, understands the multi-system implications of trauma insult, has served an apprenticeship under a more senior colleague, and is subject to continued professional appraisal.[2]

Training the Trauma Practitioner— The Art of Resuscitation

In the forward to the predecessor of this text it was emphasized that the management of victims of ballistic trauma "must not be isolated from trauma management in general."[7] By extension, the education of those

TABLE 24-1. Attributes of a general surgeon capable of managing ballistic trauma

| Knowledge | Skills | |
	Technical	Executive
Mechanics and forensic pathology of ballistic trauma of ballistic injury	ATLS® resuscitative procedures	Trauma team leadership/ interpersonal skills
Physiology of response to trauma	Surgical access to the structures of the	Trauma system management
Anatomy of trauma	neck, chest, abdomen, and limb	Decision-making skills
Planning/interpretation of investigations	Damage control surgery	Audit and research skills
Indications and limitations of selective nonoperative management	Operative skills to remove, repair, or	Education skills
Critical care: ventilatory, cardiovascular, and nutritional support, control of SIRS, sepsis and multi-organ dysfunction	reconstruct damaged tissues at the time of initial and later surgery	
Postoperative management		
Rehabilitation and psychosocial management		
Trauma systems		

managing such patients should take place within the context of trauma and critical care education as a whole, and preferably integrated within a defined system of trauma care. The initial management of patients who have suffered ballistic injury begins with the well-established resuscitative priorities of airway/breathing/circulation, and the most influential educational driver for this approach continues to be the Advanced Trauma Life Support (ATLS®) Provider course.

ATLS®

It is difficult to overstate the impact this course has had on trauma training. Advanced Trauma Life Support® was originally developed by a small cohort of surgeons and emergency physicians based in Nebraska who were aiming to improve the quality of trauma care delivered by isolated rural doctors.[8] The course was designed to provide a logical, easily remembered, and practical system of trauma management that looked no further than the "golden hour" of initial evaluation and resuscitation before definitive care. As such, ATLS® was a means of averting the one-in-three potentially preventable in-hospital deaths that occur after simple management mistakes made in the initial stages of treatment.[9]

Advanced Trauma Life Support® was innovative in a number of ways. Traditional means of medical education were dispensed with, and with the guidance of professional (non-medical) educators, a two-and-a-half–day course timetable was carefully designed to include an intense mixture of lectures, workshops, discussion groups, and practical skill stations. Students are given extensive feedback about their strengths and weaknesses, culminating with interactive moulage sessions that test and reinforce the candidate's trauma skills. By this manner, each of the "domains of learning" that constitute the educational process—knowledge, psychomotor skills, and motivational attitude—are instilled into course participants.[10,11] Furthermore, the traditional sequence of establishing a diagnosis via history, physical examination, and special investigations before initiation of treatment was discarded. A new philosophy of management was taught whereby patients were evaluated and treated simultaneously for life-threatening problems as they were discovered, with lack of a definitive patient history never precluding prompt intervention if required.

To teach the course, a cadre of trainers was created through the equally innovative ATLS® Instructors course. Students who achieve high test scores on their ATLS® Provider course, display enthusiasm for the tenets of ATLS®, and who possess excellent communication skills are identified and invited to apply for a place on an instructor's course. The Instructor program uses educational theory in order to train the potential instructor to teach, critique, and assess ATLS® students effectively and constructively. In this manner, the content, quality, and style of the ATLS® Provider course has been rigidly maintained and promulgated.

Under the aegis of the American College of Surgeons, the provider course has been widely disseminated and is taught in over 37 countries, with half a million doctors now having completed the course. However, its success in the trauma community has not been unaccompanied by criticism.[12] Caveats include the relative expense of the course, the fact that non-medical staff (e.g., nurses) are denied ATLS® certification (although they may attend courses as observers), the paucity of non-surgical and non-North American contributors to the ongoing development of the course, and a relative lack of robust proof for the efficacy of ATLS® as a means of improving patient outcome.[13] Despite the overwhelming acceptance of the ATLS® doctrine, there are few trials specifically examining patient outcome. Studies that have reported a significant benefit for patients managed according to ATLS® guidelines[14,15] have been criticized as poorly designed and confounded by other factors such as change in trauma demographics and concurrent improvements in trauma systems and the care of the critically ill.[11]

Advanced Trauma Life Support® courses are inherently expensive to arrange and to attend; implementation of a new course requires an established faculty. These factors mean that doctors based in developing nations are disadvantaged and are frequently unable to attend a course. For this reason, the National Trauma Management Course (NTMC™), produced under the auspices of the International Association for Trauma and Surgical Intensive Care (IATSIC), was specifically designed for trauma providers working in developing nations. This course teaches ATLS®-derived techniques, but by using a simpler administrative system, a higher pupil-to-instructor ratio, and case scenarios or demonstrations rather than skill stations, affordability is maximized. Although this results in a reduction in "hands-on" expertise, NTMC™ has proved a popular means of acquiring the principles of sound trauma management amongst providers working in developing countries such as India and Nigeria.

Relevance of ATLS® to Ballistic Trauma

Clinicians who are tasked with the care of the patients injured by ballistic trauma should undergo ATLS® training. Blunt and penetrating injuries are not mutually exclusive in victims of ballistic trauma, particularly so in patients exposed to blast, and the ATLS® course instills a thorough grounding in the assessment, investigation, and early management of both modes of wounding. Having completed the course, trainees can expect to use the system as a foundation upon which they can manage patients despite the often dramatic or unfamiliar nature of ballistic wounds, simply because the protocols of management provide initial security. Advanced Trauma Life Support®-trained personnel are endowed with a common vocabulary, and more importantly, a shared set of values that cross disciplinary, institutional, and national barriers.[16] Hemorrhagic shock is the most frequent cause of early death in missile injury, and although (at the time of writing) the course does not refer to the current trend toward permissive hypotension,[17] ATLS® candidates are taught the necessity of obtaining surgical expertise early in the resuscitation process in order to stop ongoing hemorrhage.[18] However, it is acknowledged that the substance of the ATLS® course reflects the predominately blunt pattern of trauma epidemiology currently observed in most industrialized nations. This fact, together with the deliberate absence of content regarding definitive care, limits the overall utility and relevance of ATLS® to ballistic trauma. Completion of ATLS® training should be thought of as a solid base for further trauma education rather than as an end in itself.

ATLS®—The Military Perspective

As a means of structured assessment and treatment of war wounded, the ATLS® format has been enthusiastically adapted by the military medical establishment[19,20] and military variants have been designed and used in the United Kingdom, the United States, and Israeli Armed Forces. The U.K. Battlefield Advanced Trauma Life Support (BATLS™) course has been employed operationally for over a decade[21]; indeed, operational doctrine is built around the provision of BATLS™ skills to medical service personnel.[22] The course uses the educational strengths of the ATLS® approach to deliver a similar package of resuscitation skills that have been modified for the special circumstances of conflict. Thus, the course reflects realities of war such as the greater prevalence of penetrating trauma and high-energy transfer wounds, the greater potential for mass casualty situations, the inherent danger to medical personnel, the lack of specialist equipment and expertise, and difficulties due to extended lines of logistics and delays in evacuation. Furthermore, although nurses may participate in civilian ATLS® courses as observers, BATLS™ purposefully demands a much fuller role for their military nursing and combat medical technician colleagues, as these staff are expected to begin the initial treatment of war wounded in the absence of medical officer support.

As with civilian ATLS®, there are few studies examining the efficacy of military ATLS® courses, although such evidence is especially difficult to gather in operational or field conditions. However, the *raison'd etre* of ATLS® dogma is to minimize deaths occurring in the second peak of the trimodal distribution of trauma mortality.[18,23] Studies from the Middle East conflict show that the corresponding peak for soldiers killed in warfare is significantly smaller than that observed by Trunkey, and that this occurs at the cost of a heightened prevalence of immediately fatal injuries.[24,25] Accordingly, because of the lethality of military weaponry, there is a diminished population of patients in which ATLS® skills have utility, and thus the ability of ATLS®-modeled systems to salvage patients will be lower than in the civilian setting. Additionally, concerns have been raised that ATLS® skills alone are insufficient for managing military casualties.[26,27] Despite these criticisms, ATLS® teaches a logical and thorough system of early management that can be readily applied under stress, and for this reason as much any other, militarily modified ATLS® courses have become a cornerstone of trauma training for personnel tasked with the provision of organized medical support on the battlefield.

Video Review of Trauma Resuscitation

Townsend showed that both trauma team performance—as judged by duration of resuscitation and time to theater—improved following institution of regular ongoing video audit.[28] This translated to a statistically significant increase in the number of unexpected survivors in the period when video audit was employed as an educational tool. The use of video audit facilitates identification of errors or delays in diagnosis, judgment, or technique. The particular advantage of video audit over conventional case-note review is that the former is a far more accurate record of the sequence of decisions and procedures that constitute the resuscitation process, thereby allowing for easier and fuller error analysis. Successful video audit requires dedicated equipment and the setting aside of regular sessions in the staff schedule so that trainees and experienced seniors can review tapes and discuss patient management. Furthermore, as well as facilitating improved performance of individual members of the trauma team, video audit also provides a mechanism for the identification of system errors and violations in infection-control protocol.[29]

Trauma Resuscitation Simulations

Sophisticated simulation has long been established as a principle means of training in the aerospace and nuclear industries, and is becoming a primary means of training military combatants. Likewise, the simulation of trauma casualties is an increasingly promising means of training, and interactive multimedia CD-ROMs and web-based training programs are commonly available. Typically, these programs present a number of different scenarios allowing physicians to practice triage, resuscitation, and decision-making skills.[30,31]

Refinements in technology have led to the development of life-sized human patient simulators capable of displaying a range of physical signs. Eyelid movement, pupilary response, peripheral pulses, respiratory effort, and breath sounds may be synthesized and continuously modulated in response to interventions made by trainees reacting to programmed clinical scenarios. Preliminary experience with these mannequins was with the training of anesthetists and emergency physicians in medical crisis management.[32] However, this technology has tremendous potential as a tool for trauma education.[33,34] Typically, trainees can be exposed to situations that demand prompt evaluation, good decision-making skills, and effective action in a manner similar to the ATLS® moulage. However, unlike actor-based moulage, the signs and symptoms are not verbally described—instead, the trainee must seek them out and quickly weigh up their significance as in the real world. Mistakes can be made repeatedly at no risk to patients, and immediate, detailed, and leisurely feedback supplied in a style rarely appropriate to the hurried environs of genuine trauma suites. If necessary, difficult scenarios can be repeated until proficiency is achieved and confidence instilled. In addition to their training value and team-building merit, simulators offer a reliable and reproducible means of testing the resuscitation skills of ATLS®-educated personnel.[35] The main drawback of these systems is their cost; the initial outlay for the METI human patient simulator plus ancillary equipment is in excess of $250000 dollars with an annual upkeep of $10000.[36] However, driven by the falling cost of technology and escalating litigation overheads, such simulators are likely to become commonplace; indeed, simulation may surpass the impact that ATLS® had on trauma training.

Trauma Resuscitation in the Prehospital Environment

Following the Korean and Viet Nam wars, and the attending developments in the role and technical capabilities of the combat medic, there was a manifest change in the training of civilian prehospital personnel in the United States. Before this, the main requirements of ambulance staff were a clean driving license and a variable knowledge of first aid. Since then, American emergency medical technicians (EMTs) have been trained as interventionists, with the upper level of technician (EMT-P) designated as a paramedic capable of using advanced resuscitation skills, including definitive airway management, intravenous infusion, and drug administration, at the scene of injury.[37] Use of such skills in the prehospital environment would seem advantageous as around 50 to 81% of all trauma mortality occurs before arrival at the hospital.[38] Although many of these casualties are unsalvageable, it is reasonable to suppose that early and effective use of resuscitation techniques at the scene will reduce overall mortality. This rationale underlies the Prehospital Trauma Life Support course that was enthusiastically introduced in 1984.[39] In many countries, the training of a paramedic corps capable of ATLS®-type interventions has become a hallmark of quality in emergency medical care, and industrialized nations are placing increasing emphasis on advanced prehospital life support training.[40,41] In the United Kingdom, the Royal College of Surgeons of Edinburgh offers a diploma in immediate care and has set standards of practice and training for emergency personnel working outside the hospital arena via a dedicated, multidisciplinary Faculty of Prehospital Care. Whether the first responder is an emergency technician, a nurse, or a doctor, he/she must be trained to operate safely within the frequently hazardous prehospital environment, to liaise with and understand the role of other emergency services, to triage effectively, and to understand the considerations relevant in planning patient evacuation. The Major Incident Medical Management and Support (MIMMS) course (disseminated by the United Kingdom Advanced Life Support Group) is highly desirable for personnel requiring training for multiple casualty scenarios and for responders tasked with a command role.[42]

Despite the increasing ubiquity of advanced training for prehospital personnel, there is considerable debate surrounding the utility of ATLS®-type interventions in the field,[43] and the relevancy of training prehospital personnel to perform these tasks. In particular, there is concern that prehospital attempts to gain intravenous access can prolong on-scene time and thus delay definitive treatment.[44] Even when advanced life support does not entail delay in transport, there may be no survival benefit attributable to prehospital advanced life support techniques.[45,46] Furthermore, two studies have documented the lower mortality of trauma patients transported in private vehicles to the hospital as compared to patients brought by ambulance.[47,48] This is unsurprising given the absence of proof for prehospital fluid resuscitation—a recent systematic review of six randomized controlled studies examining the use of early fluid resuscitation in uncontrolled hemorrhage could find no evidence to support this practice.[49] However, the growing acceptance of controlled, permissive hypotension as a valid management technique in penetrating trauma does not negate the need for adequately trained prehospital responders. Such personnel must be trained in advanced life support and must be able to use their generic skills where time to definitive treatment is prolonged by distance, weather, or entrapment. Presently, paramedic intervention is almost exclusively protocol driven, but with the rise of the degree course in paramedic studies, the next generation of paramedics will be trained to act with a greater degree of autonomy and flexibility according to the demands of each situation.[40,50]

The Military First Responder

In most Western Armies, the combat medic can expect to be trained in pre-hospital advanced resuscitation skills by means of militarily customized ATLS® courses. Training military medics to perform such skills has not as yet attracted the criticism that has befallen civilian paramedic training schemes, perhaps because appropriate use of these interventions is more likely to reduce mortality on the battlefield when evacuation to definitive care takes hours or days.[51] However, clinical proficiency forms only a small part of combat casualty care. In order to fulfill what is always an exceptionally demanding battlefield role, the medic must possess excellent generic soldiering skills and, most importantly, a good appreciation of immediate tactical imperatives so that the care and evacuation of wounded personnel does not conflict with mission priorities. This is particularly important on operations conducted by small teams where a single casualty may seriously affect the abilities and safety of the unit.[52] Thus, it has recently been argued that while militarily modified advanced life support courses such as BATLS™ equip the soldier medic with resuscitative skills, they do not address the tactical implications inherent in the care of the wounded on the frontline. In order to rectify this, and motivated by the lessons drawn from the Battle of Mogadishu in 1993—when U.S. forces sustained 18 dead and 73 wounded—U.S. Naval medical authorities designed and implemented a Tactical Combat Casualty Care Course (TCCC).[53] The course's curriculum aims to supplement military trauma teaching by dividing the initial medical response into three phases—Care under Fire, Tactical Field Care, and Casualty Evacuation—and the tactical and medical priorities in each stage are explored through the use of specific scenarios. This approach has been endorsed by inclusion of TCCC guidelines in the latest edition of the Prehospital Trauma Life Support Manual.[54]

Several notable differences exist between TCCC and traditional ATLS® protocols—for example, in the care-under-fire phase, the casualty is expected to return fire, if at all possible, in order to assist with the neutralization of on-going sources of further injury.

Similarly, hemorrhage control (and the use of tourniquets if required) is prioritized over airway and breathing because bleeding from extremity trauma is a chief cause of preventable battlefield mortality. Originally designed for medical personnel supporting U.S. special operations units, the course is now finding a wider utility amongst more conventional land forces. Elements of this approach have also been adopted by U.K. military medical trainers who created a specific trauma life support course for the isolated medic expected to manage casualties without outside help for several days.[55]

Frequently, the military first responder will not be a specialized medic, but the injured soldier himself or the soldier closest to him. Because of this, and because the trained medic may be distant, preoccupied by other casualties, or incapacitated by enemy action, all soldiers, whatever their skills or rank, should be taught and become proficient with the fundamentals of battlefield triage, external hemorrhage control, and basic airway management.

Training the Trauma Practitioner—The Art of Definitive Care

The mission of pre-surgical care has been described as "delivering a live patient to the surgeon." Unfortunately, if the surgeon makes poor decisions or lacks operative skills, the benefits of a well-conducted resuscitation will be forfeit. Traditionally, definitive care skills may be learned by treating injured patients while under the close supervision of experienced tutors, but in countries such as the United Kingdom, where surgeons undertake a median of three trauma laparotomies (one for penetrating injury) per year, training must be supplemented accordingly.[56] The elements that constitute surgical learning can be categorized as cognitive, attitudinal, or psychomotor.[10] Assuming surgical trainees have a mature learning attitude and are highly motivated, it follows that the primary task of trauma education is to furnish cognitive knowledge and technical ability. The former can be readily attained from individual study of print and electronic journals, authoritative texts, lectures, and the like. Acquisition of technical and decision-making skills will be facilitated by attendance on an appropriate definitive care course and further developed by secondment to a high-volume trauma center.

Definitive Surgical Trauma Care Course

The Definitive Surgical Trauma Care (DSTC™) course was developed by an international group of trauma surgeons working with the International Association for the Surgery of Trauma and Surgical Intensive Care (IATSIC). The DSTC™ course was designed to equip the "occasional" trauma surgeon with the decision-making and operative abilities required to manage injured patients beyond the resuscitation room. Piloted in Sydney in 1996, and formally introduced internationally in 1999, the course has been widely disseminated,[57] and is structured on the ATLS® model. Sixteen course participants receive a series of didactic lectures from an experienced faculty of trauma experts and explore difficult decision-making scenarios through case presentations, surgical scenarios, and group discussions. Following appropriate instruction, students undertake a full complement of core surgical skills and operative procedures on cadavers (when available), or alternatively, prosected specimens (see Appendix A). Additionally, where local regulations permit, students also are systematically exposed to a range of injuries on live anesthetized animal models.[58] A number of sessions dedicated to strategic thinking in trauma surgery and trouble shooting also are scheduled. A detailed course manual, instructional video, and interactive CD-ROM are supplied to facilitate post-course revision. Course conveners must be IATSIC members and faculty must have completed an "educator course" such as the ATLS® Instructor or Royal College of Surgeons "Train the Trainer" program. Importantly, and unlike ATLS®, a measure of flexibility is allowed in course content so that the particular needs of local surgeons may be addressed. Thus, additional course modules relating to such topics as trauma critical care, minimally invasive trauma surgery, skeletal trauma, and head trauma have been designed and taught. For military surgeons, a one-day module covering the austere conditions and specifics of military triage, command and control, ballistic wounds, and resource management has also been successfully developed.[59] The U.K. version of DSTC™ is known as the Definitive Surgical Trauma Skills Course (DSTS) and was jointly designed and implemented by the Royal College of Surgeons of England, the Royal Defense Medical College, and the U.S. Uniformed Services University.[60] The course was initially produced to meet the needs of U.K. and U.S. military surgeons lacking in trauma experience and shares much the same aims, curriculum, and instructional methodology as DSTC™. Recently, the course has been adapted for civilian surgeons and is now taught twice yearly in London.

As with ATLS®, it is desirable that all surgeons with responsibility for injured patients consider DSTC™/DSTS accreditation as mandatory. It is envisaged that future discipline-specific variants of these courses will be implemented to train anesthetists, critical care specialists, and other non-surgical clinicians in traumatology.

Trauma Fellowships

It is generally recognized that secondment to a high-volume Level One trauma center is essential if the trainee's trauma skills are to be developed and consolidated. In the United States, such secondments are usually under-taken when surgical training is nearing completion and there are around 40 programs, based in Level One trauma centers, offering over 80 fellowship positions.[61,62] Published guidelines exist that regulate the curriculum, duration, and scope of training, faculty organization, educational facilities, and trainee evaluation required of trauma fellowship programs.[63] Similarly, for-malized fellowship programs have been developed in Australia and South Africa, but in the United Kingdom and Europe, clinicians seeking additional trauma training must usually make their own arrangements in order to secure training positions within overseas centers.

Wherever the prospective trauma fellow intends to train, he/she should verify that the program ensures sufficient exposure to penetrating and ballistic trauma because centers located within developed nations may predominantly deal with blunt injury. Furthermore, as is the case with North American trauma fellowship models, the program should offer a significant period of critical care training, as this endows the surgeon with the skills required to manage patients on the surgical intensive care unit. Indeed, even in countries where such care is delivered by dedicated intensivists, a period of critical care training is highly desirable if the surgeon is to understand and manage the complex organ support therapies required in the crucial postoperative period.

Military Trauma Surgery Training

As acknowledged by Ogilvie following World War II, it is a profound error to liken the specialty of war surgery to that of trauma surgery.[64] Rignault has summarized the ways in which war surgery exists as a discrete, separate surgical discipline. These factors include the type and number of casualties presenting to the surgeon, the echelon system of care, resource constraints, and the particularities of the weapon systems used to wound and kill.[65,66] Thus, training for war surgeons must be specific and dedicated. Templates used to train civilian trauma specialists will not suffice.

As with surgical education in general, there is a dearth of evidence as to the best way to train military surgeons. This issue has attracted considerable debate, but a consensus view is emerging. Military surgeons should undertake higher training like their civilian colleagues, but with additional exposure to disciplines such as pediatric, cardiovascular, neurological, and urological surgery in order that a truly general training is undertaken.[4] Secondly, and most importantly, military surgeons should receive intensive training in civilian trauma centers.[5] The feasibility of this approach has been confirmed in a pilot project in Houston where U.S. army forward surgical teams (FSTs) are rotated through a busy Level One urban trauma center for 30 days at a time.[67] As well as being worthwhile to the surgeons, the scheme allowed combat medical technicians—who seldom encounter trauma patients in their usual peacetime duties—to gain valuable practice. Similar schemes have been introduced for British military surgeons in South African trauma centers, allowing the surgeon to practice and gain confidence in trauma surgical technique while supervised by highly experienced civilian trauma specialists. However, it is acknowledged that even these high-volume institutions do not encounter many patients whose wounds are caused by high-energy weapons or blast injury; moreover, Level One trauma centers are usually well resourced with sophisticated equipment and specialist personnel that the military surgeon will not have access to under operational conditions. Thus, while exceptionally worthwhile, such placements only partly meet the training requirements for combat surgeons. Therefore, the third phase of the military trauma specialist's education ought to be secondment to a nongovernmental organization (NGO) such as the International Committee of the Red Cross, with subsequent deployment on a humanitarian aid mission. By so doing, and working in conditions akin to those found in war zones, NGO missions will facilitate full maturation of the military surgeon's skills.

Difficulties with this training approach may be encountered. Training will depend upon the good will of civilian trauma institutions that may consider such placements subordinate to their own educational agendas; furthermore, political considerations may militate against neutral humanitarian agencies using foreign military surgeons. Such a strategy may mean a lengthier training period with less opportunity to develop an area of specialist expertise. However, this approach addresses the inadequacies of current systems that produce combat surgeons who are as skillful as their civilian colleagues in treating peacetime surgical conditions, but which comprehensively fail to train them to fulfill their primary mission: the care of wounded soldiers.

Virtual Reality and Trauma Training

Trauma mannequins and interactive CD-ROMs have been developed to allow providers to practice their triage and resuscitation skills, but the development of faithful digital simulations to facilitate training for trauma surgeons is a far more complex proposition.

The ultimate goal is to produce a sophisticated computer-generated (CG) training environment that immerses and spatially orientates the trainee—through headset and force-feedback gloves—in a high-fidelity virtual theater suite, "operating" on a virtual trauma patient.[68] The ideal system would allow the user to observe and interact with CG tissues that handle realistically, generating real-time tactile and proprioceptive (haptic) feedback in response to manipulation, thereby encouraging suspension of disbelief. However, such fully immersive systems are in their infancy; the majority of virtual surgical trainers available at present are non-immersive, having been developed to model endoscopic or laparoscopic procedures that, by their nature, lend themselves well to PC-based variations of "Screen and Joystick" technology.[69] These include recently developed computerized laparoscopic trainers like the MIST system, which have been successfully utilized to develop the psychomotor skills of surgical trainees.[70] Fully immersive virtual training requires a digitized anatomical dataset, powerful software that can render and animate the appropriate three-dimensional images, clinically valid algorithms to govern feedback and interaction, plus sophisticated image generation, orientation, and force-feedback hardware. While anatomic datasets such as the Visible Human project are readily available,[71] and computing power is increasing at a near exponential rate, the development of high-resolution haptic feedback technology capable of tracking the motion of the users hands and CG tissues is especially challenging and remains the rate-limiting step.[68] Once these substantial difficulties have been overcome, trauma surgery simulations are likely to become widespread and will offer a novel solution to the "training paradox" described in the introduction to this chapter.

Training for Ballistic Injury—The Johannesburg General Hospital Approach

Since her successful transition to democracy, South Africa has had to contend with a trauma burden of epic proportion. Much of this is borne by the residents of Johannesburg and Soweto, with injuries arising chiefly from firearm-related criminal violence and road traffic accidents. The murder rate is approximately 60 per 100 000, placing the city near the top of the international league table. The Johannesburg General Hospital Trauma Unit—conforming to the requirements for an American College of Surgeons Level One trauma center—serves as a tertiary referral center for the province of Gauteng, treats approximately 20 000 patients per annum, and has responsibility for trauma training at all levels of medical, nursing, and paramedic education. All general surgical registrars rotate twice through the unit, once as a junior and again as a senior registrar before exiting their training program.

Importantly, twenty-four–hour resident consultant cover facilitates continuous supervision and training of registrars, who each undertake around eight calls per month. Cases are reviewed at morning hand-over and all complications and mortalities are reviewed, with feedback from forensic pathologists, on a weekly basis. Resuscitations are videotaped and teaching cases presented to ensure that unit protocols are not breached. Registrars and junior medical staff are trained in resuscitative and trauma surgical skills during regularly held mortuary sessions and are given the opportunity to undertake ATLS® or DSTC™ courses if not already certified. All registrars and junior staff are allocated a period in the trauma intensive care unit to pursue critical care training. All staff are appraised at regular intervals. Experience in prehospital care is readily available and encouraged through attachment to provincial ambulance services and there are opportunities to gain flight training and serve as a flight doctor on the helicopter ambulance. The unit has attracted and continues to train military surgeons from the United Kingdom and other countries.[72]

Summary

Advance Trauma Life Support® was a great advance in trauma care and remains the gold standard for in-hospital resuscitation of critically injured patients. Modifications of the ATLS® training approach for the prehospital

TABLE 24-2. Suggested scheme of training for development of surgical competence in the management of ballistic trauma

Stage	Essential	Desirable	Courses
Senior House Officer/Junior Resident	Basic surgical training program	Attachment to surgical ICU	ATLS® provider CCrISP provider
Registrar/Resident	Higher surgical training program	Audit and research in trauma	ATLS® instructor DSTC™/DSTS provider
Senior Registrar/ Resident	Fellowship at high volume Level One trauma center	Completion of a higher degree in a trauma related topic	MIMMS
Consultant	High emergency/ trauma case-load Regular peer review and appraisal	Regular "refresher" secondments to high-volume Level One trauma center	DSTC™ /DSTS instructor RCS "Training the trainer"

Abbreviations: ATLS®, advanced trauma life support; CCrISP, care of the critically ill surgical patient; DSTC™, definitive surgical trauma care; DSTS, definitive surgical trauma skills; MIMMS, Major incident medical management and support; RCS, Royal College of Surgeons.

and military domains have been successfully developed to create a potentially seamless system of care. Unfortunately, the training of surgeons and other specialists to deliver optimal definitive treatment has not been addressed with the same vigor and remains a source of concern, particularly with regard to military providers. In countries such as the United Kingdom, where ballistic trauma is still comparatively uncommon, trauma education is centered on a small pool of military and civilian enthusiasts with little dedicated trauma training infrastructure. Prevention of loss of institutional memory will depend upon the successful uptake of the DSTC™/DSTS course amongst surgeons-in-training, together with recognition and incorporation of formalized overseas trauma training fellowships by the relevant specialist training authorities (Table 24-2). Eventually, it is likely that this problem will be partially solved—at least in countries able to afford it—by anticipated developments in simulation technology. By these means the necessary balance between educative and experiential training will be struck and the trauma practitioner adequately equipped to manage the demands of patients with ballistic injury.

References

1. Baker SP. Injuries: The neglected epidemic. Stone lecture. 1985 American Trauma Society meeting. *J Trauma.* 1987;27:343–348.

2. The Royal College of Surgeons of England and the British Orthopaedic Association. Better care for the severely injured—a joint report. The Royal College of Surgeons of England; 2000.
3. Englehardt S, Hoyt D, Coimbra R, Forthage D, Holbrook T. The fifteen-year evolution of an urban trauma center: What does the future hold for the trauma surgeon? *J Trauma.* 2001;51:633–637.
4. MacFarlane C, Ryan J. Training military surgeons: A challenge for the future. *Mil Med.* 2002;167:260–262.
5. Barker P. Trauma training and the military. *Injury.* 2003;34:1–2.
6. Bain IM, Kirby RM, Cook AL, Oakley PA, Templeton J. Role of the general surgeon in a British trauma center. *Brit J Surg.* 1996;83:1248–1251.
7. Ryan JM, Rich NM. Ballistic trauma—an overview. In: Ryan JM, Rich NM, Dale RF, Morgans BT, Cooper GJ, eds. *Ballistic Trauma. Clinical Relevance in Peace and War.* London: Arnold; 1997:3–7.
8. Collicott PE. Advanced trauma life support course: An improvement in rural trauma care. *Nebraska Med J.* 1979;64:279–280.
9. Anderson ID, Woodford M, DeDombal FT, Irving M. Retrospective study of 1000 deaths from injury in England and Wales. *BMJ.* 1988;296:1305–1308.
10. Romiszowski AJ. In: *Designing Educational Systems.* New York: Nichols Publishing; 1981:63–88.
11. Carley S, Driscoll P. Trauma education. *Resuscitation.* 2001;48:47–56.
12. Driscoll P, Gwinnutt C, McNeill I. Controversies in advanced trauma life support. *Trauma.* 1999;1:171–176.
13. Vestrup JA, Stormorken A, Wood V. Impact of advanced trauma life support training on early trauma management. *Am J Surg.* 1988;155:704–707.
14. Messic WJ, Rutledge R, Meyer AA. The association of advanced life support training and decreased per capita trauma death rates: An analysis of 12,417 trauma deaths. *J Trauma.* 1992;33:850–855.
15. Ali J, Adam R, Butler AK, Chang H, Howard M, Gonsalves D. Trauma outcome improves following the advanced trauma life support program in a developing country. *J Trauma.* 1993;34:890–898.
16. Bell RM, Krantz BE, Weigelt JA. ATLS®: A foundation for trauma training. *Ann Emerg Med.* 1999;34:233–237.
17. Revell M, Porter K, Greaves I. Fluid resuscitation in prehospital trauma care: A consensus view. *Emerg Med J.* 2002;19:494–498.
18. American College of Surgeons Committee on Trauma. *Advanced Trauma Life Support Student Course Manual.* 6th ed. Chicago; 1997:11–12.
19. Salander JM, Rich N. Advanced trauma life support: An idea whose time has come. *Mil Med.* 1983;148:507–508.
20. Schultz RJ. After triage: Lessons learned in Vietnam with military casualties. *Mil Med.* 1990;155:221–222.
21. Mahoney P, Riley B. Battlefield trauma life support: Its use in the resuscitation department of 32 Field Hospital during the Gulf War. *Mil Med.* 1996;161:542–546.
22. Hawley A. Trauma management on the battlefield: A modern approach. *J R Army Med Corps.* 1996;142:120–125.
23. Trunkey DD. Trauma. *Sci Am.* 1983;249:20–27.
24. Gofrit ON, Leibovici D, Shapira SC, Shemer J, Stein M, Michaelson M. The trimodal death distribution of trauma victims: Military experience from the Lebanon war. *Mil Med.* 1997;162:24–26.

25. Scope A, Farkash U, Lynn M, Abargel A, Eldad A. Mortality epidemiology in low-intensity warfare: Israel Defence Forces' experience. *Injury*. 2001;32:1–3.
26. Weideman JE, Jennings SA. Applying ATLS® to the Gulf War. *Mil Med*. 1993;158:121–126.
27. Baker MS. Advanced trauma life support: Is it adequate stand-alone training for military medicine? *Mil Med*. 1994;159:587–590.
28. Townsend RN, Clark RC, Ramenofsky ML, Diamond DL. ATLS® based trauma resuscitation review: Education and outcome. *J Trauma*. 1993;34:133–138.
29. Brooks AJ, Phipson M, Potgeiter A, Koertzen H, Boffard KD. Education of the trauma team: Video evaluation of the compliance with universal barrier precautions in resuscitation. *Eur J Surg*. 1999;165:1125–1128.
30. Willy C, Sterk J, Schwarz W, Gerngross H. Computer-assisted training program for simulation of triage, resuscitation and evacuation of casualties. *Mil Med*. 1998;163:234–238.
31. Leitch RA, Moses GR, Magee H. Simulation and the future of military medicine. *Mil Med*. 2002;167:350–354.
32. Issenberg SB, McGaghie WC, Hart, IR et al. Simulation technology for health care professional skills training and assessment. *JAMA*. 1999;282:861–886.
33. Mclellan BA. Early experience with simulated trauma resuscitation. *Can J Surg*. 1999;42:205–210.
34. Hammond J, Bermann M, Chen B, Kushins L. Incorporation of a computerized human patient simulator in critical care training: A preliminary report. *J Trauma*. 2002;53:1064–1067.
35. Ali J, Gana TJ, Howard M. Trauma mannequin assessment of management skills of surgical residents after advanced trauma life support training. *J Surg Res*. 2000;93:197–200.
36. Marshall R, Smith JS, Gorman PJ, Krummel TM, Haluck RS, Cooney RN. Use of a human patient simulator in the development of resident trauma management skills. *J Trauma*. 2001;51:17–21.
37. McSwain MJ, McSwain NE. Paramedic training in the USA. In: Greaves I, Ryan JM, Porter KM, eds. *Trauma*. London: Arnold; 1998:41–47.
38. Mock CN, Jurkovich GJ, nii-Amon-Kotei D, Areulaerija C, Maier RV. Trauma mortality patterns in three nations at different economic levels: Implications for global trauma system development. *J Trauma*. 1998;44:804–812.
39. Ali J, Adam RU, Gana TJ, Bepasie H, Williams JI. Effect of the PHTLS program on prehospital trauma care. *J Trauma*. 1997;42:786–790.
40. Christopher LD. Pre-hospital care in Gauteng Province, South Africa. *Prehosp Immed Care*. 1998;2:213–215.
41. Marsden AK. Paramedic training in the UK. In: Greaves I, Ryan JM, Porter KM, eds. *Trauma*. London: Arnold; 1998:48–52.
42. Hodgetts TJ, Mackway-Jones K, eds. *Major Incident Medical Management and Support, The Practical Approach*. London: BMJ Publishing Group; 1995.
43. Spaite DW, Criss EA, Valenzuela TD, Meislin HW. Prehospital advanced life support for major trauma: critical need for clinical trials. *Ann Emerg Med*. 1998;32:480–489.
44. Carley S, Mackway-Jones K. Paramedics—a step in the wrong direction. In: Greaves I, Ryan JM, Porter KM, eds. *Trauma*. London: Arnold; 1998:72–79.
45. Eckstein M, Chan L, Schneir A, Palmer R. Effect of prehospital advanced life support on outcomes of major trauma patients. *J Trauma*. 2000;48:643–648.

46. Sampalis JS, Lavoie A, Williams JI, et al. Impact of on-site care, prehospital time and level of in-hospital care on survival in severely injured patients. *J Trauma.* 1993;34:252–261.
47. Demetriades D, Chan L, Cornwell E, Belzberg H, Berne TV, Asensio J. Paramedic transportation of trauma patients. Effect on outcome. *Arch Surg.* 1996;131:133–138.
48. Lerer LB, Knottenbelt JD. Preventable mortality following sharp penetrating chest trauma. *J Trauma.* 1994;37:9–12.
49. Kwan I, Roberts I, Bunn F. Timing and volume of fluid administration for patients with bleeding following trauma. *Cochrane Database Syst Rev.* 2001;CD002245.
50. Edwards ND. B Med Sci degree course in paramedical studies at The University of Sheffield. *Prehosp Immed Care.* 1998;2:224–226.
51. Husum H. Effects of early prehsopital life support to war injured: The battle of Jalalabad, Afghanistan. *Prehospital Disaster Med.* 1999;14:43–48.
52. Butler FK, Hagmann J, Butler EG. Tactical combat casualty care. In: Butler FK, Hagmann J, eds. *Tactical Management of Urban Warfare Casualties in Special Operations. Mil Med.* 2000;165(suppl):1–48.
53. Butler FK, Hagmann J, Butler EG. Tactical combat casualty care in special operations. *Mil Med.* 1996;161(supp):3–16.
54. McSwain NE, Frame S, Paturas JL, eds. *Prehospital Life Support Training Manual.* 4th ed. Akron: Mosby; 1999.
55. Navein JF, Dunn RL. The combat trauma life support course: Resource-constrained first responder trauma care for Special Forces medics. *Mil Med.* 2002;167:566–572.
56. Brooks A, Butcher W, Walsh M, Lambert A, Browne J, Ryan J. The experience and training of British general surgeons in trauma surgery for the abdomen, thorax and major vessels. *Ann R Coll Surg Engl.* 2002;84:409–413.
57. Boffard K, ed. *Definitive Surgical Trauma Care Course Student Manual.* London: Arnold; 2003.
58. Jacobs LM, Lorenzo C, Brautigam RT. Definitive surgical trauma care live porcine session: A technique for training in trauma surgery. *Conn Med.* 2001;65: 265–268.
59. Rosenfeld JV. Training the military surgeon: Definitive surgical trauma course and the development of a military module. *ADF Health.* 2002;3:68–70.
60. Ryan JM, Roberts P. Definitive surgical trauma skills: A new skills course for specialist registrars and consultants in general surgery in the United Kingdom. *Trauma.* 2002;4:184–188.
61. Knuth TE. Trauma fellowship training: the insiders' perspective. *J Trauma.* 1993;35:233–240.
62. Gabram SG, Esposito TJ, Morris RM, Mendola RA, Gamelli RL. Trauma care fellowships: Current status and future survival. *J Trauma.* 1998;44:86–92.
63. Eastern Association for the Surgery of Trauma. Guidelines for trauma care fellowships. *J Trauma.* 1992;33:491–494.
64. Ogilvie H. General introduction: surgery in wartime. In: Cope Z, ed. *History of the Second World War: Surgery.* London: Her Majesty's Stationary Office; 1953.
65. Rignault DP. How to train war surgery specialists: Part II. *Mil Med.* 1990;155: 143–147.
66. Llewellyn CH. Education and training for war surgery. *Mil Med.* 1990;155: 192–193.

67. Schreiber MA, Holcomb JB, Conaway CW, Campbell KD, Wall M, Mattox KL. Military trauma training performed in a civilian trauma center. *J Surg Res.* 2002;104:8–14.
68. Kaufmann CR, Higgins GA, Champion HR. Trauma training—the use of virtual reality. In: Greaves I, Ryan JM, Porter KM, eds. *Trauma*. London: Arnold; 1998.
69. Savata BM. Surgical education and surgical simulation. *World J Surg.* 2001;25: 1484–1489.
70. McCloy R, Stone R. Science, medicine and the future. Virtual reality in surgery. *BMJ.* 2001;323:912–915.
71. Spitzer V, Whitlock D. Visible humans on the information super highway: How they got there and where they are going. In: *Proceedings of the Visible Human Project conference.* Bethesda, MD: Public Health Service, National Library of Medicine; 1996:17–18.
72. Bowley D, Brooks A. *Trauma experience overseas. Association of Surgeons in Training Yearbook 2001–2002.* Association of Surgeons of Great Britain and Ireland. 107–109.

Appendix A

Definitive Surgical Trauma Care (DSTC^{TM}) Course: Core Curriculum

Surgical Skills

Surgical Skills: Neck

1. Standard neck (pre-sternomastoid) incision
2. Control and repair of carotid vessels
    2.1. Zone II
    2.2. Extension into Zone III
    2.3. Division of digastric muscle and subluxation or division of mandible
    2.4. Extension into Zone I
3. Extension by supraclavicular incision
    3.1. Ligation of proximal internal carotid artery
    3.2. Repair with divided external carotid artery
4. Access to, control of, and ligation of internal jugular vein
5. Access to and repair of the trachea
6. Access to, and repair of the cervical esophagus

Surgical Skills: Thorax

1. Incisions
    1.1. Antero-lateral thoracotomy
    1.2. Sternotomy
    1.3. "Chevron" ("Clamshell") bilateral thoracotomy
2. Thoracotomy
    2.1. Exploration of thorax
    2.2. Ligation of intercostal and internal mammary vessels

2.3. Emergency department (resuscitative) thoracotomy
   2.3.1. Supradiaphragmatic control of the aorta
   2.3.2. Control of the pulmonary hilum
   2.3.3. Internal cardiac massage
3. Pericardiotomy
  3.1. Preservation of phrenic nerve
  3.2. Access to the pulmonary veins
4. Access to and repair of the thoracic aorta
5. Lung wounds
  5.1. Oversewing
  5.2. Stapling
  5.3. Partial lung resection
  5.4. Tractectomy
  5.5. Lobectomy
6. Access to, and repair of the thoracic esophagus
7. Access to and repair of the diaphragm
8. Compression of the left subclavian vessels from below
9. Left anterior thoracotomy
  9.1. Visualization of supra-aortic vessels
10. Heart repair
  10.1. Finger control
  10.2. Involvement of coronary vessels

Surgical Skills: Abdomen

1. Midline Laparotomy
  1.1. How to explore (priorities)
  1.2. Packing
  1.3. Localization of retroperitoneal hematomas—When to explore?
  1.4. Extension of laparotomy incision
   1.4.1. Lateral extension
   1.4.2. Sternotomy
  1.5. Cross clamping of the aorta at diaphragm (division at left crus)
  1.6. Damage control /Abbreviated laparotomy
2. Left visceral rotation
  2.1. Mattox maneuver
3. Right visceral rotation
  3.1. Kocher's maneuver
  3.2. Cattel and Braasch maneuver
4. Temporary abdominal closure
  4.1. Towel clips
  4.2. Bogota bag
  4.3. "Vacpac"/Sandwich technique

Surgical Skills: Esophagus

1. Abdominal esophagus
    1.1. Mobilization
    1.2. Repair
        1.2.1. Simple
        1.2.2. Mobilization of fundus to reinforce sutures

Surgical Skills: Stomach and Bowel

1. Stomach
    1.1. Mobilization
    1.2. Access to vascular control
    1.3. Repair of anterior and posterior wounds
    1.4. Pyloric exclusion
    1.5. Distal gastrectomy
2. Bowel
    2.1. Resection
    2.2. Small and large bowel anastomosis
    2.3. Staple colostomy
    2.4. Collagen fleece technique of anastomosis protection
3. Ileostomy technique

Surgical Skills: Liver

1. Mobilization (falciform, suspensory, triangular and coronary ligaments)
2. Liver packing
3. Hepatic isolation
    3.1. Control of infra-hepatic IVC
    3.2. Control of supra-hepatic IVC
    3.3. Pringle's maneuver
4. Repair of parenchymal laceration
5. Technique of finger fracture
6. Tractotomy
7. Packing for injury to hepatic veins
8. Hepatic resection
9. Non-anatomical partial resection
10. Use of tissue adhesives
11. Tamponade for penetrating injury (Foley/Penrose drains/Sengstaken tube)
12. Insertion of shunt

Surgical Skills: Spleen

1. Mobilization
2. Suture
3. Mesh wrap
4. Use of tissue adhesives

5. Partial splenectomy
   5.1. Sutures
   5.2. Staples
6. Total splenectomy

Surgical Skills: Pancreas

1. Mobilization of the tail of the pancreas
2. Mobilization of the head of the pancreas
3. Localization of the main duct and its repair
4. Distal pancreatic resection
   4.1. Stapler
   4.2. Oversewing
5. Use of tissue adhesives
6. Diverticulization
7. Access to mesenteric vessels (division of pancreas)

Surgical Skills: Duodenum

1. Mobilization of the duodenum
   1.1. Kocher's maneuver
   1.2. Cattel and Braasch maneuver
   1.3. Division of ligament of Treitz
2. Duodenal repair

Surgical Skills: Genito-Urinary System

1. Kidney
   1.1. Mobilization
   1.2. Vascular control
   1.3. Repair
   1.4. Partial nephrectomy
   1.5. Nephrectomy
2. Ureter
   2.1. Mobilization
   2.2. Stenting
   2.3. Repair
3. Bladder
   3.1. Repair of intra-peritoneal rupture
   3.2. Repair of extra-peritoneal rupture

Surgical Skills: Abdominal Vascular Injury

1. Exposure and control
   1.1. Aorta
      1.1.1. Exposure
      1.1.2. Repair

1.2. IVC
    1.2.1. Supra-hepatic IVC
    1.2.2. Infra-hepatic IVC
    1.2.3. Control of hemorrhage with swabs
    1.2.4. Repair through anterior wound
2. Pelvis
    2.1. Control of pelvic vessels
        2.1.1. Packing
        2.1.2. Suture or ligation of artery and vein
        2.1.3. Packing/anchor ligation of sacral vessels

Surgical Skills: Vascular

1. Extremities: Vascular access
    1.1. Axillary
    1.2. Brachial
    1.3. Femoral
    1.4. Popliteal
2. Fasciotomy
    2.1. Upper limb
    2.2. Lower limb

Appendix B

Useful Web Addresses

http://www.aast.org	American Association for the Surgery of Trauma site with information on U.S. trauma-related fellowship positions
http://www.alsg.org	Advanced life support group website. MIMMS course information.
http://www.apothecaries.org	Society of Apothecaries website offering information on the Diploma in Medical Care of Catastrophes.
http://www.east.org	Eastern Association for the Surgery of Trauma. Information on fellowship schemes.
http://www.facs.org	American College of Surgeons Website. Includes a master-schedule of worldwide ATLS® courses.
http://www.icrc.org	International Committee of the Red Cross site; information on ICRC war surgery courses.
http://www.rcsed.ac.uk	Royal College of Surgeons of Edinburgh website. Details of pre-hospital trauma training.

http://www.rcseng.ac.uk	Royal College of Surgeons of England website. Lists DSTS course schedules.
http://www.redcross.org.uk	British Red Cross site with information on their surgical training initiative for surgeons wishing to work in austere environments.
http://www.roysocmed.ac.uk	The Royal Society of Medicine Conflict and Catastrophes section holds regular meetings dealing with all aspects of the care of patients injured during war and civil strife.
http://www.trauma.org	Very useful site offering information on trauma fellowships, courses, conferences, etc.
http://www.wits.ac.za/trauma	Johannesburg Hospital Trauma Unit. Information on Fellowship positions, trauma protocols, DSTC™, NTMC, and ATLS® courses

Section 3
Resource Limited Situations

Introduction

In resource-limited situations such as disaster or conflict, external factors will influence the type of care that can be given.

This is a real culture shock for people on their first military or non-govermental organization (NGO) deployment.

The authors in the following section have all deployed widely and give clear guidelines on how to manage these situations.

25
Hospital and System Assessment

JENNY HAYWARD-KARLSSON

Introduction

The majority of weapon injuries occur in countries where resources for provision of health care are limited.[1] Many of these are countries where weapon wounded are the result of armed conflict. More than 85% of the major conflicts since the World War II have occurred in poor countries.[2]

War disrupts the normal function of all systems, be they education, logistics, or health care, by diverting already scarce resources to the conflict, by the physical disruption of supply lines, and through damage to health infrastructure and the referral system.

In armed conflict, the additional burden of weapon wounded often presents serious problems to health systems and personnel already struggling to provide an acceptable level of care.

The wounded need *access* to a *safe place* supplied with *water* and *power* where they can receive *safe anaesthesia, competent surgical treatment* and *good nursing care* within a *well-organized system* that receives *adequate supplies*."[3]

At the best of times, hospitals providing surgical care are expensive to run. They depend on a minimum of infrastructure, equipment, expertise (surgery, anesthesia, nursing care, good management, medical support services, X-ray, lab, non-medical support, that is, laundry, kitchen, cleaning, and maintenance of infrastructure). Reliable logistics are vital for medical and non-medical supplies, and adequate financial resources must be assured. All these elements must be present in both sufficient *quantity* and *quality*.

Health systems and services, especially tertiary level facilities, can be very vulnerable in resource-limited situations, and especially during armed conflict. The challenge facing medical, nursing, and hospital management personnel in such situations should not be underestimated.

Assessing the capacity of the health care system in general or of individual hospitals to provide adequate care for weapon wounded must be done carefully and with attention to detail in order assure that any support provided for these facilities is appropriate and targeted correctly.

This chapter aims to give some pointers to assess the capacity of health care systems and individual hospitals to provide this care in resource-limited situations.

Health System Assessment

An assessment of the health system should aim to identify any imbalance between the health needs of the population—in this case access to care for weapon wounded—and the local resources available to address those needs.

The provision of care for weapon wounded involves a chain of events from the moment of wounding to the rehabilitation of the wounded person into society. All links of this chain should be assessed as a first step to see how the steps fit into the health system in question and to identify weak or missing links in the chain.

Many wounded people ultimately require hospital care, but individual hospitals cannot function with complete independence from the overall health system.[4] A good understanding of how the health care system functions is vital in order to identify weak points and to develop a strategy for assistance that is appropriate and that aims to strengthen the existing system rather than to set up parallel or unsustainable systems.

Key points to consider:

System structure:
– the role of the Ministry of Health both nationally and regionally,
– involvement of the private sector,
– national health planning and policies,
– other actors involved in providing care for wounded—the military medical services; international agencies; nongovernmental organizations (NGOs), both nationally and internationally,
– Is there an established chain of health care for wounded from point of injury to definitive care?

Prehospital care for wounded:
– What is the first point of access to care for the wounded? Have any elements of the population received training in First Aid?
– Is the National Red Cross or Red Crescent Society active in the field of First Aid?
– First Aid posts: Do they exist? How well do they function? Are they organized? Do they have adequate supplies?
– Health centers: Are they equipped to receive wounded and provide first treatment?
– Ambulance system: Does it exist? Does it function everywhere or just in urban areas? Is it properly resourced?

The number and location of structures performing surgery:
- What surgical services are provided? Is specialized surgery available? What is the referral system? What is the quality of surgical care? (see below, *Individual Hospital Assessment*)

Funding:
- What are the main sources of funds for the health sector—Ministry of Health, cost recovery/cost sharing, NGOs?
- Is this organized on a central, regional, or local basis?

Human resources for health:
- Number of doctors, nurses, and other health care professionals in the country
- Training, qualifications, and experience of professional staff
- Staff salaries: Salary scale for different classes of health workers—are salaries paid regularly and on time?
- Do health professionals expect to receive payment from patients in addition to their salary?

Logistics:
- For patient referrals—ambulance service, private transport.
- For medical and non-medical supplies—into the country and distribution within the country.

Security:
- Does lack of security have an impact on the health system?
- What is the pattern of armed violence? (drug-related crime, gangs, bandits, domestic violence)
- Is there an on-going conflict? (what is the nature of the conflict, the presence or absence of antipersonnel land mines, moving front lines, curfews)

Access to health care:
- Do all population groups have access to health care?
- Are there actual or potential problems related to ethnicity, tribal loyalties, or conflicts?
- Is there economic, religious or geographic discrimination?

Epidemiology:
- What population does the health system serve?
- What are the main health problems?
- Seasonal patterns of disease.

The national Ministry of Health is also an important source of information for the country concerned. In countries in conflict or during emergencies, national health staff, international and local nongovernmental organizations (NGOs), and humanitarian organizations such as the components of the Red Cross Movement (the National Red Cross or Red Crescent Society, the International Federation of Red Cross and Red Crescent Societies, and the International Committee of the Red Cross) often have regular coordination meetings during emergencies for all actors in the health sector that provide an opportunity to exchange information. These meetings also provide an opportunity to establish a standard approach towards the provision and monitoring of health services.

Visits to health structures, discussions with medical, nursing and management staff, and the patients themselves are invaluable to gain an insight into the actual activities, needs, and performance of the health system.

Individual Hospital Assessment

Once an accurate assessment of the overall health system has been made, attention can be turned to individual hospitals providing care for weapon wounded.

It is important to remember that hospitals in resource-limited situations may be the only place to provide the whole chain of health care for weapon wounded, from first aid to definitive surgical care and rehabilitation. It may be the only point where first aid can be provided; evacuation or onward referral to specialist medical treatment is often difficult or even impossible. This is where the treatment of weapon wounded in civilian health structures in times of war differs from the military medical services where onward evacuation of the wounded out of the conflict area is the aim. The capacity of the hospital to provide definitive care will have an effect on the way any assessment is made (see Chapter 28 and Section 4).

Assessment of individual hospitals must focus on the hospital as a whole entity. There is no point in looking only at the quality of surgical or nursing care in isolation from the other essential elements. These can be grouped into the following categories:

– Security—of the hospital, staff, and patients
– Infrastructure—buildings, water and sanitation, electricity, maintenance
– Equipment—medical and non-medical
– Supplies—consumable supplies, both medical and non-medical
– Expertise—hospital management, surgery and anesthesia, nursing and support staff
– Funding and finance

All the above are interdependent and the quality and quantity of each has an impact on the overall capacity of the hospital to respond to the needs of the wounded; for example:

– If salaries are insufficient or not paid regularly, staff will be obliged to take second jobs, find alternative employment or other means of maintaining their family income.
– The best surgeon cannot operate without an appropriate range of surgical instruments that are properly sterilized.

- Good postoperative nursing care is impossible without lights going 24 hours in the wards and a basic minimum of equipment and medical supplies.
- The patient's wounds will not heal if they do not receive an adequate diet.
- Little will be possible if the hospital staff cannot work under secure conditions.

Thus, an assessment of the capacity of an individual hospital to provide correct care for wounded must consider all of these elements.

Hospital assessments of this kind must be done by experienced health professionals who have both an appreciation of the complexity and corresponding fragility of tertiary level health facilities in resource-limited situations together with professional knowledge of the basic health-care needs of the wounded. This requires both experience and a pragmatic approach towards what represents safe, appropriate, and realistic care.

It is difficult to get an accurate picture of the capacity of a hospital and the professional skills of the medical and nursing staff without spending a significant period of time working in the hospital and gaining the trust and confidence of the staff and patients. Visiting assessment teams may be perceived as intrusive and inquisitive, access to information may be difficult, hospital records may not be accurate, data about the number and type of casualties may be regarded as confidential, and information given verbally or in reports may not necessarily conform with what is seen to be happening. The conclusions of any assessment in this context will necessarily depend largely on the experience and judgement of the individuals involved.

However, if a systematic approach is adopted for an initial assessment where each of the elements essential to enable the hospital to function are examined by experienced people, enough information should be obtained to allow a conclusion to be drawn and an appropriate response to be planned. These essential elements are examined below.

Security and Protection of the Hospital

Hospital staff must be allowed to carry out their work and patients recover from their injuries in a safe environment. In areas of armed conflict, this becomes the primary consideration. This includes the protection of the hospital under international humanitarian law and measures taken to physically protect the hospital infrastructure, patients, and staff.

Protection under International Humanitarian Law

In situations of armed conflict, international humanitarian law limits the use of violence and protects those who are not or no longer taking part in the hostilities (civilians, wounded and sick combatants, prisoners of war). The Four Geneva Conventions of 1949 and the two Additional protocols of 1977 contain rules applicable in international and internal armed conflicts. Almost all States are bound by the Geneva Conventions.

The main aim of humanitarian law is to protect the civilian population from the effects of war. Civilians therefore enjoy a far-reaching immunity. In particular, they must not be attacked and are entitled to receive assistance if they lack essential goods indispensable to their survival, such as foodstuffs and medical supplies.

The International Committee of the Red Cross (ICRC), as a neutral and independent institution, has the task of monitoring the implementation of humanitarian law. In addition, the ICRC brings protection and assistance, without adverse discrimination to the victims of armed conflict and disturbances.

Humanitarian law specifically protects medical transports and civilian and military medical units, in particular hospitals: they must be respected at all times and must not be the object of attack.

All the wounded and sick and the medical personnel caring for them must also be respected and protected.

Medical units enjoy neutral status as long as they are not used to commit acts harmful to the enemy such as sheltering able-bodied combatants, storing arms and ammunition or being used as military observation posts; otherwise their protection ceases and they become legitimate military targets. This is why strict controls must be established in order to safeguard the protected status of medical units and transports.

To enhance the protection of medical units and medical transports, they should be clearly marked by the Red Cross or Red Crescent emblem, of the largest possible size. The emblem is the visible sign of the protection conferred by the Geneva Conventions and their Additional Protocols.

During armed conflicts, only the following may use the Red Cross or Red Crescent emblem as a means of protection:

- the medical units of the armed forces
- hospitals, other medical units and medical transports that have received special permission to use the emblem
- the medical personnel, medical transports and material that a National Red Cross or Red Crescent Society has put at the disposal of the medical service of the armed forces.

In order to ensure effective protection in wartime, use of the emblem must be strictly controlled in peacetime.

In peacetime the emblem may only be used by:

- the medical services of the armed forces
- National Red Cross or Red Crescent Societies, in order to indicate that persons or goods have a connection with the Society in question (here the emblem must be of a small dimension)
- Exceptionally, ambulances and aid stations exclusively assigned to the purpose of giving free treatment to the wounded and sick, with the authorisation of a National Society.

The ICRC and the International Federation of Red Cross and Red Crescent Societies are authorised to use the emblem for all their activities.

The number of cases of misuse of the emblem is unfortunately very high. In peacetime, hospitals, clinics, doctors, pharmacies, ambulances, NGO's and commercial companies tend to use the emblem in order to benefit from its reputation, even though they are not entitled to do so. This creates problems, as it clearly weakens the protective value of the emblem in wartime.

Any case of misuse of the emblem should be reported to the relevant National Red Cross or Red Crescent Society, the ICRC or the International Federation of Red Cross and Red Crescent Societies. *Source:* International Committee of the Red Cross, 1998[3]

In order to provide adequate physical protection of the hospital infrastructure, staff, and patients from the effects of working in a potentially insecure environment, certain measures should be in place.

- Is the hospital clearly identifiable as such—by day and night?
- Is it possible to restrict access to the hospital and control crowds, especially during an influx of wounded?
- Are weapons carried openly within the hospital?—This may compromise the identity of the hospital as a neutral area that is afforded protection under international humanitarian law. The presence of weapon carriers inside the hospital may also compromise the safety of the staff and patients.

Hospital Infrastructure

The infrastructure of the hospital should ensure a safe and secure environment for patients and that permits the hospital staff to carry out their work. The hospital will not function without water or electricity. Regular maintenance of the infrastructure is essential to ensure that all services are available when required.

The buildings should include these essential departments:

Medical: Admission/emergency room, operating theater, sterilization, intensive nursing ward, surgical wards, laboratory, X-ray, pharmacy, physiotherapy, nursing administration.

Non-medical: Hospital administration, kitchen, laundry/tailor, stores, construction/maintenance workshop, transport.

In addition, in areas of armed conflict, the hospital may have to increase its capacity very quickly to accommodate large numbers of wounded. The size of the compound should be able to accommodate additional space for triage and surgical wards if necessary.

Buildings:
- Is the construction of the buildings appropriate for the climate and for their intended use?

- What is their state of repair—are they weatherproof and clean?
- Can access be restricted to clinical areas such as the operating theater?
- Is there enough space within the hospital compound to increase the hospital capacity?
- Are the operating theaters and wards accessible without dependence on electricity (elevators)?

Water:

The hospital will not function without an adequate water supply.
- Absolute minimum supply—100 liters/patient/day, desirable—300 liters/patient/day (hospitals in developed countries with intensive care units and dialysis services may require 1000 liters/patient/day)
- External sources of water can easily be disrupted—does the hospital have an independent supply?
- Is there emergency storage capacity for enough water for 48 hours?

Electricity:

The hospital will not function without a guaranteed electricity supply.
- Essential for operating theater lights, refrigeration (of drugs, reagents and blood), sterilization, X-ray, general lighting, and power points.
- Does the hospital have a back-up generator in case of disruption of mains supply?
- Is there a stock of fuel for the generator?
- Is emergency lighting available in critical areas (emergency room, operating theater, wards)?

Sewage and sanitation:
- Is the system functioning and adequate to ensure a hygienic environment for the patients?

Waste disposal:
- Is there a functioning incinerator for sharps and contaminated waste?
- Is there a functioning system for the routine collection and disposal of garbage?

Maintenance:
- Is there a hospital maintenance team to ensure the functioning of essential services 24 hours/day?
- Is there a system for the regular maintenance of essential equipment?
- Are the wards and departments clean?

Equipment

A basic minimum of equipment, both medical and non-medical, is required for the surgical treatment and care of wounded.

- Medical equipment:

- Complete lists of equipment and instruments required for the operating theater are well-documented.[4]
- Medical equipment should be of good quality, robust, easily repaired and maintained. Sophisticated equipment and high technology do not often transfer successfully into resource-limited situations.
- Donations of medical equipment must be very carefully considered—the hospital must have staff that understands how to use, maintain, and repair donated equipment. Adequate funds must be available for their continued use.
- Non-medical equipment:
  - Beds for patients, stretchers, kitchen and laundry equipment, ward furniture, etc. should also be robust, easily maintained, and repaired.
  - It is more appropriate to find a local supplier for these items wherever possible—they will conform to local norms of quality and cultural acceptability.

Consumable Supplies

The basic surgical treatment and care of wounded can be managed with a limited range of consumable medical and non-medical supplies. In the absence of the possibility to refer patients for specialized surgery, treatment focuses on life- and limb-saving interventions, the basic surgical principles of which are well established.[5] The consumable supplies for this surgical care can be restricted to the basic essentials. The same as for equipment, consumable supplies do not have to be sophisticated, but should be of good quality.

Disposable presterilized supplies, including surgical linen, are expensive, often difficult to source a resupply, and thus usually unsustainable in resource-limited situations. Reusable surgical drapes and gowns are preferred, These can usually be made on the spot if a supply of good-quality cotton cloth can be identified. A functioning hospital laundry is essential, but requires a minimum of water and manpower (or, more usually, womanpower).

Prepacked dressing sets, or sets for specific interventions are also prohibitively expensive and may be misused by through attempts to reuse the material.

In countries with limited resources for health, the purchase of drugs is a major item of expenditure. The quality of all medical supplies, including drugs, must be assured. The WHO List of Essential Drugs and the Guidelines for Drug Donations should be followed. The Red Cross and Red Crescent movement Standard Item Catalogue[6] gives specifications for individual items and the consumable supplies required for first aid posts, hospitals, and other health structures. Many items in this catalogue are presented in kits giving the quantity of consumables required for 100 wounded. This represents a good approximation of what is needed for the treatment of wounded because of conventional warfare (shooting, bombing).

Non-medical supplies include fuel, food, hygienic supplies (soap, washing powder), stationery, and spare parts for maintaining equipment. Any or all of these may be in short supply where priority is often given to providing essential medical supplies, but their importance to the functioning of the hospital should not be underestimated.

Key points:

- Does the hospital have sufficient quantity and quality of consumable supplies for the actual or potential workload?
- Are the sources of supply reliable?
- Is the logistic supply chain secure?
- Does the hospital have an emergency stock of consumable supplies—for how many patients, for how long?
- Are medical consumable supplies stored in correct conditions?—in a secure, weatherproof environment, refrigerated correctly where necessary?
- Do hospital staff have access to additional supplies in case of emergencies out of normal working hours?
- Are proper records kept of supplies received, stock levels, supplies distributed, quantities consumed?

Expertise

The capacity of a hospital to provide treatment and care for wounded depends very much on the motivation, professional skills, and experience of the hospital staff. A range of both skilled and non-skilled staff is needed, from surgeons and nurses to hospital administrator, physiotherapist, and laboratory and X-ray technicians to cooks, cleaners, and drivers. Everyone working in this team must understand their role, how they fit into the system and how the system works. This needs organization, management, and coordination. It is also the most difficult area to assess when considering the potential that the hospital has to ensure safe and appropriate treatment for wounded.

It is in this area that it is essential that any assessment is carried out by health professionals who have experience in managing wounded in resource-limited situations. These people should appreciate that it is possible to maintain professional standards while providing safe and acceptable care under very basic conditions.

Hospital Management

No hospital can function without coordination and management of all activities. This includes overall planning, financial management, and accountability, ensuring that there is enough staff, with contracts, job descriptions, and regularly paid salaries to cover all the essential services, maintaining an overview of essential supplies and ensuring that the hospital is a safe working environment.

Key points:

- There must be someone in a position of authority who has the overview of all hospital activities, who has the capacity to lead the hospital team and maintain contact with authorities outside the hospital.
- This person must also be flexible enough to adapt their management to a rapidly changing situation and ensure the most efficient use of limited resources.
- Does the hospital have an emergency or major incident plan that anticipates the steps necessary to admit large numbers of wounded into the hospital?
- Does this plan allow for keeping track of the patients during an influx of wounded?
- Is there an organized system for the reception, admission, and registration of patients?
- Is there an on-call system to provide emergency services 24 hours?
- Do standard treatment and nursing protocols exist and are they applied?

Medical and Nursing Staff

The quality of care provided in the hospital depends largely, although not entirely, on the training, experience, and motivation of the health professionals delivering that care. Sheer numbers of doctors and nurses present in a hospital does not always mean that the quality of care is acceptable. The presence of a few well-trained, experienced, and motivated individuals may make all the difference.

A limited number of surgeons and nurses in Western civilian practice have experience of managing weapon wounds, especially those resulting from armed conflict.

Assessing the capacity of surgical teams and nurses to safely manage wounded patients is the most complex and difficult area to address when making an assessment of an individual hospital. Comparison with one's own clinical practice is unavoidable and requires experience and sound judgement.

Do not forget that an apparent lack of quality of surgical or nursing care may be due to factors beyond the control of the doctors or nurses working in the hospital—lack of salaries, lack of essential supplies, the absence of an organized system all contribute towards an environment that is not conducive to providing quality care.

However, much can be achieved with relatively little and there are some basic observations that can be made that give pointers towards the factors determining the delivery of safe, basic surgical and nursing care.

Key points:

- Are weapon wounds safely managed by applying the basic principles of wound management (adequate wound excision followed by delayed primary closure)?
- Is there an accurate operating theater register? What is the number and type of operations recorded?
- Is laparotomy performed safely with a trained anesthetist giving a suitable anesthetic? (endotracheal intubation, inhalational or intravenous anesthesia, muscle relaxation and assisted ventilation)
- Are patients undergoing laparotomy (or other major surgical procedures) supervised by nursing staff 24 hours postoperatively in a room with light where they can receive intravenous fluids?
- Can five or more laparotomies be performed in 24 hours under the above conditions?
- Is there 24-hour nursing supervision on the wards?
- Is there a system of recording medical orders, patient's observation (vital signs), and drugs ordered and given?

Standardization and simplification of treatment protocols, nursing care, and drug regimes, together with regular ward rounds and a clear system of information exchange will go a long way towards enabling the surgical and nursing teams to work effectively for the benefit of all patients.

The key to this is the existence of an organized system of hospital and patient management. This requires leadership and teamwork.

Clinical Services

A hospital providing surgical care for weapon wounded should have access to a functioning laboratory that can ensure safe blood for transfusion. Supplies of blood may be limited. Suitable blood donors may be difficult to find, either for cultural reasons or according to the general health status of the population. It is essential, in the light of the HIV/AIDS pandemic, that all blood is tested for HIV, as well as hepatitis B and C, syphilis, and malaria where appropriate.

Physiotherapy is essential to ensure both the general mobilization of the patient and the restoration of limb function. This must be integrated with the surgical and nursing care, but is often lacking. Patients whose limbs have been amputated should be referred to a limb-fitting service.

A functioning X-ray service is useful as an aid to precise diagnosis, but is not indispensable in the treatment of weapon wounds. Equipment should be robust and regularly maintained to ensure a minimum level of safety for the staff and patients.

Finance and Funding

Hospitals are expensive to set up and expensive to run.

Even in situations where funds are in short supply, a system of basic book-keeping accounting must be in place. The hospital administrator should know what the annual budget for the hospital is; he/she should also be able to estimate the running costs of the hospital on a monthly or annual basis and identify expenditure for specific items such as fuel, food, salaries, medical supplies, etc.

Sources of funding are often complex, with funds coming from central or local government, contributions in cash or kind from NGOs or international organizations, or medical supplies provided directly from a central pharmacy.

A system of cost sharing or cost recovery may be in place, with patients paying for drugs and/or services. Ideally, the most vulnerable in society should be exempt from some or all of these charges in order to ensure that everyone has access to emergency care.

Assistance to Hospitals in Resource-Limited Situations

The assessment of an individual hospital should identify specific areas where appropriate assistance can be targeted effectively in order to allow the provision of safe care for weapon wounded. This may be in any or all of the areas described above.

However, the aim of any assistance should be to support the existing system and build local capacity wherever possible, whether this means financial support, repair, or rehabilitation of infrastructure, the provision of medical equipment or supplies, or support and training for hospital staff in any field of expertise.

It must be emphasized that all of the essential elements are interdependent, and that systems put in place must be sustainable. Sophisticated surgery is unsustainable without corresponding expertise in nursing. Any rehabilitation of infrastructure must be accompanied by a sustainable program of regular maintenance. Supplies provided should match those that can be afforded and supplied in the longer term.

Sensitivity to different cultures is vital; systems of hospital and patient management that work well in western developed societies do not always transfer automatically into other cultures and should not be introduced without discussion and agreement with all concerned.

Be aware that assistance to hospitals in resource-limited situations may prove to be an expensive and require long-term commitment, especially with training programs.

In the absence of any functioning structure, setting up a new hospital may have to be considered. "Field hospitals" may serve a purpose in the short term to address a specific problem with a limited duration, but often develop into longer-term projects and do little to develop local capacity. A separate hospital with the specific task of treating weapon wounded may serve to relieve the existing health system of the additional burden of these patients, but setting up parallel systems of health-care needs very careful considera-tion. One of the most important consequences of this may be a "brain drain" of the better trained and experienced health professionals who will be attracted by higher salaries and better working conditions offered by the organization setting up the hospital; this should be avoided at all costs.

Whatever type of assistance is planned, the personnel selected to imple-ment the assistance must be experienced professionals able to apply prin-ciples of good, safe care without dependence on sophisticated equipment and systems and recognize that training will inevitably be a large part of their workload. They should also be able to communicate well, be flexible enough to adapt to different cultures and changing situations, and able to work as part of a team. A large dose of common sense and a sense of humor are distinct advantages.

References

1. *Global Burden of Disease Estimates*. Geneva: World Health Organization; 2000.
2. Machel G. Impact of armed conflict on children. Report of Graca Machel, expert of the Secretary General, August 26, 1996.
3. Hayward-Karisson J, Jeffery S, Kem A, Schmidt H. *Hospitals for War Wounded*. Geneva: International Committee of the Red Cross; 1998.
4. *The Hospital in Rural and Urban Districts*. Report of a WHO Study Group on the Functions of Hospitals at First Referral Levels. Geneva: World Health Orga-nization; 1992. Members of the study group were Dr MEK. Adibo, Prof. Awad Mohamed Ahmed, Prof. JH. Brynat, Miss M. Cheeseborough, Dr Karjadi Wirjoamodjo, Dr NA. Kimathi, Ms O. Nastalkova, Prof. PES. Palmer, Dr O. Periquet, Prof. A. Velez-Gil.
5. Authors of "Surgery for Victims of War"—Bertrancourt B, Dufour D, Kromann Jensen S, Friberg O, Lounavaara A, Owen-Smith M, Salmela J, Silvonen E, Stening GF, Zetterström B. First edition edited by D. Dufour, Second edition edited by R. Gray, Third edition revised and edited by Asa Molde MD. *Surgery for Victims of War*. 3rd ed. Geneva: International Committee off the Red Cross; 1998.
6. International Committee of the Red Cross and International Federation of Red Cross and Red Crescent Societies. Emergency Items Catalogue 2002. Available at: http:ww.icrc.org and http://www.ifrc.org. Accessed.

Further Reading

There are a number of useful sources of information on which to base an assess-ment of the health system. The World Health Organization offers a range of documents and guidelines on health systems and specific country health data on their website (http://www.who.int), as does the World Bank (http://www.worldbank.org).

26
Triage

ADRIAAN HOPPERUS BUMA and WALTER HENNY

Introduction

Traditionally, *triage* refers to a situation in which a medical system receives large numbers of casualties over a short period of time and is in danger of getting overwhelmed. This context originates from military and disaster medicine: the "most experienced surgeon" was supposed to sort the casualties into priority groups, deciding at what stage they should receive operative care.

Over the years, the term triage gradually developed to setting priorities repetitively from the point of wounding until the final treatment.

Nowadays, triage is performed whenever there is a discrepancy between the number of casualties and the available medical assets. Triaging is the sorting of patients into priority groups with the aim to do the best for most. It should be understood that the principles of triage apply to both military and civilian circumstances.

Given its repetitive character, any medical worker (medics, ambulance personnel, nurses, and doctors) can be called upon to perform triage. Triaging requires training; it is not something that can be done spontaneously. Although the technical aspect is not too difficult to master, it should be realized that triage has a considerable emotional impact. The process seems to go against the grain because the most serious casualty is not always cared for first. Recently, the word triage has been used increasingly to describe a method for managing every-day flow of patients in emergency departments. The latter is not the subject for this chapter. It starts with a historical overview, which is followed by an explanation about the different triage techniques.

Historical Overview

Situations in which medical personnel have been confronted with overwhelming numbers of casualties are from all ages. An important example is the horrible experience for Henri Dunant after the battle of Solferino in

1859, where he saw thousands of casualties on the battlefield with minimal resources available. This event led to the start of the International Red Cross Organization.

The French military surgeon Larrey, who served under Napoleon in the early nineteenth century, is attributed with the introduction of triage as a technique to do the best for most. Based on his vast surgical experience, he sorted the casualties into priority groups for treatment. Interestingly, he treated the lightly wounded first because they were the most likely to survive. Triage relates to the French word *trier*, meaning to sort or to sift.

Initially, the process was predominantly based on the expected outcome of surgical treatment. Later, due to a better understanding of pathophysiology, triage shifted towards a method aiming at improved survival, taking into account physiological parameters such as heart rate, perfusion, and mental status. Furthermore, it became obvious that triage should be an ongoing process from the point of wounding until the final treatment. Additional factors, such as survivability, type of injury, and distance (time) of evacuation, are also considered. Although triage has been adapted over the years, the aim has remained the same: to do the most for the most. Triage has become a well-known technique for all medical personnel involved in disaster and military medicine.

The Techniques of Triage

Triage Systems

Many systems for triage have been developed over the years, with the obvious disadvantage that different people working in the same medical chain may use different systems; this will lead to confusion. The differences may consist of different definitions of triage categories and/or different criteria attached to each category. It is impossible to describe "everything that's on the market," but a strong plea should be made for national and international standardization. An effective triage system should enable the person performing triage to expeditiously define the casualties' condition. At present, systems using physiological parameters seem to be better suited than systems using anatomical descriptions.

Two triage systems have received much attention. The P (priority) system is to be used in situations in which each casualty is expected to receive all necessary treatment. It defines 3 categories: P1(immediate), P2 (urgent), and P3 (delayed).

P1 casualties need instant treatment because of "ABC" instabilities.
P2 casualties are ABC stable, but they need surgical treatment as expeditiously as possible.

Treatment of P3 casualties, who are always ABC stable, can be deferred for a longer time if necessary.

The T (triage) system is to be used in mass casualty situations. It defines 4 categories: the first three categories are basically identical to the P groups, but a fourth group ("expectant") encompasses casualties "who are not expected to survive." The latter is politically very sensitive.

Within the P system, a further subgroup ("P1 Hold") has come into use (which is basically the same as T4).

The text below has been written "from a military perspective"; on closer inspection, it will become obvious that, as far as triage is concerned, there are many similarities between the military and civilian arenas.

Considerations

Triage is usually thought to be a consequence of situations in which there are multiple casualties. It becomes operational as soon as there is a mismatch between demand for and availability of care. Furthermore, it is a dynamic process that is to be repeated at all instances when choices have to be made; for example, who will be transported first, who can withstand postponement of surgical treatment etc., *depending on the casualties' condition amongst others.*

It is also possible that triage should not be performed, that is, when the environment is too dangerous: being under fire, obvious threat of explosions, etc. The best approach then is to get out or to get the upper hand.

There is a strong relationship between triage and treatment (or lack thereof); the assigned triage category directs the desired treatment (which may or may not be then performed, depending on extraneous factors) and the treatment given also influences subsequent triage decisions.

The more experienced the triaging person is, the more they may use intangible factors to decide on the casualty's triage category. The level of an individual's formal education does not necessarily equate with competence to perform triage; it is an art that can and should be learned by all medical personnel.

Effective triaging is much more than assigning casualties into categories based on physiological parameters. The person responsible for triage should also take into account issues such as:

Extraneous Factors
- location [in the field, on entering a medical treatment facility (MTF), in a preoperative holding area, after receiving medical care, etc.]
- number of casualties
- number and competencies of available medical personnel
- availability of equipment
- tactical situation (insecure; secure; MTF expected to move on short notice, etc.)
- type and availability of transportation
- transportation times

- capabilities and assets of MTFs
- required time for (operative) treatment
- salvageability of casualties

Casualty-Related Factors
- type of injury
- location of injury

Sometimes all relevant factors are known; under austere conditions, they usually are not. Sometimes decisions need to be made in seconds. Consequently, all these factors need to have been considered before triage starts. An explanation of the different triage techniques follows next.

A Tiered Approach

Considering the fact that there is a variety of circumstances in which triage may be performed, we present a tiered approach. These tiers are just an indication; the person performing triage should be able and willing to adapt triage to the actual circumstances. Generally speaking, the more austere the environment is, the quicker and simpler triage should be.

Unsafe Environment "Under Fire"

By far the best approach is "to get the upper hand or to get out."
    No triage is to be performed. Treatment should be kept to the barest minimum (stanching external hemorrhage, if possible).

No Direct Threat, But Away from Medical Facility: Small Number of Casualties Closely Together

Attention should be directed first to those casualties who are "silent." They are either dead, "unhurt," or have a real problem. The remaining casualties can then be triaged.
    During triage, intervention should be restricted to opening the airway and, if applicable, having external bleeding stanched by a "third party" (somebody who is not injured or possibly some other casualty who is still "vocal" and able to walk).
    After triage, further first aid measures should be instituted as circumstances and available assets allow.

No Direct Threat, But Away from Medical Facility: Larger Number of Casualties Dispersed

It is extremely important to obtain an overview first. Those people who are able to walk are asked to gather at an easily recognizable location. They are by definition categorized as P3. The remaining casualties are then addressed. Those who do not respond are turned into the recovery position. External bleeding is stanched, if possible, but by someone other than the person doing the triage. Those who do respond are assessed for external bleeding, which should be stanched, preferably by the casualty himself.

Only if time and circumstances allow, a second round is made in which all non-walking casualties are further triaged and treatment instituted.

Outside MTF, Aid Becoming Organized, Environment Secure

When casualties have been removed from the site of wounding or from the site of the accident and when aid is becoming organized, one person should assess all casualties (for condition). An effective method is to use the *sieve* algorithm, as depicted below. This algorithm uses simple physiological parameters and defines three categories: P1, P2, and P3. The criteria are indicated in the Figure 26-1.

Depending on the circumstances (darkness, low ambient temperature), the refill criterion for circulation may be replaced by pulse rate. A pulse rate of less than 120 per minute leads to a classification of P2; a rate of 120 per minute or higher is classified as P1. Treatment (i.e., first aid measures) is instituted as circumstances and available assets allow.

Algorithm Triage Sieve

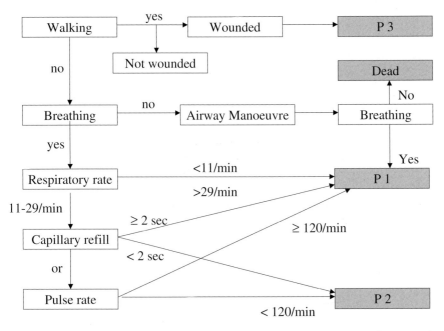

FIGURE 26-1. The algorithm triage sieve chart. BATLS manual (2nd Edn) D/AMD/113/23 Army Code No 63726 (2000). Advanced Life Support Group Major Incident Medical Management and Support (2nd Edn), London: BMJ Books; 2002 with permission.

The general principle is to have P1 casualties transported first, P2 casualties next, and finally P3 casualties. Decisions of whether or not to institute "treatment" on the spot and when to transport the casualties to which destination are also influenced by the extraneous factors, as far as they are applicable in the actual situation. For instance, if transport distance and time are short, it may be better to "scoop and run."

On Arrival at the MTF

Re-triage is performed by using the *sieve* algorithm. If the person performing triage is experienced, casualties will occasionally be assigned to a higher category than the actual physiological parameters warrant because of expected developments based on his/her experience and clinical judgement.

In case of multiple casualties arriving over a short period of time, a "P1 Hold" group may be instituted. P1 casualties are then resuscitated following the Advance Trauma Life Support (ATLS) protocol. "P1 Hold" casualties should be reviewed and resuscitated, if appropriate, as soon as all "original" P1 casualties have been treated.

Within the MTF

Further care can be either within the MTF (including operative treatment) or at some other facility. Within the facility it may be appropriate to use the methodology of the triage *sort*, as shown in Figure 26-2. This system is based on the Revised Trauma Score. It defines four categories: T1–T4. The criteria are indicated in the figure.

Those in T4 should be re-triaged as T1 as soon as all "original" T1 casualties have been treated.

The decision when to operate upon the casualty also may be influenced by the type and location of the injury. Again, only experienced personnel will be able to include these considerations in their decision-making process. The decision when and where to send the casualty (inside or outside the MTF) is also influenced by extraneous factors, as far as they are applicable in the actual situation.

Conclusions

In conclusion, triage means sorting casualties into priority groups with the aim to do the most for most. It should be performed whenever there is a discrepancy between the number of casualties and the medical assets. The technique itself is straightforward. However, it should be adapted continuously to the actual circumstances; they are often complex and therefore dictate the final outcome.

Methodology for Triage Sort based on Revised Trauma Score

Respiratory rate (breaths/min)	score
10 - 29	4
> 29	3
6 - 9	2
1- 5	1
0	0

Systolic blood pressure (mmHg)	score
> 90	4
75 - 90	3
50 - 74	2
1 - 49	1
0	0

Glasgow coma scale (EMV)	score
13 - 15	4
9 - 12	3
6 - 8	2
4 - 5	1
3	0

Scores converted to Triage Groups

Total score	Triage Group
4 - 10	T 1
11	T 2
12	T 3
1 - 3	T 4
0	Dead

FIGURE 26-2. The methodology for triage sort chart. BATLS manual (2nd Edn) D/AMD/113/23 Army Code No 63726 (2000). Advanced Life Support Group Major Incident Medical Management and Support (2nd Edn), London: BMJ Books; 2002 with permission.

Further Reading

Ryan J, Mahoney PF, Greaves I, Bowyer G. *Conflict and Catastrophe Medicine*. London: Springer-Verlag; 2002.

Driscoll P, Skinner D, Earlam R. *ABC of Major Trauma*, 3rd ed. London: BMJ Books; 2000.

Student Manual, Battlefield Advanced Trauma Life Support, 2nd ed. Ash Vale: Director General Army Medical Services; 2000.

Subcommittee on Trauma. *Manual Advanced Trauma Life Support*, 6th ed. Chicago: American College of Surgeons; 1997.

Advance Life Support Group. *Major Incident Medical Management and Support*, 2nd ed. London: BMJ Books; 2002.

Caroline NL. *Emergency Care In The Streets*, 5th ed. Boston: Little, Brown and Company; 1995.

Bellamy RF, Zajtchuk R. *Conventional Warfare: Ballistic, blast and burn injuries. Textbook of Military medicine Part 1, vol. 5.* Washington DC: WRAMC/WRAIR; 1991.

Butler FK, Hagmann J, Butler E. Tactical combat casualty care in special operations. *Milit Med.* 1996;161(Suppl. 3):3–16.

Burkle FM, Orebaugh S, Barendse BR. Emergency medicine in the Persian Gulf—Part 1: Preparations for triage and combat casualty care. *Ann Emerg Med.* 1994;23:742–747.

Burkle FM, Newland C, Orebaugh S, Blood CG. Emergency medicine in the Persian Gulf—Part 2: Triage methodology and lessons learned. *Ann Emerg Med.* 1994;23:748–754.

27
Managing Ballistic Injury in the Military Environment: The Concept of Forward Surgical Support

Donald Jenkins, Paul Dougherty, and James M. Ryan

Introduction

In this chapter, the emphasis is on surgical management in the austere environment of the battlefield. A key difference in management in the *military* environment is the need to pre-place field medical facilities providing lines or *echelons* of care.

This is in contrast to the nongovernmental organization (NGO) situation where evacuation may not be possible and all types of procedures are done in the same institution (for more detailed discussion, see Chapter 28).

Lines or Echelons of Care

The nature of war imposes unique considerations upon medical care. In short, care of the wounded in war requires constant backwards evacuation from point of wounding to medical units of increasing sophistication in rear areas.

First aid, care under fire, and tactical field care are considered in the Pre-hospital Care chapter.

Following stabilization, the casualty is evacuated to a regimental or battlegroup aid post and for the first time will come under the management of a doctor-led team in a purpose-built medical facility.

This historically is 1st Line or 1st Echelon care, but the term "Role 1" is now more commonly used (see below). The time from point of wounding to care at this level will vary with the nature of the battle, terrain, distance, and mode of evacuation—it may take minutes or hours; the objective, however, is to achieve this as fast as possible within the constraints described.

Wound care here consists of application of a sterile field dressing, if not already in place. If in place, it is not removed, as infection rates increase with each time the wound is exposed for examination.

The objective is immediate and continued control of hemorrhage, wound stabilization, and pain reduction. If bony injury is suspected, formal limb splintage, including traction splints, may be applied. As all war wounds are heavily contaminated, systemic antibiotics are commenced to delay the onset of wound infection. The choice of agent will be determined by the estimated clinical risk. In the case of the limbs, the most common infecting organisms in the initial stage are gram positive cocci and clostridial species—in upper thigh and buttock wounds, gut organisms may be present in addition.

> Antibiotics are not a replacement for correct surgical wound management.

Once stabilized, the casualty is now moved, by land or air transport to a 2nd Echelon medical facility or Role 2 medical facility.

Care at 2nd and 3rd Echelon/Role 2 & 3

Historically, care at 2nd Echelon or Role 2 consisted of further stabilization and evacuation by priority to a field surgical facility for life- and limb-saving surgery (3rd Echelon/Role 3).

This rather rigid arrangement developed in the days of static general wars. Modern war, characterized by maneuver, mobility, and blurring of forward and rear, has demanded a more flexible approach, taking resuscitative surgical capability forward to 2nd Echelon/Role 2, and even further forward in exceptional circumstances. Therefore, care at 2nd Echelon/Role 2 in modern war may include surgical intervention where there is a threat to life or limb.

Less seriously injured casualties are typically reassessed and moved rearward, which might involve evacuation to a role 3 hospital and subsequently to a role 4 in the home base or host nation.

In summary, a much more flexible approach is emerging to deal with the problems of the modern nonlinear battlefield. The basic principles of echeloned care are retained, but new terms and concepts are emerging. Note, however, that the principles underpinning the practice of war surgery have not altered.

Current Doctrine—Forward Surgery

The concept of proximity of surgical support is not new. In World War II, the formation of allied mobile tactical forces such as airborne and special forces units required the development of complementary medical support.

Surgical teams and personnel were deployed by parachute, glider, or by sea, usually alongside combat teams. Subsequent operations where surgical teams have provided close support to U.S. and U.K. forces include the Falklands war, both Gulf Wars, Afghanistan, and Sierra Leone. Each conflict and deployment has generated lessons about equipment and procedures, as have previous reviews of this subject.

Medical facilities in support of operations in modern war need to be mobile and easily deployable by air (using helicopter, fixed wing aircraft, or parachute) and by road. The equipment has to be robust and meet laid down restrictions of dimension, volume, and weight.

The same constraints apply to the equipment and supplies needed by the Surgical Teams.

This has resulted in the replacement of the terms "Lines" or "Echelons" by the term "Role (s)."

Medical facilities in the United States and British Military Medical System are classified into "roles" according to their equipment, manpower, and training:

- Role 1 is care under the direction of a doctor (such as a Regimental Aid Post),
- Role 3 provides hospital-level care,
- Role 4 is usually care provided away from the conflict, (e.g., care in Continental United States [CONUS] or the UK National Health Service [NHS] and associated military facilities).
- Role 2 provides additional care and acts as the link between Roles 1 and 3. A Role 2 facility with integral surgical teams is described in U.K. military terminology as "Role 2+." This consists of all or elements of a Medical Regiment with added Field Surgical Teams (FSTs) (Forward Surgical Teams in the USA). The terminology can become confusing as some North Atlantic Treaty Organization (NATO) forces "Role 2" units have integral surgical support as standard.

It is important to look at the basic "building blocks" of surgical care and review what can realistically be achieved at each level.

Structure of the FSTs

Personnel

An FST consists of one or more surgeons, one or more anesthetists, and a variable number of operating department practitioners (ODPs) or theater nurses. When two FSTs deploy together, this provides the option of:

- 24-hour surgical care.
- Broad surgical expertise (pairing general and orthopedic surgeons).
- Simultaneous resuscitation and anesthesia.
- An immediate medical response team while still maintaining a surgical capability.

Field Surgery 2004 & Beyond

Field surgery is not a new concept, and good outcomes have been described with very limited equipment and resources. In his report of guerrilla surgery, Goulston (see reading list) gives particular credit to the non-medical personnel who were able to administer anesthesia, assist at surgery, sterilize instruments, and provide a certain level of nursing care.

Current medical doctrine, however, aims to provide standards of care as close to peacetime standards as possible (allowing for battlefield conditions) and delivered within defined clinical timelines.

In military conflicts, the high incidence of penetrating trauma results in significant chest, head, and abdominal injuries and highly contaminated limb injuries. Early surgical intervention, particularly in those who initially survive wounds to critical areas, results in reduced mortality and morbidity.

The availability of blood is essential if forward, life-saving surgery is contemplated. During the Falklands Campaign, 600 units of blood were administered, with an average of 5 units per patient on the hospital ship Uganda. Paired UK FSTs generally deploy with 50 units.

The developing fields of damage control surgery have major implications for equipment and resources, as does Field Intensive Care (Chapters 10 and 22). The damage control surgery patient will need intensive care management postoperatively and probably during early evacuation as well. To meet these needs and the desired civilian standards is time and resource intensive. Time and resources are in short supply in the rapidly changing military environment. Reconciling these conflicting needs will be a major challenge, but essential to allow advances in the care of military patients to mirror those in the management of civilian trauma.

Surgical Management—General Principles

Adherence to stringent surgical technique and good communication are the keys to the successful use of the echelons or roles of care system for wartime surgical patients. Strict application of the surgical techniques described in earlier chapters is a safe, time-tested way to promote successful outcomes in wartime. Recent experience proves these concepts in modern warfare. Personal experience of two U.S. military surgeons at the outset of Operation Enduring Freedom's ground campaign was a wound infection rate of 0% over 48 hours using the principles of war surgery (outlined in Chapter 9). These cases included numerous open fracture cases, despite average presurgical evacuation time (wounding to surgery) of more than 10 hours. Communication includes not only providing adequate documentation of the care provided for the medical teams further down the echelons, but also

TABLE 27-1. Anatomical distribution of penetrating wounds (as a percent)

Conflict	Head & Neck	Thorax	Abdomen	Limbs	Other
World War I	17	4	2	70	7
World War II	4	8	4	75	9
Korean War	17	7	7	67	2
Vietnam War	14	7	5	74	
Northern Ireland	20	15	15	50	
Falkland Islands	16	15	10	59	
Gulf War (UK)**	6	12	11	71	(32)*
Gulf War (US)	11	8	7	56	18†
Afghanistan (US)	16	12	11	61	
Chechnya (Russia)	24	9	4	63	
Somalia	20	8	5	65	2†
Average	15	9.5	7.4	64.6	3.5

* Buttock and back wounds and multiple fragment injuries not included.
† Multiple wounds.
** 80% caused by fragments; range of hits 1–45, mean of 9.

includes keeping track of evacuation routes and times, the capability of advancing the casualty care en route, and then carefully planning the timing of and need for operations and re-operations.

Wounding Demographics and Effects in War

Just as with any medical topic, surgeons must understand the pathophysiology of war wounds in order to best care for the patient.

> The most common pattern of injury seen on a conventional battlefield is the patient with multiple small fragment wounds of the extremity. Table 27-1 illustrates this point well.

Summary

War and conflict pose unique problems when providing care for the wounded—this is all the more so when considering surgical care. Lessons, usually hard learnt, have resulted in the evolution of novel concepts, both in terms of underpinning doctrine and surgical practice.

Reading List

Bowley DMG, Barker P, Boffard KD. Damage control surgery—concepts and practice. *J R Army Med Corps*. 2000;146:176–182.

Clasper JC, Jeffrey PA, Mahoney PF. The forward deployment of surgical teams. *Curr Anaesthes Intensive Care*. 2003;14:122–125.

Gabriel RA, Metz KS. *A history of Military Medicine*, Vol II. Greenwood Press; 1992:253.

Goulston E. Guerilla surgery. *Med J Australia*. 1942;Aug 22:134–136.

Roberts MJ, Salmon JB, Sadler PJ. The provision of intensive care and high dependency care in the field. *J R Army Med Corps*. 2000;146:99–103.

28
Managing Ballistic Injury in the NGO Environment

Ari K. Leppäniemi

Introduction

There are tens of thousands of nongovernmental organizations (NGOs) operating today in most countries, with their scope varying from large, Northern-based charities to community-based self-help groups in the South. The World Bank defines NGOs as "private organizations that pursue activities to relieve suffering, promote the interests of the poor, protect the environment, provide basic social services or undertake community development." With increasing globalization, NGOs have become more influential in world affairs, and it has been estimated that over 15% of total overseas development aid are channeled through NGOs. These organizations are not directly affiliated with any national government, but often have a significant impact on the social, economic, and political activity of the country or region involved.

The most prevalent form of conflict in the post-cold war era is the occurrence of local or regional low-intensity conflicts, such as civil wars, guerrilla warfare, terrorism and counter-insurgency operations. In the 12-year post-cold war period 1990–2001, there were 57 different major armed conflicts in 45 different locations. All but three of the major conflicts were internal—the issue concerned control over the government or territory of one state. Other states contributed regular troops to one side or the other in 15 of the internal conflicts. As the historian Samuel Huntington has pointed out, communal conflicts between states or groups from different civilizations, or fault line conflicts, are likely to increase in the future. They tend to be protracted by nature, and when they are intrastate, they tend to last on average six times longer than interstate wars. Because of their protracted character, the fault line wars tend to produce a large number of casualties and refugees (see Table 28-1 for casualty figures).

With increasing erosion of nation-states, especially among the developing countries, many states are sliding into anarchy and ungovernability caused by scarcity of resources, overpopulation, refugee migration, tribal-

TABLE 28-1. Casualty figures from fault-line wars in the early 1990s

50000 in the Philippines,
50000–100000 in Sri Lanka,
20000 in Kashmir,
0.5–1.5 million in Sudan,
100000 in Tajikistan,
50000 in Croatia,
50–200000 in Bosnia,
30000–50000 in Chechnya,
100000 in Tibet,
200000 in East Timor,
The number of injured victims being multiple times higher than those killed.

ism, disease, environmental degradation, uncontrolled crime, and the empowerment of private armies, security firms, and international drug cartels.

Future wars will be associated with a large number of factors that have a major impact on the conditions of the affected people living in the conflict areas, and include population expansion, poverty, the AIDS epidemic, shortage of water and agricultural land, post-cold war availability of arms, megacities, drug trafficking (de facto governments), violent transnational groups and countries protecting them, rapid communications and travel, and recruitment of child-soldiers.

With increasing frequency of less-defined states between peace and war and risk of collapsing infrastructure, including medical facilities in the affected countries, the type of medical challenges to the local and international community is likely to involve more frequently humanitarian and peace-keeping type of missions, as well as providing surgical care for the war wounded under less-than-optimal conditions. It can be even more difficult when an internal war is combined with a total collapse of the country's infrastructure (failed states) and mass movements of people, as witnessed recently in western and central Africa. The care of the wounded under these extreme conditions has to be limited to the very basic with maximal use of the limited resources (see Triage, Chapter 26).

A major conventional war could require mobilization of surgical teams with relatively little experience in managing mass casualties (see Training, Chapter 24). This creates an enormous challenge to peacetime training of the medical personnel. In spite of recent progress of minimally invasive surgical techniques, a surgeon in a twenty-first century conflict must have the capability to adequately assess the wounded patient and perform major conventional surgery under adverse conditions with very limited resources using different techniques and approaches depending on the available resources and overall situation.

There are several organizations directly participating in the patient care of wounded civilians and soldiers in conflicts around the world, especially in developing countries. One of the best-known delivering medical care to victims of war on a large scale and with established and published management guidelines is the International Committee of the Red Cross (ICRC). Based on the mandate of the ICRC to bring protection and assistance to the victims of international and non-international armed conflicts and internal disturbances and tensions, it deploys surgical teams for the treatment of victims of armed conflicts. Surgical care is promoted by placing teams in preexisting hospitals or establishing independent ICRC surgical hospitals. First aid posts near the conflict areas usually serve these hospitals.

This review is based on published reports of surgical care from ICRC and other NGO hospitals and the personal experience of the author while working as field surgeon in an ICRC hospitals in Khao-I-Dang on the Thai–Cambodian border, in Lokichokio in northern Kenya–South Sudan and in Peshawar, Pakistan.

NGO Hospital Environment and Facilities

A health care system is one of the earliest casualties of the social and economic disruption of a country in conflict. Hospital doctors and nurses may not be able to perform their normal duties, they may not be paid or able to reach the hospital, or they might be discriminated against for working. Medical teams from humanitarian agencies who step in trying to work in these conflicts may do so in danger. There is little or no discipline among those who have the weapons, and one side of the conflict may target the agencies because they are perceived as aiding the other. With the prolongation of the conflict, the local health care facilities have little chance of reestablishing themselves, and there will be increasing demands on the NGO hospital to take care of the non-combat-related medical problems of the affected population. Occasionally, the organized management of patients is made more difficult by accompanying relatives and friends who may be armed and try to hasten treatment with threats.

The majority of NGO field hospitals can be compared with civilian hospitals, which are isolated in an area of conflict. They differ from typical military hospitals because they are not a part of echeloned care, but work, at the same time, as hospitals of first contact and referral hospitals, implying that both primary surgery, secondary surgery, and basic reconstructive

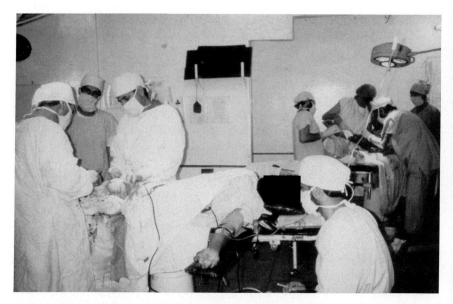

FIGURE 28-1. Operation room in the ICRC hospital in Peshawar, Pakistan, with two teams working parallel performing acute and planned surgery, respectively.

surgery are conducted in the same hospital (Figure 28-1). This poses great challenges to personnel working under these conditions because they must have broad knowledge and experience in all areas of surgical care, including wound surgery, amputations, fracture management, craniotomies, thoracotomies, vascular procedures, laparotomies, management of burns, and basic plastic surgical techniques.

Although there is great variation in the level of equipment, most NGO-run hospitals have limited availability of blood, no ventilatory equipment, minimal laboratory services, and only plain radiography. Because of the limitations and special conditions in these field hospitals, the planning of surgery is of utmost importance, and the restrictions encourage the use of simple methods of treatment and improvisation to provide adequate care. In addition, the geographical, climatic, cultural, and social environment imposes limitations and constraints, making adaptation to the environment essential. Local skills and materials should be used as much as possible. Sanitation and nutrition should be adapted to local needs and customs. The effects of endemic diseases such as malaria should be taken into account, especially in the early postoperative phase in a febrile patient. And finally, the surgical treatment should be conducted with the aim of minimizing blood loss and the need for blood transfusions, as well as optimizing the chances of postoperative recovery without the facilities for intensive care, total parenteral nutrition, and use of sophisticated and expensive medication.[1,2]

Patient Characteristics in an NGO Hospital

A large number of wounded patients brought to an NGO field hospital are civilians, defined as women and girls, boys (under 16 years of age), and men of 50 or more. Of the 18877 patients injured by bullets, bombs, shells, mortars, or mines and admitted to ICRC hospitals in 1991 through 1998, about 28% were civilians. The proportion of civilians injured by fragments and mines is larger than those injured by bullets, most probably because weapons that fragment can easily injure more than one person, and because mines remain after the conflict, both increasing the likelihood of civilian injuries. Overall, in most published reports from ICRC hospitals, fragments account for the majority of wounds, followed by bullets and mines.

Many of the wounded civilians, especially in developing countries, may not be optimal candidates for surgery because of preexisting malnutrition, chronic infections, and parasites.

The vast majority of wounded patients treated in NGO hospitals suffer from extremity injuries, with lower extremities being injured more often than upper extremities. The proportion of potentially life-threatening injuries of the head, neck, and torso is about 10 to 30%, but can be as low as five percent if there is lack of appropriate surgical attention and evacuation facilities in the field *because many of these patients die before receiving care.*

Prehospital Care

Under conditions where most NGO hospitals work, the prehospital care is poorly organized if at all. The often-chaotic conditions, collapse of infrastructure, and mass movements of population prevent or pose enormous challenges in creating a functional and adequate prehospital care system. Sometimes, when an ICRC hospital has been located inside a border of a neighboring country not participating in the conflict, first aid posts in or near the conflict areas have served the hospitals.

In most cases, patients are brought to the hospital by relatives and friends using all available means of transport. The delay from the moment of wounding can be anything from a few minutes to several days. Because it has an effect of the method of treatment, it is important to try to find out the time of injury in spite of occasional difficulties of gaining adequate information due to language problems or because the information might be politically or militarily sensitive.

Triage

In most mass casualty situations encountered in NGO hospitals, the conventional military type of triage process of categorizing patients according to the urgency of treatment can be applied.

Sometimes, however, the extent of work requires modification of the conventional approach, as described by Robin Coupland while working in ICRC hospital in Kabul, Afghanistan in 1992.[3]*

I was a team surgeon in one of four teams when we received roughly 600 new casualties over a period of six days. Most were civilians from the vicinity of the hospital. About 250 with small soft tissue wounds were sent home with antibiotic tablets after having received tetanus prophylaxis. They had instructions to return if they developed problems; few did. This was in keeping with a non-operative policy for small soft tissue wounds, but the extreme circumstances did not allow the patients to remain in hospital for observation. We were able to admit all patients with larger wounds to dress the wound and give fluids intravenously, benzylpenicillin, tetanus prophylaxis, and analgesia. Owing to fatigue and the proximity of the battle we were able to operate only for some hours each day and those with abdominal wounds had priority. The perioperative mortality was high. Those who were rushed into the operating theatre because of the severity of their wounds usually died during or soon after surgery because the admission procedure had become so disrupted that many arrived on the operating table having received insufficient intravenous fluid replacement. After surgery more died through lack of postoperative supervision. Much valuable surgical time and energy was wasted. The patients with abdominal wounds who survived were those who required laparotomy for perforation and not for bleeding. The few patients admitted with thoracic wounds whose condition was not stabilised by fluid resuscitation and chest drainage died before they could reach the operating theatre. Most patients with severe wounds of the limbs that required amputation or wound excision had to wait three or four days for their surgery; only those with massive multiple wounds died in the meantime.

Based on this experience in Kabul, three lessons were learned:[3]*

1. Intravenous fluids and antibiotics buy time for most patients.
2. Patients with severe life threatening injuries die despite treatment unless resources, the number of nursing staff, and the organization of the hospital infrastructure are adequate.
3. When the hospital infrastructure is disrupted, surgical resources are easily wasted by operating on patients whose prognosis is hopeless—underlining the importance of realistic triage for treatment—and the death rate is unacceptably high among those who should survive.

Thus, under extreme conditions, the traditional approach to triage and major surgical intervention can be challenged by an epidemiological

---

* From reference 3, page 1693, with permission.

approach, where less emphasis is placed on the more spectacular aspects of surgical care that benefit only a few, in favor of some effective care reaching many more with emphasis on adequate first aid and delayed surgery directed at casualties who would die of infective complications if surgery was not performed.

Airway protection, fluid resuscitation, arrest of accessible hemorrhage, and tube thoracostomy could prevent early deaths. Later deaths could be avoided by prevention of infective complications with antibiotics, wound excision, correct amputation, and laparotomy for perforation alone.

Surgery in an NGO Hospital

General Comments

The majority of surgical procedures carried out for wounded patients in NGO hospitals include wound surgery in different stages, amputations, and treatment of open fractures and abdominal surgery. Table 28-2 lists surgical procedures performed in one ICRC hospital.

In most cases, a NGO hospital is the sole provider of surgical care in the conflict area with no possibility of transferring patients to better-equipped hospitals for secondary surgical procedures, such as reconstructive plastic surgical procedures or correction of badly healed fractures. In addition, the local conditions to which patients return after being discharged may be challenging in terms of access to rehabilitation, prosthetic equipment, and disposable items, such as urine bags, colostomy equipment, and even gauze material. Finally, the social security network and means of surviving economically after a bilateral lower extremity amputation, for example, can in some societies and under times of conflict be almost non existent. All these

TABLE 28-2. Surgical procedures performed by a New Zealand Red Cross surgical team in the ICRC hospital in Kabul during a six month period in 1990 ($n = 1017$)

Debridement	240
Wound revision	364
Delayed primary closure	145
Split skin graft, flaps	30
Amputation	37
External fixation	31
Steinman pins	16
Laparotomy	70
Closure of colostomy	10
Hemothorax	26
Craniotomy	24
Maxillofacial, eyes	14
Vascular	8
Laminectomy	2

factors have to be considered when surgical intervention is performed for victims of armed conflicts in a NGO environment, and the surgical procedure chosen must be the most appropriate for that patient under those circumstances.

Damage Control

Successful damage control surgical approach requires access to adequate postoperative care facilities with expertise and equipment for invasive and aggressive hemodynamic monitoring, ventilatory management, correction of coagulation factors, and other procedures usually performed in a well-equipped intensive care unit (ICU). On most occasions, the NGO environment does not have the resources to establish an effective ICU, which would make a traditional damage control approach for patients with severe physiological derangement undergoing just the necessary procedure to stop hemorrhage and control contamination inappropriate. As discussed above in the triage section, most of the severely ill patients treated under extreme conditions die anyway, stressing the importance of adequate triage, concentrating the use of scarce resources to patients with a reasonable chance of survival under those conditions.

Diagnostic Equipment

Under the most primitive conditions, physical examination is the only available method of assessing the patient after appropriate history from the patient or accompanying persons. In most NGO hospitals, however, basic laboratory and radiological equipment for plain X-rays are available, although the reading of the X-ray results has to be carried out by the clinician without the support of a trained radiologist. Occasionally, simple surgical procedures, such as diagnostic peritoneal lavage with macroscopic assessment of the lavage fluid, can be performed to aid decision making.

Antibiotics

All war wounds are contaminated with bacteria and eventually will become infected. Although non-surgical treatment might be appropriate in some cases, antibiotics are not an alternative to proper wound surgery in grossly contaminated or old wounds in the presence of dead tissue because gas gangrene and tetanus are real threats in patients with inadequately managed wounds. Nevertheless, antibiotic prophylaxis with penicillin and adequate measures for tetanus prophylaxis should always accompany the surgical management of war wounds.

In patients with head wounds, penicillin should be combined with another antibiotic that, in resource-limited situations, could be chlorampenicol or trimethoprim-sulphametoxazole.

Bowel injuries are very common in penetrating abdominal war wounds, and a sufficiently broad-spectrum antibiotic with activity against anaerobic bacteria or an additional antibiotic with such activity should be given as early as possible to all abdominal casualties. A cephalosporin–metronidazole combination would probably be most effective, but with limited financial and logistical resources, other cheaper antibiotics such as crystalline penicillin or chloramphenicol could be well justified.

Anesthesia

A range of anesthetic methods can be used for surgery of war wounds, and the method of choice depends on many variables, including the available expertise, equipment and drugs, circumstances, urgency, and postoperative monitoring capabilities. A trained anesthesiologist is an integral part of most NGO hospital teams, but occasionally the surgeon has to be his own anesthetist, using methods that are familiar, safe, and applicable in conditions where the surgeon is operating and can not dedicate his full time to monitor the anesthesia.

Anesthetic methods that can be administered with relative safety by doctors not formally trained in anesthesia, but with some previous practical experience, include topical anesthesia (eyes, mucosal surfaces), local infiltration anesthesia, digital and axillary nerve blocks, spinal or epidural anesthesia, and ketamine anesthesia with spontaneous ventilation.

Blood Transfusions

Frequently, during war, the requirement to produce large quantities of blood often exceeds the ability to collect, prepare, and distribute sufficient quantities of donated blood. This is even truer in the NGO environment, where blood products are seldom available in large quantities. In a study of the use of blood products in ICRC hospitals, the average units per patient transfused were 2.9. The quantity of blood required for every 100 patients was 44.9 units. The low consumption of blood is probably related to long evacuation times, the availability of blood, and the strict ICRC criteria for transfusion.

Until oxygen-carrying blood substitutes are added to the everyday use in civilian hospitals and would be logistically and economically manageable under field conditions, there will be a constant shortage of blood products available to surgeons working in field hospitals. With appropriately measured surgical interventions, strict indications for blood transfusions, and meticulous attention to surgical technique to reduce blood loss, the blood transfusion requirements can be kept as low as possible and save the available blood for those benefiting most from it.

Surgical Management

The principles of management of war wounds in NGO hospitals differ little from the general guidelines followed in regular military hospitals and will not be reviewed here in detail. The basic principles of wound excision, delayed primary closure, external fixation of fractures, etc. apply to most NGO conditions as well. There are, however, some adjustments required in managing ballistic trauma in a typical NGO hospital and environment; these will be emphasized below.

In addition to the previously mentioned lack of echeloned care and possibility of transferring patients to receive secondary surgical treatment in better-resourced facilities, the most typical feature is the common encounter of old (days, or even weeks) or neglected wounds. Their surgical management must be flexible to take into account the wound changes this delay produces. The wound may require more aggressive surgery because of putrefaction or gangrene. Alternatively, the wound assessment may reveal that the wound has started to heal and so a less-aggressive surgical approach may be taken. Intraoperative blood loss when excising an old wound may be great because the surgeon is working through edematous and inflamed tissue, and it can be difficult to identify viable muscle and vital anatomic structures under these circumstances.[4]

Under some conditions, another characteristic of an NGO hospital environment is the admission of patients who have had a front-line treatment by local providers, including suturing of wounds, splinting of fractures, or even a front-line laparotomy. These patients sometimes arrive with pus, feces, urine, or bile leaking from wounds, incisions, or drain sites. After rehydration, antibiotics, and correction of anemia, a second operation might reveal grossly infected tissues, and in case of a relaparotomy, missed perforations, leaking anastomoses or repairs, and retained surgical compresses.

Wound Surgery

The majority of wound surgery is performed on limbs, and the application of a pneumatic tourniquet before the removal of field dressing can be helpful in initial surgery of the distal limb wounds to minimize blood loss and create a bloodless operative field, especially in patients with traumatic amputations.

Longitudinal skin incisions are usually most appropriate in extremity wounds and the surgical wound should always be larger than the initial wound, although as little skin as possible is removed. After managing the skin lesion, the wound is thoroughly exposed and debrided layer by layer by dissecting individual muscles and tendons bluntly and excising their damaged parts until healthy tissue is encountered. When a muscle group is injured, only those individual muscles that are partially divided are visible in the wound. Those muscles, completely transected, contract away from the wound. Their devitalized ends must be exposed by adequate skin incisions and dissection to achieve complete removal of dead muscle tissue. With through-and-through wounds, the skin incisions and dissection are based on both entry and exit wounds and, if possible, should meet.

Those foreign materials that could cause severe infection, such as mud, pieces of shoe, or cloth, must be meticulously removed. When the wound includes a fracture, that part of the bone must be exposed. Small and un-attached bone fragments are removed and curettage is performed to remove exposed medullary bone back to firm marrow.

The fascial compartments, especially below the knee, are prone to the compartment syndrome (Figure 28-2), and the surgeon should be prepared to perform an open fasciotomy at the time of wound excision, if needed.

After securing hemostasis with sutures and other surgical means, the wound is liberally washed with saline and then left open by packing it not too tightly with dry gauze in sufficient quantities so that blood and serum will be taken up. Gauze moistened with normal saline can be applied over exposed joints and tendons.

Exceptions to the delayed primary closure method include wounds of the face, scalp, dura, joint capsules, and serous cavities, which are closed at initial wound surgery.

After wound excision the operative dressing is left for 4 or 5 days and removed in the operating theater with the patient under general anesthesia. The state of the dressings is no indicator of the state of the wound, especially in a field hospital in a hot country. If the muscle adheres to the adjacent gauze and contracts away as the dressing is gently peeled off—

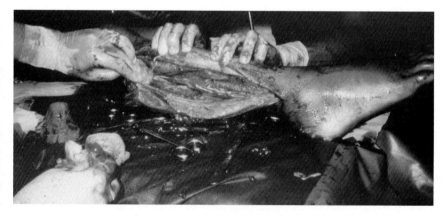

FIGURE 28-2. Compartment syndrome following a gunshot wound of the leg with necrotic muscle being excised from all compartments (ICRC hospital in Khao-I-Dang, Thailand).

sometimes with the help of saline irrigation—and the wound is clean with a reddish healthy surface, the wound excision has been adequate and it can be closed without tension using appropriately placed interrupted sutures (Figure 28-3). A large wound may require split skin grafting, which usually requires a longer period before the graft will be accepted.

If the patient's general condition is not improving after initial surgery, if there is temperature, excessive pain, and purulent discharge to the dressings, the wound requires reassessment in the theater and removal of remaining dead tissue, followed by open treatment with gauze dressings.

If the wound fails to heal after several days or even weeks, or if there is visible bone, more soft tissue usually has to be removed. A degree of healing will have occurred around the wound, which remains a cavity containing nonviable tissue, bone fragments, or protruding ends of fractured long bones. The treatment includes reincising of the skin, curettage of the cavity, and excision of the dead bone ends. When reexcision is complete, digital examination confirms a smooth cavity free of bone ends and fragments, and it will slowly heal by secondary intention, and ultimately callus will form across it.[4]

Amputations

Irreparable damage to the soft tissues or arteries of the extremities and significant bone loss are usually best treated with amputation with the primary intention of saving life by preventing infection and gas gangrene. Antipersonnel mines are, by design, intended to disable rather than kill, and the victim receives a typical pattern of injuries in which the foot, which triggers the weapon, is blown off, mud or earth, fragments of mine, shoe, or foot are blown up into genitals, buttocks, the contralateral arm and leg. When the lower tibia is shattered by explosive injury, there is considerable proximal soft tissue damage, with the muscles of the anterior, lateral, and deep anterior fascial compartments being severely contused and contaminated.

Preservation of a functional knee joint is of paramount importance for the rehabilitation of lower limb amputees, even more so in developing countries where resources are limited for the manufacturing and maintenance of prosthesis. The level of amputation is determined by the extent of the original injury, but if a below-knee amputation stump becomes severely infected postoperatively, the consequence will often be an above-knee amputation, which is much more devastating.

Depending on the level of traumatic amputation and the degree of the soft tissue damage, the surgical amputation may resemble a thorough excision of the original wound or a formal amputation with planned skin and muscle flaps. Guillotine amputations should be avoided. With the help of a pneumatic tourniquet in the proximal limb, only damaged skin is removed and devitalized and contaminated muscle is excised. The optimal lengths of amputations are:[1]

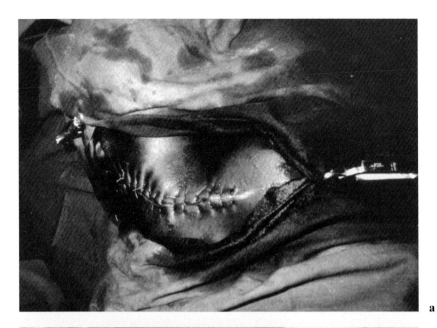

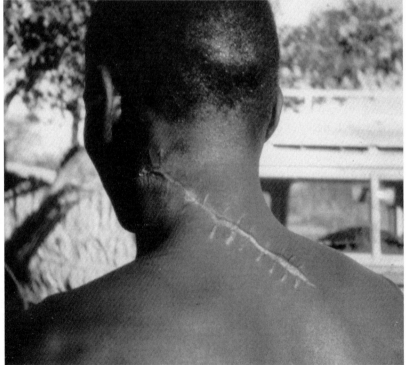

FIGURE 28-3. High-energy gunshot wound through the neck treated with wound excision, followed by delayed primary closure five days later (a) and seen at two months (b) (Lokichokio, Kenya).

- tibia: 12 to 14 centimeters from the tibial tuberosity (minimum five centimeters);
- femur: 25 to 28 centimeters from the top of the great trochanter (minimum 10 centimeters);
- arm: six to eight centimeters above the elbow (minimum 2.5 centimeters of ulna beyond the anterior axillary fold);
- forearm: six to eight centimeters above the wrist (minimum 2.5 centimeters of ulna beyond the prominence of the biceps tendon when the elbow is flexed).

It is rare to be able to perform a below-knee amputation with a long posterior myocutaneous flap, and equal skin flaps are usually the sole option. After transfixing the principal vessels with sutures, hemostasis must be secured after release of the tourniquet.

The amputation stump is left open and delayed closure is performed after four to six days. Because of the retraction of the skin and swelling of the muscle, the stump might need trimming before closure can be achieved. A suction drain can be placed under the skin flaps during delayed closure.

In an analysis of 111 below-knee amputations performed mostly for mine injuries in the ICRC hospital in Peshawar, Pakistan in 1989, the closure was performed after an average of 6.4 days, with re-amputation above the knee being required in only one case due to wound sepsis. The best results were obtained when the stump closure was performed within one week after the amputation. Overall, 84% of the stumps healed without problems, and there were no patients with gas gangrene or tetanus.

Fractures and Vascular Injuries of the Extremities

A wound with bone injury is treated with the same principles as any other ballistic wound, with careful removal of devitalized tissues including bone fragments. Fractures can be stabilized with skeletal traction, plasters, or external fixation, and the wounds are left open for delayed primary closure.

The optimal method of fracture stabilization depends on the circumstances, available equipment, surgical expertise, type and location of the fracture, degree of soft tissue injuries, and the presence of associated injuries. In general, external fixation is preferred in long bone fractures with large soft tissue injuries in adults, traction can be used with children, and plaster in cases with less degree of soft tissue injury.

In analysis of more than 200 high-velocity missile injuries treated in ICRC hospitals in Afghanistan and northern Kenya, the conclusion was that in an environment where facilities are limited and surgeons have only general experience, very careful initial wound excision is the most important factor determining outcome. Femoral fractures were treated either by traction or external fixation with identical positional outcome in both groups, but the patients treated with external fixation remained in the hospital longer than those treated with traction. In tibial fractures, the external fixator was only of extra benefit in those of the lower third when compared with simple plaster slabs, unless more-complex procedures such as flaps or vascular repair were to be performed. In complex humeral fractures, external fixation resulted in long stays in the hospital and a large number of interventions when compared with simple treatment in a sling.[5]

Because of the limited diagnostic equipment in most NGO hospitals, the diagnosis of extremity vascular injuries is based on a high index of suspicion, location of the missile track, local signs of major hemorrhage, and careful assessment of the circulatory status of the injured limb. If distal pulses remain absent after adequate fluid resuscitation, or if other signs indicating major vessel damage are present, rapid surgical exploration at the injury site for possible vascular injury is warranted. In addition to arterial transection or laceration, a possible arterial contusion has to be recognized and repaired early. Occasionally, a major vascular injury is presented as a false aneurysm or arterio-venous fistula.

The repair of vascular injuries is performed according to the established principles described elsewhere. In general, direct repair is preferred in small lacerations, but narrowing has to be avoided or prevented by using a vein patch. End-to-end anastomoses should be reconstructed without tension. Large segment damage of a major artery requires repair with a saphenous vein graft. Before completing any arterial repair, free forward bleeding and adequate back flow from the distal segment has to be established, and, if needed, distal embolectomy performed with a Fogarty balloon catheter. A repaired artery should be flushed with heparinized saline (5000 international units per 100 milliliters of saline) injected into the distal arterial tree, but no heparin should be given after operation. Injuries to major concomitant veins should be repaired if possible. All vascular repairs should be covered with viable muscle, although the wound itself is left open. Stabilization of associated fractures should not create tension to a vascular anastomosis.

Under circumstances with long evacuation times, vascular repair is not always possible and appropriate, and an amputation to save life over limb can be a better option. Among 23 consecutive patients with combat wounds from the Afghan conflict treated at the ICRC hospital in Peshawar, the mean delay from injury to treatment was 34 hours. The overall amputation rate was 65%, but only 22% for patients revascularized within 12 hours from injury in contrast to the 93% amputation rate in patients undergoing surgery more than 12 hours after injury.

Abdominal Injuries

The proportion of external war wounds located in the anterior abdomen, flanks, and back is 10 to 20%, and the proportion of casualties with abdominal injuries is 11 to 14%. Small bowel, colon, and the liver are the most commonly injured organs. The ICRC wound database carries basic information of more than 25000 war-wounded persons admitted to ICRC hospitals in different locations. Of the 7479 patients with sufficient data, 15% had abdominal wounds, and eight percent had wounds of the buttocks or pelvis. Of these, 335 had only abdominal wounds and 195 had only pelvic wounds. Of these 530 wounds, 257 (49%) did not penetrate the peritoneum or cause abdominal organ injury.

In the NGO environment, a substantial number of patients with abdominal injuries may arrive relatively late, even days after the injury. Among the 70 patients undergoing laparotomy for abdominal trauma in the ICRC hospital in Kabul from 1989 to 1990, 48 patients arrived within 12 hours from injury, and the remaining 22 arrived one to four days later.

The value of mandatory laparotomy for all abdominal casualties can be questioned when some of the patients arrive several days after injury, resulting in natural triage with the more severely injured unlikely to reach the hospital alive. Among 17 patients with abdominal injuries treated at the ICRC hospital in Quetta in 1985, 12 were managed operatively, most of them suffering from intestinal perforations and operated on within 48 hours from the injury. In five patients (29%), penetrating foreign bodies could be demonstrated radiologically to be intraperitoneal. As these injuries were several days old and the patients had no clinical signs of continuous bleeding or infection, they were managed nonoperatively with good results.

Experience from another ICRC hospital at the Thai–Cambodian border showed that when the influx of wounded overwhelms the capacity for timely surgical management of all patients, those with severe injuries and little chance of survival, such as severe thoracoabdominal injuries requiring thoracolaparotomy (Figure 28-4) should not have priority unless several surgical teams are available and one team can be sequestered for several hours in an attempt to save some of these patients.

It is of note, however, that even under the most primitive circumstances such as described by De Wind from an Ugandan mission hospital, good results can be achieved with determined efforts. Out of 19 patients with penetrating abdominal and/or thoracic injuries, only two patients (11%) died; one from irreversible shock due to extensive blood loss and the other from multiple intestinal perforations and extensive contamination leading to death on the operating table.

In summarizing his extensive experience from treating abdominal war wounds in ten ICRC hospitals, Robin Coupland concluded:

(a) assuming competent surgical care, energy transfer from the missile to tissue is the most important factor determining the mortality associated with abdominal war wounds,

(b) outside a conventional military context, the focus of surgical resource and competence should always be on the majority with intestinal perforation only, who need surgery to save life but not necessarily on an urgent basis and who have a good chance of survival,

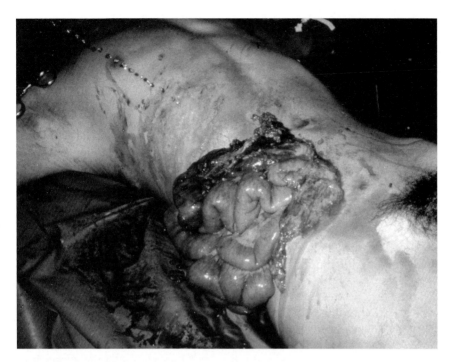

FIGURE 28-4. A soldier with multiple intrathoracic and intra-abdominal organ injuries (after detonating a mine with a jeep), exsanguinating on the operating table (Khao-I-Dang, Thailand).

(c) in modern wars, civilian casualties predominate and military forces are likely to be used in a United Nations context, and the wounded cannot travel along a conventional chain of evacuation, and

(d) a surgeon receiving wounded who have had a front-line laparotomy where the level of surgical competence or ethics is in doubt, should consider a routine second-look laparotomy to prevent death for those who have been subjected to an incompetent laparotomy and who have not yet become seriously ill through prolonged sepsis.[6]

A midline laparotomy incision is widely used due to its speed, wide exposure, and flexibility. The general conduct of trauma laparotomy depends on the surgeon's experience and preferences and should always be conducted with the time factor and overall triage situation in mind. Upon entry into the abdomen, all four quadrants should be rapidly packed to control bleeding. The importance of reducing blood loss and the need of blood transfusions while working under austere conditions can not be overemphasized. After packing, all four quadrants should be rapidly inspected for ongoing major hemorrhage. Once all major sites of hemorrhage have been identified, they should be controlled. Bleeding from venous injuries, which can initially be overlooked, can usually be controlled by packing, allowing time for volume restoration. This is also true of many arterial injuries and injuries of the liver.

After controlling major hemorrhage, gross contamination from hollow viscus injury is prevented by closing bowel injuries temporarily with clamps or sutures. Careful inspection of the small bowel and the colon, including mobilization of the retroperitoneal portions of the colon, should be performed.

After major bleeding and gross contamination have been taken care of, the abdomen can be examined in greater detail one quadrant at a time, not forgetting the lesser sac and rectum. All injured organs are repaired and the abdominal cavity is irrigated with warm saline and closed with a single-layer mass closure. Skin is closed separately; grossly contaminated skin incision wounds should be left open (see Chapter 10 and Chapter 14).

The techniques of individual organ repair are summarized below. Under field conditions, simple, quick, reliable, and established war surgical methods of organ repair should be applied. The majority of patients have multiple gastrointestinal tract perforations and relatively minor (non-bleeding) liver injuries. Among 70 patients undergoing laparotomy for abdominal trauma in the ICRC hospital in Kabul from 1989 to 1990, the most commonly injured organs were the colon and rectum (35 patients), the small bowel in 33 patients, the liver in 17 patients, and the stomach in 10 patients. There were no major vascular or pancreatic injuries.

A short list of the main principles in managing individual abdominal organ injuries in the NGO environment is presented below. Obviously, the circumstances, the skill and experience of the surgeon, and the condition of the patient have to be taken into consideration during the intraoperative decision-making process.

- liver: non-bleeding injuries need no sutures; save blood, avoid extensive procedures; careful debridement of devitalized tissue and selective hemo-static suturing or ligation of bleeders; use perihepatic tamponade for severe bleeding from multiple lacerations; use intrahepatic balloon tamponade (not suturing entry and exit holes) for bleeding through-and-through injuries; anticipate bile leak by inserting a perihepatic drain;
- extrahepatic bile ducts: cholecystectomy for gallbladder injuries; suture repair and/or T tube drainage for partial common bile duct injuries without tissue loss; in extensive common bile duct injuries Roux-en-Y hepaticojejunostomy or with less experience, a Roux-en-Y cholecystoje-junostomy or ligation of the distal common bile duct and temporary external biliary drainage with subsequent reconstruction at a later stage;
- spleen: non-bleeding injuries need no sutures; splenectomy for severe injuries; drain the splenic bed;
- stomach: two-layer suture closure; explore posterior wall; decompress with a nasogastric tube;

- duodenum: Kocher mobilization, two-layer suture closure, decompress with a nasogastro-duodenal tube with extra side holes, always insert external, periduodenal drainage; for injuries with tissue loss, Roux-en-Y duodenojejunostomy; repair of extensive injuries secured with pyloric exclusion;
- pancreas: enter lesser sac if pancreatic injury suspected, Kocher mobilization of the duodenum and head of pancreas; distal pancreatectomy with splenectomy for distal main duct injury; other injuries treated with hemostatic sutures and external drainage only;
- small bowel: suture repair in two layers; resection and primary end-to-end anastomosis in extensive injuries with multiple closely located perforations or devascularizing injury;
- intraperitoneal colon: excision of devitalized tissue and primary repair if colon wall looks healthy; otherwise colostomy, aim for colostomy closure within two to four weeks;
- rectum: suture repair (if visible without extensive mobilization) and mandatory proximal colostomy;
- kidney: hemostatic sutures; severe injuries require nephrectomy (confirm existence of contralateral normal-sized kidney);
- ureter: primary repair over stent; ureteroneocystostomy for distal injuries; nephrectomy (confirm existence of contralateral normal-sized kidney) for severe renal pelvic or proximal ureteric injuries;
- urinary bladder: two-layer suture closure with bladder decompression (transurethral or suprapubic catheter); perivesical drainage;
- urethra: primary repair if possible; otherwise suprapubic cystostomy;
- retroperitoneal hematoma and abdominal vascular injuries: explore a hematoma if expanding or large following penetrating injury; secure proximal and distal control of potentially injured vessels; repair vessel if possible, consider temporary shunting and planned re-operation or packing if impossible; second-look laparotomy if intestinal ischemia risk after repair;
- diaphragm: closure in two layers with nonabsorbable sutures; treat pneumothorax.

In order to outline the most common procedures and the every day conditions in managing abdominal injuries in the NGO environment, some published reports from ICRC hospitals are summarized herein:

Of 17 patients with liver injuries treated in the ICRC hospital in Kabul, five required no surgical intervention, seven were managed with debridement and suture, and three by debridement and omental pack. Two patients exsanguinated during operation from extensive parenchymal disruption. Morris and Sugrue managed 33 small bowel and mesenteric injuries in the ICRC hospital in Kabul with suture repair, resection of the involved segment, and primary anastomosis, or combination of these two procedures without any complications.

Of 29 patients with colon injuries treated in the ICRC hospital in Kabul from 1989 to 1990, primary suture repair or resection and primary anastomosis was performed in 16 cases, including four transverse and five left-sided colon injuries, with no mortality, no abscesses, and no fistulas. A series from the ICRC hospital in Kabul during 1990 through 1992 reported 73 patients with colon injuries, of which all underwent primary repair (resection and anastomosis in 52 and suture repair in 21) with an overall mortality rate of six percent. One patient had a fecal fistula treated conservatively and one colostomy was performed as a precaution in a patient undergoing relaparotomy for intra-abdominal abscess.

Of five patients with renal injuries treated at the ICRC hospital in Kabul from 1989 to 90, four were managed conservatively and one with a lower pole partial nephrectomy. In the ICRC hospital in Kabul, one patient with a posterior urethral injury was treated with railroading catheters, leaving urethral and suprapubic catheters in place, suturing down the prostate to the perineum, and paravesical drainage.

In the ICRC hospital in Kabul, Morris and Sugrue successfully managed three patients with injuries to the inferior mesenteric vessels by ligation, whereas two patients with injuries of the portal vein and iliac artery and vein, respectively, died.

Thoracic Injuries

More than 90% of all chest injuries can be managed initially by conservative measures, including chest tubes, without thoracotomy. A properly placed chest tube is life saving and should be inserted as soon as possible. Indications for thoracotomy include massive bleeding, persistent bleeding or air leak, mediastinal injury, and major defect in the chest wall.

Entrance and exit wounds of the chest wall are excised, intercostal vascular bleeding is treated with suture ligation, and the pleura and deep muscle layer are closed to ensure an airtight seal, leaving the outer layers open for delayed primary closure.

In thoracoabdominal injuries, separate incisions should be used when possible. A chest tube should be inserted routinely in all thoracoabdominal wounds, especially those requiring laparotomy.[1]

Head and Neck Injuries

A large part of penetrating ballistic head injuries are fatal, but at times low-energy bullets or fragments, especially if tangential or in the frontal lobe of the brain, can cause injuries that are not immediately fatal. The aims of surgical treatment in these injuries include evacuation of intracranial hematomas, debridement of dead brain tissue, and closure of the wounds to prevent infection.

A burr hole is placed close to the bone defect and the craniectomy is performed by enlarging the hole towards the area of damage with bone nibblers until healthy dura around the damaged part is encountered. If not opened by the missile, the dura is opened in a stellate manner; all bone fragments, accessible foreign bodies, and dead brain tissue is debrided with careful use of forceps, low-pressure suction, and irrigation. Hemostasis is secured with accurate use of cautery and other topical hemostatic measures. Watertight closure of the dura is important. If not possible, the dural defect can be closed with a fascial graft from the temporalis muscle or fascia lata. It is important to elevate the dura with sutures to the skull to prevent the formation of hematomas compressing the brain. Large depressed bone fragments should be elevated, or if removed during craniectomy, replaced in situ. The bone should be covered with skin using rotation flaps if needed. Chloramphenicol should be added to the antibiotic treatment.

A penetrating ocular injury should be suspected in every wound around the eye and upper part of the face. Unless it is obvious that disruption of the globe is total, the possibility of salvaging the eye should be considered, and every effort should be made to get the patient to an ophthalmologist, even after delay. Although rare, the development of sympathetic ophthalmia (angry red eye or the quiet iridocyclitis) after a penetrating eye injury is a real threat under difficult circumstances and requires prompt treatment. Extensive corneoscleral lacerations with either prolapse or loss of the intraocular contents require early excision of the eye by complete evisceration of the contents of the eye (Figure 28-5).

In patients with facial wounds, establishing and securing the airway is most important, followed by control of hemorrhage (Figure 28-6). Soft tissue injuries are carefully debrided and can usually be closed primarily including approximation of the subcutaneous tissue. Fixation of fractures with wiring requires some experience, but those of the mandibula with associated soft tissue injuries are usually stabilized with external fixation.

Any penetrating neck wound deeper than the platysma requires surgical exploration, which usually is performed through an incision along the anterior border of the sternocleidomastoid muscle. Small pharyngeal or esophageal lacerations are debrided and sutured; larger injuries may require a cervical esophagostomy and closure at a later time. Small tracheal injuries can often be suture repaired, more severe injuries require a tracheostomy. In most cases, injuries to the carotid arteries require vascular repair. One-sided injuries of the internal jugular vein can be ligated.

Burns

Burns are not uncommonly encountered during conflicts. They require prompt correction of the hypovolemia, adequate pain control, and accurate estimation of the depth and extent of burn injury as a percentage of the total body surface. Subsequent fluid-replacement therapy calculations are based on the burn area. Under a typical NGO environment, closed treatment of the burn injury with a two-component dressing (inner dressing

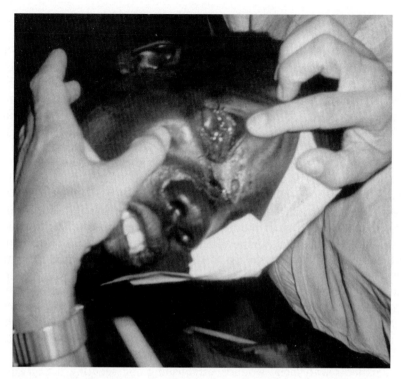

FIGURE 28-5. Penetrating eye injury leading to excision of the eye (Lokichokio, Kenya).

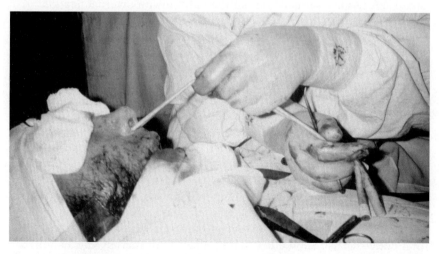

FIGURE 28-6. Mine blast injury of the face with posterior nasal hemorrhage controlled with Foley catheters and traction (Peshawar, Pakistan).

applying an antibacterial agent to the wound and an outer dressing absorbing the exudate and protecting the wound) is appropriate, although open treatment with topical antibacterial agents can also be used. One percent of silver sulphadiazine in a water-soluble cream base should be applied liberally to the wound and repeated twice daily. The definitive treatment includes excision of the dead tissue or eschar, followed by skin grafting.

Postoperative Care and Casualty Transfer

Ideally, most war-wounded patients treated in the NGO hospital should undergo two operations: wound excision and other early surgery on admission and delayed primary closure about five days later. Unless contraindicated, patients should have normal oral intake of food started as soon as possible after the first operation. Even in patients with maxillofacial, cervical, or abdominal injuries, oral intake of liquids and subsequently food should be started as soon as possible. In unconscious patients, establishing a route for gastric or enteral feeding should be anticipated early if the patient has a favorable prognosis within a reasonable time and the hospital has other facilities to treat unconscious patients. One of the most important things in postoperative care is to avoid a vicious circle of repeated surgical interventions with the patient being nil-by-mouth every other day and rapidly getting malnourished, accompanied by poor wound healing and infectious complications, which emphasizes the importance of adequate wound surgery at the initial operation and adherence to the established principles of war surgery, especially to delayed primary closure of excised wounds and amputation stumps.

In patients with fractures treated with external fixation, the fixator can be replaced with plasters as soon as the wounds are healing, enabling the patients to be more easily discharged for further follow up. Sometimes there is no possibility to organize the follow up by local providers, and the recovery and rehabilitation phases have to be completed in the NGO system. In most cases, there are NGOs specialized in rehabilitation working in the same conflict area, and close cooperation between different agencies and organizations is of utmost importance in order to provide the patient with a best possible follow-up care available.

Although occasionally (and often with the help of the media), selected patients will be provided the opportunity for advanced reconstructive procedures abroad, most other patients with persisting postoperative problems have no place to go for more advanced treatment. Therefore, at every stage beginning with the triage and admission phases, the overall perspective has to be kept in mind and the patient's treatment planned and calibrated in a way to achieve the best possible long-term outcome in those particular circumstances. In some cases, this might require unconventional solutions and even unpleasant decisions made by the surgeon in charge of the patient's overall care, but profound understanding of surgical principles, good communication with the patient, relatives, and the hospital staff, familiarity with the available resources, measured optimism, determination, and common sense are the guidelines by which everybody working in the NGO environment can do the most good to most injured people who often have nowhere else to go.

References

1. Dufour D, Kroman Jensen S, Owen-Smith M, Salmela J, Stening GF, Zetterström B. *Surgery for Victims of War.* Geneva: International Committee of the Red Cross; 1988.
2. Ryan J, Mahoney PF, Greaves I, Bowyer G, eds. *Conflict and Catastrophe Medicine. A Practical Guide.* London: Springer-Verlag Limited: London, 2002.
3. Coupland RM. Epidemiological approach to surgical management of the casualties of war. *BMJ.* 1994;308:1693–1697.
4. Coupland RM. Technical aspects of war wound excision. *Br J Surg.* 1989; 76:663–667.
5. Rowley DI. The management of war wounds involving bone. *J Bone Joint Surg [Br].* 1996;78-B:706–709.
6. Coupland R. Abdominal wounds in war. *Br J Surg.* 1996;83:1505–1511.

Further Reading

Bhatnagar MK, Smith GS. Trauma in the Afghan guerrilla war: Effect of lack of access to care. *Surgery.* 1989;105:699–705.

Bowyer GW. Afghan war wounded: Application of the Red Cross wound classification. *J Trauma.* 1995;38:64–67.

Bowyer GW. Management of small fragment wounds: Experience from the Afghan border. *J Trauma.* 1996;40:S170–S172.

Coupland RM, Korver A. Injuries from antipersonnel mines: The experience of the International Committee of the Red Cross. *BMJ.* 1991;303:1509–1512.

Coupland RM, Samnegaard HO. Effect of type and transfer of conventional weapons on civilian injuries: Retrospective analysis of prospective data from Red Cross hospitals. *BMJ.* 1999;319:410–412.

De Wind CM. War injuries treated under primitive circumstances: experiences in an Ugandan mission hospital. *Ann R Coll Surg Engl.* 1987;69:193–195.

Eshaya-Chauvin B, Coupland R. Transfusion requirements for the management of war injured: The experience of the International Committee of the Red Cross. *Br J Anaesth.* 1992;68:221–223.

Gosselin RA, Siegberg CJ, Coupland R, Agerskov K. Outcome of arterial repairs in 23 consecutive patients at the ICRC-Peshawar hospital for war wounded. *J Trauma.* 1993;34:373–376.

Huntington SP. *The Clash of Civilizations.* London: Simon & Schuster UK, Ltd.; 1997.

Husum H, Sundet M. Postinjury malaria: A study of trauma victims in Cambodia. *J Trauma.* 2002;52:259–266.

Leppäniemi A. Medical challenges of internal conflicts. *World J Surg.* 1998;22: 1197–1201.

Morris D, Sugrue W. On the border of Afghanistan with the International Committee of the Red Cross. *N Z Med J*. 1985;98:750–752.

Morris DS, Sugrue WJ. Abdominal injuries in the war wounded of Afghanistan: A report from the International Committee of the Red Cross hospital in Kabul. *Br J Surg*. 1991;78:1301–1304.

Morris D. Surgeons and the International Committee of the Red Cross. *Aust N Z J Surg*. 1992;62:170–172.

Pesonen P. Pulse oximetry during ketamine anaesthesia in war conditions. *Can J Anaesth*. 1991;38:592–594.

Rautio J, Paavolainen P. Afghan war wounded: Experience with 200 cases. *J Trauma*. 1988;28:523–525.

Simper LB. Below knee amputation in war surgery: A review of 111 amputations with delayed primary closure. *J Trauma*. 1993;34:96–98.

SIPRI Yearbook 2002: Armaments, Disarmament and International Security. Oxford: Oxford International Press; 2002.

Strada G, Raad L, Belloni G, Setti Carraro P. Large bowel perforations in war surgery: One-stage treatment in a field hospital. *J Colorectal Dis*. 1993;8:213–216.

Trouwborst A, Weber BK, Dufour D. Medical statistics of battlefield casualties. *Injury*. 1987;18:96–99.

Section 4
Expert Tutorials and Hard Lessons

Introduction

Conflict and Catastrophe Medicine (Ryan J, Mahoney PF, Greaves I, Bowyer G, eds., *Conflict and Catastrophe Medicine: A Practical Guide*. Springer Verlag; 2002) included a section entitled "Hard Knocks and Hard Lessons". The aim was to illustrate problems that occur again and again on humanitarian deployments, to forewarn people, and to let them benefit from the sometimes grim experience of others.

The feedback from readers for this was positive.

The aim here is similar. We have brought together accounts by a number of different authors writing from very different backgrounds. Some have a story to share. Others have made critical observations on deployment that either confirmed or challenged previous teaching and practice.

All bring hard experience from the field.

A
Ballistic Missile Injuries in the Siege of Sarajevo 1992–1995

John P. Beavis

To describe ballistic missile wounds without considering the environment in which they occur is incomplete and fallacious. The physics of ballistic missile injuries do not vary with geography, but the biological consequences for each victim will vary depending on the circumstances in which the injury occurs and the availability of treatment resources. The effects of war are multiple and it is impossible to separate the physical, and indeed the psychological, trauma caused by the overall environmental problems (Figure A-1).[1]

Sarajevo was subjected to the longest siege in modern history, lasting from April 1992 until the latter part of 1995. Most of the casualties were sustained within the first two years, but there was a continuous war of attrition that left the medical facilities severely depleted and the hospitals badly damaged (Figure A-2).

The close proximity of the attacking units to the besieged citizens meant that civilian casualities outnumbered the military casualties (Figure A-3).[2]

As in previous wars, the majority of surviving injured suffered wounds to their limbs (Figure A-4). In Sarajevo, sniper-fire wounds outnumbered those from mortar or shells by a ratio of two to one.

For much of the winter, the roads were impassable and re-supply was entirely dependent on an airlift that was subjected to vagaries of the climate. This led to gradual starvation of the citizens, and effects on various vulnerable groups—infants, lactating and pregnant women, and the elderly—soon became apparent.[3] There is no doubt that severely wounded individuals representing 93% of the hospital population were also particularly at risk from malnutrition.

It is worth recording the reasons that wounded patients are so susceptible to the effects of malnutrition and to relate it to special circumstances of Sarajevo.

1. Poor supply of essential nutrients to hospital and the rest of the city.
2. Increased requirement for protein, carbohydrates, and micronutrients because of obligatory catabolic response to trauma and surgery.

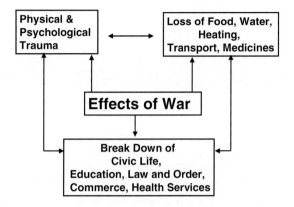

FIGURE A-1. Effects of war.

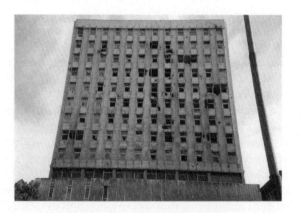

FIGURE A-2. Sarajevo State Hospital.

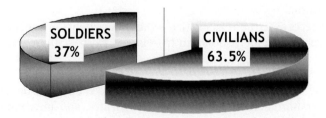

FIGURE A-3. Ratio of civilian to military casualties.

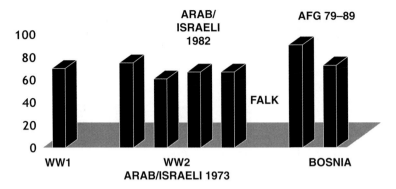

FIGURE A-4. Percentage of limb injuries in previous wars.

3. During the winter there is an increased requirement for endogenous heat production because of inadequate heating of the wards—five-percent increase for every ten-degree drop in temperature. The ambient temperature in Sarajevo can often fall to minus fifteen degrees in winter.
4. Increased demand for nutrition for wound healing and infection—ten percent rise in calorie requirement for each one-degree rise in body temperature. (There is the paradox that the cause and effects are reciprocal, that is, poor nutrition causes infection and wound dehiscence).
5. In war, the majority of wounds are extensive and polytrauma is common.
6. The poor circumstances of the patients caused anorexia and depression, leading to refusal of food.
7. Poor quality food was presented because of the limited recipes and the lack of fuel for cooking. It was unpalatable and frequently rejected.

In the winter of 1993 to 1994, a survey was undertaken of the dietary status of hospital patients.[4] It was possible to demonstrate that not only was the dietary status of hospital patients inadequate, but there was a significant increase in pin track infection when reviewing individuals whose fractures had been treated with an external fixator (State Hospital Sarajevo, unpublished data, 1992–1994) (Figure A-5).

The city suffered from continued bombardment and, effectively, all within its confines can be considered as combatants. Despite the overall susceptibility of the Sarajevan civilians, the aid distribution as derived from a cohort study of war wounded indicated that young men were the most susceptible group (Figure A-6).

War injuries are inevitably substantial and more often than not result in multiple wounds requiring immediate resuscitation because of Grade 3 hemorrhage. During the war it was found that maintaining a relative hemodilution when compared with pre-war levels was entirely satisfactory.

The long-established methods of the management of war wounds were proved essential. This involved wide excision of related tissue and removal

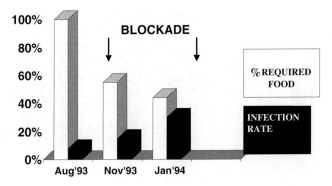

FIGURE A-5. Relationship between reduction in available food for the wounded patients in the State Hospital Sarajevo and the pin track infection from August 1993 to January 1994.

of all foreign and dead material. Fasciotomy was considered imperative, along with external fixation of fractures and immediate repair of major arteries where necessary. Nerve injuries were never primarily repaired.

The initial onslaught on the city was so great that within days external and internal fixation devices were exhausted and no more were forthcoming. This led to the development of the external fixator known as Sarafix. Just under 4000 patients were treated with this apparatus, with results that indicate that, even in extreme conditions, development of such a device is possible and allows adequate treatment of complex fractures (Figure A-7a).

A full study of the use of this device will never be possible because of the population drift that occurred in association with evacuation of seriously ill individuals, but a cohort review of 300 patients who remained

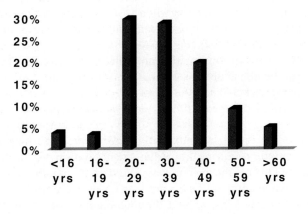

FIGURE A-6. Demography of wounds on the basis of age throughout the war.

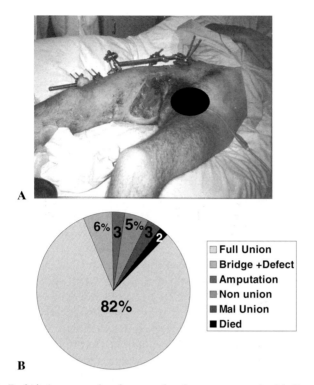

A

B

FIGURE A-7. (A) An example of a complex fracture treated with Sarafix. (B) Percentage complications in 300 patients.

within the city showed that the complications of flexion deformities, pseudoarthrosis, osteomyelitis, and persistent pain occurred. The massive soft tissue injuries accounted for most of these complications (Figure A-7b).

The limited resources available led to the adaptation of surgical techniques with penetrating abdominal wounds. In particular, because of the lack of colostomy bags, primary suture of colonic injuries was undertaken. A retrospective study of this work indicated that while *solitary colonic injuries* could be satisfactorily treated in this way, both *multiple colonic injuries* and *multiple intra-abdominal injuries with peritoneal soiling* (and persistent shock) were associated with breakdown of the anastomosis (State Hospital Sarajevo, unpublished data, 1992–1994). Therefore defunctioning colostomy is recommended under circumstances other than solitary colonic injury (Fig A-8).

The long-term consequences of ballistic missiles wounds on both the individual and their society are often overlooked. In a small study undertaken

* Solitary injury - Resected or Sutured - no colostomy (11) -1 leak (0.99%)
* Multiple injuries - Resected - no colostomy (55) - 6 leaks (10.9%)
* Multiple injuries - Resected with colostomy (30) -2 leaks (6.6%)

FIGURE A-8. Study of immediate colon repair in 394 penetrating abdominal wounds.

in Sarajevo involving 48 patients, persistent abnormality of gait and pain was recorded and over 50% of individuals had failed to return back to work because of the injuries sustained during the war.

Summary of Advice and Lessons Learned from Sarajevo Siege

The devastating effect of war should not just be analyzed in terms of the specific injuries that occur. The war-wounded patient must subsequently compete in a society which has itself been wounded in such a way that employment is reduced and the way of life remains adverse long after the missiles have ceased to fly. Unfortunately, after the initial flurry of interest, these societies and their wounded individuals are left to fare for themselves (Figure A-9).

Finally, a note of caution to all surgeons and anesthetists who seek to assist their hard-pressed and overworked colleagues in war zones. The normal peacetime standards of surgery must be aimed for and clinicians must be prepared to work in an environment that is not only hostile, but one in which adaptation to a lack of resources is essential. Transporting specialists' elective skills such as arthroscopy to a war zone will seldom, if ever, be useful, and a strong background in general traumatic surgery is essential. All volunteers should be trained to the Advanced Trauma Life Support (ATLS) standard for resuscitation and immediate care. In an attempt to

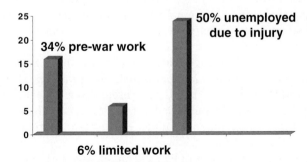

FIGURE A-9. Pre- and post-war working pattern in injured Sarajevo patients.

counteract the effects of early specialization, the International Committee of the Red Cross organizes excellent surgical courses that will, in many ways, compensate for the limited spectrum of skills and help volunteers to appreciate the problems that they will encounter. A besieged city, or any other war zone, is no place for medical tourists.

It is recommended that those medical professionals who are interested in treating war wounds in conflict zones should consider it their obligation to maintain an interest in post-war reconstructive surgery, education, and continued persuasion of politicians and industrialists to assist the recovery of the damaged society. In this way, those who have been severely injured and have persistent disability will be best assisted towards a reasonable way of life.

References

1. Beavis JP. Hunterian lecture. London: Royal College of Surgeons. December 16, 2003.
2. Djozic S. *A Study of a Cohort of Severe Limb Injuries from High energy Missile Wounds* [master's thesis]. Sarajevo: University of Sarajevo; 2002.
3. Vespa J, Watson F. Who is nutritionally vulnerable in Bosnia—Herzegovina? *BMJ*. 1995;311:652–654.
4. Beavis JP, Harper S. Hospital patients in Bosnia are nutritionally vulnerable. *BMJ*. 1996;312:315.

B
Vascular Injuries in the Groin

DAVID J. WILLIAMS

Penetrating wounds to the groin are usually below the inguinal ligament (Figure B-1), and so can be approached by a standard vertical incision with control of the proximal and distal vessels (Figure B-2). In the author's experience, if one can place one's fingers between the site of femoral injury and the inguinal ligament, then the dissection should be possible. This allows the common, superficial, and profunda femoris vessels to be looped, bleeding controlled, and repair or ligation performed. If the injury extends unexpectedly proximally, the inguinal ligament can be cut vertically to allow access to the distal external iliac; however, one must be careful not to divide the bridging vein, which is just under the ligament, or there tends to be additional bleeding.

If the femoral injury is high, a direct approach may not be possible; the options then are to either laparotomize and approach the aorta-iliac segment or to perform an extraperitoneal approach to the external iliac (the author's favored technique). This can be performed reasonably swiftly and does not affect gut function in the same way a laparotomy would. An oblique iliac fossa incision is made four finger widths above the inguinal ligament (Figure B-3); the external oblique aponeurosis is split in the line of the fibers and the underlying muscle split to reveal the peritoneum (Figure B-4). The peritoneum is full of the gut and is gently shifted upward to reveal the external iliac vessels, which can then be controlled.

While more technically difficult then a laparotomy, this technique has the advantage of allowing speedy access and good recovery of gut function.

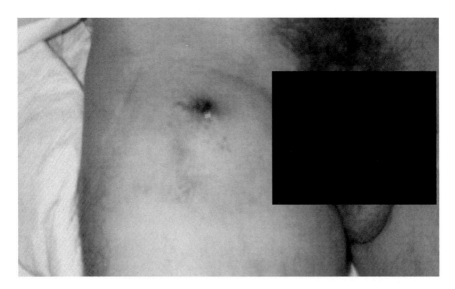

FIGURE B-1. False femoral aneurysm.

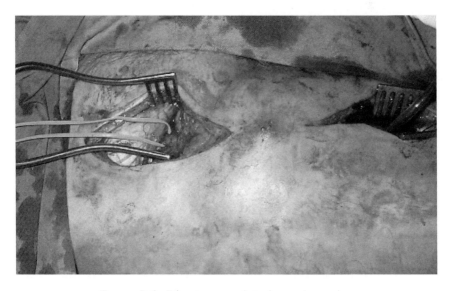

FIGURE B-2. Direct approach to femoral vessels.

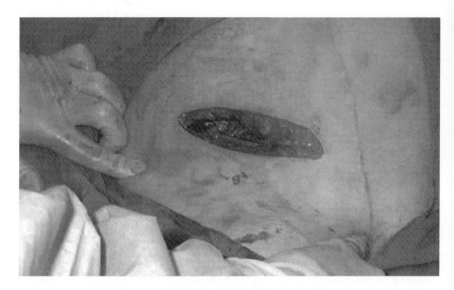

FIGURE B-3. Skin incision, iliac approach.

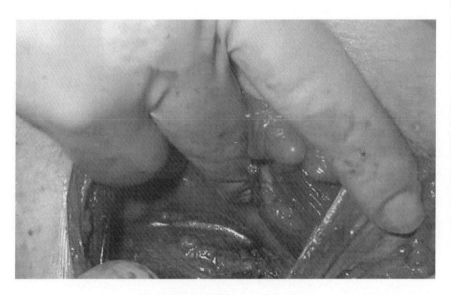

FIGURE B-4. Division of muscles.

C
Conflict Surgery

DAVID J. WILLIAMS

The difficulties that any surgeon encounters in the management of a surgical case in the well-equipped situation of a first-world hospital will also be experienced in the environment of a conflict zone, but additionally, they are compounded by a combination of environmental, logistical, and cultural factors unique to the geographical area where one is working.

The following "tips"—some clinical, some not—may help. The most important, though, is not to put yourself in a situation where you are isolated from senior support and expected to deal with an array of problems unless you are happy to do so.

Pre Deployment

Research the country to which you are being sent regarding the temperature range, weather patterns, and range of local diseases/parasites. Purchase appropriate clothing and ancillaries to increase your comfort and reduce the chance of becoming a thermal casualty, but most importantly to ensure that you are as comfortable as possible. Ensure all immunizations have been administered and malaria prophylaxis (if needed) has been commenced in a timely fashion. If the water supply locally is of unknown quality, take enough sterilizing tablets to easily see you through the duration of your stay.

Liaise with the team with whom you are to be deployed; discuss potential scenarios and iron out any disagreements in management well before any casualties arrive. Check the kit list and make sure you are happy with all the items to be taken—once you are deployed, it is too late to rectify any deficiencies. Decide who is the lead clinician in the case of a clinical dilemma.

579

Deployment

Stay happy! Integrate with all the tasks, especially if they are mundane, physically hard, and dirty (such as digging latrines). You earn an infinite amount of respect if you are seen to be doing crap jobs as readily as everyone else.

Share any luxury items with everyone—we had a "comfort box" where one put in anything that was nice, and then it would be opened intermittently and shared out. This is fantastic for morale after a bad day.

Nip any disagreements in the bud, clear the air and start fresh the next day; several weeks of festering animosity is likely to lead to major dysfunction in the team.

Look out for colleagues; the most unlikely people can prove to be the most robust, while those whom one imagines to be tough may break down after a short while.

Debrief wherever possible after a case; be constructive with the aim of increasing everyone's knowledge, improving the care of the next casualty, and (in case of a poor outcome) ensuring that no team member feels that they are to blame.

Scenarios—Routine Traffic Accidents

Even in a war, people crash vehicles!

Road Traffic Accident 1

Twenty-year-old male, driving, left-sided impact resulting in # left humerus, ruptured spleen, # femur (open), # tib/fib (open).

Investigations—blood count, U&E, X match, X-ray, ultrasound scan (USS),

Treatment—cast for # humerus, tibial traction pin, and Thomas splint post debridement and washout for # femur, ex fix post debridement, and washout for tib/fib and laparotomy/splenectomy.

Discussion

1. The above case showed the value of portable ultrasound. Clinically, this man's abdomen was not one that required a laparotomy, and without the FAST USS we would not have explored it, with the likelihood that he would have continued to bleed and have had a poorer outcome.

2. Bottled mineral water was used for washouts rather than intravenous (IV) fluids. The rationale for this was that the IV fluids were at a premium while drinking water was continually replaced and so we could be more liberal with the irrigation.

3. Traction pins and Thomas splints are rarely used in modern health services, but they are fantastic in austere environments and allow for pain

relief, hemorrhage control, and easier transfer of the patient. In combination with skeletal traction, they are life- and limb-saving devices.

4. The modern treatment of splenic injury by serial USS, High Dependency Unit care, and a wait-and-see policy does not apply to the conflict area. The patient must not be allowed to bleed for long periods otherwise hypothermia, coagulopathy, and potential for renal dysfunction will occur. Additionally, the opportunity to do a laparotomy may not occur again due to factors such as more casualties arriving or the need to move the medical facility.

5. At laparotomy, save the patients life and only commit them to another operation if absolutely necessary. An injured spleen can be wrapped and left in situ in a modern hospital where the patient can be monitored and returned to the theater if required; in the middle of a war, do a splenectomy and thereby complete the treatment. Ensure this fact is documented, commence prophylactic antibiotics, and arrange immunization against encapsulated organisms.

Road Traffic Accident 2

Twenty-eight-year-old male ejected from a vehicle at a speed of approximately 30 miles per hour. Admitted with open-book pelvic fracture (Figure C-1) and hemorrhagic shock. Ascending urethrography demonstrated disrupted urethra/bladder. Patient was treated by external fixation of pelvis with initial transient response. Clinically, he had ongoing bleeding, so

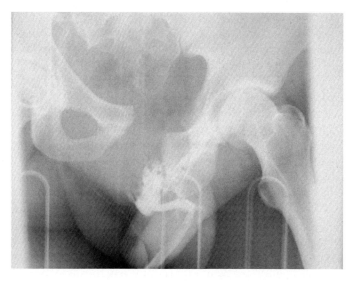

FIGURE C-1. X-ray demonstrating open book pelvic fracture.

laparotomy performed. No clotting factors held in forward facility, so unit members donated nine pints of whole fresh blood.

At laparotomy, resuscitative aortic cross-clamping was performed to arrest uncontrollable pelvic bleeding. The pelvis was packed, large volume transfusion was given to replace losses, and the aortic clamp was released after twenty minutes. Further bleeding occurred and so the aortic clamp was reapplied, followed by selective dissection and clamping of the common iliacs; this demonstrated the source of the bleeding to be on the right. The right internal and external iliac were dissected and right internal iliac tied off with Nylon.

Post operatively the patient was in a coagulopathy but after a delay of 4 hours from time of request, clotting factors including recombinant activated factor VII arrived at our location and were administered.

Discussion

1. Most pelvic fractures will be adequately treated by an external fixator, but if one has to perform a laparotomy, it is difficult because the fixator remains in place and blocks access; in addition, there is a very large pelvic hematoma (similar to a pregnant uterus) distorting tissue planes. Additionally, there is the anxiety of an exsanguinating patient. Make a generous laparotomy, if necessary, up to the xiphisternum because good access will speed the surgery.

2. STAY CALM. Pack the pelvis and apply pressure, usually the bleeding is venous and this should reduce it dramatically. If this does not work, do not spend further time on fruitless exploration in a large hematoma/fracture site; dissect out the abdominal aorta and apply a vascular clamp.

3. Having obtained control, leave the packs in situ and check the rest of the abdomen for signs of injury.

4. TALK TO THE ANESTHETISTS AND DO NOT REMOVE THE CLAMP UNTIL THEY HAVE CAUGHT UP WITH LOSSES, RECLAMP IF THEY ASK YOU TO.

5. At clamp release, there will be two events, little bleeding or much bleeding. The latter indicates major vessel disruption and may require arterial ligation as above. If you are not an experienced arterial surgeon, the safest way to dissect out the iliacs is to remain on the surface of the aorta and slowly move down to the bifurcation, do not migrate off into other tissue planes otherwise injury to ureters, bowel, or pelvic veins may occur.

6. Fresh blood was, in this case, donated by members of our unit, but it can be obtained from friends or relatives of the patient; it has the advantage of being warm, of normal biochemistry, platelet- and clotting-factor rich, and with a normal 2,3-diphosphoglycerate (2,3-DPG) content.

7. If another facility has items you require, ask for them as early as possible due to the logistical problems with delivery.

Scenarios—Pediatrics

Children do not know the difference between toys and munitions, and they play with them. Modern munitions are often scattered during a conflict and may find their way into areas where children play or work. Do not let the fact that the patient is a child change your management from the basic principles of dealing with the war wounded; their outcome is likely to be worsened by inappropriate treatment.

Pediatric 1

Fourteen-year-old boy, picked up unexploded ordnance with non-dominant hand, leading to a hemi-amputation (Figure C-2). Intravenous antibiotics and tetanus immunoglobulin given. The patient was taken to theater post X-ray, where debridement and washout was performed. Although having a vascular supply, the extensive skin loss and exposure of bone and tendon meant that the chance of keeping the hand was slight. Transfer to Plastics team arranged for attempt at flap.

Discussion

1. The definitive treatment of this injury was beyond the skills contained in our facility. If we had not had a Plastics unit available, we would have treated the wound by the same initial procedure, but at second look at 48 hours would have prepared the family for an amputation.

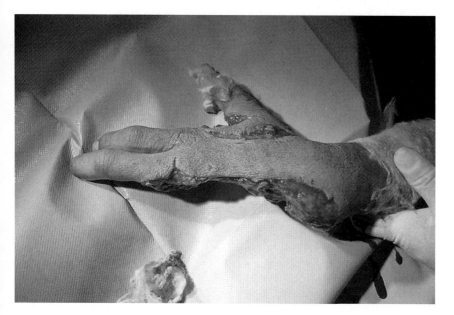

FIGURE C-2. Traumatic hemi-amputated hand in a child.

2. Desire to keep soft tissues must be tempered with the need to remove all debris and nonviable areas.
3. If there had be a lack of vascular supply or gross contamination, a primary amputation would have been performed (see Pediatric 2).

Pediatric 2

Seven-year-old boy playing with his brother encountered unexploded ordnance which he kicked, resulting in traumatic amputation of his foot, shrapnel damage to his remaining foot, and bilateral open tib/fib fractures for his brother, who was standing next to him at the time. Both children were taken to theater that night; the child with the traumatic amputation received a below-knee amputation, which was left open to be re-inspected and closed in three to five days time, with debridement and washout of the remaining foot. His brother had debridement and washout for his open fractures followed by application of plaster of paris because the external fixators were not appropriate for a child.

Discussion

1. The decision to remove a child's leg is not one that is made easily, but leaving a child with a non-healing severely injured limb is inappropriate.

2. At completion of amputation, one might be tempted to close the wound primarily if it looked clean to avoid the need for a second operation; this would almost certainly lead to deep infection and the requirement for revision amputation.

3. The child with open fractures lost large fragments of his tibia; these had periosteal stripping and were devitalized; if left in situ, they would become a focus for infection. Removal leaves a cavity that, when clean, can be bone grafted and covered with a muscle flap at a further operation.

D
Surgery in the Camps

Pauline A. Cutting

In the late 1980s, I worked for 18 months as a surgeon in the Bourj al Borajneh Palestinian refugee camp in Beirut, Lebanon, during the 15-year-long Lebanese Civil War. We were caring for more than 1200 war-injured patients during two periods of fighting—one of six weeks and one of six months.[1] During this time, the camp was attacked and surrounded. These circumstances presented various issues including:

1. Limited resources, no special tests, and no specialists;
2. Availability of blood;
3. Working extremely close to the front fighting line;
4. Austere conditions.

Limited Resources, No Special Tests, and No Specialists

To manage victims of ballistic trauma, one would ideally like to have the support of modern medical facilities with I.T.U., computed tomography, magnetic resonance imaging (MRI), image intensifiers, laboratory support, and specialist opinions, as described in the Royal College of Surgeons document, *Better Care for the Severely Injured* (see Further Reading). However, in war, this is rarely the case, and many wars are fought where the medical services are, at best, basic, inaccessible, or at a distance—sometimes several days travelling from the fighting line. War injured may be of any age, from the very young to the very old, and any or all body areas may be injured. Even in less-than-ideal conditions with limited resources and no specialists, much can be done and good surgical care provided by a surgeon with general surgical and trauma experience if sound surgical principles are followed.[2]

In the Palestinian refugee camp in Beirut, I worked in a small war-damaged field hospital that functioned as a general and emergency medical and surgical hospital. It was situated inside the refugee camp, staffed by a small team of local doctors and nurses, with a few Europeans like myself recruited by nongovernmental organizations (NGOs).

TABLE D-1. Wounding missiles %

Missile	World War II	Vietnam	Northern Ireland	Bourj al Barajneh
Bullets	10	52	55	20
Fragments	85	44	25	60
Other or unclassified	5	4	20	20

The basement and ground floor had been converted into an emergency care complex consisting of:

- an emergency room;
- a small operating theater with one anesthetic machine and one table;
- a pharmacy;
- an X-ray room with a portable machine, which worked intermittently;
- a laboratory with facilities limited to hematocrit, blood group, and cross-match (on a tile), and occasionally urine and stool microscopy, depending upon the availability of slides; and
- wards housing 30 to 40 beds.

Surgery was performed with a general surgical set. There were some orthopedic instruments, including a Gigli saw for amputation, vascular instruments, skin graft knives, and craniotomy burrs. Usually, one operation was carried out at a time, or on occasions with many seriously injured, we squeezed in another couch, brought in a desk lamp, and operated in two teams in cramped conditions, sometimes cleaning and sharing instruments.

General anesthetics were nitrous oxide and Fluothane with or without intubation and muscle relaxation, or intravenous anesthetics with patients manually ventilated on air; Ketamine in combination with Diazepam was used often.

In these circumstances, 1276 war injured were managed—all injured by conventional weapons (Table D-1), age range 2 months to 100 years, 55% men, 45% women and children with a whole spectrum of injuries from patients with serious multi-system injury to minor soft tissue wounds (Table D-2).

Injuries operated on (Table D-3) were mostly soft tissue, following the traditional time-tested treatment of primary wound excision followed by

TABLE D-2. Distribution of missile wounds (%)

Location	World War II	Vietnam	Northern Ireland	Bourj al Barajneh
Head and neck	4	14	20	11.5
Chest	8	7	15	16
Abdomen	4	5	15	18
Limbs	75	54	50	45.5
Other	9	20	—	9

TABLE D-3. Types of injury operated on

Injury	No.
Soft tissue	900
Chest, penetrating	67
Abdomen, penetrating	69
Peripheral, vascular	21
Orthopedic	112
Brain	5

delayed primary closure at about five days or left open to close by secondary intention.

There were no specialists and it was not possible to evacuate patients. I was the only doctor with a surgery qualification (F.R.C.S.), but had no war surgery experience. Amongst the Palestinian doctors, two were surgeons in training, with little formal training, but much experience. The other doctors were juniors and generalists who assisted in theater, and we trained them to put in chest drains and perform primary wound excision. None of us were orthopedic surgeons, nor did we have cardiothoracic or neurosurgical experience.

Orthopedic injuries were managed with plaster of paris and splintage, and occasionally, external fixators were used for lower leg fractures and associated extensive soft tissue loss. Fractured femurs were managed with Steinman pin traction with sandbag weights or skin traction for young children. Even patients with orthopedic injuries and requiring vascular repair were treated in this way. For non-orthopedic surgeons, I believe this approach has been supported by the work of Professor Rowley, who has shown that in similar conditions good, if not better, results can be achieved with these methods of treatment than those achieved with more intervention and use of external fixation.[3] However, that is not to say that fully trained orthopedic surgeons could not achieve better results.

All penetrating chest injuries were treated with a wide-bore basal chest tube that was connected to an underwater sealed drain and inserted in the fifth or sixth intercostal space anterior to the mid axillary line. No thoracotomies were performed.

All those with abdominal injuries suspected to be penetrating underwent laparotomy. The most devastating and difficult to deal with were those produced by multiple large fragments, and these were often associated with injuries to other body areas and with a high mortality. High-velocity bullet injuries were often complicated as expected and injured organs were removed or repaired. Mortality was related to the number of injured organs. Survivors averaged 2.1 injured organs while non-survivors averaged 3.7 injured organs.

Craniotomies for penetrating brain injuries were performed by enlarging the skull defect with bone nibblers, extracting bone fragments, accessible metal fragments, and pulped brain with low-pressure suction. There was no ventilator for postoperative ventilation. Tackling these patients with no senior or specialist opinion was daunting. Advice came from the theater nurse, who had worked in neurosurgery and gave tips on exposure and hemostasis.

There was no rearward evacuation of patients after initial surgery. The management of patients with postoperative complications was particularly difficult, with no back-up services, such as laboratory investigations, ultrasound, CT, or MRI. Even fluid balance charts were not reliable, as some nurses had little or no training. However, clinical assessment of patients took place every morning. Thus, in these conditions with limited equipment, a great deal can be done and good care provided by a surgeon with sound surgical training adhering to time-tested surgical principles.[2]

Availability of Blood

One crucial factor in caring for the patients with serious multiple injuries is the availability of blood. It is hopeless to operate on such patients without any blood. We were lucky that the population, family, and friends were ready and willing to donate blood. There was a large supply of citrated blood bags. Crossmatch was performed on a white tile. As the camp was surrounded and the whole population nearby and many people living in the hospital, there was on most occasions a ready supply of fresh blood for transfusion. This did not always help the triage decisions, and I believe we made some naive decisions and took patients to the operating theater with a poor prognosis. However, the effect on morale of labeling patients hopeless is significant, and with a short evacuation time, good initial assessment and resuscitation, and the availability of fresh blood, you get a "few good saves." Patients can recover fully, which lifts morale amongst patients, care givers, and the community alike.

Operating Very Near the Front Line

Medical facilities situated very close to or in the front line result in patients arriving alive with severe complicated multi-system injury, including major vessel injury. These patients consume a great deal of resources and only a few survive. The hospital—Haifa Hospital—was inside the Palestinian refugee camp of Bourj al Barajneh. The camp was on a slope measuring about 400 by 500 meters and housed 9000 people. During the periods of fighting, the camp was surrounded and attacked on all sides with guns, rocket-propelled grenades, mortars, and tanks. The wounded were all carried to the hospital on stretchers, and the distance from the place of wounding to the hospital was no more than a few 100 meters in any direction. The evacuation time for most was extremely short—only minutes. One patient arrived alive with a fragment injury transecting his spinal cord at C2.

A short lag time between injury and definitive surgery increases the overall mortality within the medical facilities, but improves the outcome for the individual.[1] At the other end of the scale, as the hospital was so close by, many patients came with relatively minor wounds and some with multiple superficial soft tissue wounds—sometimes tens or even hundreds of small fragment wounds. There was not much in the literature concerning these so-called "pepper pot" wounds, but it was clear that it was neither feasible, nor practical, nor necessary to perform a wound excision on all these wounds. These "pepper pot" wounds were given tetanus prophylaxis, penicillin if available and felt to be necessary, and the wounds themselves cleaned, sometimes with not much more than a good wash. A few developed focal infection, but there were no deaths in the patients whose only wounds were uncomplicated soft tissue wounds. I believe there is now supporting literature for this approach, using the International Committee of the Red Cross (ICRC) wound classification, these being the small-grade VO fragment wounds. It also has been shown that fragments transfer the maximum amount of their energy at or very close to the surface,[4] such that if the entry wound is small, there will be no hidden area of damage due to temporary cavitation.

Being very close to or in the fighting zone raises issues of safety and security of patients and health care personnel. Although the Geneva Convention sets out the rights and duties of the health care personnel in war and that hospitals and ambulances should be respected, this is not always adhered to and medical facilities may be damaged by inadvertent or intended bombardment.

Haifa Hospital, initially a five-story building, was hit hundreds of times by bombs and mortars and the two top floors were demolished piecemeal (Figure D-1). The emergency care complex was situated in the basement and there were wards in the basement and on the ground floor. Medical and nursing personnel ventured out of the hospital rarely or not at all during periods of fighting, sometimes lasting weeks on end.

One may have to face the decision of whether (as foreign personnel) to be evacuated or not. In our position, evacuation would have been extremely difficult and, in any case, we chose to remain.

Austere Conditions

There are certain basic essentials for the provision of surgical care for the victims of war. "The wounded need access to a safe place, supplied with water and power, where they can receive competent surgical treatment, backed up by good nursing care, within a well organised system, which

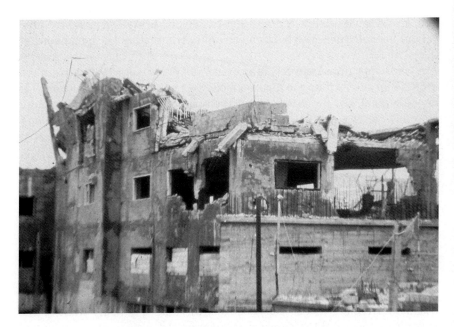

FIGURE D-1. The hospital after the battles.

receives adequate supplies."[5] The surgeon and the anesthetist may not be the most important aspect of providing care, and if the infrastructure breaks down, then proper surgical care may no longer be possible. During the six-month period of fighting around Bourj al Barajneh, the camp was under siege. There was no evacuation of patients and no replenishing of supplies, requiring rationing of resources. Disposable items were reused after cleaning. Many wounds were left open after primary wound excision, to be closed by secondary intention, thus preserving anesthetic and suture material for life- and limb-saving surgery. Patients managed their own wounds by keeping them mechanically clean by washing and applying dressings, if necessary. The increased morbidity of leaving wounds open was difficult to quantify, but no patient died whose only injury was soft tissue. Antibiotics were used sparingly. Gas gangrene was seen when we had run out of penicillin.

"The hospital will not function without water and electricity."[5] The electricity was cut off from the camp early. The generators at the hospital were used and run only for emergency use. The water tank on the roof was damaged and had to be resituated on the first floor behind reinforced walls. Fatigue and exhaustion were eventually compounded by hunger and starvation when food stores ran low. Under-nourished patients had more complications. The future looked bleak and "burnout" was seen amongst hospital staff. One doctor disappeared from the hospital for several days after a particularly difficult case and returned to work, but remained a recluse. These were not military personnel, who might be more disciplined, but civilians. Generally, the hospital staff worked well as a team, importantly supporting each other through difficult times. Small acts of generosity, such as families bringing in food for the staff from their own meager stores, were vitally important for morale when faced with hunger. Battlefields and conditions change rapidly, and just when everything appeared hopeless with starvation and threat of mass slaughter, the overall political situation changed; the Syrian Army intervened and the fighting ended, allowing for replenishing of supplies and eventual evacuation of patients still requiring further care.

References

1. Cutting PA, Agha R. Surgery in a Palestinian refugee camp. *Injury*. 1992; 23:405–409.
2. Jackson DS, Batty CG, Ryan JM, McGregor WSP. The Falklands War; Army field surgical experience. *Ann R Coll Surg Engl*. 1983;65:281–285.
3. Rowley DI. *War Wounds with Fractures: A Guide to Surgical Management*. Geneva: International Committee of the Red Cross; 1996.
4. Bowyer GW, Cooper GJ, Rice P. Management of small fragment wounds in war: Current research. *Ann R Coll Surg Engl*. 1995;77:131–134.
5. Hayward-Karlsson J, Jeffery S, Kerr A, Schmidt H. *Hospitals for War-wounded*. Geneva: International Committee of the Red Cross; 1998.

Further Reading

Better Care for the Severely Injured: A Joint Report from The Royal College of Surgeons of England and the British Orthopaedic Association. July 2000.
Coupland RM. Epidemiological approach to surgical management of the casualties of war. *BMJ*. 1994;308:1693–1697.
Coupland RM. *The Red Cross Wound Classification*. Geneva: International Committee of the Red Cross; 1991.
Coupland RM. *War Wounds of Limbs: Surgical Management*. Oxford: International Committee of the Red Cross; 1993.
Kirby GK, Blackburn G. *Ministry of Defence: Field Surgery Pocket Book*. London: HMSO; 1981.
Sellier KG, Kneubuehl BP. *Wound Ballistics and the Scientific Background*. Amsterdam: Elsevier; 1994.

Editors' note. We also recommend you read Pauline Cutting's autobiographical account *Children of the Siege*. At time of writing this is out of print, but is available second hand from internet book sellers.

E
Ballistics—Lessons Learned

MALCOLM Q. RUSSELL

The patient was an adult male who had been shot twice with high-velocity 7.62-millimeter ammunition. He was injured in an austere environment as evening fell, with temperatures not far above freezing and falling. His work colleagues gave him first aid, including the administration of intramuscular (IM) morphine.

On handover to the medical team around 30 minutes after the injury, we were told that he had an abdominal wound and an injury to his lower right leg. ABCs were rapidly assessed; he had a radial pulse of just over 100 beats per minute and delayed capillary refill time. He had an entry wound above his left superior anterior iliac spine, but his abdomen was soft. Exposure of his right leg revealed no obvious wound. Treatment at this stage was oxygen, intravenous (IV) access, and administration of ketamine (the morphine had produced little effect). Good pain relief was achieved and he was packaged for helicopter transport. His findings were put down to a combination of pain, cooling, and early shock secondary to a developing abdominal injury.

During his flight to a surgical facility (approximately 40 minutes away), he lay on the floor of a CH-47 Chinook helicopter with reasonable space, a lot of noise and vibration, and minimal (green) lighting. The only monitoring that functioned was electrocardiograph (ECG), which, despite artifact, was the only way his heart rate could be measured (no pulses palpable with the vibration present, blood pressure (BP), and SpO$_2$ modalities not functioning, auscultation impossible). The patient made intermittent eye contact, but communication was otherwise impossible.

The patient's heart rate steadily climbed while his abdomen remained surprisingly soft. There was nothing to suggest increasing pain as a cause and it became clear that the primary source of blood loss had not been found. Reassessment of ABCs including further exposure showed a distended left thigh with a small entry wound at the knee and minimal external blood loss. He had a closed fracture of his femur and the round had ruptured his femoral vein internally.

A traction splint was applied, two units of O Rh negative packed cells given, and his pulse stabilized. On arrival at the surgical facility, damage control surgery was carried out; he required 35 units of blood in the first 48 hours and extensive surgery later, but ultimately had a good outcome.

The lessons learned from this experience were:

1. Do not assume that comments during handover are accurate, particularly in a hostile environment.

2. Exposure of the patient must be sufficient to detect important injuries, but balanced against the risks from environmental cooling. It is easy to miss significant penetrating wounds. Expose as much as is necessary and be prepared to explore further if the condition of the patient fails to match your findings and expectations.

3. Even during transfer in a dedicated medical helicopter, interventions can be difficult to perform and monitoring often functions inadequately. These problems are amplified by the necessity to transfer patients in a general support helicopter as dictated by operational circumstance. Improvisation is important; therefore, consider putting an end-tidal CO_2 probe into an oxygen mask to gauge respiratory rate (and even just to confirm the patient is still breathing). Listen to your clinical instincts—they may be the most important alarm function you have. If you have the feeling something is not right, do something about it fast!

F
African Education

ADAM J. BROOKS

In 1997, as a junior Surgical Registrar, I headed back to Johannesburg, South Africa, to take up a post at Baragwanath and later Helen Joseph Hospitals. I had previously spent a year working in the emergency room at Johannesburg Hospital Trauma Unit.

My first night on call quickly dispelled my confidence; my first case was a patient who had been shot through the right lung, diaphragm, stomach, small bowel, descending colon, tail of pancreas, and finally left ureter. I had more questions than answers:

– Exteriorize or repair the colon?
– But what about the proximity of the pancreatic injury?
– How do you repair a ureteric injury?
– What do I do about the ongoing bleeding from the chest?

I quickly learned that a ballistic injury crosses junctional boundaries and has no respect for traditional surgical territories or comfort zones.

Two other cases stand out from my time in South Africa. Both taught me valuable lessons that I will never forget.

The first case involves my first two trauma thoracotomies. Both were on the same night, only a few hours apart and, unfortunately, both were on the same patient. My first penetrating wound of the heart and, as the patient's vital signs deteriorated, I was not sure who had more adrenaline in their system. A small easy-to-suture laceration rapidly turned into a larger "star"-shaped hole as suture after suture cut through the myocardium.

Lesson one was *use pledgets when suturing the heart*.

Eventually the hole was repaired, the bleeding stopped, and the chest closed. Hypotensive and on significant amounts of inotropes, the patient went to the intensive care unit. Three hours later, nearly 1300 milliliters of blood had been collected in the chest drain bottles and the patient remained unstable. Back to the theater, this time to repair the wound in the posterior aspect of the heart from the through-and-through injury.

Lesson two was, *with penetrating wounds, think pairs, think entry and exit*.

There may not be more than one wound, but by thinking about the possibility and looking, you are less likely to miss injuries.

The second case occurred several months later.

I was operating on a gunshot wound to the groin with a femoral artery transection; the procedure was going well, with the vessel controlled proximally and distally and a vein graft going in. The patient remained unstable and the anesthetist did not seem to be winning. On closing the groin and removing the drapes, the reason became all too apparent, as the abdomen was grossly distended. On "closer" examination, there was a small entrance wound deep in the umbilicus, obscured by what I had assumed was dried blood from the femoral wound.

Laparotomy revealed a gunshot wound to the liver in a now cold, coagulopathic patient.

Lesson three has been learned repeatedly by many surgeons operating on gunshot victims. *Look for wounds in inaccessible locations such as the axillae, between the buttocks and under the hairline.*

G
The Role of Intensive Care in the Management of Ballistic Trauma in War

MATTHEW J. ROBERTS

Critical care is an area that has changed beyond recognition since the 1991 Gulf war, in terms of equipment, staffing and clinical practice. The latest field intensive care modules are a compromise between sophistication and practicality.

Practicality requires items to be robust where possible, to have flexibility in power supply and not to put great demands on the medical supply organization.

Versions of these up to date field intensive care facilities have been deployed on a small scale on recent peace support operations but casualty numbers were usually low and the experience did not inform as to the extent of intensive care utilization that could be expected in warfare.

This lesson had to be learned at the outset of the 2003 conflict in Iraq.

The casualty mix on operations other than warfighting tends to be dominated by road accidents, medical admissions, burns and the occasional mine strike. Large numbers of ballistic injuries are not seen so forecasts as to the requirement for intensive care for this conflict had to be based on estimation and assumption.

It was assumed that the number of casualties reaching the field hospital with penetrating limb injuries would by far out way those with abdominal or thoracic trauma, as a result of the lethality of high velocity wounds to the trunk, the self selection of survivable injuries and the wearing of body armor.

This proved to be correct.

It was assumed that limb injuries would be resuscitated pre and peroperatively, would have relatively short operating times and be transferred to the general wards.

In the event this assumption, partly based on the templates long used on medical exercises, proved to be less accurate.

Prior to the outset of hostilities the intensivists at 202 Field Hospital anticipated being relatively underemployed and so decided on an "out reach" policy whereby a consultant would attend each major resuscitation in the A + E department and also "trawl" the operating theatres for patients who might benefit from a period of intensive or high dependency care.

However as the casualties began to arrive it soon became apparent that there would be no difficulty in filling the beds. The main concern was evacuation from the hospital.

During the war fighting phase (17 March–30 April), the largest patient group by far requiring intensive care at 202 Field Hospital were those with ballistic trauma; bullets and fragments accounted for 55% of ICU admissions, more than twice the second group, burns with 27%.

Another assumption—that the unit would be primarily a high dependency ward—also had to be discarded as 45.5% of ICU patients required tracheal intubation and ventilation.

Many patients were admitted from theatre having undergone extensive debridement for multiple fragment injuries, perhaps prolonged attempts at limb salvage, successful or otherwise. They had received multiple unit blood transfusions and continued to bleed either because of a coagulopathy or the nature of their surgery. They were acidotic and frequently, despite the environmental conditions, hypothermic.

It is easy to imagine why in the major conflicts of the last hundred years early amputation might have been viewed as the better course of action than a prolonged, physiologically disturbing and potentially futile salvage procedure where postoperative facilities were limited.

The role of the intensive care unit in the field hospital consists primarily of either continued *resuscitation* (leading to early extubation and transfer to the general ward) or preparation for *repatriation* by a critical care transfer team.

This template does not take into account the management of enemy prisoners and civilians where transfer out of country is not a possibility; over 80% of patients on the 202 Field Hospital intensive care unit were Iraqi.

The resulting length of stay on intensive care for Iraqi patients was between 2 and 3 times as long as for coalition troops with an obvious impact on bed occupancy.

It is clear that the intensivist cannot entirely avoid having to manage the later complications of severe injury by counting on early transfer out. Equipment and drug scales need to take this requirement into account.

The presence of well staffed and equipped intensive care units during this conflict no doubt influenced the morbidity and mortality of casualties with ballistic trauma, but it had another more visible effect:

The ability to act as an extension to A + E, the operating theatres and the recovery ward, admitting patients from these departments for further resuscitation and monitoring, helped to maintain flow through the field hospital and allow the surgical teams to move rapidly on to the next cases.

The very low number of patients who needed admission to the unit from the general wards was testament to the effectiveness of the policy of proactive intensive care.

Only 4.6% of 202 Field Hospital patients passed through the intensive care unit.

The ability to concentrate these, the sickest patients in the hospital, in one area with a high level of technology and a wealth of medical and nursing critical care experience, improved their chance of survival and no doubt allowed for better care of other patients on the general wards.

H
Survivors and Shooters

IAN P. PALMER

This chapter is a personal view written from a British perspective. It is the product of 28-years experience as an Royal Army Medical Corps (RAMC) Medical Officer and Psychiatrist and historical study as the Tri Service Professor of Defense Psychiatry.

Shooters

Thou shalt not murder

Shooters are a unique band of humans. In war at least, they are sanctioned to kill without legal censure. The First World War was perhaps the last, and possibly only, war of the modern era in which soldiers faced soldiers and civilian casualties were limited. During all subsequent conflicts, civilians have endured death and injury, generally resulting from air attack. This chapter focuses on "military-on-military" action.

Although killing in war is premeditated and may reflect extreme self-interest, it is not generally a psychopathic act. Unless truly sociopathic, self-examination is an inevitable consequence, for all who kill will be changed by their experience. The true "psychopath" has little place in an army, as by definition they are too self-referential and absorbed to be able to fit into a body of men where reciprocity of interest and self-sacrifice is a key part of the "warrior" ethos.

Within Her Majesty's Forces, there are many methods of delivering death, and these may be classified by the distance from release to point of impact. Unlike soldiers, sailors and airmen seldom see the result of their handiwork to the extent that their killing would seem to have achieved the status of a computer game. Distance affords emotional protection, as does the incomprehensibility of large numbers killed, even when viewed in the media. However, only when the reality of death is visited upon ships or aircraft are shot down will unconscious defense mechanisms be challenged or abruptly removed, and only at this time are sailors and airmen likely to endure a soldier's experience of combat.

Issues of class, opaque yet inherent, are involved in this process and reflected in the language used by Navies and Air Forces who have always attracted the "brighter" sections of society's youth. They use terms that reflect the "precision" involved in their technocratic structure; they talk of "surgical' strikes and compare them, favorably, with the 'butchery' of combat. However, it could be argued that a soldier is actually more surgical and much less likely to kill civilians than their naval or air force counterparts. Therefore, this chapter is related to the more intimate forms of killing undertaken by soldiers.

There is an ancient "martial" code within soldiery. Many nations have demanded that their young men prove themselves in combat or other trials of strength derived, in the West at least, from chivalric codes of combat between equals. Perhaps the "idealized" duel between equals lives on most vividly in the Royal Air Force (RAF) in the "dog fight." In some societies, killing may be seen as the "ultimate" male experience in contrast with birth being the "ultimate" female experience. It has long been held that it is easier to kill your enemy if you hate him, but there are few soldiers who despise their enemy unless they have transgressed the code of combat and behaved despicably towards comrades or civilians. Interestingly, it is easier to loathe your enemy the further you are away from them, and efforts to engender "blood lust" were spectacularly unsuccessful in the Second World War.

For many years and many reasons, British society has remained ambivalent towards those soldiers who undertake its dirty work. Soldiers are soon forgotten, marginalized, or quarantined after combat in order that society is not infected by what these merchants of death have done and seen. I have met few real combat veterans who like to talk of their experiences other than with their comrades. Most fear distressing those they love by telling their tales, and all loathe those in society who wish to vicariously and voyeuristically see action by association.

Few soldiers kill without weapons. I have seldom encountered these cases professionally or socially. Hand-to-hand combat is a struggle to the death that when the soldier subsequently cogitates upon it might engender regret, but regret tempered by the innate drive to survive in a life-or-death situation.

Weapons protect individuals by inserting distance into the equation of killing, most noticeably in air- and sea-delivered modes of death. Combat and killing can only partially be prepared for in peace, and despite the media's perception, it is my clinical experience that the events combatants encounter are a problem for only a few. This is because psychological reactions, short of psychosis (which is rare in combat), are multifactorial in genesis and meaning is integral to etiology. Such reactions are the product of an interaction between the individual, the event, the environment at the time and after, and the culture from which the individual hails and to which he returns. Meaning is generated from within individuals from all their experiences and, therefore, where they are in their life cycle; no one is a tabula rasa. The most difficult cases I have seen have nearly always had problematic issues and experiences earlier in life that have only surfaced *after* combat exposure.

Killing is an experience that requires assimilation and accommodation. Most soldier's internal dialogue will at some stage search for understanding, whether consciously or unconsciously, and seek to find some reason for what happened. These may include social and religious values such as good versus evil, necessary evil, just war, super-ordinate national goals and interests, and to save my life or that of my comrades. In these intra-psychic debates, rationalizations will alter with the level of threat at the time and where the individual is in their life cycle. Many live fulfilling lives after combat, but are troubled by their experiences in later life when their faculties fail and they sustain losses such as the bereavement of a partner and the like. Do individuals need to seek help? I would counsel against it unless symptoms are intrusive, distressing, and interfering with relationships or the ability to function in other areas of life.

Society wants demonstrable remorse in those who kill for it. It strikes me that society may have more of a problem with the fact that most individuals can kill in combat without remorse or intra-psychic distress. While talking is believed to be beneficial, there are costs to the individual, including shame and guilt at sins of omission or commission. To tell of killing also runs the risk of "abusing" the listener, which may engender feelings of being an abuser (repeating the killing); feeling different and alienated; anger by talking, especially when the listener is shocked, distressed, rejecting or pejorative in their reaction[s]. Even pride and self-esteem may be undermined when listeners do not understand what the soldier went through. But who is listening? Are they loved ones whom you do not want to turn against you, which they would "if they knew exactly what I'd done," my "guilty secret". Does the listener have an agenda (such as media, pressure groups, inexperienced "counselors," etc.)? While others may think about killing, to have actually done it sets one apart. Inexperienced therapists may feel scared, as may the individual who knows what it is like to take another's life; could they do it again? Other emotions include feelings of vulnerability when telling an emotionally charged story; how can grown men who have killed receive warmth and "holding" from loved ones? As few civilians will understand soldiers' experiences, they may either be over-solicitous or over-protective and run the risk of pitying, demeaning, or patronizing soldiers, thus setting the scene for regression and dependency. Alternatively, they may protect themselves by distancing themselves from listening. As talking is generally not a socially sanctioned behavior in young males, it may engender mixed feelings of impotent, inexpressible rage and helplessness and having faced and dealt death, risk-taking and tempting fate is possible and not uncommon.

Survivors

You never hear the bullet that kills you

What is it like to be shot? A veteran of World War I once told me it was "like being hit with a crow-bar, it f*****g well smarts." Others feel nothing until later. Some stoically remain silent while others scream terribly.

Fear is endemic in combat,[1,2] especially for "combat virgins". Experience brings understanding and calm, but later, superstitions come to the fore and luck may be felt to be running out for some. Consequently, anxiety rises. Sequelae are physical, psychological, and sociocultural. How do individuals come to terms with being a target, being singled out for death?

Injuries survived may be a badge of honor or courage, and the Americans have gone as far as honoring an injury with a medal, the Purple Heart. Like scars won in a duel, they may tell of heroism and may mark the survivor out as having cheated death. A wound, honestly obtained, is an honorable *hors de combat* removing the soldier from danger. It may serve the survivor as a reminder of painful memories, of potential loss, or of insights gained into the meaning of life. "True" soldiers are able to draw upon their military codes to remain steadfast in adversity and to continue the fight towards health and return of function. Others are less fortunate, but as in service, a "can do" mentality helps mental health when allied to support from comrades. Many find charity demeaning and counter to their military mores. As with most cases, pre-morbid personality is a potent predictor of post-trauma outcomes.

Some injuries have organic psychiatric problems such as head injury. However, most, if not all, will have to adjust to altered body image, limitation of function, and revise their spiritual beliefs. Many who survive when others have died see it as their duty to continue in life, to count their blessings, and to honor the memory of those who lost their lives.

Postcombat Mental Health Outcomes

While *everyone* involved in combat will be changed, such change may be positive, negative, or a mixture of both.[3,4] Furthermore, only a minority of those exposed to the same event will develop a mental disorder; the following may explain why. Post-traumatic mental disorders are multifactorial in origin, that is, the product of an interaction between the following, largely uncontrollable variables: The Individual—strengths and vulnerabilities [genetic, physical, cognitive, emotional, social, cultural]; The Event—threat [through personal meaning], severity, duration; The Environment—before, during and after; The Culture of the individual and group—shared cultural values, mores, and support. The same mental disorders

TABLE H-1. Postcombat, mental-health outcomes

Mental health
  Grief reactions
  Post-traumatic stress reactions (PTSR)
Mental illness
  Mental disorder
     i. Depression
    ii. Anxiety
   iii. Post-traumatic Stress Disorder
    iv. Phobias
     v. Substance misuse/abuse
  Adjustment reactions to physical injury, disfigurement, and
    disability
  Medically unexplained symptoms—War syndromes
  Personality change

and illnesses may occur in both shooters and survivors; such disorders are seldom psychotic. Mental illness and disorders may present with psychological and/or physical symptoms. Somatic preoccupation may lead to unnecessary investigation and possible iatrogenic harm, especially when no cause can be found for the individual's complaints—so called medically unexplained symptoms.

Psychological problems include Post-traumatic Stress Disorder (PTSD) (which is not as common as the media would have us believe) and Post-traumatic Stress Reactions (PTSR), which are common.

Post-traumatic Stress Reactions may be erroneously diagnosed as PTSD, as their symptoms are similar, varying only in degree, duration, and context. They are probably ubiquitous and a normal psychological response in a way similar to grief reactions. Post-traumatic Stress Disorder is only one metal-health outcome and should not be considered synonymous with postcombat mental disorder (Tables H-1 and H-2). It should only be diagnosed following expert assessment when an individual has been exposed to exceptionally life-threatening events *and* the symptomatology interferes significantly in numerous areas of their life.

TABLE H-2. War syndromes

Nostalgia
Rheumatism
Disordered Action of the Heart
Effort Syndrome
Neurocirculatory Asthenia
Dyspepsia
Agent Orange Syndrome
Gulf War Syndrome

Source: Adapted from Jones E, et al., Reference 1.

The cardinal symptoms of the PTSR and PTSD are re-experiencing, avoidance, and arousal phenomena with their associated behaviors.

- *Re-experiencing*: Recurrent, unwanted, intrusive thoughts, images, sounds, smells. Triggers leading to distress and physical arousal, Nightmares, "As if" phenomena or "flashbacks."
- *Avoidance*: Avoiding thoughts and things associated with the event, Feeling emotionally isolated, Loss of interest in things previously enjoyed.
- *Arousal*: "On edge," unable to relax, Irritable and aggressive, Difficulty in sleeping and concentrating, Forgetfulness.
- *Associated behaviors*: Substance abuse, especially drinking, Relationship problems, Risk-taking activities and impulsivity, Survivor guilt, Depression.

Like grief, PTSR usually settle within six to twelve weeks, or sooner, but are problematic for some individuals. Indeed, grief is a good simile, as coming to terms with the psychological impact of traumatic events is like a mourning process.

Post-trauma mental illness may reveal itself in many ways and at varying times after an incident. Those closest to the individual are usually the first to notice any change, as relationship problems are common. If work is suffering, it is important for work mates and management to encourage individuals to seek help.

Some changes are fundamental to our being and may alter our schemata for world and self-view, challenging our beliefs about our invulnerability, the predictability and order of daily life, etc. The personal meaning of traumatic events is idiosyncratic and may cause more problems in rehabilitation than any physical injuries. Some will feel guilty about sins of omission or commission, and where there is abnormal or delayed coping, individuals may fail to acknowledge, accept, assimilate, and accommodate to change or loss, which may lead to avoidance and maladaptive behaviors.

Prevention is only possible if exposure is prevented, but this is impossible for soldiers if they are to engage in combat; however, unnecessary exposure can often be minimized without damage to the mission. There is little one can do about the individuals exposed to trauma other than to ensure they are well trained, briefed, supported, led, and not exposed unnecessarily. Generally, nothing can change the traumatic event at the time, but it is possible to alter the environment in which soldiers operate—before, during, and after exposure to reinforce mutual support and help inculcated through training and shared hardships.

Individuals should be allowed to talk about their experiences *when* they want to. They should not be forced, as there is no evidence that shows this prevents post-trauma mental illness or disorder; indeed, interventions such as Critical Incident Stress Debriefing may actually be harmful if instituted too early or inappropriately.

For those suffering mental illness, psychiatric interventions work. However, as the genesis of post-trauma mental illness is complex, some individuals will require in-depth or long-term help—they will be the minority. Any assessment should search for treatable mental disorder; appropriate medication must be prescribed and followed-up vigorously. Cognitive, behavioral, and imaging techniques will be required to aid an individual to gain control over their symptoms and to help them address, assimilate, and accommodate to the changes wrought in them and their social world in order to get on with their life. Such processing requires time and effort and is similar to grief "work." Individuals who become preoccupied with blame and remain angry have a poorer prognosis.

Somatic problems may be part of a mental disorder such as depression; while they improve as the disorder is treated, other cases are no so straightforward. Medically unexplained symptoms are numerous and vague in nature for which no "organic" cause can be found. Patients are usually subject to batteries of tests, generally in increasing order of risk without result; this can lead to a souring of the doctor–patient relationship, which may become adversarial. Patients may become even more focused on an organic etiology and may believe the doctor is withholding information or is not doing the right tests, etc. The doctor, on the other hand, may see the case in increasingly psychological terms, usually vigorously resisted by the patient on the subtext that "you thought it was physical, now you think I'm mad!" Until the inevitable impasse, both parties have been stuck in Cartesian Dualism, and to relinquish such beliefs may lead to loss of face for one party. This is counter-therapeutic, but not an uncommon situation. Without acceptance, overt or covert, of the psychological dimension by the sufferer, treatment is difficult.

Such conditions are common after all combat and have been seen since wars began. They have attracted the sobriquet of War Syndromes and reflect the current societal health preoccupations of each generation.

References

1. Jones E, Hodgins-Vermaas R, McCartney H, Everitt B, Beech C, Poynter D, Palmer I, Hyams K, Wessely S. Post-combat syndromes from the Boer war to the Gulf war: A cluster analysis of their nature and attribution. *BMJ*. 2002: 324:321–324.
2. Palmer I. The emotion that dare not speak its name? *Br Army Rev*. 2003: 132;31–37.
3. Palmer I. War based hysteria—the military perspective. In Halligan P, Bass C, Marshall JC, eds. *Contemporary Approaches to the Study of Hysteria—Clinical and Theoretical Perspectives*. Oxford: Oxford University Press; 2001.
4. Palmer I. Malingering, shirking & self-inflicted injuries In: Halligan P, Bass C, Oakley D, eds. *The Military in Malingering and Illness Deception*. Oxford: Oxford University Press; 2003.

I
Rectal Examination Revisited

RICHARD A. DONALDSON

Digital Rectal Examination (DRE)

Digital rectal examination (DRE) is undoubtedly a very important part of the examination and assessment of most casualties, but one must be aware of its limitations.

Recently, a soldier with a gunshot wound (GSW) was admitted to a Field Hospital. He had a small entry wound over the left femoral triangle and a large open exit wound in the upper part of the right buttock, with a fist-sized cavity in the gluteal muscles. There was no evidence of any neurovascular damage to the left leg. Digital rectal examination by an experienced A&E consultant revealed no abnormality, especially no "blood on glove." Catheterization was straightforward, with clean urine obtained. Ultrasound scan (USS) revealed a slight increase in intraperitoneal-free fluid.

Laparotomy revealed a small amount of intraperitoneal bleeding with all intraperitoneal structures intact. The blood in the peritoneal cavity was assumed to be the result of transudation from a large pelvic hematoma. On exploration of the exit wound, a strong smell of feces was noted. The wound was extended to allow exploration of the rectum and a two-centimeter laceration of the rectum was found. The rectum was repaired and a de-functioning colostomy was carried out.

One would normally expect to find at least a trace of blood macroscopically in cases of rectal injury, although a tear in the rectum could not be palpated. In this case, it seemed so unlikely that a projectile could have traversed the extraperitoneal pelvis without damage to at least one important structure in that area such as the urethra or rectum.

Lesson Learned

In cases of pelvic injury with a high index of suspicion of rectal damage and where DRE is normal, it would be worthwhile to carry out a Fecal Occult Blood Test, followed by proctoscopy if positive.

"High Riding" Prostate

It is taught, and it is a misconception, that the prostate can be felt "riding high" on DRE in cases of pelvic fracture with associated transection of the supra-membranous urethra and dislocation of the prostate gland.

It is not a common injury, and in 30 years of urological practice, I have seen but four or five cases in the presenting stage.

In such cases, the dislocated prostate becomes absorbed into a "boggy" pelvic mass consisting mainly of bladder and hematoma and cannot be felt as a separate entity. What one feels on DRE is a space where the prostate should normally be located, and possibly the symphis pubis.

Section 5
And Finally

Where a Trauma Surgeon Can Go Ballistic?

Michael E. Sugrue

Introduction

The treatment of blunt trauma patients is the focus in the delivery of trauma care worldwide, particularly in Europe and Australasia. The probabilities and nature of injury in blunt mechanisms are very different when compared to penetrating mechanisms. This may challenge the trauma surgeon, especially one who infrequently participates in the management of ballistic injuries. Optimum ballistic trauma care can be difficult to deliver due to the infrequent nature of the injuries seen. The trauma surgeon, while predominantly empowered to treat the blunt multi-system patient, needs to have a consistent and rational approach to the management of specific penetrating injuries.

This chapter will deal with some of the issues that are faced by surgeons who otherwise have limited exposure to ballistic types of injuries. It will focus on some of the errors encountered and suggest a strategy to reduce these mistakes. A key to improving, overcoming, and reducing complications, even in advanced mature trauma services, lies in providing safety and reducing errors.[1]

Prehospital Care

The outcome of trauma care is only as good as the weakest link. The first challenge we face as surgeons is to recognize that more than surgeons treat trauma patients and that a team approach is required.[2]

The trauma surgeon managing penetrating injury must ask: Is our prehospital system adequately prepared to deal with patients with penetrating trauma?

To be more specific, a number of key questions need to be answered:

– What is the communication system from the scene to the resuscitation room?

– What quality assurance and performance improvement mechanisms are in place with the ambulance and retrieval service?
– What are the errors that are going to be made by prehospital care providers?

A prehospital response for penetrating trauma should be significantly quicker or have a greater degree of urgency, in general, than for blunt trauma. In an environment where blunt trauma is the predominant source of injury, a consistent and optimum approach to penetrating trauma may not be available due to lack of appropriate guidelines. In addition, there may be a relative lack of experience in prehospital care providers due to the lack of exposure.

Errors in prehospital management of penetrating injury can result in prolonged scene times, inappropriate fluid resuscitation, and poor prehospital to resuscitation room communication. It is hard to see any justification, outside a mass casualty situation, where there is a scene delay while the first ambulance waits for a more senior second responder to arrive and then take the patient to the hospital. This is not an uncommon scenario in Europe and Australia.

The definitive care of penetrating trauma should be based upon probabilities and decision-making.[3] Information relating to the vital signs of a patient are crucial, especially in the presence of prehospital hypotension with a systolic blood pressure of less than 90 millimeters of Hg in a penetrating trauma patient, as it invariably equates with the need for emergency surgery.[3] Emergency surgery will be required within the first hour of arrival in over half of these patients. Failure to obtain adequate information will put the surgeon at a significant disadvantage, potentially resulting in prolonged times in the resuscitation room, poorer preparation, and longer times to definitive arrest of hemorrhage. Recent suggestions that each three-minute delay in the resuscitation room will result in an increase in mortality of approximately one percent in a patient with significant bleeding are a potent reminder of the importance of timely care.[4]

Occasionally, the prehospital information may not be precise or doubt exists as to whether the patient has been shot. Coupled with a lack of exposure in the emergency staff to penetrating injuries can result in missed or delayed diagnosis. Patients may also come by private transport, which can make prehospital information unreliable, as can be seen in the case of a young man being treated by the emergency registrar for herpes zoster after he told them he had blurred vision and spots, only to have a television-channel enquiry about a young male who was shot in the head (Figure S5-1). In societies where gunshot wounds are infrequent, it is not uncommon for patients to imagine that they may have been assaulted with a blunt instrument or deny that they have been shot, posing challenges for the emergency department triage. Very careful inspection will give an indication that the patient has been shot rather than stabbed or hit with a blunt object, as seen in Figure S5-2. Telltale marks can include the jagged nature of the wound and the presence of burning or powder residue.

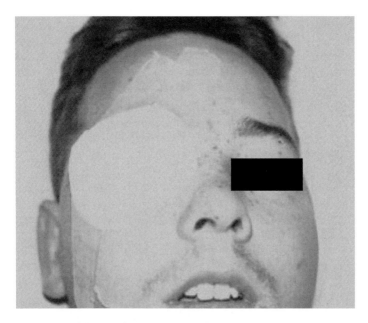

FIGURE S5-1. Patient who was being treat as herpes zoster.

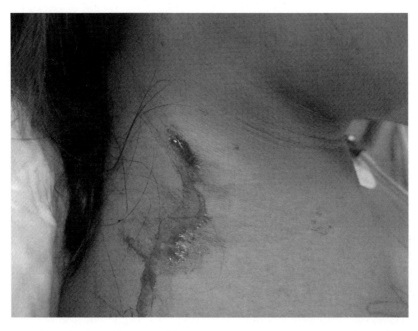

FIGURE S5-2. Patient who was said he fell on a stick, but who chest X-ray showed a bullet in the upper mediastinum.

Challenges in Thoracic Trauma

For the "blunt" trauma surgeon dealing with gunshot wounds to the chest, the majority will have been inflicted with a low-velocity handgun. There are a number of key questions that will be faced:

- For lateral chest injuries, what is optimal management?
- Can I send the patient home after six hours?
- Is there pleural penetration and should I explore the chest with my finger?
- What is optimal management of injuries in the "box"?
- What is optimal management of a thoracoabdominal injury?
- What should I do with a transcervical or transmediastinal gunshot wound into the thoracic inlet?
- When should an emergency room thoracotomy versus an urgent operating room thoracotomy be performed?

The infrequent exposure to specific scenarios makes decision-making difficult. While we are all fairly well versed with guidelines for the management of blunt aortic injury and have had the opportunity of dealing with multiple scenarios, the challenge of penetrating trauma may not be as well informed.

Additionally, gunshot and shrapnel injuries to the lateral chest wall can pose a challenge for the blunt trauma surgeon.

- Do I debride?
- Do I resect?
- Does the patient need a chest tube for through-and-through injuries?
- Do these patients need other special investigations?

An example is shown in Figure S5-3 of a patient with shotgun injury to the left chest. The young lady was shot at about 4 meters with a shotgun. Having sustained significant soft tissue injuries to her left breast and chest, the surgeon opted to perform a debridement, which amounted to almost a partial mastectomy. This was on the basis that there was some non-confluent areas of skin loss. This is probably unnecessary. There is a tendency for over resection of wounds following handgun and shotgun injuries by surgeons not familiar with ballistic injury. On the other hand, with infrequently seen high-velocity injuries, there is often a reluctance to undertake aggressive debridement of devitalized tissue.

The principles of management of a lateral chest injury should be in keeping with Advanced Trauma Life Support (ATLS) and the Definitive Surgical Care Course principles.[3]

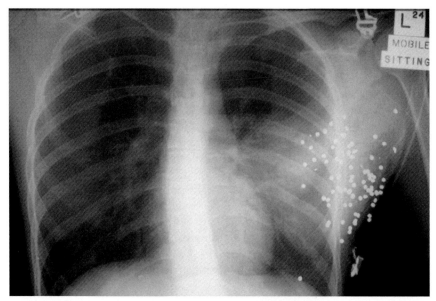

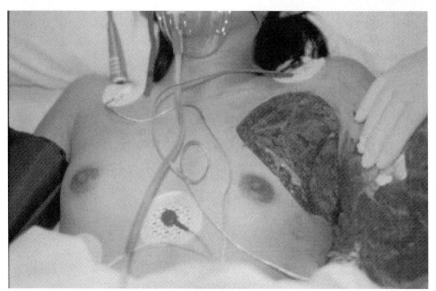

FIGURE S5-3. A shotgun injury to the anterior chest wall resulting in major debridement. (a) CXR showing shot gun pellets and underlying injury. (b) Post debridement.

- There should be no digital probing of the penetrating lateral chest wound, as seen in Figure S5-4, as this will only induce a pneumothorax, cause bleeding, or introduce exogenous infection.
- A chest tube should be inserted in the presence of a hemothorax or a pneumothorax.
- Antibiotic coverage should be administered at the time of chest tube insertion.[5]
- A computed tomography (CT) scan of the chest may be helpful in determining the missile trajectory and, if there is any doubt as to a possible cardiac injury, an echocardiogram or transesophageal echo should be performed. Detection of a septal defect in the presence of penetrating trauma, especially a stab wound, should not be attributed to a congenital defect. Missed injuries must be avoided[6] and assessment of the diaphragm should be undertaken where the entry point is in the region of the thoracic abdomen. This can be undertaken ideally with laparoscopy or alternatively with thoracoscopy. A CT scan of the abdomen or thorax is not as reliable for determining diaphragmatic injury.

With transmediastinal gunshot wounds, the indications for surgery follow basic principles of penetrating injury care; firstly, hemodynamic instability equals immediate operation. In the stable patient with injury to the bronchus, esophagus, major vessels or thoracic ducts, it is important that appropriate investigations are ordered to evaluate these structures. It is also important that these evaluations be undertaken in the first six hours of the

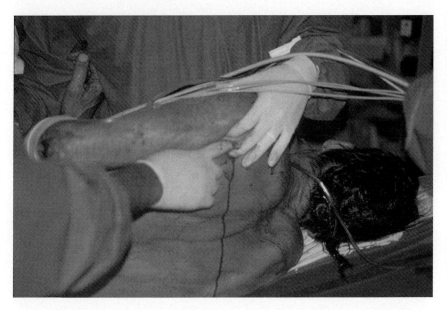

FIGURE S5-4. Craniodigital reflex. The desire to stick a finger in every hole.

patients' presentation to the hospital, not the following morning. Failure to detect an esophageal injury in the first twelve hours may result in mortality or significant morbidity. Inability to primarily repair the esophagus will doom the patient to a staged esophageal repair and a complex protracted intensive care unit (ICU) and hospital course.

The initial management of patients who have sustained gunshot wound or penetrating shrapnel injury to the chest, sometimes coupled with a blast injury, will pose a challenge for the blunt trauma surgeon who, under normal circumstances, would rarely perform an emergency room thoracotomy (ERT). To psyche one's self up from the usual of nonoperative management to an emergency room thoracotomy, while seemingly straightforward, can be psychologically challenging.

While the patient who arrives in the resuscitation room talking is very unlikely to need an emergency thoracotomy, a patient who is profoundly hypotensive with a penetrating chest injury needs an immediate ERT in the emergency department.

Further challenges facing the blunt trauma surgeon include the location of the incision, (often made too low); the type of incision (often not converted to a clamshell for rapid access to both sides of the chest), deciding which side to enter first (occasionally entering the wrong side), positioning of the equipment (incorrect positioning of the chest retractor as seen in Figure S5-5, with the bar across the center of the chest instead of laterally), attempting to cross-clamp the aorta first instead of checking for a pericardial tamponade and finally having a stepwise plan of action prior to incision. Failing to make the right incision can pose challenges in terms of access, as shown in Figure S5-6. While this patient's anterolateral thoracotomy has obviously resulted in the patients' survival, the incision is too low and would be difficult to convert into a clamshell incision.

Challenges in the Abdomen

What could be less challenging than the abdomen, where the trauma surgeon is usually the king? In reality, decision-making and operative technique has a major impact on outcomes. Key errors in ballistic trauma to the abdomen can be made in the following situations in particular:

– Failure to institute damage control principles in appropriate patients with major abdominal injury where technically brilliant surgery may directly contribute to the death of the patient because of the length of time required. The presence of hypothermia (<34°C), acidosis, and massive transfusion should prime the surgeon about the need to abbreviate any surgical procedure once the site of surgical bleeding has been controlled.

The patient in Figure S5-7 had a shotgun wound to the mid abdomen and demonstrated some classic provider-related errors with failure to perform

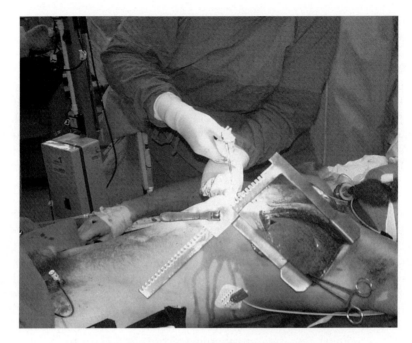

FIGURE S5-5. Incorrect positioning of chest retractors.

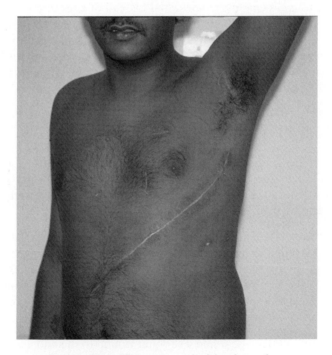

FIGURE S5-6. Thoracotomy incision is too low.

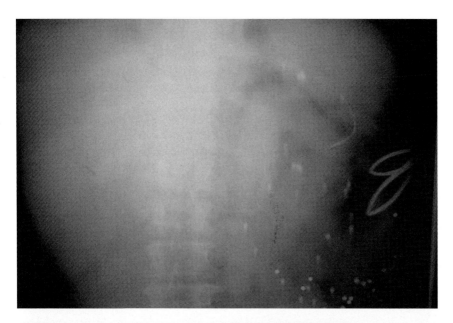

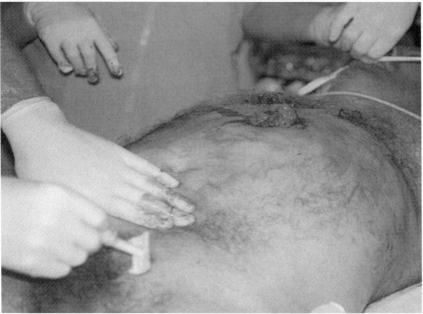

FIGURE S5-7. Shotgun injury to mid abdomen.

damage control surgery, proceeding instead to complex gastric surgery performed along with three small bowel resections and anastomoses over a four-hour period.[7,8] The patient died of exsanguination from coagulopathy in ICU two hours after surgery. He was profoundly hypothermic with a temperature of 32.8°C and a base excess of –12, having received 18 units of blood.

While this case was undertaken in the late 1980s, before damage control was popularized, it highlights the effect of inappropriate and prolonged surgery. Although this case was treated 15 years ago, for many surgeons damage control and the abdominal compartment syndrome still remain a mystery despite many recent advances.[9,10]

It is vital that surgeons do not delay transfer to the operating theater in a patient with obvious indication for laparotomy. In no situation should the patient be placed in a holding pattern, circulating in the radiology department between CT scanning and/or angiography while the surgeon organizes other commitments or displays indecision.

Failure to thoroughly evaluate the rectum for injury after a transpelvic gunshot wound (Figure S5-8) is a serious mistake. Failure to diagnose a pen-

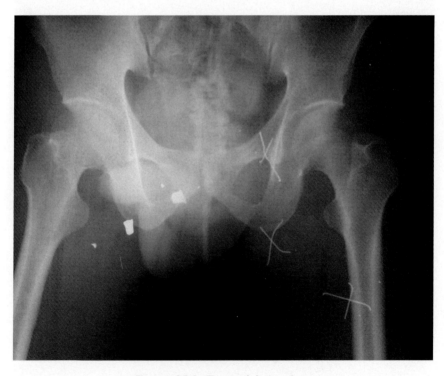

FIGURE S5-8. Transpelvic gunshot.

etrating rectal injury at first laparotomy in a trans-abdominal, pelvic gunshot, or shrapnel injury will result in secondary peritonitis and a high mortality. The surgeon must also resist the temptation to suture shrapnel injuries to the buttock and perineum. These wounds should be examined under anesthesia, debrided appropriately, and left open.

Challenges in the Head and Neck

Rarely, if ever, do we operate in the neck in blunt trauma patients. Decision-making and prioritization are very challenging with ballistic injuries to the head and neck, as seen in Figure S5-9. Obviously, the principles are somewhat similar, with attention to the airway, and in this particular case, a successful oral intubation was not secured and had to be followed by immediate cricothyroidotomy. With the increasing tendency towards non-operative management of penetrating neck injuries, there is almost some surgical guilt when undertaking surgery in this region. It is important for

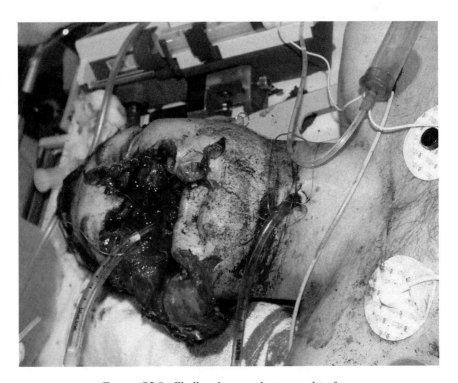

FIGURE S5-9. Challenging gunshot wound to face.

the blunt trauma surgeon to reduce potential errors in judgment by avoiding sending patients of borderline hemodynamic stability with Zone 1 neck injuries to the radiology department. A patient with a major vascular injury at the root of the neck is a time bomb, and ideally, radiological procedures should be done in an operating room environment. While this is not possible in most hospitals, facilities for urgent intervention should always be available; certainly, patients should not be transferred without a surgical presence to angiography. There are times when *"cold steel"* (size 10 or 20 scalpel) is preferable to *"coiled steel"*.

A transcervical gunshot wound poses many challenges, as often the path of the bullet may deflect, and in the stable patient without airway compromise, a CT scan may provide a useful trajectogram. It is important at the outset, especially with non-English speaking patients, to realize that gunshot wounds, especially handgun wounds to the neck, may present as apparent stab wounds.

Another challenge or pitfall in ballistic trauma is the high probability of through-and-through injuries. Figure S5-10 shows a young male who had arrested after arrival in emergency following an anterior abdominal stabbing and went immediately to the operating room. At first, a medial visceral

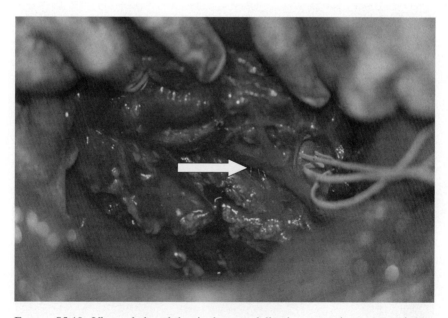

FIGURE S5-10. View of the abdominal aorta following posterior surture (white arrow) during a medical visceral rotation. However, the anterior aortic injury was not inspected.

rotation was performed with a beautiful repair of the posterior aorta. One would think, to put it *"bluntly,"* that the surgeon would have thought of the anterior wall. Well . . . that was fixed the following day when there was persistent bleeding!

Challenges in Limb Trauma

Penetrating limb trauma, particularly lower limb trauma, can create some challenging decision-making and prioritization. This is particularly so when the patient does not have an obvious life-threatening injury. This is not the case in Figure S5-11, however, where an unfortunate male suffered a cardiac arrest in the emergency department after being brought in by ambulance from a nearby park. The patient was initially semiconscious, uncooperative, and arrested some fifteen minutes after arrival. During cardiopulmonary resuscitation (CPR), it was noted he had some blood through his trousers posteriorly, where eventually a bullet wound was found, and while he made it to the operating theater, he eventually died from multi-organ failure. At

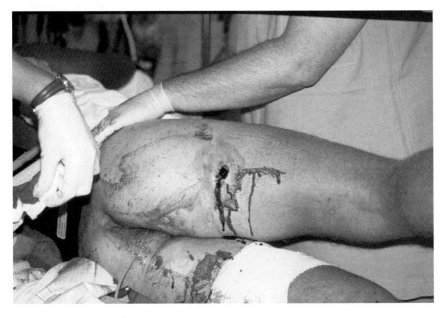

FIGURE S5-11. Potential pitfalls of an undiagnosed gunshot injury in patient who eventually died.

post-mortem he was shown to have transected the profunda femoris artery. This is a chilling reminder of the importance of thorough physical examination and the challenges of secondary survey. It should always be remembered that tertiary surveys should supplement the initial secondary survey and help reduce delayed diagnosis of injuries.

In the emergency department, faced with a simple bullet wound and normal pulses, there is an overwhelming desire to digitally explore wounds. This is an unnecessary evil in the majority of ballistic wounds to the limb. Invariably, the wounds do not need to be excised, as there is little cavitation and necrosis of the skin. With the presence of pulses and a normal ankle/brachial index, with the exception of shotgun wounds or small shrapnel injury, there is little indication for further investigation. Care must be particularly exerted where there is swollen calf or pain out of proportion to signs, as a compartment syndrome may go undiagnosed. It should be remembered, however, that injuries in the region of vessels, even of small caliber, run the risk of developing pseudoaneurysms and arterio-venous fistulae. Shotgun injuries have the potential for bullet embolisation, and this is where decision-making and thought process need to change mode from management of blunt trauma to avoid making mistakes. So if your young patient has been shot in the abdomen with a shotgun, the risk of embolisation distally must be considered, especially in the presence of dusky legs. Clinical examination supplemented by arterial dopplers and plain radiography will demonstrate emboli, as shown in Figure S5-12. Delay to theater would result in loss of limb, potentially loss of life. and even though fasciotomies are performed (as shown in Figure 12), this may be too late.

Conclusion

While the blunt and penetrating trauma surgeons are equally well trained, sharing in the skills of trauma and surgery, it is the decision-making and judgment that is paramount in penetrating trauma. The desire to stop the bleeding, the use of judicious investigations supplemented with cold steel and/or angiography for that urgent hemorrhage control, as well as with the principles of damage control, all of which essential components of care. These principles of care are clearly dealt with in the Definitive Surgical Trauma Core Course.

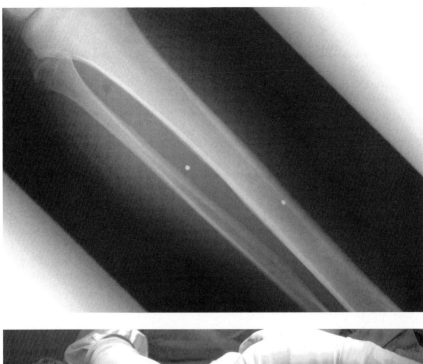

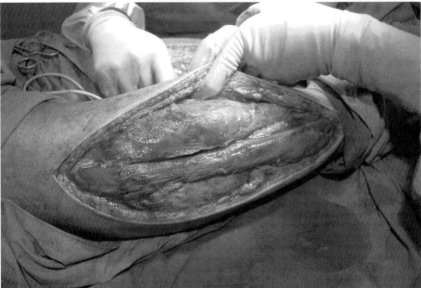

FIGURE S5-12. Pellet emboli and subsequent delayed fasciotomy with eventual amputation.

References

1. Hoyt DB, Coimbra R, Potenza B, Doucet J, Fortlage D, Holingsworth-Fridlund P, Holbrook T. A twelve-year analysis of disease and provider complications on an organised level 1 trauma service: As good as it gets? *J Trauma*. 2003;54:26–27.
2. Sugrue M, Seger M, Kerridge R, Sloane D, Deane S. A prospective study of the performance of the trauma team leader. *J Trauma*. 1995;38(1):79–82.
3. Clarke JR, Trooskin SZ, Doshi PJ, Grenwald L, Mode CJ. Time to laparotomy for intraabdominal bleeding from trauma does not affect survival for delays up to 90 minutes J Trauma 2002, 52:420–425.
4. Sugrue M , Danne P, D'Amours SK. *Definitive Surgical Trauma Care Course Manual*. Sydney: University New South Wales; 2001.
5. Eastern Association Surgery Trauma. Available at: http://www.east.org/tpg.html. Accessed June 6, 2003.
6. Janjua KJ, Sugrue M, Jones F, Deane SA, Bristow P, Hillman K. Prospective evaluation of early missed injuries and the role of the tertiary trauma survey. *J Trauma*. 1998;44;1000–1007.
7. Offner PJ, de Souza Al, Moore Ee. Avoidance of abdominal compartment syndrome in damage control laparotomy after trauma. *Arch Surg*. 2001;136: 676–681.
8. Hoey BA, Schwab CW. Damage control surgery. *Scand J Surg*. 2002;91(1): 92–103.
9. Balogh Z, McKinley BA, Holcomb JB, Miller CC, Cocanour CS, Kosar RA, Valdivia A, Ware DN, Moore FA. Both primary and secondary abdominal compartment syndrome can be predicted early and are harbingers of multiple organ failure. *J Trauma*. 2003;54:848–861.
10. Ivatury RR, Porter JM, Simon RJ. Intra-abdominal hypertension after life threatening penetrating abdominal trauma: prophylaxis, incidence, and clinical relevance of gastric mucosal pH and abdominal compartment syndrome. *J Trauma*. 1988;44:1016–1023.

Index

Coventry University